A *Textbook of Clinical Pharmacology*

Dedication

This book is dedicated to the memory of Professor Howard Rogers, the instigator of the previous editions

A *Textbook of Clinical Pharmacology*

Third Edition

James M. Ritter
MA, DPhil, FRCP
Professor of Clinical Pharmacology, United Medical and Dental Schools,
Guy's and St Thomas' Hospitals, London, UK

Lionel D. Lewis
MA, MD, MRCP
Assistant Professor of Medicine and Pharmacology,
Dartmouth–Hitchcock Medical Center, Lebanon NH, USA

Timothy G. K. Mant
BSc, FFPM, FRCP
Medical Director, Guy's Drug Research Unit, Guy's Hospital, London, UK

A member of the Hodder Headline Group
LONDON • SYDNEY • AUKLAND
Co-published in the USA by Oxford University Press, Inc., New York

First published in Great Britain 1981
Third edition 1995
Second printing by Arnold, a member of the Hodder
Headline Group, 338 Euston Road, London NW1 3BH

Copublished in the United States of America by
Oxford University Press, Inc.,
198 Madison Avenue, New York, NY10016
Oxford is a registered trademark of Oxford University Press

British Library Cataloguing in Publication Data
A catalogue record for this book is available from the
British Library

ISBN 0 340 55864 4

Typeset by Scribe Design, Gillingham, Kent.
Printed and bound in Great Britain by Bath Press
Colourbooks, Glasgow

Contents

Foreword   vii
Preface   viii
Acknowledgements   ix

PART I   GENERAL PRINCIPLES   1

1   Introduction to therapeutics   3
2   Mechanisms of drug action
     (pharmacodynamics)   9
3   Pharmacokinetics   19
4   Drug absorption and routes of
     administration   29
5   Drug metabolism   41
6   Renal excretion of drugs   51
7   Effects of disease on drug
     disposition   55
8   Therapeutic drug monitoring   67
9   Drugs in pregnancy   73
10   Drugs at extremes of age   83
11   Adverse drug reactions   93
12   Drug interactions   107
13   Pharmacogenetics   119
14   Introduction of new drugs and
     clinical trials   131
     with Paul J. Morrison

PART II   THE NERVOUS SYSTEM   145

15   Hypnotics and anxiolytics   147
     with Roy G. Spector
16   Schizophrenia and behavioral
     emergencies   159
     with Roy G. Spector
17   Mood disorders   169
     with Roy G. Spector
18   Movement disorders   181
19   Anticonvulsants   193
20   Migraine   205

21   Anesthetics and muscle
     relaxants   211
     with Mark Edwards
22   Analgesics and the control of
     pain   227

PART III THE MUSCULOSKELETAL
          SYSTEM   245

23   Anti-inflammatory drugs and the
     treatment of arthritis   247

PART IV   THE CARDIOVASCULAR
          SYSTEM   261

24   Prevention of atheroma: lowering
     plasma cholesterol and other
     approaches   263
25   Hypertension   279
26   Ischemic heart disease   307
27   Anticoagulants and antiplatelet
     drugs   321
28   Heart failure   337
29   Cardiac arrhythmias   349

PART V   THE RESPIRATORY SYSTEM   373

30   Asthma and other respiratory
     disorders   375

PART VI   THE ALIMENTARY SYSTEM   393

31   Alimentary system and liver   395
     with Dipti Amin
32   Vitamins and other nutrients   425

PART VII   FLUIDS AND
            ELECTROLYTES   435

33   Drugs and the renal and
     genitourinary systems:
     fluid and electrolyte disorders   437

PART VIII   THE ENDOCRINE
            SYSTEM   455

     with Anne Dornhorst
34   Diabetes mellitus   457
35   Thyroid   469
36   Calcium metabolism   477
37   Adrenal hormones   485
38   Reproductive endocrinology   497
39   Pituitary   509

PART IX   SELECTIVE TOXICITY   515

40   Antibacterial drugs   517
41   Mycobacterial infections   541
42   Fungal and viral infections   551
43   HIV and AIDS   565

44   Malaria and other parasitic
     infections   577
45   Cancer chemotherapy   585

PART X   HEMATOLOGY   613

46   Anemia and other hematological
     disorders   615

PART XI   IMMUNOPHARMACOLOGY   629

47   Clinical immunopharmacology   631

PART XII   THE SKIN   651

48   Drugs and the skin   653

PART XIII   CLINICAL TOXICOLOGY   665

49   Drug and alcohol abuse   667
50   Drug overdose and poisoning   685

Appendix   Legal aspects of
           prescribing   695

Index   699

Foreword

Since the last edition of this book clinical pharmacology has continued to play a vital role in undergraduate and postgraduate medical education. The majority of doctors will prescribe throughout their medical careers and it is essential, therefore, that they have knowledge and a clear understanding of the drugs which they use.

Professor Ritter and his team have undertaken a radical revision and have produced what is essentially an entirely new text. This has been necessary, not only because many new facts have emerged and new drugs have been introduced, but also because whole fresh concepts of drug action, approaches and therapy have occurred.

The textbook contains all the clinical pharmacology that the undergraduate should know without being overloaded with unnecessary detail, but is comprehensive enough to be used for revision or reference by postgraduate students and practising doctors.

Increasingly, those working in the pharmaceutical sciences are becoming involved in the use of drugs. In particular, pharmacists and those in the pharmaceutical industry will find that this book has a useful place in their studies. Nurses may well become limited prescribers in the future and are also ideally placed to note and record the effects, both beneficial and adverse, of drug treatment; a copy of this book should be available in every nursing school library.

I have little doubt that the 'new look' Textbook of Clinical Pharmacology will prove to be widely popular and will make a considerable contribution to the understanding and teaching of the subject.

Professor J.R. Trounce

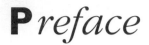Preface

Clinical pharmacologists are concerned with the use of drugs in humans. Surgeons, obstetricians and physicians of every subspecialty prescribe drugs for their patients on a daily basis to prevent and treat illness. Whilst the therapeutic possibilities have increased dramatically over the last 50 years, so has the potential for iatrogenic disease. A greater understanding of the principles of clinical pharmacology and the use of drugs can significantly improve our care of patients. It is primarily to medical students and junior doctors that this book is addressed. Our aim has been to provide an account of the general principles of the subject, and of how these are applied in the management of common clinical conditions.

The first section deals with general aspects including pharmacodynamics, pharmacokinetics and the various factors that modify drug disposition and drug interactions. Recognition and monitoring of adverse effects and the introduction of new drugs are also discussed. Pharmacokinetic descriptions are very 'model dependent' and are somewhat arbitrary. In the present edition we have avoided detailed algebraic formulations, concentrating instead on the practical utility of concepts such as half-life, clearance and volume of distribution in deciding such things as dose interval or the need for a loading dose.

Later parts of the book address treatment of common diseases of major organ systems (nervous, cardiovascular, etc.) and of diseases that influence multiple systems (infectious diseases, cancer, clinical toxicology, immune disorders, etc.). Basic pathophysiology, which is essential to understanding the approach to treatment, is described briefly, followed by principles of management and an account of the most important drugs used. In discussing individual drugs emphasis is given to clinical use and benefits, mechanisms of action, adverse effects and contraindications, and clinically important drug interactions. Special situations (e.g. the use of drugs at extremes of age, in pregnancy, or in patients with coexisting disease of major organ systems) are considered separately where relevant. We hope that this part of the book will be read by students undertaking clinical work as they encounter particular diseases and the drugs used to treat them, and that they will thereby achieve a secure background in therapeutics. We would emphasize that learning clinical pharmacology can only be effective if accompanied by clinical experience for, despite initial impressions, this is a practical subject and, just like clinical medicine, the patient is the best teacher. It is our experience that attempts to learn the subject in isolation from clinical work fail.

Although this book, with its emphasis on the application of the principles of clinical pharmacology to the practical management of patients, has been written for medical students and junior doctors, we hope that it will also be useful to scientists in the pharmaceutical industry and academic departments whose first discipline is in some quite different area but whose professional interests have moved towards the use of drugs in humans.

Acknowledgements

We would like to thank many colleagues who have helped us with advice and criticism. Their expertise in many specialist areas has enabled us to emphasize those factors most relevant. In particular, we are grateful to Professor Roy Spector (Professor Emeritus of Applied Pharmacology), Professor John Trounce (Professor Emeritus of Clinical Pharmacology, UMDS, Guy's Hospital), Dr John Henry (Consultant Physician, Poisons Unit, Guy's Hospital), Dr Robin Stott (Consultant Physician, Lewisham Hospital), Dr Piotr Bajorek (Consultant Anesthetist, East Surrey Hospital), Mr Paul Morrison, Miss Susanna Gilmour-White (Drug Information, Pharmacy, Guy's Hospital), Dr Peter Loynds, Dr Dipti Amin MRCGP and Dr Mark Edwards FRCAnaes (Guy's Drug Research Unit), Dr William van't Hoff (Hospital for Sick Children, Great Ormond Street) and Dr Anne Dornhorst. We would also like to thank the Southwark and North Lewisham Formulary Committee for permission to publish their guide to the use of antibiotics in modified form.

General Principles

I

Introduction to Therapeutics

1

Use of drugs **4**

Adverse effects and risk/benefit **4**

Drug history and therapeutic plan **5**

Formularies and restricted lists **6**

Scientific basis of use of drugs in humans **7**

*U*SE OF DRUGS

People consult a doctor to find out what (if anything) is wrong (the diagnosis) and what should be done about it (the treatment). If they are well, they may nevertheless want to know how future problems can be prevented. Depending on the diagnosis, treatment may consist of reassurance, physical therapy, surgery, radiotherapy, psychotherapy and so on. Drugs are very often either the primary therapy or an adjunct to another modality (e.g. the use of analgesic and anesthetic drugs in patients undergoing surgery). Sometimes contact with the doctor is initiated because of a public health measure rather than because of symptoms of disease, for example through contact tracing from an index case with an infectious disease, or through a screening program intended to identify individuals at increased risk of malignant or cardiovascular disease. Again drug treatment is sometimes needed, often as a supplement to advice regarding personal habits. Consequently, practicing doctors of nearly all specialties use drugs extensively, and need to understand something of the scientific basis on which their use is founded.

A century ago, physicians had at their disposal only a handful of effective drugs (e.g. morphia, quinine, ether, aspirin and digitalis leaf), and even these were used less than optimally. In the ensuing decades, potent new drugs (e.g. thiamine, insulin, sulfonamides and antibiotics, synthetic antimalarials, anticonvulsants, cortisol, diuretics, antipsychotics and antidepressants, antimetabolites and alkylating agents, contraceptives, β-blockers, H_2-blockers, converting enzyme inhibitors, calcium channel blockers, drugs that lower cholesterol, fibrinolytics and antivirals) have been introduced. New drugs are fundamental to advances in medicine, and the ingenuity of pharmaceutical chemists is continuing to pay dividends in terms of discovery of improved drugs and drugs for new indications. Indeed, with advances in genetic engineering and in basic understanding of chemical mediators in biological control systems (witnessed by the introduction of such products as genetically engineered hepatitis vaccine, erythropoietin and monoclonal antibodies directed against interleukins and their receptors among others), to say nothing of the experimental use of gene therapy in genetic disorders such as adenine deaminase deficiency, familial hypercholesterolemia and cystic fibrosis, it is likely that the pace of change will accelerate further in the next few years. Changes in therapeutics that will be seen by a physician newly qualified today will consequently be at least as great, and probably far greater, than those of the last 40 years. Medical students and doctors in training therefore need to learn something of the *principles* of therapeutics. These are discussed in the first part of this book, while systematic considerations and current approaches to treatment of common diseases are the subject of the second part, together with specifics relating to selected important therapeutic drugs.

*A*DVERSE EFFECTS AND RISK/BENEFIT

Medicinal chemistry has contributed immeasurably to human health and happiness, but the alleviation of suffering brought about by effective drugs has not come without a price. Consequently, these advances have been paralleled by a necessary change in philosophy of the medical profession, and somewhat later of the public, towards therapeutics. A physician in Osler's day could safely adhere to the Hippocratic principle 'first do no harm', because the opportunities for doing good were so limited. The discovery of new drugs has transformed this situation, but unfortunately only at the expense of very real risks of doing harm. This is particularly striking in the case of cancer chemotherapy, where great advances (e.g. cures of leukemias, Hodgkin's disease and testicular carcinomas) have come through a preparedness to accept a limited degree of containable harm to the patient in a tightly controlled setting, but similar considerations also apply in other fields of medicine as well as oncology.

Indeed, almost all (if not all) effective drugs can have adverse effects, and therapeutic judgments based on risk/benefit ratios now permeate all fields of medicine, even if the arguments are seldom formalized and may not be rehearsed consciously. This is unfortunate: drugs are the physician's prime therapeutic tools, just as diathermy and the scalpel are those of the surgeon, and just as a scalpel misplaced can spell disaster so can a thoughtless prescription. Some of the more colorful and dramatic instances of such catastrophes make for gruesome reading in the annual reports of the medical defense societies, but perhaps as important is the morbidity and expense caused by less dramatic but more common errors.

How are prescribing errors to be minimized? By combining *general* knowledge of the disease to be treated and of the drugs that may be effective for that disease with *specific* knowledge about the particular patient. Dukes and Swartz in their valuable work *Responsibility for Drug-induced Injury* list eight basic duties of prescribers:

1. **Restrictive use** – to take a proper decision that drug therapy is warranted rather than other therapy or to 'wait and see'.
2. **Careful choice** of an appropriate drug, dosage and scheme of treatment with due regard to the likely risk/benefit ratio, to the alternatives available, and to the patient's needs and susceptibilities.
3. **Consultation and consent** – wherever possible the patient should be consulted about the proposed treatment, and should give informed consent to it.
4. **Prescription and recording** – to prescribe appropriately and with care and to record what is prescribed.
5. **Explanation** to the patient of how the treatment will be given and what his or her role in it will be.
6. **Supervision** of the course of therapy, observing developments and adapting it as necessary.
7. **Termination** of therapy in an appropriate manner when it is no longer needed.
8. **Conformity with the law** relating to the prescribing and use of medicines.

The following should be considered in deciding on a therapeutic plan:

1. The patient's age.
2. The possibility of coexisting disease, especially renal impairment, liver disease and cardiac or respiratory failure.
3. The possibility of pregnancy now or during treatment.
4. The patient's drug history.
5. What is the best that can reasonably be hoped for in this individual patient?

DRUG HISTORY AND THERAPEUTIC PLAN

A reliable drug history involves questioning the patient (and sometimes the family, neighbors, other physicians etc.) about a number of issues. What prescription tablets, medicines, drops (eye, nose or ear), contraceptives, creams, suppositories or pessaries are being taken? What over-the-counter remedies? Has the patient suffered from drug-induced rashes or other allergies, or other serious reactions? Has the patient ever been treated for anything similar in the past, if so with what and did it do the job, or were there any problems? Has the patient ever had an anesthetic, and if so were there any problems? Have there ever been any serious drug reactions in a close family member or other familial disorders?

Taking these specifics into account, a therapeutic plan is formulated. At this stage, it is crucial that the potential prescriber is both meticulous and humble, especially when dealing with a situation he does not encounter every day. Checking contraindications, special precautions and doses in a formulary such as the *British National Formulary* (BNF) is the minimum that is needed. Where practicable, the proposed therapeutic plan is discussed with the patient, including consideration of the various options available, the goals of treatment, possible adverse effects and their likelihood and measures to be taken if these arise. It is crucial that the patient understands what

is intended, and is happy as to the means proposed to achieve these ends. (This will not, of course, be possible in demented or delirious patients, or in some other severely ill individuals, where discussion will be with any available family members.) Risks of causing harm can be minimized in this way, while increasing the likelihood that the patient will comply with the treatment plan that is finally agreed on.

If the therapeutic plan includes the use of drugs, a prescription must be written clearly and legibly, conforming to legal requirements. In general this should include the generic name of the drug, dose, frequency and duration of treatment, and be signed. It is wise in addition to print the prescriber's name, address and telephone number to facilitate communication from the pharmacist should there be a query. Appropriate follow-up must be arranged. Unfortunately there are still patients who believe that chronic conditions such as severe hypertension are treated by a 'course' of tablets, only to re-present months or years later with a stroke, heart attack or renal failure.

*F*ORMULARIES AND RESTRICTED LISTS

Historically, formularies listed the multiple ingredients commonly prescribed as mixtures by physicians up until the second world war. The perceived need for hospital formularies disappeared transiently when such mixtures were replaced by proprietary products of consistent quality prepared by the pharmaceutical industry. The *British National Formulary* (British Medical Association and Royal Pharmaceutical Society of Great Britain 1994) is updated regularly and contains information about all such preparations currently available in the UK. Because of the bewildering array of

licensed products, many of which are alternatives to one another, many hospitals have reintroduced formularies that are essentially a restrictive list of the drugs stocked by the hospital pharmacy, from which doctors are encouraged to prescribe. The objects of such formularies are to encourage rational prescribing, to simplify purchasing and storage of drugs and to obtain the 'best buy' among alternative preparations. Such formularies have the advantage of encouraging consistency, and when decided with input from local consultant prescribers are usually well accepted.

SCIENTIFIC BASIS OF USE OF DRUGS IN HUMANS

The scientific basis of our understanding of drug action is provided by the discipline of pharmacology. Clinical pharmacology is the branch of pharmacology that deals with effects of drugs in humans. It entails study of the interaction of drugs with their receptors, the transduction (second messenger) systems to which these are linked and the changes that these bring about in cells, organs and the whole organism. These processes ('what the drug does to the body') are sometimes grouped together as 'pharmacodynamics'. The predictive value of animal pharmacology and toxicology studies is limited. Species differences, and the fact that much *in vivo* animal pharmacology is necessarily carried out in anesthetized animals, make human studies absolutely essential, although modern methods of molecular and cell biology are permitting expression of human genes, including those coding for receptors and key signal transduction elements, in non-human cells and in transgenic animals, and seem likely to revolutionize our knowledge of these areas within the next few years. Hopefully this will improve the yield of relevant information from preclinical pharmacology and toxicology studies before the introduction of drugs in humans.

It is necessary to appreciate that drug effects that are important in humans do not necessarily occur in other species. For example, one of the early β-blocking drugs (practolol) had to be withdrawn because it causes adverse effects on the eye, skin and peritoneum. It proved impossible, however, to produce an animal model of these toxic actions. Consequently, when drugs are introduced into use in humans after animal studies have demonstrated potentially useful actions, considerable uncertainties remain regarding effects (especially subjective effects that determine whether or not the drug is well tolerated) and dose–response relationships. Such early phase human studies are usually carried out in healthy volunteers, except when near-inevitable toxicity is anticipated as for many antineoplastic drugs.

Basic pharmacologists can study isolated preparations in which the concentration of drug in the microenvironment of the receptors can be controlled fairly precisely, but such preparations are often stable only for a few minutes or hours. In therapeutics drugs are administered to the whole organism by a route that is as convenient and safe as possible for the patient (usually by mouth), often for periods of days, weeks or more. Consequently, drug concentration in the vicinity of the receptors is usually unknown, and long-term effects involving alterations in receptor density or function or the activation or modulation of homeostatic control loops may be of overriding importance. The processes of absorption, distribution, metabolism and elimination ('what the body does to the drug') determine the drug concentration–time relations at the receptors. These processes are sometimes collectively known as 'pharmacokinetics'. There is considerable interindividual variation in these processes due both to inherited and acquired factors, notably disease of the organs responsible for drug metabolism and excretion. Prescribers therefore need to understand the principles of pharmacokinetics in order to plan a rational therapeutic regime. Pharmacokinetic principles are described in chapter 3 from the point of view of a prescriber rather than of a scientist involved in drug development or studying drug metabolism. Genetic influences on pharmacodynamics and pharmacokinetics ('pharmacogenetics') are discussed in chapter 13; effects of disease in chapter 7; and the use of drugs in pregnancy and at extremes of age in chapters 9 and 10.

There are no entirely satisfactory animal models of most important human diseases (e.g. atheroma, the major cause of death in western societies). Consequently, the only way to ensure that a drug with promising pharmacological actions (e.g. a new drug that lowers plasma cholesterol) is effective in treating or preventing disease (e.g. hyperlipidemia, coronary artery disease) is to perform a clinical trial. It is important for prescribing doctors to understand the strengths and limitations of such trials, the principles of which are described in chapter 14. Prescribers can then evaluate critically and objectively papers published in the literature on the new drugs that will certainly be introduced during their professional lifetimes.

Ignorance of the principles of clinical trials leaves the physician at the mercy of sources of information that are biased by commercial interests. Sources of up-to-date and unbiased information include Dollery's encyclopedic *Therapeutic Drugs* (Churchill-Livingstone, 1991) which is an invaluable source of reference. Publications such as the *Adverse Reaction Bulletin, Prescribers Journal* and the succinctly argued *Drug and Therapeutics Bulletin* provide up-to-date discussions of therapeutic issues of current importance.

Mechanisms of Drug Action (Pharmaco-dynamics)

Introduction   **10**

Receptors and signal transduction   **11**

Agonists   **14**

Competitive antagonists   **14**

Partial agonists   **16**

Slow processes   **17**

Non-receptor mechanisms   **18**

INTRODUCTION

Pharmacodynamics is the study of effects of drugs on biological processes. For example, studies of the time course of the effect of a dose of warfarin on prothrombin time, or of ranitidine on gastric acid secretion or of atenolol on heart rate are described as pharmacodynamic studies. The term 'pharmacodynamics' implies a process that changes with time, but in practice studies that concentrate on the effect of a drug at a single time after administration (e.g. the effect of a defined dose of aspirin on bleeding time 24 hours after the dose) are also referred to as pharmacodynamic studies. Many endogenous hormones, neurotransmitters and other mediators exert their effects as a result of high-affinity binding to specific macromolecular protein or glycoprotein receptors in plasma membranes or cell cytoplasm, and many therapeutically important drugs cause their effects by combining with these receptors and either mimicking the effect of the natural mediator (in which case they are called agonists) or blocking it (in which case they are antagonists). Examples include estrogens (used in contraception and hormone replacement therapy) and antiestrogens (used in treating breast cancer), α- and β-adrenoceptor agonists and antagonists (used in treating hypertension and other cardiovascular and respiratory diseases), opioids, benzodiazepines, antihistamines and others.

Not all drugs work via receptors for endogenous mediators, and many therapeutic drugs exert their effects by combining with an enzyme, transport protein or other cellular macromolecule (e.g. DNA), and interfering with its function. Examples include inhibitors of acetylcholinesterase (used in treating myasthenia gravis and to reverse the effects of neuromuscular blocking drugs after anesthesia), monoamine oxidase inhibitors (used in Parkinsonism and some patients with depression) and cardiac glycosides such as digoxin which inhibit Na^+/K^+ adenosine triphosphatase (ATPase). Some authorities reserve the term 'receptor' exclusively for receptors of endogenous mediators. This restricted sense has not been generally adopted, however, and a broader definition of receptor is 'a macromolecule which is the primary site of action of a drug or naturally occurring substance, usually a smaller molecule, that binds to it'. This broader usage includes receptors for naturally occurring substances that do not have mediator functions, such as adhesion molecules and low density lipoprotein (LDL). Some diseases are caused by abnormalities in receptors. For example, myasthenia gravis is an autoallergic disease caused by increased acetylcholine receptor turnover secondary to cross-linking of adjacent nicotinic acetylcholine receptors at the neuromuscular junction by specific antibodies; patients with familial hypercholesterolemia lack functional LDL receptors and suffer from severe premature atheromatous disease as a result; and patients with X-linked nephrogenic diabetes insipidus have a mutation in the gene for the V_2 receptor which is the site of action of vasopressin (antidiuretic hormone) in the kidney and consequently have impaired ability to form concentrated urine.

Whether the site of action of a drug is a receptor for an endogenous mediator or an enzyme or ion channel the binding is usually highly specific with precise steric recognition between the small molecular ligand and the binding site on its macromolecular target. The binding forces are usually a combination of several weak interactions: electrostatic, dipole–dipole, hydrogen bonding, van der Waals' forces and others. Occasionally, strong covalent bonds are formed as in the acetylation of a serine residue in the active site of cyclo-oxygenase by aspirin (acetylsalicylic acid) which prevents subsequent binding of substrate as a result of steric hindrance, or the alkylation of bases in DNA by cytotoxic drugs such as phosphoramide mustard, the active metabolite of cyclophosphamide.

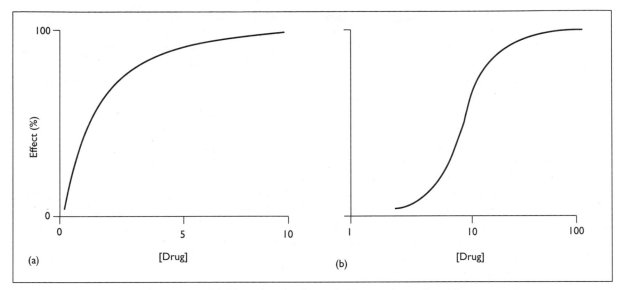

Fig. 2.1 Dose–response curves plotted (a) arithmetically and (b) semi-logarithmically.

Most drugs produce graded dose-related effects, which can be plotted as a dose–response curve. Such curves are often approximately hyperbolic (Fig. 2.1a), and can be conveniently plotted on semi-logarithmic paper to give the familiar sigmoidal shape (Fig. 2.1b). This method of plotting dose–response curves facilitates quantitative analysis (see below) of full agonists, which produce graded responses up to a maximum value; antagonists which produce no response on their own but reduce the response to an agonist; and partial agonists, which produce some response but to a lower maximum value than that of a full agonist and antagonize full agonists (Fig. 2.2). In the clinical situation dose–response curves are influenced by many factors including genetic as well as acquired sources of variation including age, weight, nutrition and other

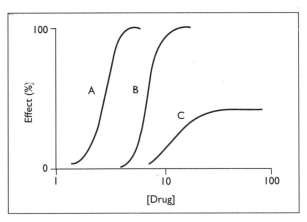

Fig. 2.2 Dose–response curves of two full agonists (A,B) of different potency, and of a partial agonist (C).

drugs as well as psychological and social factors that strongly influence compliance and placebo response.

*R*ECEPTORS AND SIGNAL TRANSDUCTION

Drugs are often potent (i.e. produce effects at low concentration) and specific (i.e. small changes in structure lead to profound changes in potency or cause a change from agonist to antagonist). High potency is a consequence of high affinity for specific macromolecular receptors. Receptors were classified originally by reference to the relative potencies of agonists, and antagonists on preparations containing different receptors. A familiar example is the order of potency of isoprenaline > adrenaline > noradrenaline on tissues rich in β-receptors such as the heart contrasted with the reverse order in α-receptor-mediated responses such as vasoconstriction in resistance arteries supplying the skin. Quantitative potency data are best obtained from comparisons of different competitive antagonists, as explained below. Such data are supplemented, but not replaced, by radiolabeled ligand binding studies. In this way adrenoceptors were divided first into α and β, then subdivided into α_1/α_2 and β_1/β_2. Many other useful receptor classifications including those of cholinoceptors, histamine receptors, serotonin receptors, benzodiazepine receptors, glutamate receptors and others have been proposed on a similar basis. Labelling with irreversible antagonists permitted receptor solubilization and purification using affinity chromatography. Partial sequencing of the

amino acid sequence then enabled oligonucleotide probes based on the deduced sequence to be used to extract the full length DNA sequence coding for different receptors. As receptors are cloned and expressed in cells in culture the original functional classifications have been supported and extended, and further developments are to be expected. Different receptor subtypes may be thought of as analogous to different forms of isoenzymes.

Receptors exist in four 'superfamilies' linked to distinct types of coupling mechanism (Fig. 2.3). Three families of receptor are located in the cell membrane, while the fourth is intracellular (e.g. steroid hormone and thyroxine receptors). In each of the three membrane families hydrophobic α helical regions form membrane spanning domains. These link an extracellular binding domain with the effector domain. One family of receptors for fast neurotransmitters (e.g. glutamate, nicotinic acetylcholine receptors) is linked directly to a transmembrane ion channel; a second family of receptors for slow neurotransmitters and hormones (e.g.

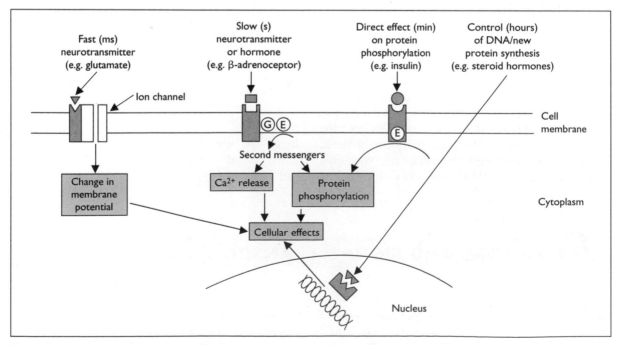

Fig. 2.3 Receptors and signal transduction. G = G-protein. E = enzyme. Ca = calcium.

muscarinic acetylcholine receptors, β-adreno-ceptors) is linked to an intracellular G-protein coupling domain; and the third family is coupled directly to the catalytic domain of an enzyme on the inner membrane (e.g. insulin coupled to tyrosine kinase, atrial natriuretic hormone coupled to membrane-bound guanylyl cyclase). Precisely what distin-guishes agonists from antagonists is not yet understood, but there have recently been great advances in understanding the events that link receptor activation with cellular response. These are termed signal transduc-tion processes. They include:

1. Direct linkage to receptor-operated ion channels (e.g. for potassium or calcium ions). These processes operate rapidly (micro- to millisecond range) and their study has been greatly facilitated by the technique of patch clamping.

2. Linkage via guanosine triphosphate (GTP)-binding proteins (G-proteins) to adenylyl cyclase which catalyzes synthesis of cyclic adenosine monophosphate (cAMP) or to other enzymes that catalyze the synthesis of second messengers. Cyclic AMP is an intracellular second messenger whose actions are terminated by degradation by specific phosphodiesterase enzymes that are themselves targets of drug action. The G-proteins are heterotrimers (α, β and γ subunits) with stimulatory or inhibitory α subunits (termed respectively α_s or α_i) that dissociate on combination of the receptor with agonist, and activate or inhibit the cyclase, operating on a time-scale of seconds to minutes. An uncommon disease, pseudohypoparathyroidism is caused by a genetic defect in the α_s subunit of the G-protein controlling adeny-lyl cyclase; consequently, although the circulating concentration of parathyroid hormone is high, responses to it are blunted with reduced phosphate excretion by the kidney and skeletal abnormalities. Some endocrine disorders are caused by somatic mutations in genes encoding proteins in the cyclase/G-protein complex that result in the enzyme operating 'full tilt' even in the absence of the hormonal agonist. Examples are an unusual form of hyperthyroidism due to hyperfunctioning adenomas in which the cells behave as though maximally stimulated by thyrotropin, and an unusual form of male sexual precocity in which Leydig cells in the testis behave as though maximally stimulated by luteinizing hormone.

3. Activation of one of several phospholipase enzymes. Phospholipase A_2 initiates the arachidonic acid cascade and also synthe-sis of lyso-PAF, which is the precursor of platelet-activating factor (PAF). Several of the eicosanoid products of arachidonic acid as well as PAF are believed to have intracellular messenger functions in addition to mediating actions via surface receptors on neighboring cells. A specific phospholipase C attacks inositol phospho-lipid, liberating diacylglycerol which diffuses in the lipid phase of cell membranes and activates membrane-bound protein kinase C. The highly polar second messenger 1,4,5-phosphatidyl inositol *bis* phosphate (inositol trisphos-phate, ITP) is formed simultaneously and diffuses through the cytoplasm and regulates release of calcium from intracel-lular stores and calcium entry via the plasma membrane.

4. Combination of drugs or hormones with cytoplasmic receptors is followed by combi-nation via a DNA binding domain (contain-ing zinc fingers) with a specific DNA receptor and derepression of transcription of messenger RNA with consequent new protein synthesis. Such effects (e.g. result-ing from steroid receptor occupation) occur over a time course of minutes to hours.

AGONISTS

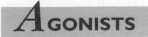

As explained above, it is useful to distinguish between drugs that act on receptors for endogenous mediators and those that do not, because only in the case of the former does it make sense to speak of agonists. For instance, it would be meaningless to talk of an agonist at the dihydrofolate reductase enzyme or at the voltage-dependent sodium channel, even though both of these are targets of drug action (e.g. of methotrexate or lignocaine, respectively), whereas it is useful to classify salbutamol as an agonist at the β_2-adrenoceptor. Agonists produce their effects by combining with and activating specific receptors for endogenous mediators. The process of activation depends on the signal transduction pathway to which the receptor is linked. The effect may be excitatory (e.g. adrenaline increases cardiac contractility) or inhibitory (e.g. dopamine relaxes renovascular smooth muscle, salbutamol relaxes airway smooth muscle). Agonists such as succinyl-choline cause a seemingly paradoxical inhibitory effect (neuromuscular blockade) by causing long-lasting depolarization at the neuromuscular junction and hence inactivation of the voltage-dependent sodium channels that initiate the action potential.

Endogenous ligands have sometimes been discovered long *after* other drugs that act on their receptors. Endorphins and enkephalins (endogenous ligands of morphine receptors) were discovered many years after morphine, which is now recognized as an agonist at opioid receptors. Evidence is currently accumulating that membrane Na^+/K^+ ATPase is the receptor of an endogenous natriuretic hormone with ouabain-like properties and there has been speculation as to the possible existence of an endogenous agonist for voltage-dependent calcium channels, so views on drugs acting on these and other targets will continue to develop as their physiology is understood more completely.

COMPETITIVE ANTAGONISTS

Competitive antagonists combine with the same receptor as an agonist (e.g. ranitidine at histamine H_2-receptors), but fail to activate it, presumably because they do not provoke the conformational changes in the receptor that lead to activation of its signal transduction pathway. When combined with the receptor they prevent access to it of its natural agonist/mediator. The complex between competitive antagonist and receptor is reversible. Consequently, in the presence of antagonist, a higher dose of agonist is needed to produce the same effect as in its absence. However, provided the dose of agonist is increased sufficiently, a maximal effect can still be obtained, i.e. the antagonism is *surmountable*. The dose of agonist needed to produce the same effect in the presence of a fixed concentration of competitive antagonist as in its absence is a constant multiple, known as the *dose ratio*. This results in the familiar parallel shift to the right of the log dose–response curve, since the addition of a constant length on a logarithmic scale corresponds to multiplication by a constant factor (Fig. 2.4a). Examples of competitive antagonists include H_1 and H_2 antagonists, β-adrenoceptor antagonists and neuromuscular-

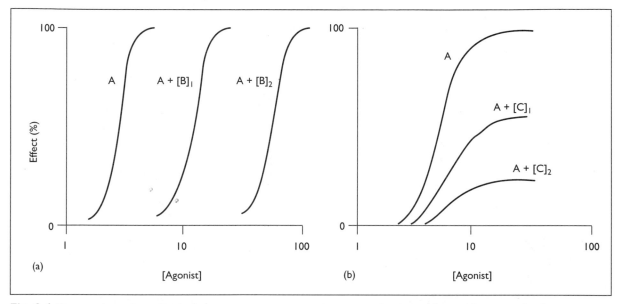

Fig. 2.4 Drug antagonism. Control dose–response curves to an agonist A together with curves in the presence of (a) a competitive antagonist B and (b) a non competitive antagonist C. Increasing concentrations of the competitive antagonist ([B]$_1$, [B]$_2$) cause a parallel shift to the right of the log dose–effect curve (a), while the non-competitive antagonist ([C]$_1$, [C]$_2$) flattens the curve and reduces its maximum (b).

blocking drugs like pancuronium. By contrast, antagonists that do not combine with the same receptor (non-competitive antagonists), or drugs that combine irreversibly with their receptors (such as phenoxybenzamine, an irreversible α-receptor antagonist used in preparing patients with pheochromocytoma for surgery), reduce the slope of the log dose–response curve and depress its maximum (Fig. 2.4b).

The relationship between concentration of a competitive antagonist [B], and dose ratio (*r*) was worked out by Gaddum, and by Schildt, and is:

$$r - 1 = [B]/K_B$$

where K_B is the dissociation equilibrium constant of the reversible reaction of the antagonist with its receptor. K_B has units of concentration and is the concentration of antagonist needed to occupy half the receptors in the absence of agonist. The lower the value of K_B the more potent is the drug. If several concentrations of a competitive antagonist are studied and the dose ratio measured at each concentration, a plot of (*r* − 1) against [B] yields a straight line through the origin of slope 1/K_B (Fig. 2.5a). Values of K_B estimated in this way often agree well with measurements of binding affinity using radiolabeled ligand, and are needed to confirm that high-affinity binding sites correspond to the receptor rather than to some other binding site such as a degradative enzyme or clearance mechanism. Schildt pointed out that if (*r* − 1) is plotted against [B] on log–log coordinates, a straight line results with a slope of unity and intercept −log K_B, which he referred to as pA$_2$, by analogy with the logarithmic pH scale. The larger the numerical value of pA$_2$, the more potent is the drug. This kind of plot (known as a Schildt plot, Fig. 2.5b) provides a means of quantifying the potencies of competitive antagonists. Such measurements provided the means of classifying and subdividing receptors in terms of the relative potencies of different antagonists.

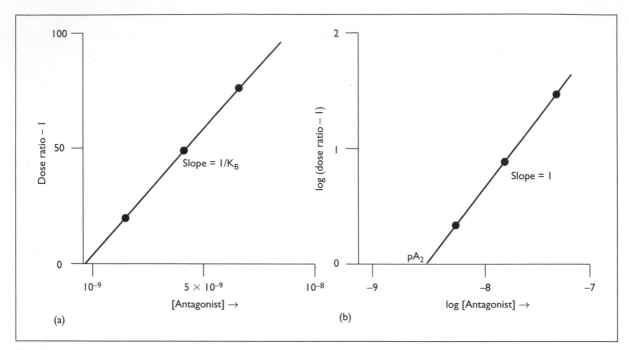

Fig. 2.5 Competitive antagonism. (a) A plot of antagonist concentration versus (dose ratio − 1) gives a straight line through the origin. (b) A log–log plot (a Schildt plot) gives a straight line of unit slope. The potency of the antagonist (pA_2) is determined from the intercept of the Schildt plot.

*P*ARTIAL AGONISTS

Some drugs combine with receptors and activate them, but are incapable of eliciting a maximal response, no matter how great their concentration. These are called partial agonists and are said to have low efficacy. Efficacy is a factor that can be ascribed a numerical value of 0 for a competitive antagonist, 1 for a full agonist and a value between 0 and 1 for a partial agonist, although this begs the question (for which there is currently no adequate answer) of what it is at the molecular level that determines whether or not a drug will activate a receptor having occupied it. Several partial agonists are used in therapeutics, including buprenorphine (a partial agonist at morphine μ-receptors) and oxprenolol and pindolol (partial agonists at β-adrenoceptors).

Full agonists are sometimes capable of eliciting a maximal response when only a small fraction of the receptors is occupied (a situation sometimes described by saying that there are 'spare receptors'), but this is not the case with partial agonists, where a substantial fraction of the receptors needs to be occupied to cause a response. This has two consequences of potential therapeutic importance. First, partial agonists *antagonize* the effect of a full agonist, because most of the receptors are occupied with low-efficacy partial agonist with which the full agonist must compete. Thus a partial β-agonist such as pindolol itself raises heart rate modestly, but opposes any further increase in heart rate caused by a strong agonist such as noradrenaline. Consequently, exercise-induced increases in rate, which are mediated by increased sympathetic nerve output to the heart, are abolished or blunted. A second consequence of clinical importance is that it is more difficult to reverse the effects of a partial agonist such as buprenorphine with a competitive antagonist such as naloxone, than it would be to reverse the effects of a strong agonist such as morphine with the same antagonist: a larger fraction of the receptors is occupied by buprenorphine than by morphine, and a much larger concentration of naloxone is required to compete successfully and displace buprenorphine from the receptors.

Slow Processes

Protracted exposure of receptors to agonists, as frequently occurs in therapeutic use as opposed to tissue bath experiments, can cause down-regulation or desensitization by one of several mechanisms. Desensitization is sometimes specific for a particular agonist (when it is referred to as homologous desensitization), or there may be cross-desensitization to different agonists (heterologous desensitization). Membrane receptors may become internalized and hence no longer accessible to drugs in the extracellular fluid. This occurs when low density lipoprotein (LDL) particles are taken up via specific LDL receptors on hepatocytes. Alternatively, G-protein-mediated linkage between receptors and effector enzymes (e.g. adenylyl cyclase) may be disrupted. Since G-proteins link several distinct receptors to the same effector molecule this can give rise to heterologous desensitization. Receptor desensitization is probably involved in the tolerance that occurs during prolonged administration of drugs such as morphine and the benzodiazepines (see chapter 15 on hypnotics and chapter 22 on control of pain).

Therapeutic effects sometimes depend on induction of tolerance, albeit rarely. For example, analogs of gonadotropin-releasing hormone (GnRH) such as buserelin are used in treating patients with disseminated prostate cancer. Gonadotropin-releasing hormone is released physiologically in a pulsatile manner. During continuous treatment with buserelin there is initial stimulation of luteinizing hormone (LH) and follicle-stimulating hormone (FSH) release followed by receptor desensitization and suppression of LH and FSH release. This results in regression of the hormone-sensitive tumor. During initial stages of treatment there is a risk of exacerbation of symptoms from tumor metastases which can be prevented by use of an androgen receptor antagonist such as cyproterone acetate. Once tolerance to GnRH has developed, cyproterone acetate can be stopped avoiding long-term side effects of androgen receptor blockade.

Conversely, reduced exposure of a cell or tissue to an agonist that is normally present results in increased receptor numbers and so-called up-regulation. Denervation supersensitivity to acetylcholine is a well-known example. Prolonged use of receptor-blocking drugs may produce an analogous effect. Up-regulation of receptors is important in some of the movement disorders caused by prolonged treatment with antipsychotic drugs (chapter 16). One example of clinical importance in some patients is increased β-adrenoceptor numbers following prolonged use of β-blocking drugs such as atenolol. Abrupt drug withdrawal can lead to tachycardia and worsening angina in patients being treated for ischemic heart disease. Whether receptor up-regulation also contributes to the withdrawal syndromes that occur on abrupt discontinuation of opiates, benzodiazepines, ethanol and anticonvulsants is not known.

NON-RECEPTOR MECHANISMS

By contrast to high-potency/high-selectivity drugs such as atropine or morphine that combine with specific receptors, some drugs exert their effects via simple physical properties or chemical reactions due to their presence in some body compartment. Examples of medications that work in such ways include antacids (neutralization of gastric acid), the osmotic diuretic mannitol (increasing the osmolality of renal tubular fluid), and bulk and lubricating laxatives. These agents are of low potency and specificity, and hardly qualify as 'drugs' in the usual sense at all, although some of them are very useful medicines. Oxygen is an example of a highly specific therapeutic agent that is used in high concentrations (i.e. is of low molar potency). It combines with a high-affinity binding site on a transport protein (hemoglobin) as well as dissolving in plasma, and works by promoting aerobic respiration in tissues. This is an example of a therapeutic agent of low potency but high specificity, working through a non-receptor mechanism.

Finally, metal chelating agents, which are used in the treatment of certain kinds of poisoning and of copper or iron overload in Wilson's disease or thalassemia, are examples of drugs that exert their effects through interaction with small molecular species rather than with macromolecules, yet possess significant specificity.

General anesthetics are believed to act in or on membrane lipids. They have low molar potencies determined by their olive oil/water partition coefficients, and low specificity. Debate as to whether general anesthetics may in fact after all act on specific receptors in hydrophobic regions of membrane proteins has recently been rekindled. Furthermore, some of the effects of ethanol (another drug sometimes used to exemplify non-receptor-mediated mechanisms) are partly reversed by flumazenil, a benzodiazepine receptor antagonist. The distinction between receptor-mediated and non-receptor-mediated centrally acting drugs is thus currently somewhat blurred.

Pharmacokinetics

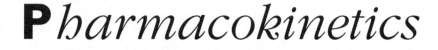

Introduction   **20**

Constant rate infusion   **20**

Single bolus dose   **22**

Repeated (multiple) dosing   **24**

Deviations from the one-compartment model with first-order elimination   **25**

INTRODUCTION

By convention, pharmacokinetics is defined as the study of the time course of drug absorption, distribution, metabolism and excretion, whereas the term pharmacodynamics refers to the corresponding pharmacological response. The magnitude of pharmacological effect usually depends directly on the concentration of the drug (or an active metabolite) in the vicinity of the receptors, although there are a few exceptions in the form of 'hit-and-run' drugs that form irreversible bonds with their sites of action so that their effects outlast their presence at these sites (e.g. aspirin, omeprazole, alkylating agents and some monoamine oxidase inhibitors). Understanding pharmacokinetic principles combined with specific information regarding the pharmacokinetic profile of an individual drug facilitates appropriate use of the drug (e.g. route of administration, dose interval) and may help explain therapeutic failure or toxicity (chapter 8). The limitations of this approach also need to be borne in mind: when pharmacokinetic parameters of a particular drug are looked up it should be appreciated that these are derived from a limited and relatively homogeneous population, usually of healthy male volunteers. Age, genetic factors, disease (especially renal or hepatic disease) or the coadministration of other drugs can markedly alter these values in an individual patient.

In view of the complexity of the human body it is inevitable that pharmacokinetic formulations must be based on drastically simplifying assumptions. Despite this such formulations are often mathematically cumbrous,

rendering the subject unintelligible to many clinicians. The object of this chapter is to introduce and explain some basic pharmacokinetic concepts by considering three clinical dosing situations: constant rate intravenous infusion, bolus dose injection and repeated dosing. For a more extended treatment the reader is recommended to read *Clinical Pharmacokinetics; Consequences and Applications* by Rowland and Tozer (Lea & Febiger, Philadelphia).

Bulk flow in the blood stream is very rapid, as is diffusion after drugs have traversed membranous barriers, so the rate-limiting step in drug distribution is usually the penetration of these barriers. This is determined mainly by the lipid solubility of the drug, highly polar water-soluble drugs being transferred slowly wherever highly lipid-soluble, non-polar, drugs are transferred rapidly across the lipid-rich membranes of cells. A few polar drugs are transported rapidly by a different mechanism, namely by combination with a specific carrier. The simplest pharmacokinetic model considers the body as a single well-stirred compartment in which an administered drug distributes homogeneously instantaneously and from which it is eliminated. Many drugs are eliminated at a rate proportional to their concentration: 'first-order' elimination. A one-compartment model with first-order elimination often approximates the clinical situation surprisingly well once absorption and distribution have occurred. We start by considering this, and then describe some important deviations from it.

CONSTANT RATE INFUSION

If a drug is administered intravenously into one arm via a syringe driven by a constant rate infusion pump, and a series of blood

samples are drawn from the contralateral arm for measurement of drug concentration, a plot of plasma concentration versus time

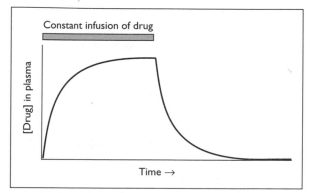

Constant infusion of drug

[Drug] in plasma

Time →

Fig. 3.1 Plasma concentration of a drug during and after a constant intravenous infusion as indicated by the bar.

can be constructed (Fig. 3.1). At time zero, just as the infusion is started, plasma drug concentration is also zero, so the curve begins at the origin. Concentration then rises, rapidly at first and then more slowly until a plateau is approached that represents a steady state. At steady state the rate of input of drug to the body (as determined by the concentration of drug in the syringe and setting of the infusion pump) equals the rate of elimination of drug from the body. Plasma drug concentration at plateau is called the steady-state concentration (C_{ss}). The steady-state concentration depends on the rate of drug infusion, and on the clearance of the drug from the body: the greater the infusion rate or the lower the clearance, the greater is C_{ss}. The clearance is the volume of plasma from which the drug is totally eliminated (i.e. cleared) per unit time. At steady state:

Administration rate = Elimination rate

Elimination rate = C_{ss} × Clearance

so:

Clearance = Administration rate/C_{ss}

Consider an example: a drug is infused at 10 mg/min, and the plasma concentration rises to a steady-state value of 2 mg/ml. At steady state the rate of elimination is the same as the rate of input, i.e. 10 mg/min. Ten milligrams of drug are contained in 5 ml

plasma (since the concentration is 2 mg/ml) so 5 ml plasma is cleared each minute (clearance = 5 ml/min).

Clearance is the best measure of the efficiency with which a drug is eliminated from the body, whether by renal excretion, by metabolism or by a combination of both. The concept will be familiar from physiology, where clearances of substances with particular properties are used as measures of physiologically important processes such as glomerular filtration rate, effective renal plasma flow or hepatic plasma flow. For instance, inulin (which is not metabolized, is filtered at the glomeruli but neither reabsorbed from nor secreted into the renal tubules) is used in this way to estimate glomerular filtration rate. In the case of therapeutic drugs, knowledge of the clearance in an individual patient helps the physician to adjust the dose accurately in such a way as to achieve a desired target steady-state concentration of drug in the patient's plasma, since:

$$\frac{\text{Required}}{\text{administration rate}} = \frac{\text{Desired } C_{ss}}{\times \text{ Clearance}}$$

This is useful in situations where therapy is guided by measurement of drug concentrations in plasma. The reason that clearance is not more used by clinicians is partly that these situations are fairly few (see chapter 8), and partly that chemical pathology laboratories often quote therapeutic ranges and report plasma concentrations of drugs in molar terms, whereas drug doses are usually given in units of mass. Consequently, one needs to know the molecular weight of the drug before one can use this method of calculating the rate of administration required to achieve a plasma concentration within the given therapeutic range.

When drug infusion is stopped, plasma concentration declines again toward zero. The time taken for plasma concentration to halve is the half-life ($t_{1/2}$). A one-compartment model with first-order elimination predicts an exponential decline in concentration when the infusion is discontinued as shown in Fig. 3.1. After a second half-life has elapsed, concentration will have halved again (i.e. to one-quarter the original concentration) and so on. The increase in drug concentration when the infusion is started is also exponential, being the inverse of the decay curve. This has a very important practical implication, namely that the half-life of a drug not only determines the time course of its disappearance when administration is stopped, but also determines the time course of its accumulation when administration is started. This is discussed again below when multiple dosing is considered.

The half-life is a very useful concept for the clinician, helping to determine a sensible dose interval, indicating the time over which drug accumulation occurs after starting a patient on a regular dose regimen and helping decide on the advisability or otherwise of a loading dose as explained below. What it is not is a direct measure of drug elimination, since differences in $t_{1/2}$ can be caused either by differences in the efficiency of elimination (i.e. the clearance) or differences in another important parameter, the volume of distribution (V_d). Clearance and not $t_{1/2}$ must therefore be used when a measure of the efficiency with which a drug is eliminated is required.

SINGLE BOLUS DOSE

The concept of apparent V_d can be understood readily in the context of the relation between the size (mass) of a bolus dose and the plasma concentration that results. Volume of distribution is a multiplying factor with units of volume relating the amount of drug in the whole body to the plasma concentration, C_p (i.e. amount of drug in the body = $C_p \times V_d$). Before addressing the biological situation consider a very simple physical analogy. By definition, concentration (c) equals mass (m) /volume (v):

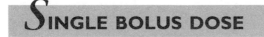

$$c = \frac{m}{v}$$

Thus, if a known mass of an inert marker substance (say 300 mg) is dissolved in a glass beaker of water of unknown volume (v), v can be estimated by measuring the concentration of substance in a sample of solution. If the concentration is 0.1 mg/ml, for instance, we would calculate that $v = 3000$ ml ($v = m/c$). This is valid unless a fraction of the substance has become adsorbed on the glass surface of the beaker, in which case the solution will be less concentrated than if all the substance had been present dissolved in the water. Say that 90% of the substance is adsorbed in this way, then the concentration in solution will be 0.01 mg/ml, and the volume will be correspondingly overestimated, as 30 000 ml in this example. Based on the mass of substance dissolved and the measured concentration we might say that it is 'as if' the substance were dissolved in 30 litres of water, whereas the real volume of water in the beaker is only 3 litres.

Now consider the parallel situation when a known mass of a drug (say 300 mg) is injected intravenously into a human. Suppose that distribution occurs instantaneously before any drug is eliminated, and that blood is sampled and the concentration of drug measured in the plasma is 0.1 mg/ml. We could infer that it is 'as if' the drug has distributed in 3 litres, and we would say that that this is the apparent volume of distribution. If the measured plasma concentration was 0.01 mg/ml we would say that the apparent volume of distribution was 30 litres, and if the measured concentration was 0.001 mg/ml the apparent volume of distribution would be 300 litres.

What does volume of distribution mean? From these examples it is obvious that it is not necessarily the real volume of a body compartment, since it may be greater than the volume of the whole body. At the lower

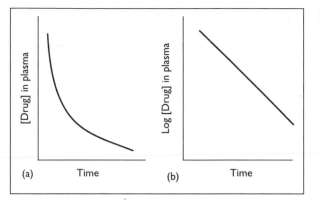

Fig. 3.2 One-compartment model. Plasma concentration–time curve following a bolus dose of drug plotted (a) arithmetically or (b) semi-logarithmically. This drug fits a one-compartment model, i.e. its concentration falls exponentially with time.

end, values of V_d are limited by the plasma volume (approximately 3 litres in an adult): this is the smallest volume in which a drug could distribute following intravenous injection, but there is no theoretical upper limit on V_d, very large values occurring when very little of the injected dose remains in the plasma, most being taken up in fat or bound to tissues.

In reality, processes of elimination begin as soon as the bolus dose (d) of drug is administered, the drug being cleared at a rate Cl_s (total systemic clearance). In practice a series of blood samples are obtained at intervals starting shortly after administration of the dose. If the one-compartment, first-order elimination model holds, there is an exponential decline of plasma drug concentration, just as at the end of the constant rate infusion (Fig. 3.2a). If the data are plotted on semilogarithmic graph paper, with time on the abscissa, a straight line with negative slope results (Fig. 3.2b). Extrapolation back to zero time gives the concentration (c_0) that would have occurred at time 0, and this is used to calculate V_d:

$$V_d = \frac{d}{c_0}$$

Half-life can be read off the graph as the time between any point (concentration c_0)

and the point at which the concentration c_t has reduced by 50%, i.e. $c_0/c_t = 2$. The slope of the line is the elimination rate constant, k_{el}:

$$k_{el} = \frac{Cl_s}{V_d}$$

$t_{1/2}$ and k_{el} are related:

$$t_{1/2} = \frac{l_n2}{k_{el}} = \frac{0.693}{k_{el}}$$

The volume of distribution is related partly to the characteristics of the drug, for example lipid solubility, and partly to patient characteristics such as body size, plasma protein concentration, body water and fat content. In general highly lipid-soluble compounds able to penetrate cells and fatty tissues have a large V_d, whereas highly polar water-soluble compounds have a smaller V_d. The volume of distribution determines the peak plasma concentration after a bolus dose, so factors that influence V_d, such as body mass, need to be taken into account when deciding on dose (e.g. by expressing dose per kg body weight). In babies (chapter 10), not only is body mass small, but body composition differs qualitatively from that in the adult, proportionately more body mass being accounted for by aqueous rather than fatty tissues. Thus, the 'standard' starting dose expressed on a 'per kg body weight' basis of a polar drug such as gentamicin is greater in babies than in adults. Conversely, in elderly people fat accounts for a greater fraction of body mass than in young adults.

Knowing V_d (or having an estimate of it) tells the physician what peak plasma concentration can be expected following a bolus dose. It is also useful to know V_d when considering dialysis as a means of accelerating drug elimination in poisoned patients (chapter 50). Drugs with a large V_d (e.g. many tricyclic antidepressants) are unlikely to be removed efficiently by hemodialysis, especially if they are also highly bound by plasma protein, becase only a small fraction of the total drug in the body is present in unbound form in the plasma, the fluid compartment accessible to the artificial kidney.

If both V_d and $t_{1/2}$ of a drug are known (or can be estimated) in an individual subject, they can be used to calculate the systemic clearance of the drug using the expression:

$$Cl_s = 0.693 \times \frac{V_d}{t_{1/2}}$$

Note that clearance has units of volume/unit time (e.g. ml/min), V_d has units of volume (e.g. ml), $t_{1/2}$ units of time (e.g. min) and 0.693 is a constant arising because ln (0.5) = ln 2 = 0.693. This expression relates clearance to V_d and $t_{1/2}$, but unlike the steady-state situation referred to above only applies for a single-compartment model with first-order elimination kinetics.

REPEATED (MULTIPLE) DOSING

If multiple doses of a drug are administered at intervals much greater than the half-life, little if any accumulation occurs (Fig. 3.3a). Some drugs are used effectively in this way (e.g. penicillin in treating a mild infection by a susceptible organism). More often it is desirable to achieve a continuous finite plasma concentration. Figure 3.3b shows the plasma concentration–time curve that results when a constant dose of drug is administered as a bolus at intervals less than the half-life. It is apparent that the average concentration rises toward a plateau just as if the drug were being administered by constant rate infusion. That is, after one half-life the average concentration is 50% of the plateau (steady-state) concentration, after two half-lives it is 75%, after three half lives it is 87.5% and after four half-lives 93.75%. However, unlike the constant rate infusion situation, the actual plasma concentration at any time swings above or below the mean level. Increasing the dosing frequency smoothes out the peaks and troughs between doses, while decreasing the frequency has the opposite effect. If the peaks are too high toxicity may result, while if the troughs are too low there may be a loss of efficacy. If a drug is administered once every half-life the peak plasma concentration will be double the trough level; in practice this amount of variation is acceptable in many therapeutic situations, so a dosing interval is often selected that is approximately equal to the half-life.

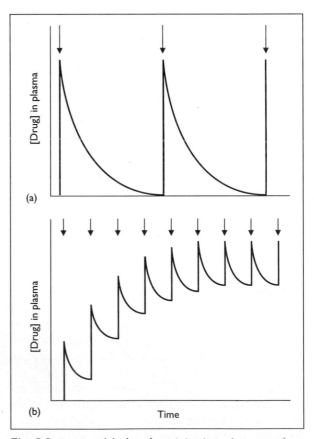

Fig. 3.3 Repeated bolus dose injections (at arrows) at (a) intervals much greater than $t_{1/2}$ and (b) intervals less than $t_{1/2}$.

Knowing the half-life of a drug alerts the prescriber to the likely time course over which it will accumulate. Drug excretion often declines with age (chapter 10), so that for a given dose higher plasma concentrations may be achieved in the elderly. A further pitfall is that several drugs have active metabolites that are eliminated more slowly than the parent drug. This is the case with several of the benzodiazepines, which have metabolites that have half-lives of many days. Consequently adverse effects such as memory impairment and ataxia, which may incorrectly be ascribed to aging or disease, may make their appearance when steady state is approached after several weeks of treatment when four to five half-lives (of the active metabolite) have elapsed. Such effects resolve only slowly (over a similar time course) when dosing is discontinued.

Knowing the half-life of a drug also helps the prescribing physician to decide whether or not to initiate treatment with a loading dose. Consider the use of digoxin (half-life approximately 40 hours) as an example. Digoxin is usually prescribed once daily, resulting in a less than twofold variation in maximum and minimum plasma concentrations, and reaching >90% of the mean steady-state concentration in approximately 1 week (i.e. four half-lives). In many clinical situations, for instance a patient with atrial fibrillation and no evidence of heart failure, such a time course is acceptable. In other cases, (for example a patient with heart failure and a ventricular rate of 155 beats/min) a more rapid response can be achieved by using a loading dose.

This loading dose strategy is not universally appropriate, however. Thus the rate-limiting step in achieving a desired therapeutic response may occur at or beyond the level of the receptor (i.e. the time course of the response may be determined by pharmacodynamic rather than pharmacokinetic processes). Examples include the use of glucocorticoids in a patient with acute severe asthma, where latency is accounted for by processes of transcription and new protein synthesis subsequent to receptor occupancy (chapters 2 and 30) or initiation of treatment with warfarin in a patient with deep vein thrombosis where latency depends on clearance from the body of preformed vitamin K-dependent coagulation factors (chapter 27).

*D*EVIATIONS FROM THE ONE-COMPARTMENT MODEL WITH FIRST-ORDER ELIMINATION

Two-compartment model

This is useful to understand a situation that often occurs following an intravenous bolus dose. Instead of a simple exponential decline in plasma concentration as predicted by the one-compartment model, what is often actually observed is a biphasic decline (Fig. 3.4). The two-compartment model (Fig. 3.5) treats the body as a smaller central compartment and a larger peripheral compartment. Again, these compartments have no precise physiological or anatomical meaning, although the central compartment is assumed to comprise blood (from which samples are taken for analysis) with the extracellular spaces of some well-perfused tissues such as heart, lungs, liver and kidneys. The peripheral compartment is due to less well-perfused tissues such as muscle, skin and fat into which drug permeates more slowly. Reversible transfer occurs between these two compartments depending on such factors as blood flow and affinity of tissues for the drug.

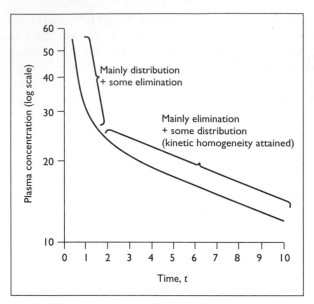

Fig. 3.4 Two-compartment model. Plasma concentration–time curve (semi-logarithmic) following a bolus dose of a drug that fits a two-compartment model.

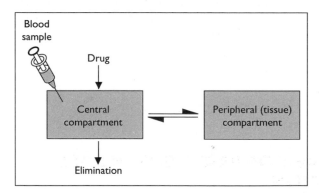

Fig. 3.5 Schematic representation of a two-compartment model.

When a drug is instantaneously introduced into the central compartment (i.e. by intravenous injection) drug concentration in plasma falls biphasically. The initial rapid fall is called the α phase and reflects mainly distribution from the central to the peripheral compartment, although elimination also starts from the moment the drug enters the body. At some point in time a pseudodistribution equilibrium is attained between the central and peripheral compartments when the ratio

of drug in each compartment approaches a constant value which is maintained during the second slower phase of decline in blood concentration, which mainly reflects elimination. This second slower phase is called the β phase, and the corresponding $t_{1/2}$ is known as $t_{1/2\beta}$. This is the appropriate value for clinical use such as estimation of need for loading dose, time to plateau, likely accumulation and time required for elimination.

For some drugs even the two-compartment model is insufficient to describe the observed plasma concentration–time curves. More complex models such as a three-compartment model with central and 'shallow' and 'deep' peripheral compartments have been used to describe the triphasic decline in the log plasma concentration versus time curves of several drugs (e.g. amiodarone). These are, however, algebraically unwieldy and seldom clinically useful and are not considered further here.

Non-linear ('dose-dependent') pharmacokinetics

Although many drugs are eliminated at a rate roughly proportional to their concentration (i.e. obey 'first-order' kinetics) there are several therapeutically important exceptions. To understand how this arises, consider a drug that is eliminated by conversion to an inactive metabolite by an enzyme, and suppose that at high concentrations the enzyme becomes saturated. Drug concentration and reaction velocity will be related by the Michaelis–Menten equation (Fig. 3.6). At low concentrations rate is approximately linearly related to concentration (first-order kinetics), whereas at saturating concentrations rate is independent of concentration (zero-order kinetics). Similar behavior is anticipated when a drug is eliminated by a saturable transport process. In clinical practice drugs exhibiting non-linear kinetics are the exception rather than the rule. This is because most

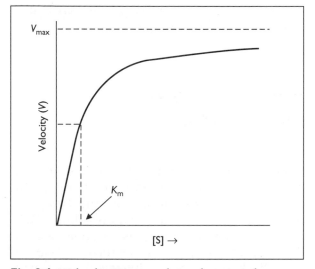

Fig. 3.6 Michaelis–Menten relation between the velocity (V) of an enzyme reaction and the substrate concentration ([S]). [S] at 50% V_{max} is equal to K_m, the Michaelis–Menten constant.

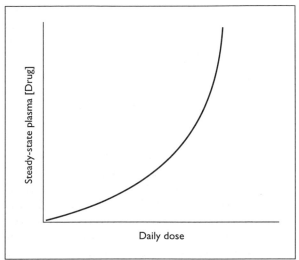

Fig. 3.8 Non-linear kinetics: steady-state plasma concentration of a drug following repeated dosing as a function of dose.

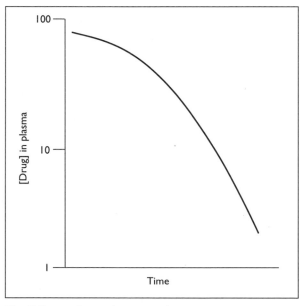

Fig. 3.7 Non-linear kinetics: plasma concentration–time curve following administration of a bolus dose of a drug eliminated by Michaelis–Menten kinetics.

drugs are used therapeutically at doses that give rise to concentrations that are well below the Michaelis constant (K_m: the concentration at which the rate of elimination

is half maximal), and so operate on the lower, approximately linear, part of the Michaelis–Menten curve relating elimination velocity to plasma concentration.

Drugs that show non-linear kinetics in the therapeutic range include salicylate, heparin, phenytoin and ethanol. Some drugs (e.g. barbiturates) show non-linearity in the part of the toxic range encountered clinically. Implications of non-linear pharmacokinetics include:

1. The decline of concentration versus time following a bolus dose of such a drug is not exponential. Instead, elimination begins slowly and accelerates as plasma concentration falls as illustrated in Fig. 3.7.
2. The time required to eliminate 50% of a dose increases with increasing dose and the concept of a constant half-life is meaningless.
3. A relatively modest increase in dose of such a drug dramatically increases the amount of drug in the body once the drug-elimination process is saturated, as illustrated in Fig. 3.8. This is very important clinically when using plasma concentrations of a drug as a guide to dosing. Consider phenytoin, with a therapeutic

range of 10–20 mg/l. If in a particular patient a dose of 200 mg/day is found to give a steady-state plasma concentration of 7.5 mg/l and phenytoin had linear kinetics, doubling the dose to 400 mg/day would double the steady-state plasma concentration to 15 mg/l, nicely in the therapeutic range. However, phenytoin does not have linear kinetics, so that doubling the dose would actually cause a proportionately much greater increase in concentration and almost certainly precipitate toxicity. A much smaller dose increment is appropriate. Moreover, because of the decreased rate of elimination at higher plasma concentrations (i.e. because of the longer apparent $t_{1/2}$) the plateau is attained only after a longer time than at the lower dose. In practice dose increments of phenytoin should therefore be small (25–50 mg/day) and the plasma concentration checked 10–14 days after increasing the dose.

Enterohepatic circulation

Interpretation of plasma concentration–time curves is complicated when there is an enterohepatic circulation of the drug in question. This occurs when drug (e.g. rifampicin, several estrogens) is conjugated in the liver and conjugate is secreted in bile but then broken down by intestinal flora with regeneration of free drug that is reabsorbed from the gut. This can result in a second peak in plasma concentration following an intravenous bolus dose.

Drug Absorption and Routes of Administration

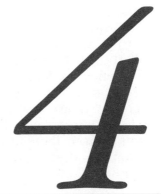

4

Introduction   **30**

Bioavailability, bioequivalence and generic versus proprietary prescribing   **30**

Prodrugs   **32**

Routes of administration   **33**

*I*NTRODUCTION

Drugs must cross several biological membranes to reach their sites of action. Drug absorption, and hence the possible routes by which a particular drug may usefully be administered in order to obtain a systemic effect, is determined by the rate and extent of penetration of such membranes. Conversely, drugs are sometimes used for their local effects, in which case systemic absorption from the site of application is a disadvantage. Most biological membranes are readily penetrated by lipid-soluble substances and low molecular weight lipid-insoluble molecules whilst presenting a barrier to larger lipid-insoluble molecules. A simple model considers such membranes as a lipid barrier containing small aqueous channels. The most convenient route of drug administration for patients is usually by mouth, and absorption processes in the alimentary tract are among the best understood.

*B*IOAVAILABILITY, BIOEQUIVALENCE AND GENERIC VERSUS PROPRIETARY PRESCRIBING

Drugs must reach the systemic circulation if they are to exert a systemic effect. When administered other than intravenously, and specifically when administered by mouth, most drugs are absorbed incompletely (Fig. 4.1). There are three reasons for this: (1) drug is inactivated within the gut lumen by gastric acid, digestive enzymes or bacteria; (2) absorption is incomplete; and (3) presystemic ('first-pass') metabolism in gut wall and liver. If hepatic metabolism is rapid and extensive, nearly all of an absorbed dose may be cleared from the portal venous blood so that little or no drug is present in hepatic venous blood (i.e. the hepatic *extraction ratio* is nearly 100%), and little drug enters the systemic circulation. Together these processes account for the fact that bioavailability of orally administered drugs (i.e. the extent to which the active component in a pharmaceutical product enters the systemic circulation in active form) is less than 100%. Drug absorption depends on the presence of drug in solution at the absorption site. Many factors in the manufacture of the dosage form influence its disintegration, dispersion and

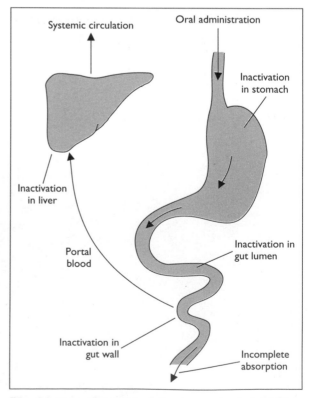

Fig. 4.1 Drug absorption following oral administration may be incomplete for several reasons.

dissolution. Pharmaceutical factors are therefore important in determining bioavailability. Tablets and capsules are complex products, for in addition to the drug there are excipients, disintegrating agents, binders, diluents, lubricants and dyes, which contribute to their performance as drug delivery systems, and influence bioavailability.

Differences in absorption from different preparations of the same drug occur, but it is important to distinguish statistically significant from clinically important differences in this regard. The former are common whereas the latter are not. Differences in bioavailability did, however, account for an epidemic of anticonvulsant intoxication in Australia in 1968–69. This was investigated in Brisbane where affected patients were found to be taking one brand of phenytoin. It was shown that the excipient in the responsible phenytoin capsules was changed from calcium sulfate to lactose several months before the outbreak · and that this change increased phenytoin bioavailability thereby precipitating toxicity.

Similarly, an apparently minor change in the manufacturing process of Lanoxin™ (a digoxin preparation made in the UK) resulted in reduced potency due to poor bioavailability, making this comparable with the potency of most other brands. Restoring the original manufacturing conditions restored potency but led to some confusion, and considerable variation occurred in blood levels recorded in patients who changed from 'old' to 'new' Lanoxin. These events drew attention to the non-equivalence of digoxin tablets available in the UK and alerted physicians to the potential for toxicity due to treatment with different digoxin formulations. Improved manufacturing standards have now reduced these problems.

These examples raise the question of whether prescribing should be by generic or by proprietary or brand name. When a new preparation is marketed in the UK it has a proprietary name supplied by the pharmaceutical company, and a non-proprietary (generic) name supplied by the *British Pharmacopoiea*. It is usually available only from the company that introduced it until the

patent runs out. After this, other companies can manufacture and market the product, sometimes under its generic name and sometimes under their own proprietary name. At this stage hospital pharmacists usually shop around for the best buy. If a doctor in hospital prescribes by proprietary name, the same drug produced by another company may be substituted. This saves considerable amounts of money. In contrast, if a general practitioner prescribes a proprietary product, the pharmacist must dispense that product even though it may cost more than the same drug made by another company. The attractions of generic prescribing in terms of minimizing costs are therefore obvious, but there are counterarguments, of which the strongest relates to the bioequivalence or otherwise of the proprietary product with its generic competitors. The formulation of a drug (i.e. excipients etc.) differs between products, sometimes affecting bioavailability. This is especially a concern with slow or sustained release preparations or preparations to be administered by different routes (e.g. rectal versus oral preparations). Drug regulatory bodies have strict criteria to assess whether such products can be licensed without the full supporting information that would be required for a completely new product (i.e. one based on a new chemical entity).

Absolute bioavailability is determined by measuring the area under the plasma concentration–time curve (AUC) following oral and intravenous administration (100% bioavailability). The area under the concentration–time curve represents the amount of drug absorbed, so a comparison of AUC after oral administration with AUC after intravenous administration expressed as a percentage gives the percentage bioavailability following oral administration (Fig. 4.2). It will be noted that the absolute bioavailabilty of two drugs may be the same (same AUC), but that the kinetics may be very different (e.g. one may have a much higher peak plasma concentration than the other, but a shorter duration). The rate at which a drug enters the body determines the onset of its pharmacological action, and also influences the intensity and

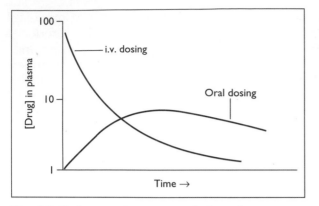

Fig. 4.2 Oral versus intravenous dosing: plasma concentration–time curves following administration of a drug intravenously (i.v.) or by mouth (oral).

sometimes duration of its action and is important in addition to the extent (completeness) of absorption.

The concept of bioavailability can also be criticized as implying a spurious precision and universality to the numerical value assigned. It must be appreciated that bioavailability will vary not only between groups of patients with different characteristics of age, gastrointestinal motility and pH, hepatic blood flow and so on, but that changes of these variables also occur within an individual so that 'bioavailability' can vary from one occasion to another. However, doctors prescribing for patients need to be confident that different preparations (branded or generic) are sufficiently similar that their substitution is unlikely to lead to clinically important alterations in outcome. Regulatory authorities have responded to this need by requiring companies seeking to introduce generic equivalents to products no longer protected by patent, to present evidence that their product behaves similarly to the one that is currently marketed. If evidence is presented that a new product can be treated as therapeutically equivalent to the current 'market leader' this is accepted as 'bioequivalence'. This does not imply that all possible pharmacokinetic parameters are identical between the two products, but that any such differences are unlikely to be of medical importance, and is a useful regulatory concept, albeit one that is hard to define quantitatively in a general (i.e. applying to different drugs) way.

It is impossible to give a universal answer to the generic versus proprietary issue for prescribing doctors. However, substitution of generic for brand-name products seldom causes problems. In addition, brand names cause confusion by creating multiple alternatives to the approved name, and unlike many approved names seldom reveal the pharmacological category of the drug (e.g. suffix -olol for β-blockers, -statin for β-hydroxymethylglutaryl coenzyme A (HMGCoA) reductase inhibitors, -opril for converting enzyme inhibitors etc.).

*P*RODRUGS

An approach to improving absorption or distribution to a relatively inaccessible tissue (e.g. brain) is to modify the drug molecule chemically to form a compound that is better absorbed and from which active drug is liberated after absorption. Such modified drugs are termed prodrugs. Examples are shown in Table 4.1.

Table 4.1 Prodrugs.

Prodrug	Product
Enalapril	Enalaprilat
Benorylate	Aspirin + paracetamol
Levodopa	Dopamine
Minoxidil	Minoxidil sulfate
Carbimazole	Methimazole
Azathiaprine	6-Mercaptopurine

ROUTES OF ADMINISTRATION

Oral

FOR *LOCAL* EFFECT

Oral drug administration may be used to produce local effects within the gastrointestinal tract. Examples include antacids, activated charcoal (given in some cases of poisoning to bind the toxic agent in the gut lumen), oral vancomycin (given to patients with pseudomembranous colitis to kill toxin-producing *Clostridium difficile* within the bowel), and sulfasalazine which delivers 5-amino salicylic acid (5-ASA) to the colon, thereby prolonging remission in patients with ulcerative colitis. Sulfasalazine commonly (5–55% of patients treated) causes adverse effects, ranging from trivial to severe. These are mainly attributable to the sulfapyridine moiety rather than the active 5-ASA, leading to the design of agents without a sulfa-based carrier. These include mesalazine and olsalazine, which have different mechanisms whereby the active 5-ASA is liberated. Mesalazine has a pH-dependent acrylic coat that degrades when the surrounding pH is greater than 7, as in the colon and distal part of the ileum. Olsalazine is a prodrug consisting of a dimer of two 5-ASA moieties joined by an azo bond that is cleaved by colonic bacteria. Olsalazine is superior to mesalazine in preventing relapses of ulcerative colitis, especially those occurring in the distal and sigmoid colon, presumably because it delivers 5-ASA more reliably than mesalazine to the distal colon.

Drugs that are not absorbed can have a systemic effect via an indirect action. Cholestyramine, a bile acid binding resin that lowers plasma concentrations of low density lipoprotein cholesterol and reduces the risk of myocardial infarction in men with hypercholesterolemia, is an example.

TO ACHIEVE SYSTEMIC EFFECTS

Oral administration of drugs is safer and more convenient than injection. There are two main mechanisms of drug absorption by the gut:

1. **Passive diffusion** is the most important mechanism. Non-polar lipid-soluble agents are well absorbed from the gut, mainly from the small intestine, because of its enormous absorptive surface area. In the case of weak acids or weak bases the non-ionized form of the drug is relatively fat soluble and thus diffuses easily. Absorption is therefore influenced by the pK of the drug and the pH at the absorption site. However, in practice, the very large surface area of the small intestine is of overriding importance. For example, if salicylate (a weak acid) is given with propantheline (which slows gastric emptying) its absorption is retarded, whereas if it is given with metoclopramide (which speeds gastric emptying) its absorption is accelerated.

2. **Active transport** which requires a specific, carrier-mediated, energy-consuming mechanism. Naturally occurring polar nutrients and aliments including sugars, amino acids and vitamins are absorbed by active or facilitated transport mechanisms. Drugs that are analogs of such molecules compete with these substrates and are transported via the carrier. Examples include L-dopa, methyldopa, some antimetabolites (such as methotrexate and 5-fluorouracil) and lithium (which competes with sodium ions for absorption).

Other factors that influence absorption from the gastrointestinal tract include:

1. **Surgical interference with gastric function** Gastrectomy reduces absorption of drugs including digoxin, levodopa, sulfonamides, ethambutol, ethionamide, iron and folic acid.

2. **Disease of the gastrointestinal tract** (e.g. celiac disease, cystic fibrosis) Effects of such disease are unpredictable, but often surprisingly minor (chapter 7).

3. **Presence of food or other substances in the gut** The timing of drug administration in relation to food can be important. Food and drink dilute the drug and can adsorb or otherwise complex with it. Food also influences the rate and/or extent of absorption by altering gastric emptying. Transient increases in hepatic portal blood flow such as occur after a meal may result in *greater* availability of drug by reducing presystemic hepatic metabolism. Plasma concentrations of propranolol and metoprolol are considerably higher when given with food for this reason.

   Conversely, most oral antibiotics should be given on an empty stomach to avoid impairment of absorption by food. Anthelmintics should also be taken similarly to maximize the concentration of drug to which the parasites are exposed, whereas indomethacin, levodopa, iron preparations, sodium valproate and other drugs likely to cause indigestion when given on an empty stomach should be taken with food.

4. **Drug metabolism by intestinal flora** may affect drug absorption and activity. The examples of sulfasalazine and olsalazine have been described above. Sulfinpyrazone is converted to an active sulfide metabolite by bacteria in the colon. Alteration of bowel flora (e.g. by concomitant use of antibiotics) can interrupt enterohepatic recycling and result in loss of activity of the low estrogen contraceptive pill (chapter 12 on drug interactions).

PROLONGED ACTION AND SUSTAINED RELEASE PREPARATIONS

Some drugs with short elimination half-lives need to be administered at inconveniently short intervals, making compliance difficult for the patient. A drug with similar actions but a longer half-life may be substituted. Examples are terazosin or doxazosin (long-acting α_1-adrenoceptor antagonists) for

prazosin, or amlodipine (a long-acting calcium channel antagonist) for nifedipine. Where no such option exists, there are various pharmaceutical means of slowing absorption of a rapidly eliminated drug. The aim of such sustained release preparations is to release a steady 'infusion' of drug into the gut lumen for absorption during transit of the small intestine. Reduced dosing frequency may improve compliance and in the case of some drugs (e.g. carbamazepine, quinidine), reduce adverse effects due to high peak plasma concentrations. Absorption of such preparations is likely to be incomplete, so it is especially important that bioavailability is established before their general introduction. Other problems associated with slow release preparations are:

1. Because transit time through the small intestine is only about 6 hours, prolongation of dosage interval from 12 to 24 hours is not reliably achieved.

2. If the gut lumen is narrowed or intestinal transit is slow, as in the elderly, there is a danger of high local drug concentrations causing mucosal damage. Osmosin™, an osmotically released formulation of indomethacin, had to be withdrawn because of bleeding and ulceration of the small intestine.

3. Overdose with sustained release preparations is difficult to treat because large amounts of drug continue to be absorbed several hours after tablets have left the stomach.

4. Reduced flexibility of dosing, since sustained release tablets should not be divided.

5. Expense.

Buccal and sublingual

Drugs are given to be retained in the mouth for local disorders of the pharynx or buccal mucosa such as aphthous ulcers (hydrocortisone lozenges or carbenoxelone gel) or thrush (nystatin lozenges).

Sublingual administration is an effective means of causing systemic effects, and has distinct advantages over oral administration (i.e. the drug to be swallowed) for drugs with pronounced presystemic metabolism, providing direct and rapid access to the systemic circulation bypassing intestine and liver. Glyceryl trinitrate and buprenorphine are given sublingually for this reason. Glycerine trinitrate is taken either as a sublingual tablet or as a spray. Sublingual administration provides short-term effects which can be terminated by swallowing the tablet. Tablets for buccal absorption provide more sustained plasma concentrations, and are held in one spot between lip and gum until dissolved.

Rectal

Drugs may be given rectally for their local effects, for example sulfasalazine or corticosteroid suppositories or retention enemas in the treatment of proctitis. Drugs are also absorbed when administered by this route, and are sometimes given rectally, a route of administration that is culturally more accepted in France and Italy than in England, for their systemic rather than their local actions. Several advantages have been claimed for the rectal route of administration:

1. Exposure to the acidity of the gastric juice and to digestive enzymes is avoided.
2. The portal circulation is partly bypassed, reducing presystemic metabolism.
3. It can be used in patients unable to swallow or who are vomiting.
4. Duration of action may be prolonged.

Rectal diazepam is useful to control convulsions when it is impossible to establish venous access during status epilepticus (as is often the case in children). Metronidazole is well absorbed when administered rectally and is less expensive than intravenous preparations. Rectal administration is occasionally used to ensure nocturnal absorption of drugs, for example indomethacin for the morning stiffness of rheumatoid arthritis, or when the drug is poorly absorbed when given by mouth, for example ergotamine during a migraine attack, but there are usually more reliable alternatives, and drugs given rectally can cause severe local irritation.

Skin

Drugs are applied topically to treat skin diseases such as psoriasis or acne (chapter 48). Systemic absorption can sometimes cause undesired effects, for example in the case of potent glucocorticoids, especially if applied to large areas under occlusive dressings, but application of drugs to skin can also be used to achieve a systemic therapeutic effect. The skin has evolved as an impermeable integument so that the problems of getting drugs through it are completely different from transport through an absorptive surface such as the gut. Factors affecting percutaneous drug absorption include:

1. **Skin condition** Injury and disease affecting the stratum corneum result in shunts across the horny layer allowing greater penetration. The penetration of isotopically labeled hydrocortisone increases from 1–2% to 78–90% after removal of the stratum corneum by repeated stripping with cellophane tape.
2. **Age** Infant skin is more permeable than adult skin.
3. **Region** Skin sites differ in permeability (plantar < anterior forearm < scalp < scrotum < posterior auricular skin).
4. **Hydration** of the stratum corneum is one of the most important factors which increases the passage of all substances that penetrate skin. Under plastic-film occlusion (sometimes employed by dermatologists) the stratum corneum changes from a tissue normally containing very little (10%) water to one containing up to 50% water with increased permeability. Penetration of corticosteroids into the skin is increased up to 100-fold by occlusion and systemic side effects occur more commonly.

5. **Vehicle** Little is known about the importance of the various substances which have over the years been empirically included in skin creams and ointments. The physical chemistry of these mixtures may be very complex and change during an application, for example evaporation of water from an ointment may cause phase reversal from a suspension of oil in water to a suspension of water in oil with resulting changes in the solubility and partitioning of drug within the ointment.

6. **Physical properties of the drug** As with other biological membranes penetration of drugs through skin increases with increasing lipid solubility of the drug. When compounds are relatively insoluble reduction of particle size in the cream or ointment enhances absorption and solutions penetrate best of all. As expected, the rate of drug absorption increases as drug concentration in the preparation is increased.

7. **Surface area to which the drug is applied** This is especially important when treating infants who have a relatively large surface area to volume ratio.

Transdermal absorption is sufficiently reliable to enable systemically active drugs (e.g. glyceryl trinitrate, estradiol, hyoscine, nicotine) to be administered by this route in the form of patches to be applied to the skin. As with injection or buccal administration, transdermal administration bypasses presystemic metabolism in gut wall or liver. Patients should be told to apply each dose to the same general anatomical area (e.g. chest for glyceryl trinitrate, buttock for estradiol, behind the ear for hyoscine), but to a different spot for successive patches, to minimize local irritation. Patches are more expensive than alternative preparations, and are justified only if a particular patient prefers them substantially or in some instances of poor compliance.

Gels or creams are sometimes rubbed in to skin overlying a tender muscle or joint. This may influence symptoms by: (1) placebo effect; (2) mechanical effects of rubbing/ massage on underlying blood vessels and other structures; (3) a so-called 'counterirritant' effect, by which is meant the relief of discomfort in a deep structure by stimulating pain fibers in the skin by some irritant such as capsaicin (the irritant from red pepper); or (4) absorption of a non-steroidal anti-inflammatory drug such as piroxicam. Although small amounts of piroxicam are absorbed transdermally, this does not lead to higher concentrations in the underlying joint than elsewhere in the body and the efficacy of such gels is not great.

Lungs

Drugs, notably steroids, β_2-adrenoceptor agonists, muscarinic receptor antagonists and sodium cromoglycate, are inhaled as aerosols or particles for their local effects on bronchioles. Nebulized antibiotics are also sometimes used in children with cystic fibrosis and recurrent *Pseudomonas* infections. Drug absorption in these circumstances can give rise to unwanted systemic effects. Physical properties that limit systemic absorption are therefore desirable. Ipratropium, for example, is a quaternary ammonium ion analog of atropine which is highly polar by virtue of the charged quaternary ammonium N^+ group, and is consequently poorly absorbed and has fewer atropine-like side effects than would a more lipid-soluble muscarinic receptor-blocking drug. A large fraction of an 'inhaled' dose of salbutamol is in fact swallowed; however, the bioavailability of swallowed salbutamol is low due to inactivation by sulfation in the gut wall so systemic effects such as tremor are minimized in comparison with effects on the bronchioles.

The lungs are ideally suited for absorption from the gas phase since the total respiratory surface area is about 60 m² through which only 60 ml blood is percolating in the capillaries, thus presenting an enormous absorptive surface area. This is exploited in the case of volatile anesthetics as discussed in chapter 21.

Nose

Drugs such as steroids and sympathomimetic amines may be administered intranasally for their local effects on nasal mucosa. Systemic absorption may result in undesirable effects, such as loss of control of blood pressure by antihypertensive medication, in such circumstances.

Nasal mucosal epithelium has remarkable and potentially very valuable absorptive properties, notably the capacity to absorb intact complex peptides that cannot be administered by mouth because they would be digested. This has opened up an area of therapeutics that was previously limited by the inconvenience of repeated injections. At present drugs administered by this route include desmopressin (DDAVP: an analog of antidiuretic hormone) for patients with diabetes insipidus and buserelin (an analog of gonadotropin-releasing hormone) for patients with prostate cancer, but there is great interest in this area and every reason to hope for new indications for intranasal administration.

Eye, ear and vagina

Drugs are administered topically to these sites for their local effects, for example chloramphenicol eye drops for purulent conjunctivitis, sodium bicarbonate ear drops for softening wax and nystatin pessaries for treating *Candida* infections. Occasionally, they are absorbed in sufficient amount to have unwanted systemic effects such as worsening of asthma caused by timolol (a β-adrenoceptor antagonist) eye drops given for open angle glaucoma, or diarrhea caused by a prostaglandin E_2 pessary administered to induce therapeutic abortion. However, such absorption is not sufficiently reliable to make use of these routes for therapeutic ends.

Systems have been developed to apply drugs locally using rate-controlling membranes, for example the pilocarpine 'Ocusert' system for glaucoma. This is a flat flexible elliptical-shaped device consisting of a drug reservoir core containing pilocarpine enclosed in two outer plastic polymer membranes. These membranes give a zero-order release rate of pilocarpine, i.e. release is at a constant rate and does not decrease as the reservoir empties. The device is small enough to insert comfortably into the lower conjunctival sac and can remain there releasing drug for several days. This may improve compliance since the alternative is to use pilocarpine drops several times daily, and also provides smoother control of intraocular pressure with a reduced total pilocarpine dosage.

Intramuscular injection

Lipid-soluble drugs diffuse freely through capillary walls and are well absorbed when administered intramuscularly. Polar drugs can also be absorbed rapidly, providing they are of low molecular weight. However, polar drugs of high molecular weight are only absorbed slowly, via the lymphatics.

Rate of absorption is also governed by the total surface area available for diffusion and is increased when the solution is distributed throughout a large volume of muscle. Dispersion of the solution is enhanced by massage of the injection site. Transport away from the injection site is governed by muscle blood flow and this varies from site to site (deltoid > vastus lateralis > gluteus maximus). Blood flow to muscle is increased by exercise and absorption rates are increased in all sites after exercise and conversely shock, heart failure or other conditions reducing muscular blood flow reduce absorption.

The drug must be sufficiently water soluble to remain in solution at the injection site until absorption occurs. This is a problem for some drugs including phenytoin, diazepam and digoxin: crystallization and/or poor absorption occurs when these are given by intramuscular injection, which should therefore be avoided. Slow absorption is useful in some circumstances where appreciable concentrations of drug are required for prolonged periods. For example benzathine penicillin is a suspension for deep intramuscular injection of value in treating late latent syphilis which is caused by sensitive slowly dividing organisms (penicillin works by inhibiting bacterial cell wall synthesis in dividing organisms, see chapter 40). Depot intramuscular injections are also used to improve compliance in psychiatric patients, for example the decanoate ester of fluphenazine which is slowly hydrolyzed to release active free drug.

Intramuscular injection has a number of disadvantages:

1. Pain: muscle is poorly innervated with pain fibers compared to skin but distension with large volumes is painful and injected volumes should usually be no greater than 5 ml.
2. Sciatic nerve palsy following injection into the buttock is avoided by injecting into the upper outer gluteal quadrant.
3. Sterile abscesses at the injection site (e.g. paraldehyde).
4. Elevated serum creatine phosphokinase due to enzyme release from muscle can cause diagnostic confusion.
5. Severe allergic reactions (e.g. anaphylaxis) may be protracted because there is no way of stopping absorption of the drug.
6. The intramuscular route is not always more effective or rapid than the oral route, for example for diazepam or chlordiazepoxide oral administration requires a lower dose of drug and produces a given level of sedation more rapidly than intramuscular injection.
7. Hematoma formation can occur, especially after fibrinolytic therapy.

Subcutaneous injection

This is influenced by the same factors as affect intramuscular injections. Cutaneous blood flow is lower than in muscle and therefore absorption is slower. If the skin of a limb is injected drug absorption is increased by exercise, one factor in exercise-induced hypoglycemia in insulin-dependent diabetics. Absorption is retarded by immobilization, reduction of blood flow by a tourniquet and local cooling, all of which may be used to reduce absorption in wasp stings and snake bites.

Adrenaline incorporated into an injection reduces absorption rate by causing vasoconstriction, conversely hyaluronidase increases it by spreading the injection more widely within subcutaneous tissues.

Sustained effects from subcutaneous injections are extremely important clinically, most notably in treatment of insulin-dependent diabetics. Isophane insulin is a suspension of insulin with protamine often used to initiate twice daily regimes. Insulin zinc suspension (amorphous) has an intermediate duration of action and insulin zinc suspension (crystalline) a more prolonged duration of action.

Sustained effects have also been obtained from subcutaneous injections by using oily suspensions (e.g. in the past of vasopressin, now largely supplanted by intranasal administration of desmopressin), or by implanting a compressed pellet of drug subcutaneously, for example of estrogen or testosterone for hormone replacement therapy.

Intravenous injection

This has the following advantages:

1. Rapid action (e.g. frusemide in pulmonary edema).
2. Presystemic metabolism is avoided (e.g. glyceryl trinitrate infusion in patients with unstable angina).
3. Intravenous injection is used for drugs that are not absorbed by mouth, for example gentamicin and heparin. It is also used for drugs that are too painful or toxic to be given intramuscularly, for example streptokinase or mustine. Mustine and other cytotoxic drugs must not be allowed to

leak from the vein or considerable damage and pain will result.

4. Intravenous infusion is easily controlled, enabling precise titration of drugs with short half-lives. This is essential for drugs such as sodium nitroprusside or epoprostenol (prostacyclin).

The chief drawbacks of intravenous administration are:

1. Drugs once injected cannot be recalled.
2. Very high drug levels result if the drug is given too rapidly; the right heart receives the highest concentration, possibly as a bolus, and drugs with arrhythmogenic potential such as phenytoin have caused fatal cardiac arrest when administered too rapidly by this route.
3. Embolism of foreign particles or air, sepsis or thrombosis are all possible, especially in addicts self-administering drugs of abuse. Probably the greatest hazard during legitimate use is sepsis occurring via intravenous catheters in neutropenic, immunosuppressed or debilitated patients.
4. Accidental extravascular injection or leakage of toxic drugs, for example doxorubicin and vincristine produce severe local tissue necrosis.
5. Inadvertent intra-arterial injection can cause arterial spasm and peripheral gangrene.

Intrathecal injection

This route provides access to the central nervous system for drugs that are normally excluded by the blood–brain barrier. This inevitably entails very great risks of neurotoxicity, and this route should **never** be used without adequate training. (In the UK junior doctors who have made mistakes of this kind have been held criminally as well as professionally negligent.) The possibility of causing death or permanent neurological disability is such that extra care must be taken in checking that both the drug and the dose are correct. Examples of drugs used in this way include methotrexate (to eliminate malignant cells from the central nervous system in childhood leukemias) and local anesthetics (e.g. bupivacaine) or opiates (e.g. morphine) administered by an anesthetist to produce spinal anesthesia. (More commonly anesthetists use the much safer extradural route to administer local anesthetic drugs to produce regional analgesia without depressing respiration in, for example, women during labor.) Aminoglycosides are sometimes administered by neurosurgeons via a cisternal reservoir to patients with Gram-negative infections of the brain. The antispasmodic baclofen is sometimes administered by this route.

Penicillin used to be administered intrathecally to patients with pneumococcal meningitis, because of the belief that it penetrated the blood–brain barrier inadequately. However, when the meninges are inflamed (as in meningitis) high-dose intravenous penicillin results in adequate concentrations in the cerebrospinal fluid. Intravenous penicillin should now always be used for meningitis, since penicillin is a predictable neurotoxin (it used to be used to produce an animal model of seizures), and seizures, encephalopathy and death have been caused by injecting a dose intrathecally that would have been appropriate for intravenous administration.

Drug *Metabolism*

5

Introduction **42**

Phase I metabolism **42**

Metabolism of drugs by intestinal organisms **44**

Phase II metabolism (conjugation reactions) **44**

Enzyme induction **46**

Enzyme inhibition **47**

Presystemic metabolism ('first-pass' effect) **47**

*I*NTRODUCTION

Drug metabolism is a complex and important part of biochemical pharmacology. There are considerable species variations in drug metabolism, and, at least until recently, the subject has been hindered by limited availability of human tissue. Much of our present understanding derives from analytical studies of drugs and metabolites in plasma or urine from human volunteers. The aim of this chapter is to introduce some of the basic principles of drug metabolism.

The pharmacological activity of many drugs is reduced or abolished by enzymic processes, and drug metabolism is one of the main mechanisms by which drugs are inactivated. Examples include oxidation of phenytoin and of alcohol. However, not all metabolic processes result in inactivation and drug activity is sometimes *increased* by metabolism (as in activation of prodrugs, e.g. decarboxylation of levodopa to dopamine in central neurons, and conversion of enalapril to its active metabolite enalaprilat).

Formation of polar metabolites from a non-polar drug permits efficient urinary excretion (chapter 6). Some metabolic transformations, however, result in active compounds with a longer half-life than the parent drug (e.g. diazepam has a half-life of 20–50 hours, whereas its pharmacologically active metabolite desmethyldiazepam has a plasma half-life of approximately 100 hours). Delayed effects many days after starting regular treatment with such drugs can be caused by accumulation of such long-lived metabolites.

It is convenient to divide drug metabolism into two phases (I and II) (Fig. 5.1). These sometimes, but not always, occur sequentially. Phase I reactions involve a metabolic modification of the drug: commonly oxidation, reduction or hydrolysis. Products of phase I reactions may be either pharmacologically active or inactive. Phase II reactions are synthetic conjugation reactions between the drug and a second molecule (or between a phase I metabolite of a drug and a second molecule). The products have increased polarity compared with the parent drugs and are therefore more readily excreted in the urine (or, less often, bile); they are usually, but not always, pharmacologically inactive. Molecules or groups involved in conjugation reactions include glucuronic acid, glycine, glutamine, sulfate and acetate.

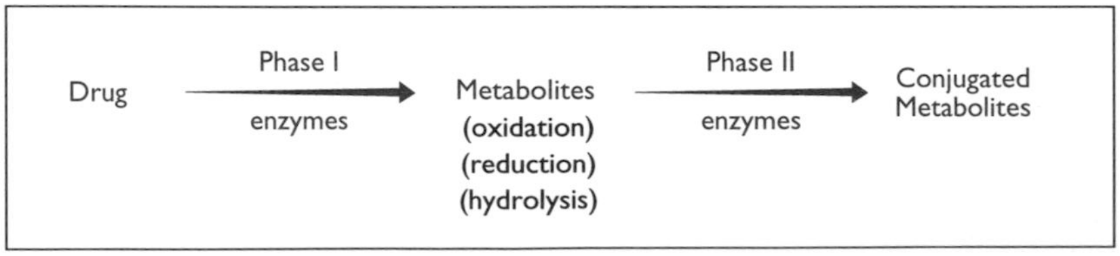

```
┌─────────────────────────────────────────────────────────┐
│                Phase I                    Phase II        │
│  Drug    ─────────────►  Metabolites  ─────────────►  Conjugated │
│          enzymes         (oxidation)     enzymes      Metabolites │
│                          (reduction)                      │
│                          (hydrolysis)                     │
└─────────────────────────────────────────────────────────┘
```

Fig. 5.1 Phase I and II of drug metabolism.

*P*HASE I METABOLISM

The liver is the most important site of drug metabolism. Hepatocyte endoplasmic reticulum is particularly important, but cytosol and mitochondria are also involved in phase I reactions.

Endoplasmic reticulum

Hepatic smooth endoplasmic reticulum contains enzyme systems that metabolize foreign substances ('xenobiotics': i.e. drugs as well as pesticides, fertilizers and other chemicals that may contaminate human food supplies). Centrifugation of hepatic homogenates yields a microsomal fraction that is rich in endoplasmic reticulum, and is used to study these metabolic processes, which include oxidation, reduction and hydrolysis.

OXIDATION

Microsomal oxidation causes aromatic or aliphatic hydroxylation, deamination, dealkylation or S-oxidation. These reactions all involve reduced nicotinamide adenine dinucleotide phosphate (NADP), molecular oxygen, mixed function oxidase and one or more of a group of cytochrome P_{450} hemoproteins. Cytochrome P_{450} (so named because it reacts with carbon monoxide to yield a pink (P) complex with an absorption peak at 450 nm) acts as a terminal oxidase in the oxidation reaction. Such reactions are generally rather non-specific as regards substrate in contrast to many enzyme-catalyzed reactions, although cytochrome P_{450} exists in several distinct isoenzyme forms each with a different, albeit often overlapping, pattern of substrate preferences (Table 5.1).

It is intriguing to speculate how humans and other species have evolved efficient methods of eliminating chemicals that have only recently been synthesized, and which our ancestors can never have encountered. Modern pharmacology owes much to the study of plant-derived products (alkaloids),

and it may be that it was of selective advantage to be able to detoxify a range of such plant poisons. The most versatile mechanism for doing so, the cytochrome P_{450} system, may have evolved from other cytochromes and cytochrome P_{450} enzyme systems involved in the oxidative biosynthesis of mediators or other biochemically important intermediates. For example, synthase enzymes involved in the oxidation of arachidonic acid to prostaglandins and thromboxanes are cytochrome P_{450} enzymes with distinct specificities.

REDUCTION

Reduction requires reduced NADP-cytochrome c reductase or reduced NAD-cytochrome b_5 reductase. Chloramphenicol is reduced by NADH and a nitroreductase in the liver by this mechanism.

HYDROLYSIS

Pethidine is de-esterified to meperidinic acid by hepatic membrane-bound esterase activity.

Non-endoplasmic reticulum drug metabolism

OXIDATION

Oxidation of alcohol to acetaldehyde and of chloral to trichlorethanol is catalyzed by a cytosolic enzyme ('alcohol dehydrogenase') whose substrates also include vitamin A and the aldehyde retinene. Diamine oxidase (DAO) and monoamine oxidase (MAO) are membrane-bound mitochondrial enzymes that oxidatively deaminate primary amines to aldehydes (further oxidized to carboxylic acids) or ketones. Monoamine oxidase occurs in liver, kidney, intestine and nervous tissue and its substrates include catecholamines (dopamine, noradrenaline, adrenaline), tyramine, phenylephrine and tryptophan

Table 5.1 Some cytochrome P_{450} isoenzymes and their substrates.

Isoenzyme	Substrate
Cytochrome P_{450} 1A2	Caffeine, theophylline
Cytochrome P_{450} 2A6	Warfarin
Cytochrome P_{450} 3A	Nifedipine, cyclosporin, erythromycin
Cytochrome P_{450} 2B6	Phenobarbitone
Cytochrome P_{450} 2D6	Debrisoquine, thioridazine, amitriptyline, codeine, timolol, metoprolol
Cytochrome P_{450} E	Ethanol

derivatives (5-hydroxytryptamine and tryptamine). Diamine oxidase has a substrate specificity overlapping that of MAO and is involved in histamine metabolism. Oxidation of purines by xanthine oxidase (e.g. of 6-mercaptopurine to inactive 6-thiouric acid) is non-microsomal.

REDUCTION

For example, enzymic reduction of double bonds.

HYDROLYSIS

Esterases catalyze hydrolytic reactions including cleavage of suxamethonium by plasma cholinesterase, an enzyme with pharmacogenetic variation (chapter 13), as well as hydrolysis of aspirin (acetylsalicylic acid) to salicylate, enalapril to enalaprilat and of many other drugs.

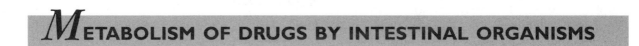

METABOLISM OF DRUGS BY INTESTINAL ORGANISMS

This is important for drugs undergoing enterohepatic circulation. Estradiol, for example, which is excreted in bile as a glucuronide conjugate, loses glucuronic acid by microbial activity so that free drug is available for reabsorption via the terminal ileum, only a small proportion (approximately 7%) being excreted in the feces under usual circumstances, although this can increase if gastrointestinal disease or concurrent antibiotic use alters the intestinal flora.

PHASE II METABOLISM (CONJUGATION REACTIONS)

Glucuronidation

Conjugations between glucuronic acid and carboxyl groups are involved in the metabolism of bilirubin, salicylate and lorazepam.

Some patients inherit a deficiency of glucuronide formation that presents clinically as a non-hemolytic jaundice due to excess unconjugated bilirubin (Crigler–Najjar syndrome). Drugs that are normally conjugated in this way aggravate the jaundice in such patients.

O-glucuronides formed by reaction with a hydroxyl group of the drug results in an ether glucuronide. This occurs with morphine, paracetamol and chloramphenicol.

Amino acid reactions

Glycine and glutamine are the amino acids chiefly involved in conjugation reactions in humans. Glycine forms conjugates with nicotinic acid and salicylate whilst glutamine forms conjugates with *p*-aminosalicylate. Hepatocellular damage depletes the intracellular pool of these amino acids, thus restricting this pathway. Amino acid conjugation is also reduced in the newborn.

Acetylation

Acetate derived from acetyl coenzyme A conjugates with several drugs including isoniazid, hydralazine and procainamide (see chapter 13 for discussion of polymorphic variation of drug acetylation). Acetylating activity resides in the cytosol and is widely distributed, occurring in leukocytes and gastrointestinal cells as well as in liver, in which it is present in reticuloendothelial rather than parenchymal cells.

Methylation

Methylation proceeds by a pathway involving S-adenosyl methionine as methyl donor to drugs with free amino, hydroxyl or thiol groups. Catechol O-methyltransferase is an example of such a methylating enzyme and is of physiological as well as pharmacological importance. It is present in cytosol and catalyzes transfer of a methyl group to catecholamines, inactivating noradrenaline and adrenaline. Phenylethanolamine N-methyltransferase is also important in catecholamine metabolism. It methylates the terminal $-NH_2$ of noradrenaline to form adrenaline in the adrenal medulla. It also acts on exogenous amines, including phenylethanolamine and phenylephrine. It is induced by glucocorticoids, and its presence in high activity in the adrenal medulla reflects the anatomical arrangement of the blood supply to the medulla which comes from the adrenal cortex and consequently contains very high concentrations of corticosteroids.

Sulfation

Sulfation of hydroxyl (alcoholic or phenolic) and amine groups occurs in cytosol via an active sulfate compound, 3'-phosphoadenosine 5'-phosphosulfate (PAPS). This system forms sulfates such as heparin and chondroitin sulfate under physiological conditions. Sulfotransferases produce ethereal sulfates from several estrogens and androgens, from 3-hydroxycoumarin (a phase I metabolite of warfarin), and from chloramphenicol. There are a number of S-transferases in liver, with different specificities.

Mercapturic acid formation

Mercapturic acid formation via reaction with cysteine in glutathione (a tripeptide) is a relatively unusual pathway. It is, however, very important in paracetamol *over*dose when the usual pathway of paracetamol elimination is overwhelmed with resulting production of a highly toxic metabolite (N-acetylbenzoquinone imine, NABQI). NABQI is detoxified by conjugation with reduced glutathione, and the availability of this is critical in determining clinical outcome. Seriously poisoned patients are therefore treated with thiol donors such as acetyl cysteine or methionine to increase the endogenous supply of reduced glutathione (chapter 50).

Glutathione conjugates

Naphthalene and some sulfonamides also form conjugates with glutathione. One endogenous function of glutathione conjugation is formation of a sulfidopeptide leukotriene, leukotriene (LT) C_4. This is formed by conjugation of glutathione with LTA_4, analogous to a phase II reaction. LTA_4 is an epoxide which is synthesized from arachidonic acid by a 'phase I' type oxidation reaction catalyzed by a lipoxygenase enzyme. LTC_4, together with its dipeptide product LTD_4, comprise the activity once known as slow reacting substance of anaphylaxis, and these leukotrienes are believed to play a role as bronchoconstrictor mediators in anaphylaxis and possibly in asthma (chapter 30).

ENZYME INDUCTION

Enzyme induction (Table 5.2) is a process in which there is enhanced enzyme activity because of increased enzyme synthesis (less often, reduced enzyme breakdown). This increased enzyme activity is sometimes accompanied by hypertrophy of the endoplasmic reticulum. There is a rise in cytochrome P_{450} content and increased cytochrome P_{450} reductase activity. The size of the liver and hepatic blood flow also increase.

There is much interindividual variability between the degree of induction produced by a given agent, part of which is inherited.

Studies of induction indicate selectivity, for example, rifampicin selectively increases N-demethylation of antipyrine relative to its 4-hydroxylation and 3-methylhydroxylation. This and other evidence suggests the existence of multiple separate isoenzyme forms of cytochrome P_{450} proteins, as mentioned above. Exogenous inducing agents include not only drugs but also halogenated insecticides (particularly chlorophenothane – DDT – and gamma benzene hexachloride), herbicides, polycyclic aromatic hydrocarbons, dyes, food preservatives, nicotine and alcohol. A practical consequence of enzyme induction is that if two or more drugs are given simultaneously, then one substance that is an inducing agent accelerates the metabolism of other drugs (see chapter 12 for a discussion of the practical consequences of this). Substrates of induced drug-metabolizing enzymes include pollutants, carcinogens and normal body constituents (e.g. steroids, bilirubin, thyroxine and fat-soluble vitamins) in addition to drugs.

Table 5.2 Examples of drugs that cause enzyme induction.

Rifampicin
Carbamazepine
Ethanol
Phenobarbitone

Tests for induction

The level of induction of liver enzymes can be assessed by measuring the clearance of a drug such as antipyrene, although this is seldom indicated clinically. Plasma levels of γ-glutamyl transpeptidase and/or the urinary concentration of 6-β-hydroxycortisol have also been used. It is unlikely that a single test will ever be reliable, since the mixed function oxidase system is so complex that at any one time the activity of some enzymes may be increased and others reduced.

Enzymes in cells (e.g. fibroblasts and lymphocytes) and tissues other than liver are also capable of undergoing induction.

Induction of drug metabolism is a model of variable expression of a constant genetic constitution. It is important in drug elimination and also in several other biological processes including adaptation to extrauterine life which involves a series of biochemical changes, delay in which is hazardous to the infant. Many of the mediators of such changes are hormones, including glucocorticoids, thyroxine and glucagon.

Neonates fail to form glucuronide conjugates because of immaturity of hepatic glucuronyl transferase. Chloramphenicol conjugation (and hence excretion) is impaired, rendering neonates at risk of 'gray baby' syndrome if treated with chloramphenicol. Defective bilirubin conjugation increases the risk of accumulation of unconjugated lipid-soluble bilirubin that can enter the brain, staining the basal ganglia ('kernicterus') and causing choreoathetosis. Another important consequence of immature enzyme systems in premature infants is a low level of lung surfactant and consequent respiratory distress. Administration of glucocorticoids as enzyme inducers to the mothers of certain high-risk babies before delivery reduces this hazard.

ENZYME INHIBITION

Several drugs including monoamine oxidase inhibitors, allopurinol, methotrexate, converting enzyme inhibitors, non-steroidal anti-inflammatory drugs and many others, exert their therapeutic effects by enzyme inhibition. Quite apart from such direct actions, inhibition of drug metabolism by a concurrently administered drug (Table 5.3) can lead to drug accumulation and toxicity. For example, cimetidine, which owes its therapeutic action to antagonism at the histamine H_2-receptor, inhibits drug metabolism by the cytochrome P_{450} system and therefore potentiates the actions of quite unrelated drugs such as warfarin (chapter 12). This kind of clinically important enzyme inhibition is, however, less common than enzyme induction.

The specificity of enzyme inhibition is sometimes incomplete, for example disulfiram, which is used to encourage abstinence in alcoholics, owes its therapeutic effect to inhibition of oxidation of acetaldehyde formed from ethanol but also prolongs

Table 5.3 Examples of drugs that inhibit cytochrome P_{450}.

Cimetidine
Erythromycin
Ciprofloxacin
Isoniazid
Chloramphenicol

antipyrine half-life and raises the steady-state plasma concentrations of warfarin and phenytoin in patients receiving these drugs. The mechanism of these last two interactions is unknown but presumably results from inhibition of microsomal drug metabolism. Warfarin and phenytoin compete with one another for metabolism, coadministration resulting in elevation of plasma steady-state concentrations of both drugs. Chloramphenicol is a non-competitive inhibitor of microsomal enzymes and inhibits phenytoin, tolbutamide and chlorpropamide metabolism. Oral contraceptives also inhibit drug metabolism, probably due to their estrogen component.

PRESYSTEMIC METABOLISM ('FIRST-PASS' EFFECT)

Metabolism of some drugs is markedly dependent on the route of administration. Following oral administration, drugs gain access to the systemic circulation via the portal vein so the entire absorbed dose is exposed first to the intestinal wall and then to the liver before gaining access to the rest of the body. A considerably smaller fraction of the absorbed dose goes through gut and liver in subsequent passes because of distribution to other tissues and drug elimination by other routes.

If a drug is subject to a high hepatic clearance (i.e. it is rapidly metabolized by the liver) a substantial fraction will be extracted

from the portal blood and metabolized before reaching the systemic circulation. This is known as presystemic metabolism. Common examples are shown in Table 5.4.

Table 5.4 Examples of drugs subject to extensive presystemic metabolism.

Glyceryl trinitrate
Propranolol
Acetylsalicylic acid
Morphine
Verapamil
Chlormethiazole

Route of administation and presystemic metabolism markedly influence the pattern of drug metabolism. For example, when salbutamol is given to asthmatic subjects the ratio of unchanged drug to metabolite in the urine is 2:1 after intravenous administration but 1:2 after an oral dose. When lignocaine is given orally the levels of the major primary metabolite monoethyl glycine xylidide (MEGX) are comparable to those of lignocaine itself, whereas after a single intravenous dose, MEGX levels are about 15–20% of those of lignocaine. Propranolol undergoes substantial hepatic presystemic metabolism, and small doses given orally are completely metabolized before reaching the systematic circulation. After intravenous administration the area under the plasma concentration–time curve is proportional to the dose administered and passes through the origin (Fig. 5.2). After oral administration the relationship, although linear, does not pass through the origin and there is a threshold dose below which measurable concentrations of propranolol are not detectable in systemic venous plasma. In patients with portocaval anastomoses bypassing the liver, hepatic presystemic metabolism is bypassed, so very small doses are needed compared with the usual oral dose.

Presystemic metabolism is not limited to the liver since the gastrointestinal mucosa also metabolizes drugs such as salbutamol, levodopa and chlorpromazine before they enter hepatic portal blood. Pronounced first-pass metabolism by either the gastrointestinal mucosa (e.g. salbutamol, levodopa) or liver (e.g. glyceryl trinitrate, morphine, naloxone) necessitates high oral doses in comparison with the intravenous route. Alternative routes of drug delivery such as rectal, buccal, sublingual, inhalation or transdermal partly or wholly bypass presystemic elimination (chapter 4).

Drugs that undergo extensive presystemic metabolism usually exhibit pronounced interindividual variability in drug disposition. This results in highly variable responses to therapy and is one of the major difficulties in their clinical use. Variability in first-pass metabolism results from:

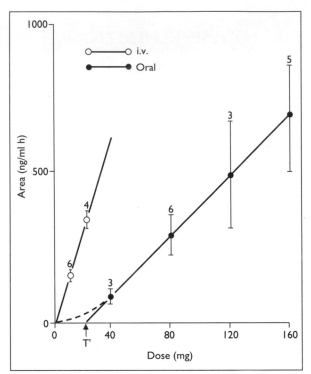

Fig. 5.2 Area under blood concentration–time curve after oral (● and intravenous (○) administration of propanolol to humans in various doses. T' is the apparent threshold for propanolol following oral administration. (From D.G. Shand and R.E. Rangno. *Pharmacology* 1972; **7**: 159. Reproduced with permission of S. Karger AG, Basle.)

1. Genetic variation, for example the bioavailability of hydralazine is about double in slow compared with fast acetylators. Presystemic hydroxylation of debrisoquine, metoprolol and encainide also depends on a genetic polymorphism.
2. Induction or inhibition of metabolic enzymes.
3. Food increases liver blood flow and can *increase* the bioavailability of drugs such as propranolol, metoprolol and hydralazine by increasing the amount of drug presented to the liver in unit time above the threshold for complete hepatic extraction.
4. Drugs that increase liver blood flow have similar effects to food, for example hydralazine increases propranolol bioavailability by approximately one-third, whereas drugs that reduce liver blood flow (e.g. β-adrenoceptor antagonists) reduce it.

5. Non-linear first-pass kinetics are common (e.g. hydralazine, propranolol, 5-fluorouracil): increasing the dose disproportionately increases bioavailability so the fraction of the dose of such a drug that reaches the systemic circulation depends dramatically on dose. When low doses of aspirin are given orally little or no acetyl salicylic acid reaches the systemic circulation, and acetylation of cyclo-oxygenase is limited to portal venous tissues and to circulating elements such as platelets. Larger doses result in appreciable systemic concentrations of aspirin, as well as its metabolite salicylate.

6. Liver disease increases the bioavailability of some drugs with extensive first-pass extraction, for example chlormethiazole and pethidine.

Renal Excretion of Drugs

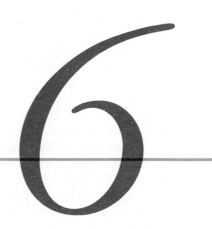

6

Introduction **52**

Glomerular filtration **52**

Proximal tubular secretion **52**

Passive tubular reabsorption **53**

Active tubular reabsorption **54**

*I*NTRODUCTION

The kidneys are involved to some degree in the elimination of virtually every drug or drug metabolite. Whether or not renal elimination is the major or only a minor contributor to total body clearance of any particular drug is determined in large part by its polarity. The kidneys receive 20% of the cardiac output and in a healthy young adult about 130 ml/min of protein-free filtrate is formed at the glomeruli. Only 1–2 ml of this filtrate finally appears in the urine. Consequently, non-polar lipid-soluble drugs are very efficiently reabsorbed down the >100-fold concentration gradient that is generated between tubular and interstitial fluids.

Non-polar drugs often have a large volume of distribution (due to partition into fat), so only a small fraction of drug in the body at any time is present in plasma where it is accessible to glomerular filtration or secretion into the tubules. Elimination of non-polar drugs therefore usually depends on metabolic conversion in liver or intestine to more polar metabolites, which are then excreted in the urine. Polar substances are eliminated efficiently by the kidneys, because they are not freely diffusible across the tubular membrane and so remain in the urine despite the concentration gradient favoring back-diffusion into interstitial fluid. Renal elimination of polar drugs or drug metabolites is influenced by several processes that alter drug concentration in tubular fluid. Depending upon which of these predominates, the renal clearance of a drug may be either an important or a trivial component in its overall elimination.

*G*LOMERULAR FILTRATION

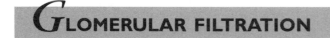

The glomerular filtrate contains similar concentrations of low molecular weight solutes as does plasma. In contrast, molecules with a molecular weight of 66 000 or above (which includes plasma proteins and drug–protein complexes) do not pass the glomerulus. Accordingly only free drug passes into the filtrate. Renal impairment (chapter 7), predictably reduces elimination of drugs that depend on glomerular filtration for their clearance (e.g. digoxin, aminoglycoside antibiotics). Drugs that are highly bound to albumin in plasma are not efficiently filtered, because only the free fraction is able to diffuse down its concentration gradient into the glomerular fluid, and this has little effect on the total concentration (bound plus free) of drug in plasma in the glomerular capillaries.

*P*ROXIMAL TUBULAR SECRETION

There are mechanisms for active secretion both of acids and bases into the tubular fluid in the proximal segment. These are relatively non-specific in their structural requirements and share some of the characteristics of transport systems in the intestine. The organic acid transport mechanism excretes hippuric acid, endogenous phenols, sulfates and glucuronides as well as acidic drugs such as probenecid, penicillin and some sulfonamides. For some acidic drugs like benzylpenicillin virtually all of the drug is excreted in this way. Para-aminohippuric acid (PAH) is excreted so efficiently by this mechanism that at appropriate concentrations it is completely extracted from renal plasma in a single pass (i.e. during intravenous infusion of PAH its concentration in renal venous blood is zero). Clearance of PAH is therefore limited by the rate at which it is delivered to the kidney, i.e. renal blood flow. Consequently PAH clearance is used as a non-invasive measure of renal blood (or more strictly renal plasma) flow.

The organic base transport mechanism contributes to the elimination of basic drugs (e.g. quinidine, cimetidine) from the body.

Each mechanism is characterized by a maximal rate of transport for a given drug so that the process is theoretically saturable although this maximum is rarely reached in practice. Because secretion of free drug occurs up a concentration gradient from peritubular fluid into the lumen, the equilibrium between unbound and bound drug in plasma can be disturbed, with bound drug dissociating from protein binding sites. Unlike glomerular filtration, tubular secretion can therefore eliminate drugs efficiently even if they are highly protein bound. Competitive effects can occur between drugs carried on these systems. Thus probenecid, a weak acid, competitively inhibits the tubular secretion of the penicillins and methotrexate whilst cimetidine competes with quinidine for the basic drug transport system.

PASSIVE DISTAL TUBULAR REABSORPTION

The renal tubule behaves like a lipid barrier separating the high drug concentration in the tubular lumen and the lower concentration in the interstitial fluid and plasma. Reabsorption of drug down its concentration gradient therefore occurs by passive diffusion. To traverse the lipid membrane of the tubule the drug must be lipid soluble, so that for highly lipid-soluble drugs such as griseofulvin, reabsorption is so effective that its renal clearance is virtually zero. Conversely polar substances, such as mannitol, are too water soluble to be absorbed and are eliminated virtually without reabsorption.

Tubular reabsorption is influenced by urine flow rate. Diuresis increases the renal clearance of drugs that are passively reabsorbed since the concentration gradient is reduced. Diuresis may be induced deliberately so as to increase drug elimination during treatment of overdose.

Reabsorption of drugs that are weak acids (AH) or bases (B) depends upon the pH of the tubular fluid, because this determines the fraction of acid or base in the charged, polar form and the fraction in the uncharged non-polar lipid-soluble form. For acidic drugs, the more alkaline the urine, the greater the renal clearance and *vice versa* for basic drugs, since:

$$AH \rightleftharpoons A^- + H^+$$

and

$$B + H^+ \rightleftharpoons BH^+$$

Thus high pH (alkaline conditions) favors A^-, the charged form of the weak acid which remains in the tubular fluid and is excreted in the urine, while low pH (acid conditions) favors BH^+, the charged form of the base. This is made use of in treating overdose with aspirin (a weak acid) by causing an alkaline urine, thereby accelerating elimination of salicylate (chapter 50).

The extent to which urinary pH affects renal excretion of weak acids and bases depends quantitatively upon the pK_a of the drug. Relatively strong acids or bases are essentially completely ionized (and therefore lipid insoluble) over the entire range of physiological urine pH, and so undergo little passive reabsorption. The critical range of pK_a values for pH-dependent excretion is about 3.0–6.5 for acids and 7.5–10.5 for bases.

Urinary pH may also influence the fraction of the total dose which is excreted unchanged. Thus about 57% of a dose of amphetamine is excreted unchanged (i.e. as the parent drug rather than as a metabolite) in acid urine (pH 4.5–5.6) compared to about 7% in subjects with alkaline urine (pH 7.1–8.0). Administration of amphetamines with sodium bicarbonate has been used illicitly by athletes to enhance the pharmacological effects of the drug on performance as well as to make its detection by urinary screening tests more difficult. The extent to which urinary pH changes alter the rate of drug elimination naturally depends upon the contribution that renal clearance makes to the total drug clearance from the body.

ACTIVE TUBULAR REABSORPTION

This is a relatively minor process in the case of most therapeutic drugs. Uric acid is reabsorbed by an active transport system which is inhibited by uricosuric drugs such as probenecid and sulfinpyrazone. Lithium, riboflavine and fluoride also undergo active tubular reabsorption. Conditions in which sodium reabsorption is enhanced, notably salt depletion, predispose to lithium intoxication.

Effects of Disease on Drug Disposition

7

Introduction   **56**

Gastrointestinal disease   **56**

Cardiac failure   **57**

Renal disease   **59**

Liver disease   **62**

Thyroid disease   **64**

INTRODUCTION

Several common disorders influence the way the body handles drugs. It is important that the possibility of such disorder is borne in mind before prescribing a course of therapy. Gastrointestinal, cardiac, renal, liver and thyroid disorders all influence pharmacoki-netics, and individualization of therapy is important in patients with such disturbances. Most of this chapter is devoted to their influence on pharmacokinetics, with a few additional comments regarding influences of disease on pharmacodynamics.

GASTROINTESTINAL DISEASE

Gastrointestinal disease alters absorption of orally administered drugs, and prescribers need to keep in mind that therapeutic failure may be a consequence of this. Alternative routes of administration (chapter 4) may be appropriate in such circumstances.

GASTRIC EMPTYING

Gastric emptying is an important determinant of the rate and, sometimes, extent of drug absorption (chapter 4). Several pathological factors alter gastric emptying (Table 7.1). There is, however, little detailed information about the effect of these on drug absorption. Absorption of aspirin (even when adminis-tered as a solution) is delayed in migraine attacks and a more rapid effect can be achieved by administering it with metoclo-pramide which increases gastric emptying. Pyloric stenosis results in impaired absorption of paracetamol and doubtless also of other drugs.

SMALL INTESTINAL DISEASE

The very large surface area of small intestine available for drug absorption provides a substantial functional reserve, so that exten-sive disease may be present without clinically important reduction in drug absorption occurring. Despite destruction of villi and microvilli in celiac disease, with consequent reduction in the area available for drug absorption, most orally active drugs are effec-tive when administered by mouth in the usual dose. Crohn's disease typically affects the terminal ileum (in contrast to celiac disease which affects the jejunum) but may involve any part of the small or large intes-tine. Absorption of clindamycin and of sulfamethoxazole *increases* in Crohn's disease, peak concentrations of the latter being approximately three times those in healthy controls. Absorption of trimethoprim is slightly reduced and hypothetically the change in the ratio of the two components

Table 7.1 Pathological factors influencing the rate of gastric emptying.

Decreased	Increased
Trauma	Duodenal ulcer
Pain (including myocardial infarction, acute abdomen)	Gastroenterostomy
	Celiac disease
Labor	
Migraine	
Myxedema	
Raised intracranial pressure	
Intestinal obstruction	
Gastric ulcer	

of co-trimoxazole (sulfamethoxazole/tri-methoprim) could influence the efficacy of this combination. In practice, trimethoprim as a single agent is now preferred in most clinical situations in any event, so this is unlikely to be a problem save possibly when co-trimoxazole is used in patients infected with *Pneumocystis carinii*.

PANCREATIC DISEASE

Pancreatic disease can produce steatorrhea and reduce absorption of highly lipophilic molecules, including the fat-soluble vitamins. Significant reductions in absorption of cephalexin have been demonstrated in cystic fibrosis, necessitating increased doses in such patients.

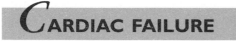

CARDIAC FAILURE

Cardiac failure affects pharmacokinetics in several ways, although the clinical importance of some of them has yet to be established. In practice the most important thing is for prescribers to be alert to the possibility that therapeutic failure is due to malabsorption, and to appreciate that the risk of toxicity is increased by reduced clearance. Consequently monitoring each patient's response to therapy and individualizing therapy accordingly are essential. The following pharmacokinetic phenomena may be abnormal in patients with heart failure.

ABSORPTION

Malabsorption of many substances, including drugs, can occur in cardiac failure because of mucosal edema. In addition, reduced gastrointestinal blood flow due to low cardiac output can reduce drug absorption. Splanchnic vasoconstriction accompanies cardiac failure as an adaptive response redistributing blood to more vital organs, and exacerbates any problem with drug absorption. Other secondary changes in gastrointestinal motility, secretion, altered pH and so on presumably also affect drug absorption adversely. However, hard data on the effects of cardiac failure on drug absorption are limited. Absorption of thiazide diuretics (e.g. hydrochlorothiazide) is reduced by 30–40% in such patients. Total availability of loop diuretics (e.g. frusemide, bumetanide) is not affected by heart failure, but absorption of frusemide is delayed, and there is a marked blunting of its diuretic effect which does not occur if it is administered intravenously.

DISTRIBUTION

Drug distribution is altered by cardiac failure. The apparent volume of distribution (V_d) of quinine and quinidine in patients with congestive cardiac failure is approximately one-third of normal. Usual doses can therefore result in elevated plasma concentrations, producing toxicity. The volume of distribution of lignocaine is also reduced by approximately 25% in heart failure, with corresponding increases in plasma concentrations. Decreased volume of distribution in patients with heart failure is probably caused by decreased tissue perfusion and perhaps in part by alteration in the partition of drugs such as lignocaine between blood and tissue components. The distribution volume of frusemide, which is largely confined to the vascular compartment, is little changed in heart failure.

Tissue injury during myocardial infarction causes a rise in erythrocyte sedimentation rate (ESR), and in plasma concentration of acute phase reaction proteins. Acute phase proteins include α_1-acid glycoprotein which binds many basic drugs (e.g. chlorpromazine, many β-adrenoceptor antagonists). Thus acute myocardial infarction is associated with increased binding of such drugs and, perhaps, reduced efficacy. A decrease of approximately 50% in free disopyramide concentration has been documented over the first 5 days following myocardial infarction and similar but less marked changes have been reported for lignocaine. The clinical significance of such changes is uncertain.

ELIMINATION

Elimination of several drugs by liver and/or kidneys is diminished in heart failure. Decreased hepatic perfusion accompanies reduced cardiac output. Drugs such as lignocaine with an extraction ratio >70% show perfusion-limited clearance and steady-state levels are inversely related to cardiac output (Fig. 7.1). Terminal half-lives of lignocaine and its two pharmacologically active metabolites monoethylglycinexylidide (MEGX) and glycinexylidide (GX) are prolonged in patients following myocardial infarction. During lignocaine infusion the steady-state concentrations are almost 50% higher in patients with cardiac failure than in healthy volunteers. The potential for lignocaine toxicity in heart failure is further increased by the accumulation of MEGX and GX which have cardiodepressant and convulsant properties.

Similar decreases in elimination occur with other drugs with high hepatic extraction ratios. Theophylline clearance is decreased and its half-life doubled in patients with cardiac failure and pulmonary edema, although interpatient variability is wide relative to these kinetic changes. If a patient with chronic stable heart failure also has severe reversible asthmatic bronchospasm, and aminophylline is used in its treatment, the above considerations indicate that the patient should receive a usual loading dose, but that plasma drug concentrations will need to be monitored especially closely subsequently in view of the possibility of excessive accumulation.

The metabolic capacity of the liver is also reduced in heart failure both by tissue hypoxia and hepatocellular damage from

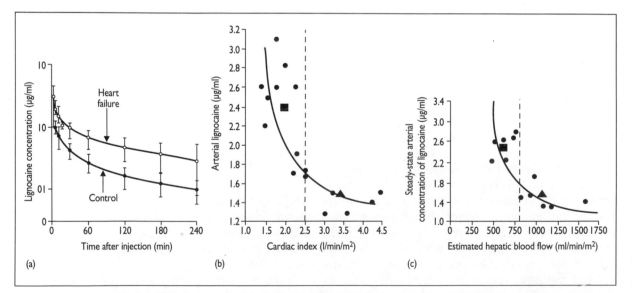

Fig. 7.1 (a) Mean (and standard deviations) of plasma lignocaine concentrations in seven heart failure patients and controls following a 50 mg intravenous bolus. (b) Relationship of arterial lignocaine level and cardiac index (dotted vertical line is lower limit of normal cardiac index, square is mean for low cardiac index patients, triangle is mean for patients with normal cardiac index). (c) Relationship of steady-state arterial lignocaine level following 50 mg bolus and infusion of 40 mg/kg/min (vertical line is lower limit of normal hepatic blood flow, square is mean for patients with low hepatic blood flow, triangle is mean for patients with normal flow). (From (a) P.D. Thompson *et al. Am Heart J* 1971; **82**: 417; (b & c) R.E. Stenson *et al. Circulation* 1971; **43**: 205. By permission of the American Heart Association Inc.)

hepatic congestion. Liver biopsy samples from patients with heart failure have reduced drug metabolizing activity.

Heart failure reduces renal elimination of drugs because of reduced glomerular filtration, predisposing to toxicity from drugs such as aminoglycosides and digoxin that are eliminated by this route.

RENAL DISEASE

Renal impairment

Renal excretion is a major route of elimination for many drugs, as described in chapter 6, and drugs and their metabolites excreted predominantly by the kidneys accumulate in renal failure. In addition to this self-evident effect on elimination, renal disease also affects other pharmacokinetic parameters (i.e. drug absorption, distribution and metabolism) in more subtle ways.

ABSORPTION

Gastric pH increases in chronic renal failure because urea is split yielding ammonia which buffers acid in the stomach. This reduces absorption of ferrous sulfate, and possibly also of other drugs. Nephrotic syndrome is sometimes associated with resistance to oral diuretics, and malabsorption of loop diuretics through the edematous intestine may contribute to this.

DISTRIBUTION

Renal impairment causes accumulation of several acidic substances that compete with drugs for binding sites on albumin and other plasma proteins. This alters the pharmacokinetics of many drugs, but this is seldom clinically important. Phenytoin is an exception, because therapy is guided by plasma concentration and routine analytical methods detect total (bound and free) drug. In renal impairment protein binding is reduced so for any measured phenytoin concentration free (active) drug is increased compared with a subject with normal renal function and the same measured total concentration. The therapeutic range therefore has to be adjusted to lower values in patients with renal impairment since otherwise doses will be selected that cause toxicity.

Tissue binding of digoxin is reduced in patients with impaired renal function, resulting in a lower volume of distribution than in healthy subjects. A smaller loading dose of digoxin is therefore appropriate in such patients, although the effect of reduced glomerular filtration on digoxin clearance is even more important, necessitating a reduced maintenance dose as decribed below.

The blood–brain barrier is more permeable in uremia. This can result in increased access of drugs to the central nervous system, an effect that is believed to contribute to the increased incidence of confusion caused by cimetidine in patients with renal failure.

METABOLISM

Metabolism of several drugs is reduced in renal failure. These include acyclovir and metaclopramide, non-renal clearance of which is reduced in patients with uremia. Conversion of sulindac to its active sulfide metabolite is also impaired in renal failure. These effects are probably of minor practical importance.

RENAL EXCRETION

Glomerular filtration and tubular secretion of drugs usually fall *pari passu* in patients with renal impairment. The decline in drug excretion is directly related to glomerular filtration rate (GFR). Some measure or estimate of GFR is therefore essential in deciding on an appropriate dose regimen in patients with impaired renal function. Radioisotope (e.g. chromium-EGTA) or inulin clearance measurement of GFR is seldom feasible in acute situations. Measurement of endogenous creatinine clearance requires accurate urine collection, which is often far from easy in ill, confused and incontinent patients. Furthermore, it is often not safe to delay treatment until the collection is complete and a result available.

Estimation of GFR from a single plasma measurement therefore has much to commend it. Blood urea is almost useless as an index of renal drug elimination since it is influenced by protein intake and metabolism, liver function, state of hydration, urine flow and other factors. However, plasma creatinine, adjusted for body weight, age and sex, is more helpful and is usually adequate for clinical purposes provided its limitations are appreciated. Glomerular filtration rate declines predictably and substantially with age but plasma creatinine concentration usually remains in the 'normal' range because creatinine production also declines in the elderly secondary to reduced muscle mass. Figure 7.2 is a nomogram for estimation of creatinine clearance given plasma creatinine, age, sex and body weight redrawn from Siersbaek–Nielsen *et al.* Alternatively some formula such as a modification of that of Cockcroft and Gault is used:

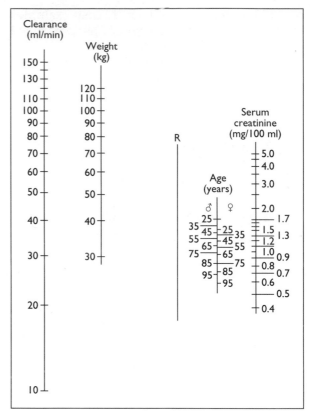

Fig. 7.2 Nomogram for rapid evaluation of endogenous creatinine clearance – with a ruler join weight to age; keep ruler at crossing point on R, then move the right-hand side of the ruler to the appropriate serum creatinine value and read off clearance from left-hand scale. (From K. Siersbaek–Nielson *et al. Lancet* 1971; **1**: 1133.)

$$\text{Creatinine clearance (ml/min)} = \frac{1.2 \times [140 - \text{Age (years)}] \times \text{weight (kg)}}{\text{Plasma creatinine } (\mu\text{M})}$$

Estimated creatinine clearance is used to adjust the dose regimen for drugs with a low therapeutic index that are eliminated mainly by renal excretion.

The main limitation of plasma creatinine as a means of estimating GFR is in acute renal failure. Plasma creatinine reflects renal function accurately in *chronic* renal failure unless severe, but only increases after an acute reduction in renal function after a lag of several days: plasma creatinine would be normal immediately after bilateral nephrectomy, even though GFR was zero. A normal creatinine therefore does *not* mean that usual doses can be assumed to be safe in a patient who may have suffered an *acute* renal insult such as an episode of severe hypotension during septicemia, injury or other such conditions.

Adjustment of dose regimens in patients with renal impairment must be considered for drugs that are eliminated >50% by renal excretion. The *British National Formulary* tabulates drugs to be avoided or used with caution in patients with renal failure. Common examples are shown in Table 7.2.

Table 7.2 Examples of drugs to be used with especial caution or avoided in renal failure.

Aminoglycosides	Captopril
Digoxin	Enalapril
Lithium	Allopurinol
Amphotericin B	Atenolol
Metformin	Ciprofloxacin
Ethambutol	Trimethoprim
Azathioprine	Methotrexate

Detailed recommendations as to dosage reduction are contained in textbooks of nephrology. These are useful in getting treatment under way but, although precise, such recommendations are inevitably based only on effects of reduced renal function on drug elimination in 'average' populations. Individual variation is substantial and therapeutic monitoring of efficacy, toxicity and sometimes of drug concentrations is essential in patients with impaired renal function.

There are two ways of reducing total dose to compensate for impaired renal function. Either each dose can be reduced, or the interval between each dose can be lengthened. The latter method is useful when a drug must achieve some threshold concentration to produce its desired effect, but does not need to remain at this level throughout the dose interval. This is the case with aminoglycoside antibiotics. Therapy with these drugs is appropriately monitored by measuring 'peak' levels (in blood sampled at a fixed brief interval after dosing, sufficient to permit at least partial tissue distribution) which indicate whether the dose is large enough to achieve a therapeutic plasma concentration, and 'trough' levels immediately before the next dose (chapter 4). If the peak level is satisfactory but the trough level is higher than desired (i.e. toxicity is present or imminent), the dose is not reduced but the interval between doses is increased.

RENAL HEMODYNAMICS

Patients with mild renal impairment depend on vasodilator prostaglandin biosynthesis to preserve renal blood flow and GFR. The same is true of patients with heart failure, nephrotic syndrome, cirrhosis or ascites. Such patients develop acute reversible renal impairment often accompanied by salt and water retention and hypertension if treated with non-steroidal anti-inflammatory drugs (NSAIDs) because these inhibit cyclo-oxygenase and hence synthesis of vasodilator prostaglandins, notably prostaglandin I_2 (prostacyclin) and prostaglandin E_2. Sulindac is a partial exception, because it inhibits cyclo-oxygenase less in kidneys than in other tissues, although this specificity is incomplete and dose dependent.

Converting enzyme inhibitors (e.g. captopril, enalapril) can also cause reversible renal failure due to altered renal hemodynamics. This occurs predictably in patients with bilateral renal artery stenosis or with renal artery stenosis involving a single functioning kidney. The explanation is that in such patients GFR is preserved in the face of the fixed proximal obstruction by angiotensin II-mediated efferent arteriolar vasoconstriction. Inhibition of converting enzyme disables this homeostatic mechanism, and precipitates renal failure.

Nephrotic syndrome

Plasma albumin concentration is low in patients with nephrotic syndrome, resulting in increased fluctuations of free drug concentration following each dose. This could cause adverse effects, although in practice this is seldom clinically important. The high albumin concentration in tubular fluid contributes to the resistance to diuretics that sometimes accompanies nephrotic syndrome. This is because both loop diuretics and thiazides act on ion transport processes in luminal membranes of tubular cells. Protein binding of such diuretics within the tubular lumen therefore reduces the concentration of free (active) drug in tubular fluid in contact with the iontransporters on which they act.

Prescribing for patients with renal disease

1. Consider the possibility of renal impairment before drugs are prescribed.
2. Check how drugs are eliminated before prescribing them. If non-renal elimination accounts for less than 50% of total elimination then dose reduction will probably be necessary.
3. Monitor therapeutic and adverse effects and, where appropriate, drug concentrations in plasma.
4. Use potentially nephrotoxic drugs with special care (e.g. aminoglycosides, NSAIDs, converting enzyme inhibitors).

Once a potential problem has been identified there are a number of handbooks, of which the *British National Formulary* is the most concise, simple and accessible, that provide guidelines for dose adjustment in patients with renal impairment. These are useful approximations to get treatment under way, but the mathematical precision of some of the more elaborate tables of recommendations is illusory, and must not lull the inexperienced into a false sense of security: they do *not* permit a full 'course' of treatment to be prescribed safely. The patient must be monitored, and treatment modified in the light of individual responses.

*L*IVER DISEASE

The liver is the main site of drug metabolism (chapter 5). Liver disease causes multiple pathophysiological disturbances and unpredictable effects on drug handling. The precise etiology of the disease is only of limited relevance, the end stage in chronic liver disease being similar in many conditions, with a combination of hepatocyte necrosis and fibrosis. Direct portal tract to hepatic vein shunts develop, resulting in reduced presentation of hepatic portal blood to hepatocytes. Vascular resistance within the liver increases, producing portal hypertension and opening up extrahepatic collaterals between portal and systemic circulations. Initially, hepatic regeneration compensates for cell loss but with continuing damage hepatic function is compromised. This is reflected in decreased protein synthesis and reduced serum albumin and coagulation factors.

Attempts to correlate changes in pharmacokinetics of drugs with tests for derangement of liver function have been unsuccessful in contrast to the successful use of plasma creatinine in renal impairment. In chronic liver disease, serum albumin is the most useful index of hepatic drug metabolizing activity, possibly because a low albumin reflects depressed synthesis of hepatic proteins including those involved in drug metabolism. Prothrombin time also shows moderate correlation with drug clearance by the liver. However, in neither case has a continuous relationship been demonstrated and such indices of hepatic function serve mainly to distinguish the severely affected from the milder cases. Indocyanine green, antipyrine and lignocaine have also proved of little value as markers of hepatic function, although lignocaine is currently undergoing re-evaluation in this regard.

Presently, therefore, empiricism coupled with an awareness of an increased likelihood of adverse drug effects and close clinical monitoring is the best way to approach a patient with liver disease. Drugs should be used only if absolutely necessary and the risks weighed against any potential advantage. If possible, drugs that are eliminated by routes other than the liver should be employed. Some of the effects of liver disease on pharmacokinetics are described here, and some empirical 'rules' regarding prescribing for patients with liver disease laid out below.

Pharmacokinetic factors that are affected in liver disease include: absorption, distribution and metabolism of drugs.

ABSORPTION

Absorption of drugs is altered in liver disease since portal hypertension and hypoalbuminemia cause mucosal edema. Portal/systemic anastomoses allow passage of orally administered drug directly into the systemic circulation bypassing hepatic presystemic metabolism and markedly increasing bioavailability of drugs such as propranolol and chlormethiazole which must therefore be started in low doses in such patients and titrated according to effect.

DISTRIBUTION

Drug distribution is altered in liver disease. Reduced plasma albumin reduces plasma protein binding. This is also influenced by bilirubin and other endogenous substances that accumulate in liver disease, and may displace drugs from binding sites (as in renal failure). The free fraction of tolbutamide is increased by 115% in cirrhosis and that of phenytoin by up to 40%. It is particularly important to appreciate this when plasma concentrations of phenytoin are being used to monitor therapy, since unless the therapeutic range is adjusted downward toxicity will be induced, as explained above in the section on drug distribution in renal disease.

Reduced plasma protein binding increases apparent V_d if other things remain unchanged. Increased V_d of several drugs (e.g. diazepam, lignocaine, theophylline) is indeed observed in patients with liver disease. Increased V_d partly or completely explains observed changes in $t_{1/2}$ of such drugs in patients with liver disease, invalidating the interpretation of much early work where this was not appreciated. Disease-induced alterations in clearance and V_d often act in opposite directions with respect to their effect on $t_{1/2}$, probably accounting for inconsistencies in studies where $t_{1/2}$ was the only pharmacokinetic parameter estimated. Data on $t_{1/2}$ in isolation give little information regarding the extent of changes in metabolism or drug distribution which result from liver disease.

METABOLISM

Cytochrome P_{450} is reduced in patients with very severe liver disease, but drug metabolism is surprisingly little impaired in patients with moderate to severe disease. There is a poor correlation between microsomal enzyme activity from liver biopsy specimens *in vitro* and drug clearance measurements *in vivo*. Even in very severe disease the metabolism of different drugs is not affected to the same extent. It is therefore hazardous to extrapolate from knowledge of the handling of one drug to effects on another in an individual patient with liver disease. A possible explanation for this heterogeneity lies in the multiple forms of cytochrome P_{450}, some of which act on different substrates and which may be differently affected by hepatocellular dysfunction.

Prescribing for patients with liver disease

1. Risks must be weighed against possible benefit, and drugs prescribed only if the risk/benefit is judged favorable.
2. If possible, use drugs that are eliminated by routes other than the liver.
3. Response, adverse effects (and, occasionally, drug concentrations) must be monitored closely, and therapy adjusted accordingly.
4. Sedative and analgesic drugs are common precipitants of hepatic coma, probably because of a combination of pharmacokinetic and pharmacodynamic alterations, and should be avoided when possible.

5. Predictable hepatotoxins (e.g. cytotoxic drugs) should only be used for the strongest of indications, and then only with close clinical and biochemical monitoring.

6. Drugs known to cause idiosyncratic liver disease (e.g. isoniazid, phenytoin, methyldopa) are not necessarily contraindicated in stable chronic disease as there is no evidence of an increased susceptibility to further damage. Oral contraceptives are not advisable if there is active liver disease or a history of jaundice of pregnancy, but need not be withheld after recovery from acute hepatitis.

7. Constipation favors bacterial production of false neurotransmitter amines in the bowel, and drugs that cause constipation (e.g. verapamil, tricyclic antidepressants) should be avoided if possible in patients at risk of hepatic encephalopathy.

8. Drugs that inhibit catabolism of such amines (e.g. monoamine oxidase inhibitors) also provoke coma, and should be avoided.

9. Kaliuretic drugs (e.g. thiazide or loop diuretics) also provoke encephalopathy and potassium-sparing drugs such as spironolactone or amiloride are often preferable.

10. Fluid overload and ascites are exacerbated by drugs causing sodium retention (e.g. indomethacin, glucocorticoids, stilbestrol or carbenoxolone) and those containing sodium (e.g. sodium-containing antacids and high-dose carbenicillin).

11. Avoid drugs that interfere with hemostasis, such as aspirin, anticoagulants and fibrinolytics whenever possible, because of the increased risk of bleeding, especially if varices are suspected.

THYROID DISEASE

Thyroid dysfunction affects drug disposition partly by effects on drug metabolism and partly via changes in renal elimination. Existing data refer to only a few drugs, but it is prudent to anticipate the possibility of increased sensitivity of hypothyroid patients to many drugs when prescribing. Information is available regarding the following.

DIGOXIN

It has been known for many years that myxedematous patients are extremely sensitive to digoxin, whereas unusually large doses are required to control the ventricular rate in thyrotoxic atrial fibrillation. In general, hyperthyroid patients have lower plasma digoxin concentrations and hypothyroid patients higher plasma concentrations than euthyroid patients on the same dose. There is no significant difference in half-life between these groups and a difference in V_d

has been postulated to explain the alteration of plasma concentration with thyroid activity. Changes in renal function which occur with changes in thyroid status complicate this interpretation. Glomerular filtration rate is increased in thyrotoxicosis and decreased in myxedema. These changes in renal function influence elimination and the reduced plasma levels of digoxin correlate well with the increased creatinine clearance in thyrotoxicosis. In addition enhanced biliary clearance, digoxin malabsorption due to intestinal hurry and increased hepatic metabolism have all been postulated as factors in the insensitivity of thyrotoxic patients to cardiac glycosides.

ANTICOAGULANTS

Oral anticoagulants produce an exaggerated prolongation of prothrombin time in hyperthyroid patients. This is due to increased metabolic breakdown of vitamin K-dependent clotting factors rather than from changes in drug kinetics.

GLUCOCORTICOIDS

Glucocorticoids are metabolized by hepatic mixed-function oxidases which are influenced by thyroid status. In hyperthyroidism there is increased cortisol production and a reduced cortisol half-life, the converse obtaining in myxedema.

THYROXINE

The normal half-life of thyroxine (6–7 days) is reduced to 3–4 days by hyperthyroidism and prolonged to 9–10 days by hypothyroidism. This is of considerable clinical importance when deciding on an appropriate interval at which to increase the dose of thyroxine in patients treated for myxedema, especially if they have coincident ischemic heart disease which would be exacerbated if an excessive steady-state thyroxine level were achieved.

ANTITHYROID DRUGS

The half-life of propylthiouracil and methimazole is prolonged in hypothyroidism and shortened in hyperthyroidism, these values returning to normal on attainment of the euthyroid state, probably because of altered hepatic metabolism.

OPIATES

Patients with hypothyroidism are exceptionally sensitive to opioid analgesics, which cause profound respiratory depression in this setting.

Therapeutic Drug Monitoring

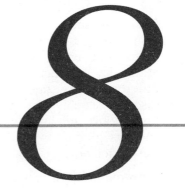

Introduction **68**

Role of drug monitoring in therapeutics **68**

Pharmacokinetic factors and drug response **69**

Practical aspects **69**

Drugs for which therapeutic drug monitoring is used **70**

*I*NTRODUCTION

The large interpatient variability in responses to drugs results from two main sources:

1. Pharmacokinetic variability in absorption, distribution, metabolism or elimination.
2. Pharmacodynamic variability in sensitivity at or beyond receptors, due to acquired differences (e.g. age, obesity or effects of disease such as hypothyroidism or myasthenia gravis), or inherited disease such as glucose-6-phosphate dehydrogenase deficiency.

Measurement of drug concentrations in the blood or plasma allows evaluation of the relative importance of these two sources of variation and in some instances facilitates adjustment of dosage to produce a desired response. Monitoring of drug therapy by clinical response has been used for many years and, where applicable, is more valuable than complex methods of drug analysis. Pharmacodynamic measures of response include clinical or laboratory measurements such as relief of pain in response to an analgesic, arterial blood pressure in patients with hypertension, peak expiratory flow rate in patients with asthma, bactericidal activity of plasma from a patient treated with antibiotics for bacterial endocarditis, or international normalized ratio (INR) in patients treated with oral anticoagulants. There is no place for routine estimation of plasma concentrations of drugs that achieve adequate concentrations in all patients without causing toxicity following a standard dose.

*R*OLE OF DRUG MONITORING IN THERAPEUTICS

Monitoring drug concentrations to assist in the therapy of an individual patient is sometimes a useful supplement to clinical monitoring. Determination of concentrations of drugs in plasma can also be useful in other ways (e.g. management of overdose, see below). Accurate and convenient assay methods are necessary. Measurement of drug concentrations in plasma are most useful when:

1. A direct relationship exists between drug (or drug metabolite) concentration in plasma or other accessible biological fluid and pharmacological or toxic effect, i.e. a therapeutic range of plasma concentrations has been established. In contrast, drugs with irreversible or 'hit and run' actions such as some monoamine oxidase inhibitors or alkylating agents are generally unsuited to this approach. The development of tolerance to drug action also restricts the usefulness of plasma concentrations.
2. The effect cannot readily be assessed by clinical observation. This is particularly the case when the clinical end point is 'quantal' (e.g. a *grand mal* seizure), and there is no satisfactory intermediate end point which is a continuous variable (such as blood pressure or INR). Plasma concentration is a useful indirect continuous variable whereby therapy can be adjusted to optimize efficacy and minimize toxicity in some such cases.
3. Interindividual variability in plasma drug concentrations from the same dose is large and unpredictable, for example phenytoin.
4. There is a low therapeutic index (i.e. ratio of toxic concentration/effective

concentration < 2). Drugs with a narrow 'therapeutic window' are particularly suitable for plasma concentration monitoring. Measuring drug concentrations helps when several drugs are being given concurrently and serious interactions are anticipated.

5. It is sometimes useful to check that replacement treatment is adequate and not excessive, and in some situations such as treatment of hypothyroidism measuring the concentration in plasma of thyroxine, for example, may be the most appropriate way of doing so. In other situations response to therapy is best monitored by a measure of drug effect (i.e. a pharmacodynamic measure). Examples are the rise in reticulocyte count and hematocrit in patients with Addisonian pernicious anemia treated with vitamin B_{12}, or those with iron deficiency treated with ferrous sulfate.

5. There are circumstances in which compliance with therapy with drugs such as theophylline, phenytoin or carbamazepine needs to be checked.

6. There are some cases of poisoning (e.g. with paracetamol or aspirin) in which knowledge of the plasma concentration can be invaluable in deciding on the need for active measures such as the use of specific antidotes.

PHARMACOKINETIC FACTORS AND DRUG RESPONSE

Pharmacokinetic factors can influence the relationship between plasma drug concentration and response: for example, the rate of change of plasma concentration determines pharmacological responses to some drugs including alcohol, amphetamine and barbiturates. There is a close relationship between pharmacological effects of amphetamine and the initial rate of entry of the drug into the circulation, but not the peak plasma level or the area under the plasma concentration–time curve (AUC).

PRACTICAL ASPECTS

Drug distribution and active metabolite formation influence the relationship between plasma drug concentration and effect, as may alterations of homeostatic mechanisms. A constant tissue to plasma drug concentration ratio only occurs during the terminal β-phase of elimination. Measurements should therefore be made when enough time has elapsed after a dose for this to have been established. Greater care is therefore required in the timing and labelling of specimens for drug concentration determination than is the case for 'routine' chemical pathology specimens.

Usually during repeated dosing a sample is taken just before the next dose to assess the 'trough' concentration and a sample may also be taken at some specified time after dosing (depending upon the drug) to determine the 'peak' level.

Given this information the laboratory should be able to produce useful information. Useful advice on the interpretation of this information is sometimes available from a local therapeutic drug monitoring service such as is provided by some clinical pharmacology and/or clinical pharmacy departments.

In general the cost of measuring drug levels is greater than for clinical chemical estimations and to use expensive facilities to produce 'numbers' resulting from analysis of samples taken at random from patients described only by name or number is meaningless and misleading, as well as a waste of money.

Analytical techniques of high specificity (often relying on high-performance liquid chromatography or radioimmunoassay) avoid the pitfalls of several of the older spectrophotometric methods for drugs such as theophylline which were influenced by inactive metabolites. Drugs administered concomitantly may interfere with assays, for example some laboratories assay antibiotics by a microbiological assay, and if the patient is given a second antibiotic concurrently results are meaningless. The clinician should always be aware of the possibility of error in laboratory data. Experience with quality control monitoring of anticonvulsant analyses performed by laboratories both in the UK and in the USA reveals that repeated analyses of a reference sample can produce some startlingly different results. The most important principle for the clinician is that plasma drug concentrations must always be interpreted in the context of the patient's clinical state.

Few prospective studies of the effects of using therapeutic drug monitoring services on the quality of patient care have been carried out. A retrospective survey carried out at the Massachusetts General Hospital showed that before the use of digoxin monitoring 13.9% of all patients receiving digoxin showed evidence of toxicity and that this fell to 5.9% following introduction of monitoring.

DRUGS FOR WHICH THERAPEUTIC DRUG MONITORING IS USED

Table 8.1 lists drugs which may be monitored.

1. **Digoxin** (therapeutic range 0.8–2 μg/l, 1–2.6 nmol/l) and other cardiac glycosides. Measuring the plasma concentration can help as a guide to individualize therapy, and may also be a useful adjunct in cases of suspected toxicity or poor compliance.
2. **Lithium** Plasma concentrations in samples obtained 12 hours after dosing of 0.75–1.25 mmol/l are usually regarded as therapeutic, although a lower range of 0.5–0.8 mmol/l has also been recommended.
3. **Aminoglycoside antibiotics. Gentamicin**: peak concentrations, measured 30 min after dosing, of 7–10 mg/l are usually effective against sensitive organisms, and trough levels, taken immediately before a dose, of 1 to not >2 mg/l reduce the risk of toxicity; **amikacin, netilmycin**: the desirable

Table 8.1 Therapeutically monitored drugs.

Drug	Therapeutic range
Digoxin	0.8–2 μg/l (1–2.6 nmol/l)
Lithium	0.5–1.25 mmol/l
Aminoglycoside antibiotics	Various*
Phenytoin	10–20 mg/l (40–80 μmol/l)
Methotrexate	Not applicable†
Theophylline	5–20 mg/l (28–110 μmol/l)
Cyclosporin	50–200 μg/l
Some antiarrhythmic drugs	Various

* Peak and trough levels needed – see text.
† Monitoring must be performed to prevent toxicity: plasma concentrations >5 μmol/l 24 hours after dosing usually require high dose leucovorin to prevent serious marrow/gut toxicity.

peak concentration is 4–12 mg/l, with a trough value not > 4 mg/l; **tobramycin** peak 4–5 mg/l, trough not > 2 mg/l.
4. **Phenytoin** (usual therapeutic range 10–20 mg/l, 40–80 μmol/l) and some other anticonvulsants including **carbamazepine**

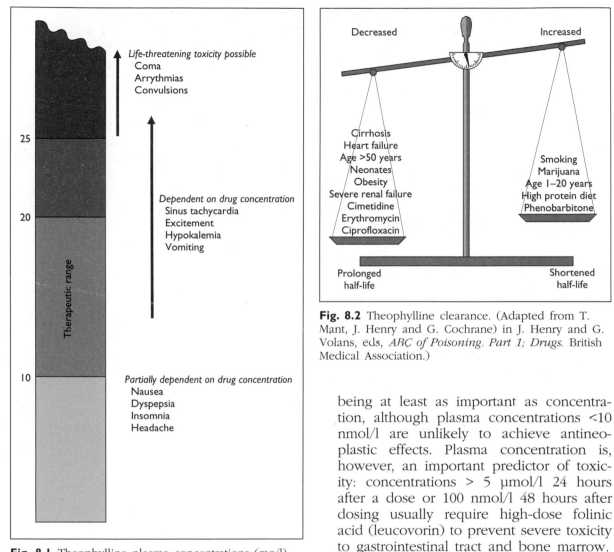

Fig. 8.1 Theophylline plasma concentrations (mg/l). NB There is a wide variety in incidence and severity of adverse effects. (Adapted from T. Mant, J. Henry and G. Cochrane) in J. Henry and G. Volans, eds, *ABC of Poisoning. Part 1: Drugs.* British Medical Association.)

Fig. 8.2 Theophylline clearance. (Adapted from T. Mant, J. Henry and G. Cochrane) in J. Henry and G. Volans, eds, *ABC of Poisoning. Part 1; Drugs.* British Medical Association.)

(approximate therapeutic range 5–10 mg/l, 20–40 µmol/l). When using the steady-state plasma concentration of phenytoin as a guide to dose adjustment, it is important to be aware of the non-linear nature of its pharmacokinetics, and of possible effects of concurrent renal or hepatic disease or of pregnancy on its distribution.

5. **Methotrexate** does not have a clear concentration/effect relationship, duration of exposure of neoplastic cells to the drug being at least as important as concentration, although plasma concentrations <10 nmol/l are unlikely to achieve antineoplastic effects. Plasma concentration is, however, an important predictor of toxicity: concentrations > 5 µmol/l 24 hours after a dose or 100 nmol/l 48 hours after dosing usually require high-dose folinic acid (leucovorin) to prevent severe toxicity to gastrointestinal tract and bone marrow.

6. **Theophylline** is an effective drug with a narrow therapeutic index (Fig 8.1) and many factors influence its clearance (Fig. 8.2). Measurement of plasma theophylline concentration can help minimize toxicity (which can be severe, e.g. unheralded cardiac arrhythmias or seizures). A therapeutic range of 5–20 mg/l is quoted. This is somewhat of an oversimplification, and plasma concentrations of 15–20 mg/l are associated with severe toxicity in neonates due to decreased protein binding and accumulation of caffeine, to which theophylline is methylated in neonates but not in older children.

7. Therapeutic ranges of plasma concentrations of several **antiarrhythmic drugs**

(e.g. lignocaine) have been established with reasonable confidence. **Amiodarone**, an effective antiarrhythmic drug, is difficult to use because of its extremely long plasma half-life and significant toxicities. The therapeutic range of plasma amiodarone concentrations for ventricular arrhythmias (1.0–2.5 mg/l) is higher than that needed for atrial arrhythmias (0.5–1.5 mg/l). It is not useful to measure the plasma concentrations of other antiarrhythmic drugs routinely, dose adjustment being made on clinical grounds. Plasma concentration determination can, however, be helpful if there is unexpected therapeutic failure or unexpected toxicity.

8. **Cyclosporin** Careful pharmacokinetic monitoring of this uniquely valuable but toxic immunosuppressant is essential. Trough plasma concentrations in the range 50–200 μg/l are usually recommended during maintenance treatment. Compliance is a particular problem in children, and deterioration in renal function can reflect either graft rejection due to inadequate cyclosporin concentration or toxicity from excessive concentrations.

Drugs in Pregnancy

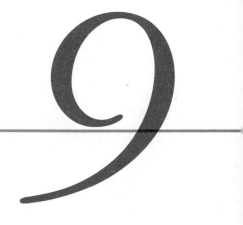

9

Introduction **74**

Harmful effects on the fetus **74**

Recognition of teratogenic drugs **75**

Pharmacokinetics in pregnancy **76**

Prescribing in pregnancy **77**

Non-therapeutic drugs **80**

INTRODUCTION

The use of drugs in pregnancy is complicated by the potential for harmful effects on the growing fetus, altered maternal physiology and the paucity and difficulties of research in this field.

HARMFUL EFFECTS ON THE FETUS

Because experience with many drugs in pregnancy is severely limited, it should be assumed that all drugs are harmful until sufficient data exist to indicate otherwise. 'Social' drugs (alcohol and cigarette smoking) are definitely harmful and their use should be discouraged.

In the placenta maternal blood is separated from fetal blood by a cellular membrane. The diffusion path is longer in early pregnancy than in late pregnancy. Drugs can cross the placenta by active transport or by passive diffusion down the concentration gradient, and it is the latter which is usually involved in drug transfer. Hence the rate of diffusion depends on (1) the concentration of free drug (i.e. non-protein bound) on each side of the membrane; and (2) the lipid solubility of the drug, which is determined in part by the degree of ionization. Diffusion occurs if the drug is in the unionized state. Placental function is also modified by changes in blood flow, and drugs which reduce placental blood flow can reduce birth weight. This may be the mechanism which causes the small reduction in birth weight following treatment of the mother with β-blockers in pregnancy. Early in embryonic development, exogenous substances accumulate in the neuroectoderm. The blood–brain barrier to diffusion is not developed until the second half of pregnancy, and the susceptibility of the central nervous system (CNS) to developmental toxins may be partly related to this. The human placenta possesses multiple enzymes that are primarily involved with endogenous steroid metabolism but may also contribute to drug metabolism and clearance.

The stage of gestation influences the effects of drugs on the fetus. It is convenient to divide pregnancy into four stages: fertilization and implantation (<17 days), the organogenesis/embryonic stage (17–57 days), the fetogenic stage and delivery.

Fertilization and implantation

Animal studies suggest that interference with the fetus before 17 days' gestation causes abortion, i.e. if pregnancy continues the fetus is unharmed.

Organogenesis/ embryonic stage

At this stage the fetus is differentiating to form major organs and this is the critical period for teratogenesis. Teratogens cause deviations or abnormalities in the develop-

Table 9.1 Some drugs that are definitely teratogenic in humans.

Thalidomide	Androgens
Cytotoxic agents	Progestogens
Alcohol	Diethylstilbestrol
Warfarin	Radioisotopes
Retinoids	Some live vaccines
Most anticonvulsants	Lithium

Table 9.2 Adverse effects of drugs on fetal growth and development.

- Drugs used to treat maternal hyperthyroidism can cause fetal and neonatal hypothyroidism
- Tetracycline antibiotics inhibit growth of fetal bones and stain teeth
- Aminoglycosides cause fetal VIIIth nerve damage
- Opioids and cocaine taken regularly during pregnancy can lead to fetal drug dependency

ment of the embryo that are compatible with prenatal life and are observable postnatally. Drugs that interfere with this process can cause gross structural defects, for example thalidomide phocomelia.

Some drugs are confirmed teratogens (Table 9.1), but for many the evidence is inconclusive. Thalidomide was unusual in the way in which a very small dose of the drug given on only one or two occasions between the fourth and seventh weeks of pregnancy produced serious malformations. Despite its wide use it was nearly 4 years before these adverse effects were recognized.

Fetogenic stage

In this stage the fetus undergoes further development and maturation. Even after organogenesis is almost complete drugs can have significant adverse effects on fetal growth and development (Table 9.2).

Delivery

Some drugs given late in pregnancy or during delivery may cause particular problems. Pethidine, regularly administered as an analgesic can cause fetal apnea (which is reversed with naloxone). Anesthetic agents given during Cesarian section may transiently depress neurological, respiratory and muscular functions. Warfarin given in late pregnancy causes a hemostasis defect in the baby and predisposes to cerebral hemorrhage during delivery.

RECOGNITION OF TERATOGENIC DRUGS

The incidence of serious congenital abnormality is about 2% of all births and a small but unknown fraction of these are due to drugs. Two principal problems face those who try to determine whether a drug is teratogenic when it is used to treat disease in humans:

1. Many drugs produce birth defects when given experimentally in large doses to pregnant animals. This does not necessarily mean that they are teratogenic in humans in therapeutic doses. Indeed the metabolism and kinetics of drugs in high doses in other species is so different from humans as to limit seriously the relevance of such studies.

2. Fetal defects are common (2%). Consequently if the incidence of drug-induced abnormalities is low, a very large

number of cases has to be observed to define a significant increase above this background level. Effects on the fetus may take several years to become clinically manifest, an example being diethylstilbestrol which was widely used in the late 1940s for preventing miscarriages and preterm births (despite little evidence of efficacy). In 1971 an association was reported between adenocarcinoma of the vagina in girls in their late teens whose mothers had been given diethylstilbestrol during the pregnancy. Exposure to stilbestrol *in utero* has also been associated with a T-shaped uterus, and other structural abnormalities of the genital tract and increased rates of ectopic pregnancy and premature labor.

The tragedy of thalidomide and the sinister delayed presentation of diethylstilbestrol toxicity, illustrate the absolute necessity for meticulous data analysis of drug administration in pregnancy – assessing efficacy and both short- and long-term side effects on mothers and fetus – before the introduction of any new treatment can be recommended during pregnancy when acceptable alternatives are available.

PHARMACOKINETICS IN PREGNANCY

Ethical and practical considerations make pharmacokinetic studies in pregnancy difficult. There is no evidence however that pregnancy changes pharmacological response and known differences in drug effects are usually explained by altered pharmacokinetics.

ABSORPTION

Gastric emptying and small intestinal motility are reduced. This is of little consequence unless rapid drug action is required. Vomiting associated with pregnancy may make oral drug administration impractical.

DISTRIBUTION

During pregnancy the blood volume increases by a third, with expansion in plasma volume (from 2.5 to 4 litres at term) being disproportionate to expansion in red cell mass, so that hematocrit falls. There is also an increase in body water due to a larger extravascular volume and changes in uterus and breasts.

Edema, which at least one-third of women experience during pregnancy, may add up to 8 litres to the volume of extracellular water. For water-soluble drugs (which usually have a relatively small volume of distribution) this increases the apparent volume of distribution and although clearance is unaltered their half-life is prolonged. During pregnancy plasma protein concentration falls and there is increased competition for binding sites due to competition by endogenous ligands such as increased hormone levels. These factors alter the total amount of bound drug and the apparent volume of distribution. The concentration of free drug however usually remains unaltered, because a greater volume of distribution for free drug is accompanied by increased clearance of free drug. Thus in practice these changes are rarely of pharmacological significance. They may however cause confusion in monitoring of plasma drug levels since these usually measure total (rather than free) drug concentrations.

METABOLISM

Metabolism of drugs by the pregnant liver is increased, largely due to enzyme induction perhaps by raised hormone levels. Liver blood flow does not change. This may lead to an increased rate of elimination of those drugs, for example theophylline, where enzyme activity rather than liver blood flow is the main determinant of elimination rate.

RENAL EXCRETION

Excretion of drugs via the kidney increases because renal plasma flow almost doubles and the glomerular filtration rate increases by two-thirds during pregnancy. This has been documented for digoxin, lithium, ampicillin, cephalexin and gentamicin.

PRESCRIBING IN PREGNANCY

The prescription of drugs to a pregnant woman is a balance between possible adverse drug effects on the fetus and the risk of leaving maternal disease inadequately treated. Effects on the human fetus cannot be reliably predicted from animal studies, hence one should prescribe drugs for which there is experience of safety over many years in preference to new or untried drugs. The smallest effective dose should be used. The fetus is most sensitive to adverse drug effects during the first trimester and all women of child-bearing potential should be assumed pregnant until determined otherwise.

Delayed toxicity is a sinister problem, for example diethylstilbestrol, and the world was 'fortunate' that the teratogenic effect of thalidomide produced such an unusual congenital abnormality – phocomelia – otherwise its detection may have been delayed further. If drugs have more subtle effects on the fetus, for example minor reduction in intelligence, or cause an increased incidence of a common disease, for example atopy, it may never be detected. Many publications demand careful prospective controlled clinical trials but the ethics and practicalities of such studies make their demands often unrealistic. A more rational approach is for drug regulatory bodies, the pharmaceutical industry and drug information agencies to collaborate closely and internationally to collate all information concerning drug use in pregnancy whether inadvertent or planned and associate these with outcome not only of the fetus but also the adult. This will require

significant investment in time and money as well as considerable encouragement to doctors and midwives to complete the endless forms. For now all who prescribe drugs must be aware of the potential hazard to pregnant women and judge each case on its individual merit. To do this doctors must have rapid access to clear information on the experience of drug use in pregnancy and the morbidity/mortality of untreated disease. A rational decision can then be made on which, if any, drug therapy is necessary. Doctors have a responsibility to warn patients of the risks of over-the-counter medicines, smoking and alcohol abuse in pregnancy.

Guidance to the use of drugs for a selection of conditions is summarized below. If in doubt consult the *British National Formulary*, appendix 4 (which is appropriately conservative).

Antimicrobial drugs

Antimicrobial drugs are commonly prescribed during pregnancy. The safest antibiotics in pregnancy are the penicillins and cephalosporins. Trimethoprim is a theoretical teratogen as it is a folic acid antagonist. The aminoglycosides can cause ototoxicity. There is no experience in pregnancy with the fluroquinolones such as ciprofloxacin and they should be avoided. Erythromycin is probably safe. Metronidazole is a teratogen in animals but there is no evidence of teratogenicity in humans and its benefit in serious anaerobic sepsis probably outweighs any risks. Unless there is a life-threatening infection in the mother antiviral agents should be avoided in pregnancy. Falciparum malaria (chapter 44) has an especially high mortality in late pregnancy. Fortunately the standard regimens of intravenous and oral quinine are safe in pregnancy.

Analgesics

Opioids cross the placenta. This is particularly relevant in the management of labor when the use of opioids such as pethidine depresses the fetal respiratory centre and can inhibit the start of normal respiration. If the mother is dependent on opioids the fetus can experience opioid withdrawal syndrome during and after delivery which can be fatal. In neonates the chief withdrawal symptoms are tremor, irritability, diarrhea and vomiting. Chlorpromazine is commonly used to treat this withdrawal state. Paracetamol is preferred to aspirin when mild analgesia is required. Where a systemic anti-inflammatory action is required (e.g. in rheumatoid arthritis) ibuprofen is the drug of choice.

Anesthesia

Anesthesia in pregnancy is a very specialist subject and should only be undertaken by experienced anesthetists. Local anesthetics used for regional anesthesia readily cross the placenta. However when used in epidural anesthesia the drug remains largely confined to the epidural space. Pregnant women are at increased risk of aspiration. Although commonly used, pethidine frequently causes vomiting and may also lead to neonatal respiratory depression. Metoclopramide should be used in preference to prochlorperazine (which has an antianalgesic effect

when combined with pethidine) and naloxone (an opioid antagonist) must always be available. Respiratory depression in the newborn is not usually a problem with modern general anesthetics presently in use in Cesarian section. Several studies have shown an increased incidence of spontaneous abortions in mothers who have had general anesthesia during pregnancy although a causal relation is not proven and in most circumstances failure to operate would have dramatically increased the risk to mother and fetus.

Antiemetics

Nausea and vomiting are common in early pregnancy but are usually self-limiting and ideally should be managed with reassurance and non-drug strategies such as small frequent meals, avoiding large volumes of fluid and raising the head of the bed. If symptoms are prolonged or severe drug treatment may be effective. Meclozine and cyclizine are commonly used although both have been weakly associated with an increased risk of congenital malformations. Metoclopramide is considered safe and efficacious in labor and before anesthesia in late pregnancy but its routine use in early pregnancy cannot be recommended because of lack of controlled data, and a significant incidence of dystonic reactions in young women.

Dyspepsia and constipation

The high incidence of dyspepsia due to gastro-esophageal reflux in the second and third trimesters is probably related to the reduction in lower esophageal sphincter pressure. Non-drug treatment – reassurance, small frequent meals and advice on posture

– should be pursued in the first instance particularly in the first trimester. Fortunately most cases occur later in pregnancy when non-absorbable antacids such as alginates should be used. In late pregnancy meto-clopromide is particularly effective as it increases lower esophageal sphincter pressure. H_2-receptor blockers should not be used for non-ulcer dyspepsia in this setting. Constipation should be managed with dietary advice. Stimulant laxatives may be uterotonic and should be avoided if possible.

Peptic ulceration

Antacids may relieve symptoms. There are inadequate safety data on the use of H_2-receptor blockers and omeprazole in pregnancy. Sucralfate has been recommended for use in pregnancy in the USA and is rational as it is not systemically absorbed. Misoprostol, a prostaglandin which stimulates the uterus, is contraindicated because it causes abortion.

Anticonvulsants

Epilepsy in pregnancy can lead to fetal and maternal morbidity/mortality through convulsions whilst all the anticonvulsants used have been associated with teratogenic effects, for example phenytoin is associated with cleft palate and congenital heart disease. However, there is no doubt the benefits of good seizure control outweigh the drug-induced teratogenic risk. Thorough explanation to the mother, ideally before a planned pregnancy, is essential and it must be emphasized that the majority of epileptic mothers have normal babies (>90%). (The usual risk of fetal malformation is about 2%. In epileptic mothers it is up to 10%.) In view of the association of spina bifida with sodium valproate and carbamazepine therapy it is often recommended that the

standard dose of folic acid be increased to 4–5 mg daily. Both these anticonvulsants cause hypospadias. As in non-pregnant epilepsy single drug therapy is preferable. Plasma concentration monitoring is particularly relevant for phenytoin because the decrease in plasma protein binding and the increase in hepatic metabolism may cause considerable changes in the plasma concentration of free (active) drug. As always the guide to the correct dose is freedom from fits and absence of toxicity. Owing to the changes in plasma protein binding it is generally recommended that the therapeutic range is 5–15 mg/l whereas in the non-pregnant state it is 10–20 mg/l. This is only a rough guide as protein binding varies.

Anticoagulation

Warfarin has been associated with nasal hypoplasia and chondrodysplasia when given in the first trimester and CNS abnormalities after administration in later pregnancy as well as a high incidence of hemorrhagic complications towards the end of pregnancy. Neonatal hemorrhage is difficult to prevent because of the immature enzymes in fetal liver and low stores of vitamin K. Heparin, which does not cross the placenta, is the anticoagulant of choice in pregnancy although chronic use can cause maternal osteoporosis (chapter 27). Women on long-term oral anticoagulants should be warned that these drugs are likely to affect the fetus in early pregnancy. Subcutaneous heparin (usually self-administered) must be substituted for warfarin as soon as possible, well before the critical period of 6–9 weeks' gestation. Subcutaneous heparin can be continued throughout pregnancy but due to the risk of maternal osteoporosis and thrombocytopenia warfarin may be considered as an alternative during the second trimester changing back to heparin at 36 weeks. Patients with prosthetic heart values present a special problem: in these patients in spite of the risks to the fetus warfarin is often given up to 36 weeks. The prothrombin time/international normalized ratio (INR) (warfarin) or APTT (activated partial thromboplastin time) (heparin) should be monitored closely.

Cardiovascular drugs

Hypertension in pregnancy (see chapter 25) can normally be managed with either methyl-dopa or atenolol or labetalol. Parenteral hydralazine is useful in lowering blood pressure in pre-eclampsia. These drugs have an excellent safety record in pregnancy. Diuretics should not be started to treat hypertension in pregnancy, although some American authorities now continue thiazide diuretics in women with essential hypertension already stabilized on these drugs. Angiotensin-converting enzyme inhibitors must be avoided.

Hormones

Progestogens, particularly synthetic ones, can masculinize the female fetus. There is no evidence that this occurs with the small amount of progestogen (or estrogen) in the oral contraceptive: the risk applies to large doses. Corticosteroids do not appear to give rise to any serious problems when given via inhalation or in short courses. Transient suppression of the fetal hypothalamic–pituitary–adrenal axis has been reported. Rarely cleft palate and congenital cataract have been linked with steroids in pregnancy but the benefit of treatment usually outweighs any such risk. Iodine and antithyroid drugs (iodine and radioiodine) cross the placenta as do carbimazole and related drugs and can cause hypothyroidism and goiter. Management of hyperthyroidism during pregnancy is discussed in chapter 35.

Tranquillizers and antidepressants

Benzodiazepines accumulate in the tissues and are slowly eliminated by the neonate, resulting in prolonged hypotonia ('floppy baby'), subnormal temperatures (hypothermia), periodic cessation of respiration and poor sucking. There is no evidence that the phenothiazines or tricyclic antidepressants are teratogenic. There is as yet insufficient evidence on the newer 5-hydroxytryptamine reuptake inhibitors. Lithium can cause fetal goiter and possible cardiovascular abnormalities.

NON-THERAPEUTIC DRUGS

Excessive ethanol consumption is associated with spontaneous abortion, craniofacial abnormalities, mental retardation, congenital heart disease and impaired growth. Even moderate alcohol intake may adversely affect the baby: the risk of having an abnormal child is about 10% in mothers drinking 30–60 ml ethanol per day rising to 40% in chronic alcoholics. Fetal alcohol syndrome describes the distinct pattern of abnormal morphogenesis and central nervous system dysfunction is children whose mothers were chronic alcoholics. Fetal alcohol syndrome is a leading cause of mental retardation. After birth the characteristic craniofacial malformations diminish but microcephaly and to a lesser degree short stature persist. Cigarette smoking is associated with spontaneous abortion, premature delivery, small babies, increased perinatal mortality and a higher incidence of sudden infant death syndrome (cot death). Cocaine causes vasoconstriction of placental vessels. There is a high incidence of low birth weight, congenital abnormalities and, in particular, delayed neurological and behavioral development.

Drugs at Extremes of Age

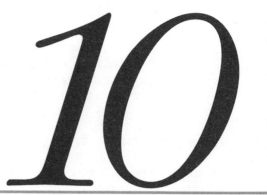

Drugs in infants and children **84**

Drugs in the elderly **86**

DRUGS IN INFANTS AND CHILDREN

Pharmacokinetics

Children are not miniature adults in terms of drug handling because of differences in body constitution, drug absorption and elimination, and sensitivity to adverse reactions.

ABSORPTION

Reduced gastric acidity in neonates results in greater oral absorption of certain antibiotics, for example amoxycillin. The major practical difference in children is the more frequent use of oral liquid preparations resulting in less accurate dosing, more rapid rate of absorption (although minimal difference in bioavailability). This can be significant for drugs with a close correlation between high peak plasma concentration and adverse effects, or low trough concentration with lack of efficacy (e.g. carbamazepine and theophylline). Infant skin is thin and percutaneous absorption is increased relative to adults, hence systemic absorption of corticosteroids from local preparations may be increased and can cause toxicity if used extensively.

DISTRIBUTION

Fat content is relatively low in children leading to a lower volume of distribution of fat-soluble drugs (e.g. diazepam) in babies. Plasma protein binding of drugs is reduced in neonates due to a lower plasma albumin concentration which is not generally of clinical significance although the danger of kernicterus caused by displacement of bilirubin from albumin by sulfonamides (chapter 12) is well recognized. The blood–brain barrier is more permeable in neonates and young children leading to an increased risk of central nervous system (CNS) adverse effects.

METABOLISM

At birth the hepatic microsomal enzyme system (chapter 5) is relatively immature (particularly in the preterm infant) but after the first 4 weeks it matures rapidly. Chloramphenicol can produce 'grey baby syndrome' in neonates due to high plasma levels secondary to inefficient glucuronidation. Drugs administered to the mother can induce neonatal enzyme activity, for example barbiturates. In children there is evidence that aspirin metabolism is relatively impaired whilst phenobarbitone metabolism is increased. This may be because of induction of hepatic enzyme activity or because the ratio of the weight of the liver to body weight is up to 50% higher than in adults.

EXCRETION

All renal mechanisms (filtration, secretion and reabsorption) are reduced in babies and renal excretion of drugs is relatively reduced in the newborn. Glomerular filtration rate (GFR) rapidly increases during the first 4 weeks of life with consequent changes in rate of drug elimination (Table 10.1).

Table 10.1

	Plasma half-life of gentamicin (hours)
Premature infant	
<48 hours old	18
5–22 days old	6
Normal infant	
1–4 weeks old	3
Adult	2

Pharmacodynamics

Documented evidence of differences in receptor sensitivity in children is lacking and the apparent paradoxical effects of some drugs (e.g. hyperkinesia with phenobarbitone, sedation of hyperactive children with amphetamine) is unexplained.

Breast feeding

Breast feeding can lead to toxicity in the infant if the drug enters the milk in pharmacological quantities. Milk concentration of some drugs (e.g. iodides) may exceed the maternal plasma concentration, but the total dose delivered to the baby is usually very small. However, drugs in breast milk may cause hypersensitivity reactions even in very low dose. Virtually all drugs that reach the maternal systemic circulation will enter breast milk, especially lipid-soluble unionized low molecular weight drugs. Milk is weakly acidic, so drugs that are weak bases are concentrated in breast milk by trapping of the charged form of the drug (cf. renal elimination, chapter 6). The resulting dose administered to the fetus in breast milk is however usually clinically insignificant although some drugs are contraindicated (Table 10.2) and breast feeding should cease during treatment if there is no safer alternative.

The infant should be monitored if β-adrenoceptor antagonists, corticosteroids or lithium are prescribed to the mother. β-adrenoceptor antagonists rarely cause significant bradycardia. In high doses corticosteroids can affect the infant's adrenal function and lithium may cause intoxication. Bromocriptine and diuretics suppress lactation but adverse effects outweigh benefits in women who chose not to breast feed. Metronidazole gives milk an unpleasant taste.

Practical aspects of prescribing

COMPLIANCE AND ROUTE OF ADMINISTRATION

Children under the age of 5 years may have difficulty swallowing even small tablets hence oral preparations which taste pleasant are often necessary to improve compliance. Liquid preparations are given by a graduated syringe. However, chronic use of sucrose-containing elixirs encourages tooth cavities and gingivitis. The dyes and colorings used may induce hypersensitivity.

Pressurized aerosols (e.g. salbutamol inhaler, see chapter 30) are usually only practical in children over the age of 10 years as coordinated deep inspiration is required, unless a device such as a spacer is used. Spacers can be combined with a face mask from early infancy. Likewise nebulizers may be used to enhance local therapeutic effect and reduce systemic toxicity.

Only in unusual circumstances, i.e. extensive areas of application especially to inflamed or broken skin, or in infants, does systemic absorption of drugs (e.g. steroids, neomycin) become significant following topical application to the skin.

Intramuscular injection should be used only when absolutely necessary. Intravenous therapy is less painful but skill is required to cannulate infants' veins (and a confident colleague to keep the target still!). Children find intravenous infusions uncomfortable and

Table 10.2 Some drugs to be avoided during breast feeding.

Vitamin A/retinoid analogs (e.g. etretinate)
Amiodarone
Stimulant laxatives
Benzodiazepines
Chloramphenicol
Ciprofloxacin
Combined oral contraceptives
Cyclosporin
Cytotoxics
Ergotamine
Octreotide
Sulfonylureas
Thiazide diuretics

restrictive. Rectal administration (chapter 4) is a convenient alternative, for example metronidazole to prevent/treat anaerobic infections. Rectal diazepam is particularly valuable in the treatment of status epilepticus when intravenous access is often difficult. Rectal diazepam may also be administered by parents. Rectal administration should also be considered if the child is vomiting.

Paramount to ensuring compliance is full communication with parents and teachers. This should include not only how to administer the drug but why it is being prescribed, for how long the treatment should continue and whether any adverse effects are likely.

DOSAGE

Even after adjustment of dose according to surface area, calculation of the correct dose must consider the relatively large volume of distribution of polar drugs in the first 4 months of life and the immature microsomal enzymes. The *British National Formulary* and specialist pediatric textbooks and formularies provide appropriate guidelines and must be consulted by physicians not familiar with prescribing to infants and children.

ADVERSE EFFECTS

Drugs in children generally have a similar adverse effect profile to adults – of particular significance is the potential of chronic corticosteroid use including high-dose inhaled corticosteroids to inhibit growth. Aspirin is avoided in those under 12 (except in specific indications) due to an association with Reye's syndrome, a rare but often fatal illness of unknown etiology consisting of hepatic necrosis and encephalopathy, often in the aftermath of a viral illness. Tetracyclines are deposited in growing bone and teeth causing staining and occasionally dental hypoplasia, and should not be given to children.

Research

Research in pediatric clinical pharmacology is limited. Not only is there concern as to the potential for the adverse effects of new drugs on those who are growing and developing mentally but there are also considerable ethical problems encountered in research involving those too young to give informed consent. New drugs are often given to children for the first time only when no alternative is available or when unacceptable side effects have been encountered in the individual with established drugs. Pharmaceutical companies seldom seek to license their products for use in children for these reasons. When drugs are prescribed to children that are not licensed for use in this age group it is important to make careful records of both efficacy and possible adverse effects.

*D*RUGS IN THE ELDERLY

The proportion of elderly people in the population of the UK is increasing steadily. The elderly are subject to a variety of complaints many of which are chronic and incapacitating, and so they receive a great deal of drug treatment. Elderly persons comprise some 12% of the population but consume about one-third of the National Health Service's drug expenditure. Adverse drug reactions become more common with increasing age. In one study 11.8% of patients aged 41–50 years experienced adverse reactions to drugs but this increased to 25% in patients over 80. There are several reasons for this:

1. Elderly people take more drugs. In one survey in general practice, 87% of patients over 75 were on regular drug therapy with 34% taking three to four different drugs daily. The most commonly prescribed drugs were diuretics (34% of patients), analgesics (27%), tranquillizers and antidepressants (24%), hypnotics (22%) and digoxin (20%). All these are associated with a high incidence of important adverse effects.
2. Pharmacokinetics change with increasing age and concomitant disease leading to higher plasma concentrations of drugs and increased liability to side effects (see below).
3. Homeostatic mechanisms become less effective with advancing age, so individuals are less able to compensate for adverse effects such as unsteadiness or postural hypotension.
4. The central nervous system becomes more sensitive to the actions of sedative drugs.
5. Increasing age produces changes in the immune response that cause an increased liability to allergic reactions.

Pharmacokinetics

ABSORPTION

Iron, xylose, galactose, calcium and thiamine absorption are reduced in old people. Most drugs are absorbed by simple diffusion down the concentration gradient and this is not impaired by age. Intestinal blood flow is reduced by up to 50% in the elderly and gastric motility is increased, probably due to the tendency towards reduced acid secretion in the old. However, unless gastrointestinal pathology is present it appears that age *per se* does not affect drug absorption to a large extent.

DISTRIBUTION

Aging is associated with loss of weight and lean body mass and an increased ratio of fat to muscle and body water. This enlarges the volume of distribution of fat-soluble drugs such as diazepam and lignocaine whereas the distribution of polar drugs such as digoxin is reduced compared with younger adults. When the dosage of a drug is critical it is important to make suitable adjustment for weight. Changes in plasma proteins also occur with aging, especially if associated with chronic disease and malnutrition with a fall in albumin and a rise in gamma globulin concentrations.

HEPATIC METABOLISM

There is a decrease in the rate of hepatic clearance of some, but not all, drugs with advancing age. Many early studies depended on demonstrating a prolonged plasma half-life (Fig. 10.1) which could be secondary to an increased apparent volume of distribution rather than reduced metabolism. Changes in clearance with age should be documented to confirm that aging reduces drug metabolism. The reduced clearance of long half-life benzodiazepines have important clinical consequences as when these are prescribed for prolonged periods, slow accumulation of drug (and active metabolites) may lead to adverse effects whose onset may be days or

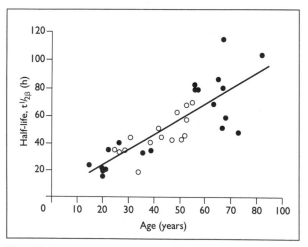

Fig. 10.1 Relationship between diazepam half-life and age in 33 normal individuals. Non-smokers (●). Smokers (○). (From U. Klotz et al. *J Clin Invest* 1975; **55**: 347.)

weeks after initiating therapy. Consequently confusion or memory impairment may be falsely attributed to aging rather than adverse drug effects.

RENAL EXCRETION

Probably the most important cause of drug accumulation in the elderly is declining renal function. In healthy individuals aged over 80 glomerular filtration rate is < 60–70 ml/min and renal disorders associated with advancing years such as prostatic hypertrophy further reduce renal function. The glomerular filtration rate falls at a rate of approximately 1 ml/min/1.73 m² each year after the age of 20. It is important to appreciate that although glomerular filtration rate declines with age this is not adequately reflected by serum creatinine which can remain within the range defined as 'normal' for a younger adult population in spite of a marked decline in renal function. This is related to the lower endogenous production of creatinine in the elderly secondary to their reduced muscle mass.

Tubular function also declines with age. These changes are reflected in the increasing plasma creatinine and urea concentrations with age. A number of dosage rules and nomograms are based upon creatinine clearance (chapter 7). Drugs that are mainly excreted via the kidney are likely to accumulate in patients in their seventies and eighties if given in doses suitable for young adults. Examples of drugs which may require reduced dosage in the elderly secondary to reduced renal excretion and/or hepatic clearance are shown in Table 10.3.

Table 10.3 Examples of drugs requiring dose adjustment in the elderly.

Aminoglycosides (e.g. gentamicin)
Atenolol
Cimetidine
Diazepam
Digoxin
Non-steroidal anti-inflammatory drugs
Oral hypoglycemic agents
Warfarin

Pharmacodynamic changes

Evidence that the elderly are intrinsically more sensitive to drugs than the young is scanty, however the sensitivity of the elderly to benzodiazepines as measured by psychometric tests is increased and their effects last longer than in the young. It is common clinical experience that benzodiazepines given to the elderly in hypnotic doses used for the young can produce prolonged daytime confusion even after single doses. The incidence of confusion associated with cimetidine is increased in the elderly. Other drugs may expose physiological defects that are a normal concomitant of aging. Postural hypotension can occur in healthy elderly people and the increased incidence of postural hypotension from drugs such as phenothiazines, β-adrenoceptor antagonists, tricyclic antidepressants and diuretics in elderly patients is not surprising. The increase in heart rate produced by isoprenaline is diminished in older patients suggesting that the sensitivity of the β-receptor response mechanism falls with age. Clotting factor synthesis by the liver is reduced in the elderly and old people often require lower warfarin doses for effective anticoagulation than younger adults.

Compliance in the elderly

Young adult patients frequently fail to take their medicines as instructed even in diseases such as tuberculosis where there should be considerable motivation towards compliance. Non-compliance is even more common (probably about 60%) in elderly people. This may be due to a failure of memory or to not understanding how the drug should be taken. In addition, patients may have previously prescribed drugs in the medicine cupboard which they take from time to time. It is therefore essential that the drug regimen be kept simple and be carefully explained. There is scope for improved methods of packaging so that over- or under-dosage is prevented. Multiple drug regimens must be avoided if possible. Not only will such regimens confuse the patient but they increase the risk of interactions (see Fig. 12.1).

Effect of drugs on some systems in the elderly

CENTRAL NERVOUS SYSTEM

Cerebral function is easily disturbed in old people resulting in disorientation and confusion. Drugs are one of the factors that contribute to this state; sedatives and hypnotics can easily precipitate a loss of awareness and clouding of consciousness. Overvigorous attempts to lower blood pressure may produce cerebral ischemia and confusion.

Night sedation

The elderly do not sleep as well as the young. They sleep for a shorter time, sleep is more likely to be broken and they are more easily aroused. This is quite normal, old people should not have the expectations of youth as far as sleep is concerned. Before hynotics are commenced other possible factors should be considered and treated if possible. They include:

1. Pain, which may be due to such causes as arthritis.
2. Constipation – the discomfort of a loaded rectum.
3. Urinary frequency.
4. Depression.
5. Anxiety.
6. Left ventricular failure.
7. Dementia.

A little more exercise may help and 'catnapping' in the day should be reduced to a minimum.

The prescription of hypnotics (chapter 15) should be minimized in the elderly.

Tranquillizers

Restlessness and agitated depression are common in old people and are associated with dementia. These states can be ameliorated by phenothiazines, for example thioridazine (chapter 16).

Of particular importance are:

1. The development of Parkinsonian symptoms, particularly slowness and rigidity, may be a problem and may require lowering the dose or stopping the drug. Concurrent use of anti-Parkinsonian drugs (e.g. muscarinic antagonists) is associated with a high incidence of adverse effects in this age group (e.g. urinary retention). The elderly are more prone to Parkinsonian syndromes and tardive dyskinesia than young people.
2. Postural hypotension.
3. Hypothermia.

Antidepressants

Although depression is common in old age and may indeed need treating, it should be remembered that the tricyclic antidepressants (chapter 17) can cause constipation, urinary retention and glaucoma (all due to their parasympathetic blocking action), and also drowsiness, confusion, postural hypotension and cardiac arrhythmias. The possibility that depression results from a drug used in the treatment of another disease (e.g. a β-adrenoreceptor antagonist) should be remembered. Tricyclic antidepressants can produce worthwhile remissions of depression but should be started at very low dosage, for example amitriptyline, 25 mg *nocte*, and only cautiously increased in dose.

Lofepramine is an alternative which has fewer of the anticholinergic side effects that are particularly troublesome in this age group.

5-Hydroxytryptamine reuptake inhibitors (e.g. fluoxetine) are as effective as the tricyclics and have a distinct side effect profile (chapter 17), but are generally well tolerated by the elderly. They are however more expensive than tricyclic antidepressants.

Anti-Parkinsonian drugs

The anticholinergic group of anti-Parkinsonian drugs (e.g. benzhexol, orphenadrine) quite often cause side effects in the elderly. Urinary retention is common in men. Glaucoma may be precipitated or aggravated and confusion may occur with quite small doses. Levodopa can be effective but it is particularly important to start with a small dose. Levodopa, 100 mg, and carbidopa, 10 mg (co-careldopa), is a suitable initial dose and can be increased gradually as needed. In patients with dementia the use of anticholinergics, levodopa or amantidine may produce adverse cerebral stimulation, leading to complete decompensation of cerebral functioning with excitement and inability to cope.

CARDIOVASCULAR SYSTEM

Hypertension

There is accumulating evidence that treating hypertension in the elderly reduces both morbidity and mortality. Treatment of hypertension in the elderly is discussed in chapter 25.

Digoxin

Digoxin toxicity is common in the elderly because of decreased renal elimination and reduced apparent volume of distribution. Confusion, toxic psychosis, depression and an acute abdominal syndrome resembling mesenteric artery obstruction are all more common features of digoxin toxicity in the old than in the young. Hypokalemia, due to decreased intake (potassium-rich foods are often expensive), faulty homeostatic mechanisms resulting in increased renal loss and the concomitant use of diuretics is commoner in the old and is a contributory factor in some patients. Digoxin is sometimes prescribed when there is no indication for it, for example for an irregular pulse which is due to multiple ectopic beats rather than atrial fibrillation. At other times the indications for initiation of treatment are correct but the situation is never

reviewed and the drug stopped. In one series of geriatric patients on digoxin the drug was withdrawn in 78% without detriment.

Diuretics

Diuretics are more likely to cause adverse effects (e.g. postural hypotension and electrolyte disturbances) in elderly patients. Too vigorous a diuresis may result in urinary retention in an old man with an enlarged prostate and necessitate bladder catheterization with its attendant risks. Brisk diuresis in patients with mental impairment or reduced mobility can result in incontinence. For many patients a thiazide diuretic is adequate. Loop diuretics should be used in acute heart failure or in low doses for maintenance treatment. Clinically important hypokalemia is uncommon with low doses of diuretics but plasma potassium should be checked after starting treatment. If clinically important hypokalemia develops a thiazide plus potassium-retaining diuretic (amiloride or triamterene) can be considered, but there is a risk of hyperkalemia due to renal impairment especially if angiotensin-converting enzyme (ACE) inhibitors are given together with the diuretic for hypertension or heart failure. Thiazide-induced gout and glucose intolerance are important side effects.

Angiotensin-converting enzyme inhibitors

This group of drugs plays an important part in the treatment of chronic heart failure as well as hypertension (chapters 25 and 28) and is effective and usually well tolerated in the elderly. Hypotension, hyperkalemia and renal failure are, however, more common in this age group. Potassium-retaining diuretics should be stopped and plasma potassium monitored when starting treatment.

Oral hypoglycemic agents

Diabetes is common in the elderly and many patients are treated with oral hypoglycemic drugs. It is best for elderly patients to be managed with diet if at all possible and to use drugs only to relieve symptoms of hyperglycemia. Chlorpropamide (half-life 36 hours) can cause prolonged hypoglycemia and is specifically contraindicated in this age group, and glibenclamide should also be avoided. Shorter acting drugs (e.g. gliclazide, chapter 34) are preferred.

Antibiotics

Antibiotics do not usually cause undue problems in old age as long as the decline in renal function is remembered when an aminoglycoside or tetracycline is used. Amoxycillin and ampicillin are the commonest causes of drug rashes in the elderly.

Practical aspects of prescribing

Improper prescription of drugs is a common cause of morbidity in elderly persons. Common-sense rules for prescribing have been suggested (and apply not only for the elderly).

1. Take a full drug history (chapter 1) which should include any adverse reactions and use of over-the-counter drugs.
2. Know the pharmacological action of the drug employed.
3. Use the lowest effective dose.
4. Use the fewest drugs a patient needs.
5. Drugs should not be used to treat symptoms without first discovering the cause of the symptoms, i.e. first diagnosis, then treatment.
6. Drugs should not be withheld because of old age, but it should be remembered that there is no cure for old age either.
7. A drug should not be continued if it is no longer necessary.
8. Do not use a drug if the symptoms it causes are worse than those it is meant to relieve.
9. It is seldom sensible to treat the side effects of one drug by prescribing another.

In the elderly it is often important to pay attention to matters such as the formulation of the drug to be used: many old people tolerate elixirs and liquid medicines better than tablets or capsules. Supervision of drug taking may be necessary since an old person with a serious physical or mental disability cannot be expected to comply with any but the simplest drug regimen. Containers require especially clear labelling and should be easy to open: child-proof containers are often also grandparent proof!

Adverse Drug Reactions

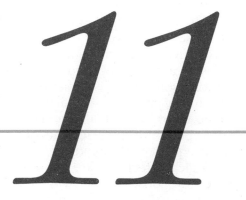

11

Introduction **94**

Adverse drug reaction monitoring/surveillance (pharmacovigilance) **95**

Allergic adverse drug reactions **100**

Examples of allergic and other adverse drug reactions **101**

Identification of the drug at fault **105**

Prevention of allergic drug reactions **105**

INTRODUCTION

Adverse drug reactions are defined as unwanted effects occurring at therapeutic doses of the drug. Drugs are great mimics of disease and adverse drug reactions present with diverse clinical signs and symptoms. The classification proposed by Rawlins and Thompson (1977) is arbitrary but has proven useful in practice. This divides reactions into type A and type B (Table 11.1).

Type A are adverse reactions which are a consequence of the drug's normal pharmacological effect and are therefore predictable; they are dose-related with a low mortality. Such reactions are usually due to incorrect dosage (too much or for too long) or to disordered pharmacokinetics, usually a failure of drug elimination. The term 'side effects' is often applied to minor type A reactions.

Type B reactions are not predictable from the drug's known action, are not dose-related and have a considerable mortality. The underlying pathophysiology of type B reactions is by definition poorly if at all understood, and may have a genetic or immunological basis. Indeed as more is known about the pharmacology of a drug, an adverse effect may have to be reclassified type B to type A. A good example of this is hemolytic anemia due to primaquine which used to be regarded as a rare type B effect of possible immune etiology until its association with glucose-6-phosphate dehydrogenase (G-6PD) deficiency was established (see chapter 13). It is now a predictable (type A) reaction in such genetically predisposed individuals. Type B reactions occur infrequently (1:1000–1:10 000 treated subjects being typical).

Adverse drug reactions due to drug–drug interactions are considered in chapter 12. Three further minor categories of adverse drug reaction have been proposed:

1. Type C: continuous reactions due to long-term use, such as tardive dyskinesia or analgesic nephropathy.
2. Type D: delayed reactions such as carcinogenesis or teratogenesis.
3. Type E: end of use reactions such as adrenocortical insufficiency following withdrawal of corticosteroids, or withdrawal syndromes following discontinuation of treatment with clonidine, benzodiazepines, tricyclic antidepressants or β-adrenoreceptor antagonists.

There are between 30 000 and 40 000 medicinal products available directly or on prescription in the UK. A random survey found that approximately 80% of adults took some kind of medication during a 2-week period. Exposure to drugs in the population is thus substantial and the incidence of adverse reactions must be viewed in this context. Adverse drug reactions are most commonly of type A (80%) causing up to 3% of acute hospital admissions and 2–3% of consultations in general practice. In hospital their incidence is estimated to be 10–20%, causing increased use of hospital resources and a mortality of 0.3–1%. They are most

Table 11.1 Some examples of type A and type B reactions.

Drug	Type A reaction	Type B reaction
Ampicillin	Pseudomembranous colitis	Interstitial nephritis
Chlorpromazine	Sedation	Hepatotoxicity
Naproxen	Gastrointestinal hemorrhage	Agranulocytosis
Practolol	Bradycardia	Oculomucocutaneous syndrome
Thiazides	Gout	Thrombocytopenia
Warfarin	Bleeding	Breast necrosis

Table 11.2 Factors involved in adverse drug reactions.

Patient factors

Intrinsic

Age – neonatal, infant and elderly

Sex – hormonal environment

Genetic abnormalities, e.g. enzyme defects

Previous adverse drug reactions, allergy, atopy

Presence of organ dysfunction – disease

Personality and habits – alcoholic, drug addict, nicotine, compliance

Extrinsic

Environment – sun

Xenobiotics (e.g. drugs, herbicides)

Malnutrition

Prescriber factors

Incorrect drug or drug combination

Incorrect route of administration

Incorrect dose

Incorrect duration of therapy

Drug factors

Drug–drug interactions (chapter 12)

Pharmaceutical – batch problems, shelf-life, incorrect dispensing

---

frequent and most severe in neonates or the elderly (>60 years), in women, patients with hepatic or renal disease, and those with a history of previous adverse drug reactions. Adverse drug reactions occur most commonly early in therapy (1–10 days), and the drugs most commonly implicated are digoxin, antimicrobials, diuretics, potassium, analgesics, sedatives and tranquillizers, insulin, aspirin, glucocorticosteroids, antihypertensives and warfarin.

Factors involved in the etiology of adverse drug reactions can be classified as shown in Table 11.2.

ADVERSE DRUG REACTION MONITORING/SURVEILLANCE (PHARMACOVIGILANCE)

The evaluation of drug safety is complex and there are many methods by which adverse drug reactions are monitored. Each of these has its own advantages and shortcomings, but no single system can offer the security that the community now demands. The ideal method would identify adverse drug reactions with high sensitivity and specificity and respond rapidly. It would detect rare adverse drug reactions but not be overwhelmed by common ones, the incidence of which it would quantify together with predisposing factors. Continued surveillance is mandatory after a new drug has been marketed since it is inevitable that the preliminary testing of medicines during drug development, although excluding many ill effects, cannot identify uncommon adverse effects. A variety of early detection methods have been introduced to discover these actions as swiftly as possible.

Phase I/II/III trials

Early (phase I/II) trials (chapter 14) are important in assessing the tolerability and dose–response of new drugs, but they are very insensitive at detecting adverse reactions because they are performed on relatively few subjects (perhaps 200–300). This is illustrated

Table 11.3 Incidence of adverse drug reactions.

Expected frequency of adverse effect	Approximate number of patients required to be exposed	
	For 1 event	For 3 events
1 in 100	300	650
1 in 1000	3000	6500
1 in 10 000	30 000	65 000

by the failure to detect the serious toxicity of several drugs (e.g. practolol, benoxaprofen or temofloxacin) before marketing. Phase III clinical trials (chapter 14) can, however, establish the incidence of common adverse reactions and relate this to therapeutic benefit. Analysis of the reasons given for dropping out of phase III trials is particularly valuable in establishing whether common events such as headache, constipation, lethargy or male sexual dysfunction are truly drug related. The Medical Research Council mild hypertension study unexpectedly identified impotence as more commonly associated with thiazide diuretics than with placebo or β-adrenoreceptor antagonist therapy in this way. Table 11.3 illustrates how difficult it is to detect relatively rare adverse drug reactions with no background incidence and positive diagnosis, with 95% confidence, at an early stage of a drug's development. Regulatory authorities may act after three or more documented events.

The problem of detection is several orders of magnitude worse if the adverse drug reaction resembles spontaneous disease in the population, such that physicians are unlikely to attribute the reaction to drug exposure.

Yellow card scheme and postmarketing surveillance

Untoward effects that have been missed in early clinical trials become apparent when the drug is used on a wider scale. Case reports in the literature, which may often stimulate further reports, remain the most sensitive means of detecting rare but serious and unusual adverse effects. In the UK, a Register of Adverse Reactions was started in 1964. Doctors and dentists were asked to report any adverse effects which they considered due to drugs. The Committee of Safety of Medicines (CSM) and the Medicines Control Agency (MCA) operate a system of spontaneous reporting by doctors on prepaid yellow postcards. The yellow card scheme consists of three stages: (1) collection of data; (2) analysis of data; and (3) feedback of information to doctors.

Such methods of surveillance have proved useful as an early warning system, but the major difficulty is underreporting. On average probably not more than 10% of adverse reactions are reported. This may be due partly to confusion about what events to report, or in deciding the precise relationship of a drug to a specific adverse event or sometimes which of several drugs being taken by the patient is responsible. A further problem is that if the drug is responsible for an increase in the incidence of some disease which is already common, for example gallbladder disease or carcinoma of the bronchus, the change in incidence must be very large before this can be detected, since cases due to drug therapy are obscured by cases due to other (often unknown) causes. Doctors are inefficient at detecting adverse reactions to drugs and those reactions reported are in general the obvious or previously described and well-known reactions. Several initiatives are currently underway to try to improve this situation by both education and involvement of specially trained pharmacists in and out of hospitals.

The CSM introduced a system of high vigilance for newly marketed drugs. Any newly marketed drug has on its data sheet and its entry in the *British National Formulary* a black triangle for its first 2 years in the general market. This conveys to the prescriber that any unexpected event occurring to a patient prescribed this drug should be reported by the yellow card system. The pharmaceutical company marketing a new drug is also responsible for obtaining accurate reports on all patients treated up to an agreed number. The scheme was successful in the case of benoxaprofen, an anti-inflammatory analgesic. Following its release, there were spontaneous reports to the CSM of photosensitivity and onycholysis. Further reports appeared in the elderly, in whom its half-life is prolonged, of cholestatic jaundice and hepatorenal failure, which was fatal in eight cases. Benoxaprofen was subsequently taken off the market when 3500 adverse drug reaction reports were received with 61 fatalities. The yellow card black triangle scheme was instrumental in the early identification of urticaria and cough as adverse effects of angiotensin-converting enzyme inhibitors. Although, potentially, the population under study by this system comprises all the patients using a drug, in fact underreporting yields a population that is not uniformly sampled and thus data that are unrepresentative and difficult to work with statistically. This accounts for the paucity of accurate incidence data for adverse drug reactions.

Systems such as the yellow card one are relatively inexpensive and easy to manage and facilitate ongoing monitoring of all drugs, all consumers and all types of adverse reaction. Reports from drug regulatory bodies of 22 countries are collated by the World Health Organization (WHO) Unit of Drug Evaluation and Monitoring in Geneva. Rapid access to reports from other countries should be of great value in detecting rarer types of adverse reaction, although the same reservations as apply to national systems apply to this register. Additionally, this database might be able to yield information concerning different prescribing habits and even differences in the pattern of untoward drug effects in different countries.

Prescription event monitoring

Successful studies have been carried out by the Drug Surveillance Research Unit at the University of Southampton using prescription event monitoring. Prescriptions for certain drugs are identified by the prescriptions pricing office in Edinburgh. These are followed up and the prescribing doctor asked to fill in a simple questionnaire recording any medical event from the patient notes. This has the advantage that the prescriber does not have to judge causality between the event and the drug. This scheme identified a new event associated with enalapril, i.e. deafness in 19/12 500. This is in excess of an expected five patients developing deafness in the general population. This needs further investigation, but highlights the potential usefulness of the approach as well as one of its main limitations, namely the absence of a control goup.

Case-control studies

One of the great difficulties in monitoring drugs for adverse effects is that if they occur relatively rarely (perhaps 1 in 1000 patients), very many patients have to be monitored before a particular side effect becomes apparent. An alternative approach is to study a group of patients who have developed a particular symptom or syndrome and to compare the frequency of exposure to possible etiologic agents with a control group. A prior suspicion (hypothesis) must exist to prompt the setting up of such a study: examples are the possible connection between irradiation or environmental pollution and certain malignancies, especially where they are observed in clusters. Although this method is comparatively easy to carry out, artifacts occur as a result of faulty selection of patients and controls, and the approach remains highly controversial among epidemiologists, public health physicians and statisticians. It has had some apparent successes, such as the linking of stilbestrol with vaginal adenocarcinoma and of lincomycin with pseudomembranous colitis, and, recently, the association between fenoterol use and an increased number of deaths in asthmatics. In its most simple form it is really an extension of the idea of the alert doctor, but with the considerable amount of data now available in such studies as the Boston Drug Surveillance Program, it should be possible to use this method on a wider scale and in a more sophisticated manner.

Patient questionnaires

Self-administered questionnaires have been used for outpatients attending hypertension and diabetic clinics and have detected previously unsuspected adverse effects, for example headache and weakness in the legs as effects of metformin. They have also been used to show an absence of effects, for example that propranolol is not associated with any of the eye symptoms caused by practolol.

Intensive monitoring

In the last few years a number of intensive monitoring programs, usually hospital-based, have been started. The Aberdeen–Dundee monitoring system abstracts data from some 70 000 hospital admissions each year, storing these on a computer file before analysis. The Boston Collaborative Drug Surveillance Program (BCDSP) which involves selected hospitals in several countries, is even more comprehensive. In the BCDSP all patients admitted to specially designated general wards are included in the analysis. Specially trained personnel obtain the following information from hospital patients and records:

1. Background information, i.e. age, weight, height, etc.
2. Patient's medical history.
3. Patient's drug exposure.
4. Side effects of drugs.
5. Outcome of treatment and changes in laboratory tests during hospital admission.

A unique feature of comprehensive drug-monitoring systems lies in their potential to follow-up and investigate adverse reactions suggested by less sophisticated detection systems or by isolated case reports in medical journals. Furthermore, the frequency of side effects can be determined more cheaply than by a specially mounted trial to investigate a simple adverse effect. Thus, for example, the risk of developing a rash with ampicillin was found to be around 7% both by clinical trial and by the BCDSP which can determine such facts almost automatically from data on its files. New adverse reactions or drug interactions are sought by multiple correlation analysis of the data. Thus, when an unexpected relationship arises, such as the 20% incidence of gastrointestinal bleeding in severely ill patients treated with ethacrynic acid compared to 4.3% of similar patients treated with other diuretics, there is little chance of bias arising from awareness of the hypothesis during data collection since the data are collected before the hypothesis is proposed. It is also possible to isolate factors predisposing patients to a particular complication; in the case of ethacrynic acid these were female sex, a high blood urea, previous heparin administration and intravenous administration of the drug. An important aspect of this type of approach is that *lack* of clinically important associations can also be detected. Thus no significant association between aspirin and renal disease was found, whereas long-term aspirin consumption is associated with a decreased incidence of myocardial infarction, an association which has been shown to be of therapeutic importance in randomized clinical trials (chapter 27). There are plans to extend intensive drug monitoring to cover other areas of medical practice.

In terms of new but uncommon adverse reactions, however, the numbers of patients undergoing intensive monitoring while taking a particular drug will inevitably be too small for the effect to be detectable. Such monitoring therefore can provide information only about relatively common, early reactions to drugs used under hospital conditions. Patients are not in hospital long enough for detection of delayed effects, which are just the reactions least likely to be recognized as such even by an astute clinician.

Monitoring from national statistics

A great deal of information is available from death certificates, hospital discharge diagnoses and similar records. It may be possible from these data to pick out a change in disease trends and relate this to drug therapy. Perhaps the best-known example of this is the increased death rate in young asthmatics noted in the mid-1960s, which was connected with overuse of bronchodilator inhalers containing non-specific β-adrenoreceptor agonists (e.g. adrenaline and/or isoprenaline). Although relatively inexpensive the difficulty of this method is obvious. Large numbers of patients must suffer before the change is detectable, particularly in diseases with an appreciable mortality. Data interpretation is particularly difficult when hospital discharges are used as a source of information, since sometimes diagnosis is provisional and changes as the patient's disease progresses.

Record linkage

Record linkage is presently under investigation as a method of monitoring adverse drug reactions and may well produce some important results. The basic idea is that the medical records from a defined population (both general practice and hospital sources) are kept from cradle to grave and analyzed. This method could be particularly useful when looking for really long-term ill effects from drugs or from other factors, for instance the increased incidence of leukemia in those receiving radiation *in utero* or the occurrence of diseases such as cancer or mental retardation in individuals whose mothers had received drugs during pregnancy. Analysis of data is becoming more sophisticated with the use of computers to store information, but one must know what information is worth storing, and ask the correct questions to avoid the well-known 'garbage in – garbage out' situation.

Two main types of inquiry can be made:

1. Follow-up of individuals who have received selected drugs to determine adverse reactions attributable to the drug. This approach is of most value when a drug is already suspected of producing some particular effect and is not particularly suited to the discovery of unexpected adverse effects. A defect is the absence of a control group. It has been convincingly demonstrated that untreated subjects or those receiving placebo often experience symptoms commonly listed as side effects of drugs. Therefore the results of such studies can be biased by the preconceived ideas of the investigator or the effects on the patient of his or her enhanced interest.
2. Follow-up of patients with specific diseases rather than those treated with specific drugs is sometimes easier to carry out since most clinicians categorize their patients under disease rather than treatment. Thus it is possible to investigate the frequency of adverse reactions to, say, phenytoin, by selecting the records of epileptics. One of the largest disease-oriented systems is that of the USA Perinatal Study which received data on drug exposure and fetal outcome from over 50 000 consecutive pregnancies. From this has come evidence linking malformations and maternal exposure to phenytoin.

Feedback

There is no use in collecting vast amounts of data on adverse reactions unless they are analyzed and important information reported back to prescribing doctors. In addition to articles in the medical press the CSM and MCA circulate to all doctors a 'Current Problems' information sheet which deals with important and recently discovered adverse reactions. If an acute and serious problem is recognized doctors will usually receive notification from the CSM and often from the pharmaceutical company involved.

ALLERGIC ADVERSE DRUG REACTIONS

Immune mechanisms are involved in a number of adverse effects caused by drugs (chapter 47). The development of allergy implies previous exposure to the drug or to some very closely related substance. Most drugs are of low molecular weight (less than 1000) and thus are not antigenic. They can, however, combine with substances of high molecular weight, usually proteins, acting as haptens so that the conjugate thus formed is antigenic.

The factors that determine the development of allergy to a drug are not fully understood. Some drugs (e.g. penicillin) are more likely to cause allergic reactions than others, and type I (immediate anaphylactic) reactions are more common in patients with a history of atopy. A correlation between allergic reactions involving immunoglobulin E (IgE) and human leukocyte antigen (HLA) serotypes have been reported and so genetic factors may also be important. There is some evidence that drug allergies are more common in older people, in women, and in those with a previous history of drug reaction. This may, however, merely represent increased frequencies of drug exposure in these groups, and prevalence figures (expressed relative to the appropriate denominator) are currently not available.

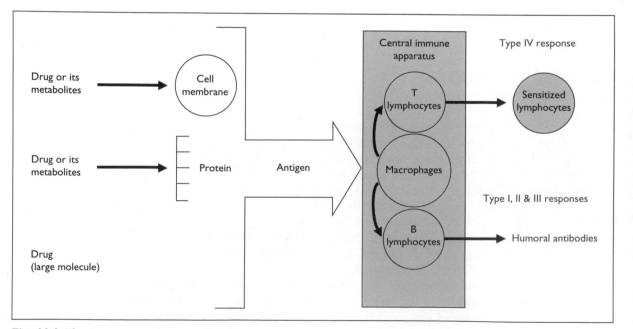

Fig. 11.1 The immune response to drugs.

Types of allergy

Drugs cause a variety of allergic responses (Fig. 11.1) and sometimes a single drug can be responsible for more than one type of allergic response.

TYPE I

Type I reactions (e.g. to penicillin) are due to the production of reagenic antibodies known to consist predominantly of class IgE. The antigen–antibody reaction on the surface of mast cells causes degranulation and release of pharmacologically active substances. It occurs commonly with foreign serum or penicillin but may also occur with streptomycin and some local anesthetics. With penicillin it is believed that the penicilloyl moiety of the penicillin molecule is responsible for the production of antibodies. Occasionally the development of symptoms is delayed for some hours after the drug has been taken. It seems probable that antigen–antibody aggregates are involved. The antibody in this mechanism consists of IgG. The therapy of anaphylactic shock is described in chapter 47.

TYPE II

These are due to antibodies of class IgG and IgM which on contact with antibodies on the surface of cells are able to fix complement, causing cell lysis, for example penicillin and methyldopa causing Coombs' positive hemolytic anemia.

TYPE III, IMMUNE COMPLEX, ARTHUS REACTIONS

Circulating immune complexes can produce several clinical allergic states including serum sickness and immune complex glomerulonephritis, and a syndrome resembling systemic lupus erythematosus. The onset of serum sickness is delayed for some days until the symptoms – fever, urticaria, arthropathy, lymphadenopathy and eosinophilia – develop. Proteinuria occurs frequently. Recovery takes a few days. Causative agents include foreign serum, penicillin, sulfonamides, streptomycin and propylthiouracil. Amiodarone lung and hydralazine induced systemic lupus syndrome are also possibly mediated by immune complex-related mechanisms, although these reactions are less well understood.

TYPE IV

Type IV are delayed hypersensitivity reactions, the classical example of which is contact dermatitis (e.g. to topical antibiotics such as penicillin). The mechanism here is that the drug applied to the skin forms an antigenic conjugate with dermal proteins, stimulating formation of sensitized T lymphocytes in the regional lymph nodes with a resultant rash if the drug is applied again. Drug photosensitivity is due to a photochemical combination between the drug (e.g. tetracycline, amiodarone) and dermal protein. Delayed sensitivity can also result from the systemic administration of drugs.

EXAMPLES OF ALLERGIC AND OTHER KINDS OF ADVERSE DRUG REACTIONS

Adverse drug reactions can be manifest in any organ system, or involve multiple organ systems, and in extraordinarily diverse forms. Specific instances are dealt with throughout this book. Some examples to illustrate the diversity of adverse drug reactions are also given here.

Rashes

These are common manifestations of drug reactions. A number of immune mechanisms may be involved which produce many types

Table 11.4 Skin reactions to some commonly used drugs.

	Acne	Alopecia	Bullous	Epidermo-necrolysis	Erythema multiforme	Erythema nodosa	Exfoliative dermatitis	Fixed	Lich-enoid	Lupus erythe-matosus	Morbilli-form	Nails	Photosensi-tivity	Porphyria	Purpura	Urticaria	Psoriasi-form
Anticonvulsants	+			+	+	+	+			+	+						
Barbiturates			+	+		+	+	+			+			+		+	
β-blockers									+	+						+	+
Chlorpropamide					+		+										
Codeine						+											
Cytotoxics		+									+	+			+		
Gold							+	+	+		+				+	+	
Griseofulvin										+			+	+			
Halides	+		+		+	+	+										
Penicillins			+	+	+	+	+	+		+					+	+	
Phenolphthalein					+		+	+				+				+	
Phenothiazines					+		+			+	+		+		+		
Phenylbutazone				+			+	+		+							
Salicylates			+		+	+		+							+	+	
Steroids	+										+						
Streptomycin										+						+	
Sulfonamides				+	+	+	+	+					+		+	+	
Tetracyclines				+				+				+	+		+	+	
Thiazides					+	+			+		+		+		+		
Thiouracils		+				+					+					+	

of rash. In some cases (e.g. ampicillin) the rash is more commonly due to non-allergic factors; in others the cause is not known (Table 11.4).

Serum sickness

This (see chapter 47) is caused by circulating immune complexes and the onset is delayed for some days until the symptoms – fever, urticaria and arthropathy develop. Proteinuria, cosinophilia and lymphadenopathy occur frequently. Recovery takes a few days. Causative agents include foreign serum, penicillin, sulfonamides, streptomycin and propylthiouracil, possibly amiodarone lung and hydralazine-induced systemic lupus syndrome.

Lymphadenopathy

Lymph-node enlargement can result from taking drugs (e.g. phenytoin). The mechanism is not known, but allergic factors may be involved. The reaction may be confused with a lymphoma and inquiry about chronic drug taking is important in patients with lymphadenopathy of unknown cause.

Blood dyscrasias

Thrombocytopenia, anemia (aplastic, iron deficiency, macrocytic, hemolytic) and agranulocytosis can all be produced by drugs.

Thrombocytopenia can occur with many drugs and in many instances it is direct suppression of the megakarocytes rather than immune processes which is important. Quinine thrombocytopenia may be an allergic phenomenon. The following are some of the drugs which most commonly cause thrombocytopenia:

- Thiazides, chloramphenicol.
- Quinidine.
- Heparin.
- Sulfonamides, quinine, gold.
- Most cytotoxic agents.

Hemolytic anemia can be caused by a number of drugs and sometimes immune mechanisms are responsible. Glucose–6-phosphate dehydrogenase deficiency (chapter 13) predisposes to non-immune hemolysis (e.g. to primaquine). Immune mechanisms include:

1. Combination of the drug with the red cell membrane with the conjugate acting as an antigen. This has been shown to occur with penicillin-induced hemolysis, and may also occur with chlorpromazine, chlorpropamide and sulfonamides.
2. Alteration of the red-cell membrane by the drug so that it becomes autoimmunogenic. This may happen with methyldopa, and a direct positive Coombs' test develops in about 20% of patients who have been treated with this drug for more than a year. In only a small proportion does hemolysis actually occur. Similar changes can take place with levodopa and mefenamic acid.
3. Causing non-specific binding of plasma protein to red cells and thus causing hemolysis. This is believed to occur with cephalosporins.

Aplastic anemia as an isolated entity is not common but may occur either in isolation or as part of a general depression of bone-marrow activity (pancytopenia); examples include chloramphenicol and, commonly and predictably, cytotoxic drugs.

Agranulocytosis can be caused by many drugs. Several different mechanisms are implicated and it is not known whether allergy plays a part. Among the drugs most frequently implicated are:

- Antithyroid drugs.
- Phenothiazines, tolbutamide, most cytotoxic agents.
- Sulfonamides, antidepressants (especially mianserin, chapter 17).
- Clozapine.

Systemic lupus erythematosus

Several drugs (including procainamide, isoniazid, hydralazine, chlorpromazine, anticonvulsants) produce a syndrome that resembles systemic lupus together with a positive antinuclear factor test. The development of this is closely related to dose, and in the case of hydralazine also depends upon the rate of acetylation of the drug, which is genetically controlled (see chapter 13). There is some evidence that the drugs act as haptens combining with DNA and forming antigens. Symptoms usually disappear when the drug is stopped, but recovery may be slow.

Vasculitis

Both acute and chronic vasculitis can result from taking drugs, and may have an allergic basis. Acute vasculitis with purpura and renal involvement occurs with penicillins and the sulfonamides. A more chronic form can occur with phenytoin.

Renal

All clinical expressions of renal disease can be caused by drugs: common culprits are non-steroidal anti-inflammatory drugs and angiotensin-converting enzyme inhibitors (which cause functional and usually reversible renal failure in susceptible patients; chapters 23 and 25). Nephrotic syndrome results from several drugs (e.g. penicillamine, high-dose captopril, gold) which cause a variety of immune-mediated glomerular injuries. Interstitial nephritis can be caused by several drugs including non-steroidal anti-inflammatory drugs and penicillins. Aminoglycoside antibiotics and vancomycin cause direct tubular toxicty. Many drugs cause electrolyte or acid–base disturbances via their predictable direct or indirect effects on renal electrolyte excretion (e.g. hypokalemia and hypomagnesemia from loop diuretics, hyperkalemia from potassium-sparing diuretics and converting enzyme inhibitors, proximal renal tubular acidosis from carbonic anhydrase inhibitors) and some cause unpredictable toxic effects on acid–base balance (e.g. distal renal tubular acidosis from amphotericin). Obstructive uropathy can be caused by uric acid crystals consequent on initiation of chemotherapy in patients with hematological malignancy, and rarely poorly soluble drugs such as sulfonamides can themselves cause clinical problems consequent on crystaluria.

Other reactions

Fever is a common manifestation of drug allergy and should be remembered in patients with fever of unknown cause.

Liver damage (hepatitis with or without obstructive features) as a side effect from drugs is important. It may be insidious, leading slowly to end-stage cirrhosis (e.g. during chronic treatment with methotrexate) or acute and fulminant (as in some cases of isoniazid, halothane or phenytoin hepatitis). Chlorpromazine commonly causes liver involvement characterized by raised alkaline phosphatase ('obstructive' pattern). Gallstones (and mechanical obstruction) can be caused by fibrates and other lipid-lowering drugs (chapter 24), and by octreotide, a somatostatin analog used to treat a variety of enteropancreatic tumors including carcinoid syndrome and VIPomas* (chapter 39). Immune mechanisms are implicated in some forms of hepatic injury by drugs, but are seldom solely responsible.

*VIP = vasoactive intestinal polypeptide.

IDENTIFICATION OF THE DRUG AT FAULT

It is often difficult to decide whether a clinical event is drug related; even when this is probable it may be difficult to determine which drug is responsible, as patients are often taking more than one. One or more of several possible approaches may be appropriate:

1. A careful drug history is essential, but may be inconclusive, because although allergy to a drug implies previous exposure the antigen may have occurred in foods (e.g. antibiotics are often fed to livestock and drug residues remain in the flesh), in drug mixtures or in some casual fashion.

2. Provocation tests. This means giving a very small amount of the suspected drug and seeing if a reaction ensues. The commonest method is skin testing, where a drug is applied as a patch, or is pricked or scratched into the skin, or injected intradermally. Unfortunately prick and scratch testing is less useful for assessing the systemic reaction to drugs than it is for the more usual atopic antigens (e.g. pollens) and both false positives and false negatives can occur. Intradermal injection can provoke serious systemic anaphylaxis and fatalities have been recorded. Patch testing is safe and is useful for the diagnosis of contact sensitivity but does not reflect systemic reactions. It may also itself cause allergy. Provocation tests can also involve giving small doses of the drug by inhalation, by mouth or parenterally and should only be undertaken under expert guidance, after obtaining informed consent, and with full facilities for resuscitation available. The initial dose should not exceed 1.0 mg by mouth or 1.0 ng by injection. The dose is increased at intervals until a therapeutic dose is reached or a reaction occurs.

3. Serological testing is rarely helpful as the demonstration of circulating antibodies does not mean that they are necessarily the cause of the symptoms.

4. Sensitized lymphocytes. The demonstration of transformation occurring when lymphocytes are exposed to a drug suggests that they are T lymphocytes sensitized to the drug, but interpretation of results can be difficult in a clinical context. In this type of reaction the hapten itself will often provoke lymphocyte transformation as well as the conjugate.

5. Often it is necessary to stop all the drugs that a patient is taking and reintroduce them one by one until the drug at fault is discovered. This should only be done if the reaction is not serious or if the drug is essential and no chemically unrelated alternative is available. Drug allergies should be recorded in the case notes and the patient informed of the risks involved in taking the drug again.

PREVENTION OF ALLERGIC DRUG REACTIONS

Although it is probably not possible to avoid allergic drug reactions completely, the following can decrease the incidence:

1. Taking a drug history is essential whenever drug treatment is anticipated, particularly with antibiotics and other

drugs with a high allergy potential. A history of atopy, although not excluding the use of drugs, should make one wary.

2. Drugs given orally are less likely to cause severe allergic reactions than when given by injection.

3. Prophylactic skin testing is not usually practicable and a negative test does not exclude the possibility of an allergic reaction. Such testing may, however, be appropriate where a suspect drug is potentially life saving and there is no equally effective alternative. It probably reduces the risk of anaphylaxis if not of other less severe reactions.

4. Desensitization (hyposensitization). This should only be used when continued use of the drug is essential. It consists of giving a very small dose of the drug and increasing the dose at regular intervals, sometimes under cover of a glucorticosteroid and β_2-adrenoreceptor agonist. An antihistamine may be added if a drug reaction occurs, and equipment for resuscitation and therapy of anaphylactic shock must be close at hand. It is often successful, though little is known of the mechanism by which it is achieved.

Reference

Rawlins MD, Thompson JW. Pathogenesis of adverse drug reactions. In: Davis DM, ed. *Textbook of Adverse Drug Reactions.* Oxford: Oxford University Press, 1977: 44.

Drug *Interactions*

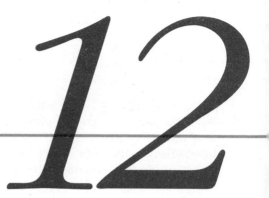

12

Introduction **108**

Useful interactions **109**

Trivial interactions **111**

Harmful interactions **112**

INTRODUCTION

Drug interaction is the modification of the action of one drug by another as a result of one or more of three kinds of mechanism:

I   Pharmaceutic
II Pharmacodynamic
III Pharmacokinetic

Drug interaction is important, because whereas judicious use of more than one drug at a time can greatly benefit patients, adverse interactions are not uncommon, may be catastrophic, yet are often avoidable. Multiple drug use ('polypharmacy') is extremely common, so the potential for drug interaction is enormous. One study showed that 14 drugs on average were prescribed to medical inpatients per admission (one patient received 36 different drugs). This undesirable state of affairs is likely to get worse, for several reasons:

1. Many drugs are not curative, but rather ameliorate chronic conditions such as cardiac failure, arthritis and so on. The populations of western countries are aging, so these diseases are progressively more likely to coexist within elderly individuals.
2. It is all too easy to enter an iatrogenic spiral where a drug (often given for uncertain or inadequate reasons) results in an adverse effect that is countered by the introduction of another drug and so on. Prescribers should heed the moral of the nursery rhyme about the old lady who swallowed the fly! Hospital admission provides an opportunity to review the medications that patients are receiving, and make sure that the overall regimen is rational.

Outpatients also often receive several drugs; sometimes these are supplemented by proprietary over-the-counter medicines, by drugs supplied by friends and relatives or by drugs prescribed by other doctors without reference to the patient's own practitioner. The greater

the number of drugs prescribed, the more likely things are to go wrong (Fig. 12.1).

Drug interactions can be useful, of no consequence, or harmful.

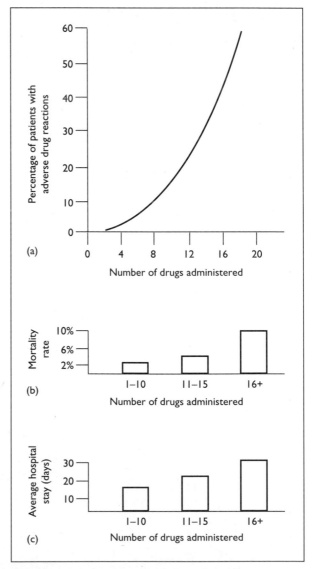

Fig. 12.1 Relationship of number of drugs administered to (a) adverse drug reactions, (b) mortality rate, and (c) average duration of hospital stay. (From J.W. Smith *et al. Ann Intern Med* 1966; **65**: 631.)

USEFUL INTERACTIONS

Increased effect

Drugs can be used in combination to enhance their effectiveness. Disease is often caused by complex processes, and drugs that influence different components of the disease mechanism may have additive effects. Myocardial infarction is usually caused by white thrombus forming on a ruptured atheromatous plaque in an coronary artery. Such thrombi consist of fibrin and platelet aggregates, and the ISIS II study showed that streptokinase (a fibrinolytic drug) and aspirin (which inhibits platelet function) each improve outcome in patients with myocardial infarction, and that the combination of aspirin with streptokinase has an additive effect. Other examples include the use of a β_2 agonist with a glucocorticoid in treatment of asthma (to cause bronchodilation and suppress inflammation, respectively), use of an H_2 antagonist with an antacid in acid peptic disease (to reduce acid secretion and buffer gastric fluid), use of a muscarinic antagonist with L-dopa in treating Parkinson's disease and so on.

Combinations of antimicrobial drugs may be required in treating chronic infections to prevent the selection of drug-resistant organisms. Tuberculosis is the best example of a disease whose successful treatment requires this approach, usually employing combinations that include isoniazid, rifampicin and pyrazinamide. Sometimes micro-organisms acquire drug resistance via synthesis of an enzyme that degrades antibiotic (e.g. penicillinase producing staphylococci). This can sometimes be countered by using a combination of the antibiotic with an inhibitor of the enzyme, for example co-amoxiclav is a combination of clavulanic acid, an inhibitor of penicillinase with amoxycillin, a semisynthetic penicillin. Clavulinic acid has no antibacterial activity on its own, but by inhibiting penicillinase makes the combination effective against organisms that would be resistant to amoxycillin alone by reason of penicillinase production. These include most *Staphylococcus aureus* as well as a fraction of Gram-negative organisms such as *Escherichia coli, Hemophilus influenzae, Klebsiella* and some anaerobes. Imipenem, a broad-spectrum thienamycin β-lactam antibiotic active against many Gram-positive and Gram-negative aerobic and anaerobic organisms, is partly inactivated by a dipeptidase in the kidney. This is overcome by administering imipenem in combination with cilastin, a specific renal dipeptidase inhibitor. This results in more prolonged plasma concentrations of imipenem.

Some combinations of drugs have a more than additive effect ('synergy'). Several antibacterial combinations are synergistic, including sulfamethoxazole with trimethoprim (co-trimoxazole). Each component acts on the folate pathway, but at different points. The combination is more effective than either component alone when tested against many micro-organisms *in vitro*. In clinical practice, however, trimethoprim is as effective as co-trimoxazole in many common infections (e.g. urinary tract infection), lacks sulfonamide-related toxicity and is less expensive. Co-trimoxazole is, however, useful in special circumstances, especially in the treatment of *Pneumocystis carinii*. Aminoglycoside antibiotics synergize usefully with penicillin in some cases of enterococcal endocarditis. It is probable that several drugs used in cancer chemotherapy are mutually synergistic.

Therapeutic effects of drugs are often limited by the activation of a physiological control loop, particularly in the case of cardiovascular drugs. The use of a low dose of a second drug that interrupts this negative feedback may therefore enhance effectiveness substantially. Examples include the combination of a converting enzyme inhibitor (to block the renin–angiotensin system) with a diuretic (the effect of which is limited by activation of the renin–angiotensin system), or of a β-hydroxymethylglutaryl coenzyme A (HMGCoA) reductase inhibitor (to block cholesterol biosynthesis) with a bile acid binding resin (which on its own has a limited effect due to increased hepatic cholesterol biosynthesis).

Sometimes a drug is in such short supply as to make it worthwhile to use a second drug to interfere with its elimination. Historically this was the case when penicillin was introduced. Probenecid, which inhibits its secretion into the renal tubules, was used to maximize the effect of small doses of the drug. It is still used occasionally to prolong the action of penicillin-related antibiotics in single dose treatment of sexually transmitted disease where non-compliance with multiple dose treatment may have serious individual and public health consequences. Zidovudine is active against human immunodeficiency virus, but is expensive. It undergoes glucuronidation and is then eliminated into the urine by tubular secretion. Probenecid blocks glucuronidation of zidovudine and impairs its secretion into tubular fluid in the kidney, offering the intriguing possibility that combining these drugs might permit a reduced dose frequency and lower cost, without loss of efficacy. The safety of such a combination has yet to be evaluated thoroughly, however, and the occurrence of fever and rashes has limited long-term use of this combination.

Minimize side effects

There are many situations, including moderate hypertension and heart failure, where low doses of two drugs may be better tolerated as well as more effective than larger doses of a single agent. To some extent this is the result of disabling physiological control mechanisms, as discussed above. Sometimes drugs with similar therapeutic effects have opposing undesired metabolic effects, which can to some extent cancel out when the

drugs are used together. The combination of a loop diuretic (e.g. frusemide) with a potassium-sparing diuretic (e.g. amiloride) provides an example of this principle, and such drug combinations are useful when hypokalemia is clinically important, as when digoxin is needed to control atrial fibrillation in a patient with heart failure.

Predictable adverse effects can sometimes be averted by the use of drug combinations. Isoniazid neuropathy is caused by pyridoxine deficiency, and is prevented by the prophylactic use of pyridoxine. When desired and adverse effects of a drug are mediated by different receptors, it may be possible to block the adverse effects without losing effectiveness. Cholinesterase inhibitors improve strength in patients with myasthenia gravis because they increase the concentration of acetylcholine at the nicotinic receptors of the neuromuscular junction. Excessive doses cause diarrhea, salivation and abdominal pain as a result of increased activation of muscarinic receptors, and these effects can be prevented by an atropine-like drug. A drug that inhibits the metabolism of another drug can be used to minimize adverse effects. An important instance is the combination of a peripheral dopa decarboxylase inhibitor (e.g. carbidopa or benserazide) with L-dopa. Carbidopa permits an equivalent therapeutic effect to be achieved by a lower dose of L-dopa than is needed when used as a single agent, while reducing dose-related peripheral side effects of nausea and vomiting (see chapter 18).

Block acutely an unwanted (toxic) effect

Reversal of the effect of one drug by another may be desirable, as for example when an anesthetist uses a cholinesterase inhibitor to reverse neuromuscular blockade or when antidotes such as naloxone or Fab fragments of digoxin antibodies are used to treat specific kinds of poisoning (chapter 50). Prevention of toxic effects may depend on binding the drug or its receptor as in the above examples or, less directly, on influencing metabolic pathways responsible for drug elimination, as in the use of acetyl cysteine in patients poisoned with paracetamol or of sodium thiosulfate in cases of cyanide poisoning. The choice of the most appropriate antagonist depends on the urgency of the clinical situation. For instance,

in a patient receiving warfarin in whom the prothrombin time is excessively prolonged and who has some gastrointestinal bleeding but is hemodynamically stable, use of vitamin K to compete with the warfarin and permit resynthesis of functional coagulation factors may be indicated. By contrast, were the same patient to be bleeding intracranially, the use of fresh plasma or factor concentrates would be required to reverse the effect of the warfarin non-competitively and immediately.

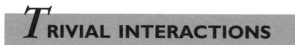TRIVIAL INTERACTIONS

Many of the interactions described in large compendia are based on animal or *in vitro* experiments, the results of which cannot be transferred uncritically to the clinical situation. Many such potential interactions are of no practical consequence. This is true especially of drugs with shallow dose–response curves, and of interactions that depend on competition for non-receptor binding sites.

Shallow dose–response curves

Interactions are likely to be clinically important only when there is a steep dose–response curve and a narrow therapeutic window between minimum effective dose and minimum toxic dose of one or both interacting drugs. This is often not the case. Penicillin, for example, when used in most ordinary clinical situations is so non-toxic that the usual dose is more than adequate for therapeutic efficacy, yet far below that which would cause dose-related toxicity. Consequently, a second drug that interacts with penicillin is unlikely to cause either toxicity or loss of efficacy.

Plasma and tissue binding site interactions

One large group of potential drug interactions that are seldom, if ever, clinically important, consists of drugs that displace one another from binding sites on plasma albumin or within tissues. This is a common occurrence, and can readily be demonstrated in plasma or solutions of albumin *in vitro*. The simple expectation that the displacing drug will increase the effects of the displaced drug by increasing its free (unbound) concentration is, however, seldom evident in clinical practice. This is because drug clearance (renal or metabolic) also depends directly on the concentration of free drug. Consider a patient receiving a regular maintenance dose of a drug. When a second displacing drug is commenced, the free concentration of the first drug rises only transiently before increased renal or hepatic elimination reduces total (bound + free) drug, and restores the free concentration to that which prevailed before the second drug was started. Consequently, any increased effect of the displaced drug is transient, and is seldom important in practice, although it must be taken into account if therapy is being guided by measurements of plasma drug concentrations since most such determinations are of total rather than free concentration (chapter 8). An exception, where a transient increase in free concentration of a circulating substance (albeit not a drug) can have devastating consequences, is provided by bilirubin in premature babies with severe jaundice, whose ability to metabolize bile pigments is immature. Unconjugated bilirubin is bound by plasma albumin, and unjudicious treatment with drugs such as sulfonamides that displace it from these binding sites may permit diffusion of free bilirubin across the immature blood–brain barrier and consequent staining of and damage to basal ganglia (kernicterus) and subsequent choreoathetosis in the child.

Instances where clinically important consequences do occur on introducing a drug that displaces another from tissue binding sites are often in fact due to additional actions of the second drug on *elimination* of the first. For instance, quinidine displaces digoxin from tissue binding sites, and can cause digoxin toxicity, but only because it simultaneously reduces the renal clearance of digoxin by a separate mechanism. Phenylbutazone displaces warfarin from binding sites on albumin and can cause excessive prolongation of the prothrombin time and bleeding, but only because it also inhibits the metabolism of the active isomer of warfarin causing this to accumulate at the expense of the inactive isomer. Indomethacin also displaces warfarin from binding sites on albumin but does not inhibit its metabolism and does not further prolong prothrombin time in patients treated with warfarin, although it can cause bleeding by causing peptic ulceration and interfering with platelet function.

HARMFUL INTERACTIONS

It is impossible to memorize reliably even the examples contained in this chapter, and prescribers should have access to suitable references (e.g. the *British National Formulary*) to check on potentially harmful interactions. There are certain drugs with steep dose–response curves and serious dose-related toxicities where drug interactions are especially liable to cause harm and where special caution is required with concurrent therapy. These include:

- Anticoagulants.
- Anticonvulsants.
- Cytotoxic drugs.
- Digoxin and other antiarrhythmic drugs.
- Monoamine oxidase inhibitors.
- Oral hypoglycemic agents.
- Xanthine alkaloids (e.g. theophylline).

The frequency and consequences of an adverse interaction when two drugs are used together are seldom known precisely. Every time a doctor prescribes a drug or drug combination he or she is in effect performing an experiment on that particular patient. Every individual has a peculiar set of characteristics that determine response to therapy. When potentially interacting drugs are prescribed adverse effects are probable but not inevitable.

Risk of adverse drug interactions

In the Boston Collaborative Drug Surveillance program 234 out of 3600 adverse drug reactions in acute care hospitals (about 7%) were identified as being due to drug interactions. In a smaller study in a chronic care setting the prevalence of adverse interactions was much higher (22%), probably because of the more frequent use of multiple drugs in elderly patients with multiple pathologies. The same problems exist for the detection of drug interactions as for adverse drug reactions. In particular, it is possible that the frequency of such interactions is underestimated due to attribution of poor therapeutic outcome to progression of underlying disease in settings where data are not being compared quantitatively. For example, graft rejection following renal transplantation is not uncommon. Historically, it took several years for nephrologists to appreciate that epileptic patients suffered much greater rejection rates than did non-epileptic subjects. These adverse events proved to be due to an interaction between anticonvulsant medication and immunosuppressant therapy, which was rendered ineffective because of increased drug metabolism. A better understanding of the potential mechanisms of such interactions should lead in future to their prediction and prevention by study in early phase drug evaluation.

Severity of adverse drug interactions

The manifestations of adverse drug interactions are diverse, including unwanted pregnancy (from failure of the contraceptive pill due to concomitant medication), hypertensive stroke (from hypertensive crisis in patients on monoamine oxidase inhibitors), gastrointestinal and other hemorrhage (aspirin with warfarin), cardiac arrhythmias (e.g. secondary to interactions leading to electrolyte disturbance) and blood dyscrasias (e.g. from interactions between allopurinol and azathioprine). Adverse interactions can be severe as well as mild in intensity: in one study of 27 fatal drug reactions nine were caused by drug interactions.

ADVERSE INTERACTIONS GROUPED BY MECHANISM

I Pharmaceutic interactions

These consist of incompatibilities that result in precipitation or inactivation when drugs are mixed. Drugs should not be added to blood or, usually, to blood products, and it is essential to check before making additions to infusions of crystalloid or dextrose solutions. Specific examples are given in Table 12.1. Drugs may also interact physically or chemically in the lumen of the gut (e.g. tetracycline with iron or aluminum; cholestyramine with digoxin or warfarin).

Table 12.1 Interactions outside the body.

Mixture	Result
Thiopentone + suxamethonium	Precipitation
Diazepam + infusion fluids	Precipitation
Phenytoin + infusion fluids	Precipitation
Soluble insulin + protamine zinc insulin	Reduced effect of soluble insulin
Heparin + hydrocortisone	Inactivation of heparin
Kanamycin + hydrocortisone	Inactivation of kanamycin
Penicillin + hydrocortisone	Inactivation of penicillin

II *Pharmacodynamic interactions*

These are the commonest drug interactions in clinical practice. Most have a simple mechanism consisting of summation or opposition of effects of drugs with similar or opposing actions initiated by combination with different receptors. Since this kind of interaction depends broadly on the effect of a drug, rather than on its specific chemical structure, such interactions are non-specific. Drowsiness caused by an H_1-blocking antihistamine and by alcohol provides an example: this occurs to a greater or lesser degree with *all* H_1-blockers irrespective of the chemical structure of the particular drug used. Patients must be warned of the dangers of imbibing concurrently when such antihistamines are prescribed, especially if they drive or operate machinery. Non-steroidal anti-inflammatory agents and antihypertensive drugs provide another clinically important example: many, if not all, antihypertensive drugs (including β-blockers, diuretics and converting enzyme inhibitors) are rendered substantially less effective by concurrent use of most non-steroidal anti-inflammatory drugs, irrespective of the chemical group to which they belong. The interaction is probably due to inhibition of biosynthesis of vasodilator prostaglandins in the kidney.

Drugs with negative inotropic effects can precipitate heart failure, and this is especially true when negative inotropes with different mechanisms are used in combination. Cardiac status and route of administration are critical. Thus β-blockers and calcium channel blockers, which may safely be given together by mouth in many patients with uncomplicated hypertension or angina pectoris, precipitate heart failure, which may be fatal, if used sequentially intravenously in patients with supraventricular tachycardia.

Warfarin interferes with hemostasis by inhibiting the coagulation cascade, whereas aspirin influences hemostasis by inhibiting platelet function. Aspirin also predisposes to gastric bleeding by direct irritation and by inhibition of prostaglandin E_2 biosynthesis in gastric mucosa. There is therefore the potential for serious adverse interaction between them. Patients anticoagulated with warfarin should be warned to avoid aspirin (outside of tightly monitored clinical trials specifically exploring this combination), as well as the many proprietory medicines that contain aspirin (e.g. Alka-Seltzer™, Lemsip™, Beecham's Powders™).

In some instances, important interactions occur between drugs acting at a common receptor. These interactions are generally useful when used deliberately, for example the use of naloxone to reverse opiate intoxication, or less directly the reversal of muscular relaxation by tubocurarine by the local increase of acetylcholine caused by cholinesterase inhibition with neostigmine alluded to above. Such actions at a common receptor, or at least on a common receptor-initiated pathway, may occasionally underlie undesired interactions. A possible example is drowsiness caused by concurrent use of alcohol and benzodiazepines. These drugs probably act on a common pathway since flumazenil, a benzodiazepine antagonist, also partly reverses sedation caused by alcohol.

One potentially important kind of pharmacodynamic drug interaction involves the interruption of physiological control loops. This was mentioned above as a desirable means of increasing efficacy in certain circumstances (e.g. diuretics with converting enzyme inhibitors in treating hypertension). However, there are also situations in which such control mechanisms are vital, and their disablement fraught with hazard. The use of β-blocking drugs in patients with insulin requiring diabetes is such a case, since such patients may depend on sensations initiated by activation of β-receptors to warn them of impending hypoglycemic coma.

Alterations in fluid and electrolyte balance constitute an important source of pharmacodynamic drug interaction (Table 12.2). Combined use of diuretics with actions at different parts of the nephron (e.g. metolazone and frusemide) is valuable in the treatment of resistant edema, but without close monitoring of plasma urea such combinations readily

Table 12.2 Interactions secondary to drug-induced alterations of fluid and electrolyte balance.

Primary drug	Interacting drug effect	Result of interaction
Digoxin	Diuretic-induced hypokalemia	Digoxin toxicity
Lignocaine	Diuretic-induced hypokalemia	Antagonism of antiarrhythmic effects
Diuretics	NSAID-induced salt and water retention	Antagonism of diuretic effects
Tubocurarine	Diuretic-induced hypokalemia	Prolonged paralysis
Lithium	Thiazide-induced reduction in renal clearance	Raised plasma lithium
Angiotensin-converting enzyme inhibitor	Potassium chloride and/or potassium-retaining diuretic-induced hyperkalemia	Severe hyperkalemia

NSAID = non-steroidal anti-inflammatory drug.

cause excessive intravascular fluid depletion and prerenal renal failure (chapter 33). Thiazide and loop diuretics commonly cause mild hypokalemia, which is usually of no consequence. However, the binding of digoxin to plasma membrane Na^+/K^+ adenosine triphosphatase (ATPase), and hence its toxicity, is increased when extracellular potassium concentration is low. Concurrent use of such diuretics therefore increases the risk of digoxin toxicity. β_2-Agonists such as salbutamol also reduce plasma potassium concentration, especially when used intravenously. Conversely, potassium-sparing diuretics may cause hyperkalemia if combined with potassium supplements and/or converting enzyme inhibitors (which reduce circulating aldosterone), especially in patients with renal impairment. Hyperkalemia is one of the commonest causes of fatal adverse drug reaction.

III Pharmacokinetic interactions

ABSORPTION

In addition to direct interaction within the gut lumen, drugs that increase or reduce the rate of gastric emptying (e.g. metoclopramide or propantheline, respectively) can alter the rate or completeness of absorption of a second drug, particularly if this has low bioavailability. More importantly, drugs can interfere with the enterohepatic recirculation of other drugs: failure of oral contraception (particularly low-dose estrogen preparations) can result from concurrent use of antibiotics as a result of this mechanism. Many different antibiotics have been implicated, although trimethoprim and co-trimoxazole are believed to be exceptions. Phenytoin reduces the effectiveness of cyclosporin A by an uncertain mechanism, possibly by reducing its absorption.

DISTRIBUTION

As explained above interactions that involve only mutual competition for inert protein or tissue binding sites seldom, if ever, give rise to clinically important effects. Examples of complex interactions where competition for binding sites occurs in conjunction with reduced clearance are mentioned in the section below on renal elimination. Effects on specific transport mechanisms may prevent drugs reaching their site of action on receptors or else prolong their effect due to slow removal from the vicinity of receptors. Tricyclic antidepressants block high-affinity amine uptake sites on presynaptic sympathetic nerve terminals, preventing the effect of adrenergic neuron-blocking drugs and prolonging the action of amines such as noradrenaline and phenylephrine whose action at the postsynaptic receptors is usually terminated by such uptake.

METABOLISM

Decreased efficacy can result from enzyme induction by a second agent (Table 12.3).

Table 12.3 Interactions due to enzyme induction.

Primary drug	Inducing agent	Effect of interaction
Warfarin	Barbiturates	Decreased anticoagulation
	Alcohol	
	Rifampicin	
Oral contraceptives	Rifampicin	Pregnancy
Prednisolone/Cyclosporin	Anticonvulsants	Reduced immunosuppression (graft rejection)
Theophylline	Smoking	Decreased plasma theophylline

Historically, barbiturates were clinically the most important enzyme inducers, but with the decline in their use, other anticonvulsants, notably carbamazepine, and the antituberculous drug rifampicin are now the commonest cause of such interactions. These necessitate special care in concurrent therapy with warfarin, phenytoin, oral contraceptives, glucocorticoids or cyclosporin.

Withdrawal of an inducing agent during continued administration of a second drug can result in a *slow* decline in enzyme activity with emergence of delayed toxicity from the second drug due to what is no longer an appropriate dose. For example, a patient receiving warfarin may be admitted to hospital for an intercurrent event and receive treatment with a drug that induces the form of cytochrome P_{450} that metabolizes warfarin. During the hospital stay the dose of warfarin therefore has to be increased so as to maintain measurements of international normalized ratio (INR) within the therapeutic range. The intercurrent problem is resolved, the inducing drug discontinued and the patient discharged taking the larger dose of warfarin. If the INR is not checked frequently, bleeding may result from an excessive effect of warfarin days or weeks after discharge from hospital as the effect of the enzyme inducer gradually wears off.

Inhibition of drug metabolism may also produce toxicity (Table 12.4). The time course of such interactions is often shorter than for enzyme induction, since it depends merely upon the attainment of a high enough concentration of the inhibiting drug at the metabolic site. Xanthine oxidase is responsible for inactivation of 6-mercaptopurine, itself a metabolite of azathioprine. Allopurinol markedly potentiates these drugs by inhibiting xanthine oxidase. Xanthine alkaloids (e.g. theophylline) are *not* inactivated by xanthine oxidase, but rather by a form of cytochrome P_{450}. Theophylline has serious (sometimes fatal) dose-related toxicities, and clinically

Table 12.4 Interactions due to enzyme inhibition.

Primary drug	Inhibiting drug	Effect of interaction
Phenytoin	Isoniazid	Phenytoin intoxication
	Cimetidine	
	Chloramphenicol	
Warfarin	Allopurinol	Hemorrhage
	Metronidazole	
	Phenylbutazone	
	Co-trimoxazole	
Azathioprine, 6MP	Allopurinol	Bone-marrow suppression
Pethidine	MAOI	Prolonged sedation
Theophylline	Cimetidine	Theophylline toxicity
	Erythromycin	
Terfenadine	Erythromycin	Ventricular tachycardia
	Ketoconazole	

MAOI = monoamine oxidase inhibitor. 6MP = 6-mercaptopurine.

important interactions occur with inhibitors of the cytochrome P_{450} system, notably cimetidine, ciprofloxacin and erythromycin. Asthmatic patients are often admitted to hospital with severe attacks of airflow obstruction precipitated by chest infections, so an awareness of these interactions before commencing antibiotic treatment is essential if aminophylline is also to be administered. Erythromycin also inhibits cyclosporin A metabolism, and can cause severe toxicity.

Enzyme inhibition also accounts for clinically important interactions with phenytoin (isoniazid, cimetidine, chloramphenicol and sulfonamides have all been implicated) and with warfarin (where cimetidine, the sulfonamides and phenylbutazone are all important, and stereoselective inhibition of the isomers of warfarin is a complicating factor). Non-selective monoamine oxidase inhibitors (e.g. phenelzine) potentiate the action of indirectly acting amines such as tyramine, which is present in a wide variety of fermented products (Camembert and other soft cheeses, yeast extract and Chianti wine amongst others), and of a number of drugs, including pethidine.

Clinically important impairment of drug metabolism may also result indirectly from hemodynamic effects rather than enzyme inhibition. Lignocaine is metabolized in the liver, and hepatic extraction ratio is high. Consequently, any drug that reduces hepatic blood flow (e.g. a negative inotrope) will reduce hepatic clearance of lignocaine and cause it to accumulate. This accounts for the increased lignocaine concentration and toxicity that is caused by β-blocking drugs. This is important following myocardial infarction, when β-blockers are administered despite diminished myocardial reserve and lignocaine is used to prevent recurrence of ventricular arrhythmias.

EXCRETION

Many drugs share a common transport mechanism in the proximal tubules (chapter 6), and can mutually reduce one another's excretion by competition (Table 12.5). The effect of probenecid on penicillin elimination is mentioned above, and sulfinpyrazone has a similar action. Aspirin and non-steroidal anti-inflammatory drugs inhibit secretion of methotrexate into urine, as well as displacing it from protein binding sites, and can cause methotrexate toxicity. Most diuretics reduce sodium absorption in the loop of Henlé or distal tubule (chapter 33); this leads indirectly to increased proximal tubular reabsorption of monovalent cations via a homeostatic control loop. Increased proximal tubular reabsorption of lithium ions in patients treated with lithium salts can cause lithium accumulation and potentially fatal toxicity. Digoxin secretion is reduced by spironolactone, by quinidine, by verapamil and by amiodarone, all of which can precipitate digoxin toxicity in consequence, although several of these interactions are complex in mechanism, involving displacement from tissue binding sites in addition to reduced digoxin elimination.

Changes in urinary pH alter excretion of drugs that are weak acids or bases, and

Table 12.5 Competitive interactions for renal tubular transport.

Primary drug	Competing drug	Effect of interaction
Penicillin	Probenecid	Increased penicillin blood level
Methotrexate	Salicylates	Bone-marrow suppression
	Sulfonamides	
Salicylate	Probenecid	Salicylate toxicity
Indomethacin	Probenecid	Indomethacin toxicity
Chlorpropamide	Phenylbutazone	Hypoglycemia
Digoxin	Spironolactone	Increased plasma digoxin
	Amiodarone	
	Verapamil	

administration of systemic alkalinizing or acidifying agents or carbonic anhydrase inhibitors change the concentrations of these drugs in plasma and urine (e.g. excretion of salicylate and of phenobarbitone is increased in an alkaline urine). Such effects are seldom of clinical significance, although they are sometimes of value in the management of overdose to increase drug elimination (chapter 50).

Pharmacogenetics 13

Introduction **120**

Mendelian traits that influence drug metabolism **121**

Inherited traits that influence drug action **124**

Inherited diseases that predispose to drug toxicity **125**

Polygenic influences on drug action **128**

*I*NTRODUCTION

Drug responses vary greatly between individuals. Such differences are due to genetic as well as to environmental effects on drug absorption, distribution, metabolism or excretion (pharmacokinetics) and on receptor or postreceptor sensitivity (pharmacodynamics). In addition, several instances of adverse reactions to drugs that had originally been attributed to idiosyncratic or immunologic mechanisms have been explained in terms of genetically determined variation in the activity of enzymes involved in detoxification or of other abnormal proteins (e.g. variants of hemoglobin) that render an individual especially susceptible to some adverse reaction such as hemolysis. The study of

Table 13.1 Variations in drug metabolism due to genetic polymorphism.

Pharmacogenetic variation	Mechanism	Inheritance	Occurrence	Drugs involved
Rapid acetylator status	Increased hepatic N-acetyltransferase	Autosomal dominant	40% whites	Isoniazid; hydralazine; some sulfonamides; phenelzine; dapsone procainamide
Suxamethonium sensitivity	Several types of abnormal plasma pseudocholinesterase	Autosomal recessive	Most common form 1:2500	Suxamethonium
Defective hydroxylation of debrisoquine	Functionally defective cytochrome P_{450} 2D6	Autosomal recessive	8% Britons; 1% Saudi Arabians; 30% Chinese	Debrisoquine; metoprolol; perhexiline; nortriptyline
Ethanol sensitivity	Relatively low rate of alcohol metabolism	Usual in some ethnic groups	Orientals	Alcohol

Table 13.2 Variations in drug response due to genetic polymorphism.

Pharmacogenetic variation	Mechanism	Inheritance	Occurrence	Drugs involved
G6PD deficiency, favism, drug-induced hemolytic anemia	80 distinct forms of G6PD	X-linked incomplete codominant	10 000 000 affected in the world	Many—including 8-aminoquinolines, antimicrobials and minor analgesics (see text)
Steroid-induced raised intraocular pressure	Unknown	Autosomal recessive (heterozygotes show some response)	5% white population	Glucocorticosteroids
Methemoglobinemia: drug-induced hemolysis	Methemoglobin reductase deficiency	Autosomal recessive (heterozygotes show some response)	1:100 are heterozygotes	Same drugs as for G6PD deficiency
Malignant hyperthermia with muscular rigidity	Unknown	Autosomal dominant	1:20 000 of population	Some anesthetics especially halothane Suxamethonium
Acute intermittent porphyria: exacerbation induced by drugs	Increased activity of δ-amino levulinic synthetase secondary to defective porphyrin synthesis	Autosomal dominant	Acute intermittent type 15:1 000 000 in Sweden; Porphyria cutanea tarda 1:100 in Afrikaaners	Barbiturates, chloral, chloroquine, ethanol, sulfonamides, phenytoin, griseofulvin (and many others)

G6PD = glucose-6-phosphate dehydrogenase.

variations in drug responses under hereditary control is called pharmacogenetics. Pharmacogenetic variation is sometimes due to the actions of a single mutant gene (as in genetic polymorphism, or Mendelian disorders that exhibit discontinuous variation). Tables 13.1 and 13.2 show examples of disorders that influence, respectively, drug metabolism and drug response. Alternatively, pharmacogenetic variation can result from polygenic influences.

MENDELIAN TRAITS THAT INFLUENCE DRUG METABOLISM

Abnormal sensitivity to a drug may be the result of an inborn error of its metabolism. Inheritance may be autosomal recessive, and such disorders are rare although they are important since they may have severe consequences. However, there are also dominant patterns of inheritance that lead to much commoner variations within the population. Genetic polymorphism is a type of variation in which individuals with sharply distinct characteristics coexist as healthy members of a population. It is probable that balanced polymorphism, when a substantial fraction of a population differs from the remainder in such a way over many generations, results when heterozygotes experience some selective advantage. Balanced polymorphisms of enzymes that are involved in drug metabolism are not uncommon, although the selective advantage conferred by heterozygosity is unknown.

Acetylator status

Administration of identical doses (per kg body weight) of isoniazid (INH, an antituberculous drug) to individuals in a population results in great variation in blood concentrations. A distribution histogram of such concentrations shows two distinct groups ('bimodal' distribution; Fig. 13.1). INH is metabolized in the liver by acetylation.

Individuals who acetylate the drug more rapidly because of a greater hepatic enzyme activity achieve lower concentrations of INH in their blood following a standard dose than do slow acetylators. Acetylator status is conveniently measured using dapsone as the test drug by measuring the ratio of monoacetyldapsone to dapsone following a test dose.

Slow and rapid acetylator status are inherited in a simple Mendelian manner. Heterozygotes as well as homozygotes are rapid acetylators because rapid metabolism is

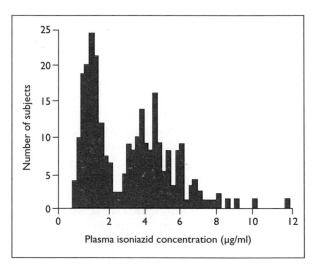

Fig. 13.1 Plasma isoniazid concentrations in 483 subjects 6 hours after oral isoniazid (9.8 mg/kg). Acetylator polymorphism produces a bimodal distribution into fast and slow acetylators. (From D.A.P. Evans *et al., Br Med J* 1960; **2**: 485. Reproduced by permission of the Editor.)

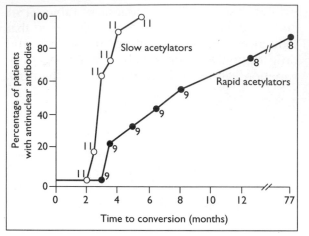

Fig. 13.2 Development of procainamide-induced antinuclear antibody in slow aceylators (○) and rapid aceylators (●) with time. Number of patients shown at each point. (From R.L. Woosley *et al.* Reprinted by permission from the *New Engl J Med* 1978; **298**: 1157.)

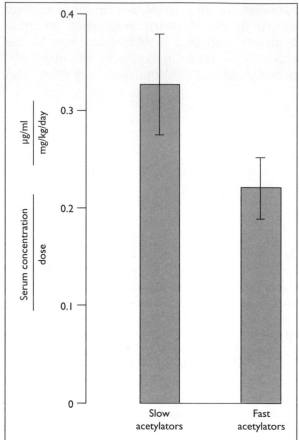

Fig. 13.3 Relationship between aceylator status and dose-normalized serum hydralazine concentration (i.e. serum level corrected for variable daily dose). Serum concentrations were measured 1–2 hours after oral hydralazine doses of 25–100 mg in 24 slow and 11 fast acetylators. (From J. Koch–Weser. *Med Clin N Am* 1974; **58**: 1027.)

an autosomal dominant. Fifty-five to sixty per cent of Europeans are slow acetylators and 40–45% are rapid acetylators. The rapid acetylator phenotype is most common in Eskimos and Japanese (95%) and lowest among some Mediterranean Jews (20%).

INH toxicity, in the form of peripheral neuropathy, occurs most commonly in slow acetylators, whilst slower response and greater risk of relapse of infection is more frequent in rapid acetylators, particularly when the drug is not given daily, but twice weekly. In addition, slow acetylators are more likely to show phenytoin toxicity when this drug is given with INH, because INH inhibits hepatic microsomal hydroxylation of phenytoin. Isoniazid hepatitis *may* be commoner among rapid acetylators but the data are conflicting.

Acetylator status affects other drugs (e.g. procainamide, hydralazine) that are inactivated by acetylation. Steady-state plasma concentrations are higher in slow acetylators during chronic dosing with these drugs. Approximately 40% of patients treated with procainamide for 6 months or more develop antinuclear antibodies. Slow acetylators are more likely to develop such antibodies than rapid acetylators (Fig. 13.2), and more slow

acetylators develop procainamide-induced lupus erythematosus. Similarly, lower doses of hydralazine are needed to control hypertension in slow acetylators (Fig. 13.3), and in these individuals high doses (above 200 mg/day) are more likely to lead to production of antinuclear antibodies and lupus syndrome.

Sulfasalazine is acetylated and treatment of ulcerative colitis with this drug causes mild hemolysis in some patients, particularly those who are slow acetylators.

Acetylation may also detoxify carcinogens: the incidence of bladder cancer in men exposed to arylamines whilst employed in the dyestuffs industry is higher in slow acetylators although there is no clear association of acetylator phenotype with sporadic bladder cancer.

Debrisoquine hydroxylation

4-Hydroxylation of debrisoquine (an adrenergic neuron-blocking drug used in the past to treat hypertension), is deficient in about 8% of the British population (Table 13.1). Hydroxylation polymorphisms explain several clinical phenomena:

- Debrisoquine: excessive hypotension (in poor metabolizers).
- Perhexiline: neuropathy and hepatotoxicity more common (in poor metabolizers).
- Nortriptyline: headache, confusion (in poor metabolizers).

Several other drugs (e.g. metoprolol, propranolol, timolol, dextromethorphan) exhibit oxidation polymorphism associated with debrisoquine-linked defective metabolism. As yet the clinical importance of this defect in these cases is not established.

Sulfoxidation

Sulfoxidation shows polymorphism. There is approximately a 100-fold difference between individuals with respect to the amount of sulfoxide metabolites in the urine following a dose of carbocysteine. Sulfoxidation is inherited autosomally and is incompletely recessive. It is apparently independent of the nitrogen oxidation ('debrisoquine') system. It is not yet known whether this genotype controls oxidation of other sulfur-containing drugs (e.g. phenothiazines, thioxanthines) but an association has been demonstrated between impaired sulfoxidation and an

increased incidence of adverse reactions to penicillamine therapy for rheumatoid arthritis.

Alcohol dehydrogenase

Not all enzyme variants produce clinical effects. Alcohol dehydrogenase in human liver exists as an atypical variant with a specific activity about five times higher than the normal enzyme. This occurs in approximately 20% of Londoners. Despite the high specific activity of the atypical enzyme, alcohol oxidation *in vivo* is no higher than normal in individuals possessing this variant because alcohol dehydrogenase is not the rate-limiting step in ethanol elimination.

Slow metabolism of tolbutamide

This pharmacogenetic variant was described following the finding of a nine-fold variation in the interindividual rate of tolbutamide elimination. Inactivation of this sulfonylurea oral hypoglycemic drug is largely genetically determined, by autosomal transmission. The primary site of genetic control is at the level of oxidation to hydroxytolbutamide. The clinical implication is that a fixed dose regime should not be applied indiscriminately.

Suxamethonium sensitivity

The usual response to a single intravenous dose of suxamethonium is muscular paralysis for about 6 min. The effect is brief because suxamethonium is rapidly hydrolyzed by plasma pseudocholinesterase. Occasional individuals show a much more prolonged response and may remain paralyzed and require artificial ventilation for 2 hours or more. This results from the presence of an aberrant form of plasma cholinesterase. The commonest variant which causes suxamethonium sensitivity occurs at a frequency of around 1 in 2500. Heterozygotes are unaffected carriers and comprise about 4% of the population.

INHERITED TRAITS THAT INFLUENCE DRUG ACTION

Familial hypercholesterolemia

Familial hypercholesterolemia (FH) is an autosomal disease in which the ability to synthesize receptors for low density lipoprotein (LDL) is impaired. Low density lipoprotein receptors are needed for hepatic uptake of LDL, and individuals with FH consequently have very high circulating concentrations of LDL, and suffer from atheromatous disease at a young age. Homozygotes completely lack the ability to synthesize LDL receptors and may suffer from coronary artery disease in childhood, whereas the much commoner heterozygotes have intermediate numbers of receptors between homozygotes and healthy individuals and commonly suffer from coronary disease in young adulthood. β-Hydroxy-β-methylglutaryl coenzyme A (HMGCoA) reductase inhibitors (an important class of drug for lowering circulating cholesterol) work largely by indirectly increasing the number of hepatic LDL receptors. Such drugs are especially valuable in treating heterozygotes with FH, because they restore hepatic LDL receptors toward normal in such individuals by increasing their synthesis. In contrast, they are completely ineffective in homozygotes because such individuals lack entirely the genetic material needed for LDL receptor synthesis.

Glucocorticoid-induced raised intraocular pressure

In some individuals steroid eye drops (e.g. 0.1% dexamethasone) cause a reversible increase in intraocular pressure. This response is inherited in a simple Mendelian manner. Populations can be divided into individuals who produce little or no (<5 mmHg) rise in pressure, those whose pressure rises by 5–15 mmHg and those with rises >15 mmHg. The clinical importance of this has been determined by observing the risk of developing open angle (simple) glaucoma in individuals with the various allelic pairs. Heterozygotes have 18 times the risk of developing glaucoma compared to those homozygous for low pressure response to steroids, whilst homozygotes for high pressure response have 101 times the risk of those homozygous for low pressure response. Furthermore, steroid eye drops precipitate glaucoma in some such individuals.

Warfarin resistance

This has been observed in very few pedigrees in humans, but has become common in rats, where the selective advantage is obvious. (Warfarin has been widely used as a rat poison.)

Angiotensin-converting enzyme gene polymorphism

There is a genetic polymorphism involving the angiotensin-converting enzyme (ACE) gene. This involves a deletion in a flanking region of DNA that controls the activity of the gene. Recent evidence has indicated that the double deletion genotype is a strong independent risk factor for coronary artery disease, especially in individuals who lack other conventional risk factors such as hypertension or hypercholesterolemia. If this is confirmed it suggests the possibility of using drugs that act on the renin–angiotensin system (such as ACE inhibitors) in genetically defined individuals at high risk of heart disease.

INHERITED DISEASES THAT PREDISPOSE TO DRUG TOXICITY

Glucose-6-phosphate dehydrogenase deficiency

Glucose-6-phosphatase dehydrogenase (G6PD) catalyzes formation of reduced nicotinamide adenine dinucleotide phosphate (NADPH), which maintains glutathione in its reduced form (Fig. 13.4). The gene for G6PD is located on the X chromosome so deficiency of this enzyme is inherited in a sex-linked fashion. Glucose-6-phosphate dehydrogenase deficiency is common, especially in Mediterranean peoples, those of African or Indian descent and in the Far East. Reduced enzyme activity results in methemoglobinemia and hemolysis when red cells are exposed to oxidizing agents, for example as a result of ingestion of broad beans (*Vicia fava*), naphthalene or one of several drugs.

There are over 80 distinct variants of G6PD, but not all produce hemolysis: the lower the activity of the enzyme the more severe the clinical disease. The following drugs can produce hemolysis in such patients:

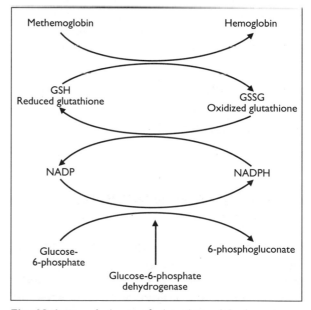

Fig. 13.4 Site of glucose-6-phosphate dehydrogenase deficiency.

1. Analgesics: aspirin.
2. Antimalarials: primaquine, quinacrine, quinine.
3. Antibacterials: sulfonamides, sulfones, nitrofurantoin, chloramphenicol.

4. Miscellaneous: quinidine, probenecid, vitamin K.

Patients with G6PD deficiency treated with an 8-aminoquinoline (e.g. primaquine) should spend at least the first few days in hospital under supervision. If acute severe hemolysis occurs primaquine may have to be withdrawn and blood transfusion may be needed. Cortisol, 100–200 mg, is given intravenously and the urine is alkalinized to reduce the likelihood of deposition of acid hematin in the renal tubules.

The high incidence of this condition in some areas is attributed to a balanced polymorphism, i.e. to a selective advantage conferred on heterozygotes. It is hypothesized that this selective advantage is due to a protective effect of partial enzyme deficiency against falciparum malaria. This is supported by the observation that in Sardinia there is a positive correlation between genes for both thalassemia and G6PD deficiency and previous malarial endemicity. Resistance may arise because parasites survive less well in enzyme-deficient cells because these are more rapidly removed from the circulation.

Several other enzymic defects in the glutathione-generating system have been discovered which lead to hemolysis when oxidizing drugs are taken.

Methemoglobinemia

Several compounds oxidize hemoglobin to methemoglobin. These include nitrates, nitrites, chlorates, sulfonamides, sulfones, nitrobenzenes, nitrotoluenes and anilines. In certain hemoglobin variants (e.g. HbM, HbH) the oxidized (methemoglobin) form is not readily converted back into reduced, functional hemoglobin. Exposure to the above substances causes methemoglobinemia in individuals with these hemoglobin variants.

Similarly nitrites, chlorates, dapsone and primaquine can cause cyanosis in patients with a deficiency of NADH-methemoglobin reductase.

Other hemoglobin variants

Hb Zurich causes acute hemolytic reactions when sulfonamides are administered. HbH is a relatively common variant in the East (1/300 births in Bangkok). Oxidants cause acute hemolysis in homozygotes, similar to that occurring in patients with G6PD deficiency.

Malignant hyperthermia

This is a rare but potentially fatal complication of general anesthesia. The causative agent is usually halothane or suxamethonium. Sufferers exhibit a rapid rise in temperature and (usually) increasing muscular rigidity, tachycardia, sweating, cyanosis and rapid respiration. There are several forms, one of the more common of which (characterized by halothane-induced rigidity) is inherited as a Mendelian dominant. The frequency of this phenotype is 1:20 000.

Several separate underlying muscle diseases predispose to malignant hyperthermia, including myopathies and myotonia congenita. Serum creatine phosphokinase is sometimes elevated in such individuals but a more accurate prediction of susceptibility can be made by muscle biopsy: muscle from affected individuals is abnormally sensitive to caffeine *in vitro*, responding with a strong contraction to low concentrations. (Pharmacological doses of caffeine release calcium from intracellular stores and cause contraction even in normal muscle in high enough concentration.) Affected muscle responds similarly to halothane or suxamethonium.

Acute porphyrias

This group of diseases comprises acute intermittent porphyria, variegate porphyria and hereditary coproporphyria. In all three

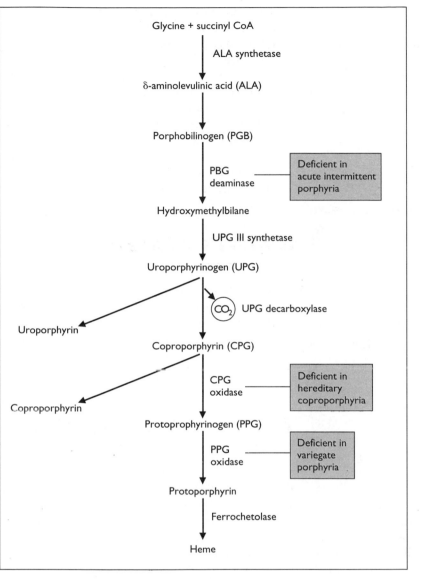

Fig. 13.5 Porphyrin metabolism showing sites of enzyme deficiency in the porphyrins.

varieties acute illness is precipitated by drugs because of inherited enzyme deficiencies in the pathway of heme synthesis (Fig. 13.5). Drugs do not precipitate acute attacks in porphyria cutanea tarda, a non-acute porphyria, although this condition is aggravated by alcohol, estrogens, iron and polychlorinated aromatic compounds.

Drug-induced exacerbations of acute porphyria (neurological, psychiatric, cardiovascular and gastrointestinal disturbances that are occasionally fatal) are accompanied by increased urinary excretion of 5-aminolevulinic acid (ALA) and porphobilinogen. An extraord-

inarily wide array of drugs can cause such exacerbations. Most of the drugs that have been incriminated are enzyme inducers that raise hepatic ALA synthetase levels. These drugs include phenytoin, sulfonylureas, ethanol, griseofulvin, sulfonamides, sex hormones, methyldopa, imipramine, theophylline, rifampicin, pyrazinamide and chloramphenicol. Often a single dose of one drug of this type can precipitate an acute episode, but in some patients, repeated doses are necessary to provoke a reaction.

These patients used to fare considerably better *before* the therapeutic advances of the twentieth century, and it behoves clinicians to consider the possibility of this diagnosis, and, having made it, to minimize drug treatment and seek specialist advice before prescribing *any* medication. A useful list of drugs unsafe for use in acute porphyrias is included in the *British National Formulary*.

Down's syndrome

Children with trisomy 21 show excessive sensitivity to antimuscarinic drugs.

Gout

Some forms of gout are inherited in an autosomal dominant manner. In other cases there is evidence of polygenic inheritance. Gout is aggravated by:

1. **Ethanol** This is metabolized by oxidation and simultaneous formation of NADH from NAD$^+$. NADH favors conversion of pyruvate to lactate which impairs renal excretion of urate.
2. **Diuretics** (both thiazides and loop diuretics) These reduce renal excretion of uric acid and consequently increase plasma urate concentration. As a result they precipitate gout in susceptible individuals.
3. **Allopurinol** This reduces the frequency of acute gouty attacks by inhibiting xanthine oxidase which converts xanthine to uric acid. Allopurinol also inhibits total synthesis of purines. In a small fraction of

patients (<1%) with reduced hypoxanthine–guanine phosphoribosyltransferase (HGPRT) activity, this second action of allopurinol does not operate and the drug can, rarely, cause xanthine renal stones to form in such individuals. Activation of 6-mercaptopurine and azathioprine, purine antimetabolites, depends on HGPRT. Consequently, the therapeutic effects of these drugs are not attained in patients lacking this enzyme (e.g. children with Lesch–Nyhan syndrome).

Gilbert's disease

This is a benign chronic form of hyperbilirubinemia due to an inherited lack of a hepatic conjugating enzyme (glucuronyl transferase). Estrogens impair bilirubin uptake and aggravate the jaundice in patients with this condition, as does fasting.

Transketolase deficiency

It has been found that some individuals inherit an abnormal form of transketolase with reduced avidity for its cofactor, thiamine pyrophosphate, inheritance being autosomal recessive. If dietary thiamine is reduced because of chronic alcoholism the activity of transketolase becomes compromised. It is hypothesized that this explains why only some alcoholics develop Wernicke–Korsakov syndrome whereas others with similar degrees of malnutrition are unaffected.

POLYGENIC INFLUENCES ON DRUG ACTION

The above are examples of *discontinuous* variations in drug response, usually due to the effects of variations in a single allele. The response to most drugs in a population demonstrates continuous variation and is the result of multiple genetic and environmental factors. Twin studies have been used to investigate the role of genetic influences

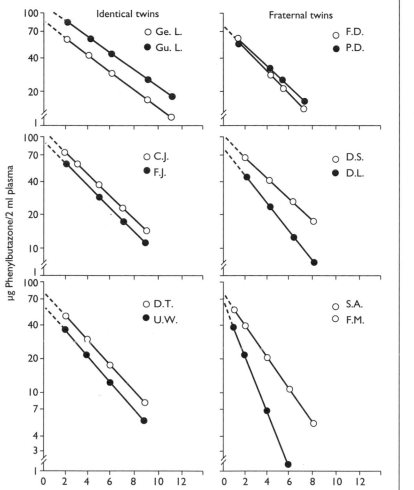

Fig. 13.6 Decline in plasma phenylbutazone concentrations following a single dose of 6 mg/kg to three sets of identical and three sets of fraternal twins. (From E.S. Vesell and J.G. Page. *Science* 1968; **159**: 1479. Copyright 1968. American Association for the Advancement of Science.)

acting in this type of distribution. There is much greater similarity between identical twins than between fraternal twins as regards disposition of many drugs including ethanol, phenytoin, halothane and nortriptyline (Fig. 13.6). Family studies have confirmed this type of inheritance despite complications arising from differences in drug disposition according to age, sex, disease and exposure to chemicals in the environment. Thus, like blood pressure and height, which are also under polygenic control, the patterns of metabolism of these drugs in offspring tend to lie between those of the parents.

Estimates of heritability (H = 1 implying complete hereditary control; H = 0 implying no hereditary control) for antipyrine and ethanol metabolism have been put as high as 0.98 and 0.99, respectively, for identical twins and 0.47 and 0.38 for fraternal twins. Large interindividual differences in rates of elimination of these drugs are apparently remarkably free from environmental influences, at least under the environmental conditions in which these studies were undertaken.

Drugs whose metabolism is mainly influenced by variations in a single gene may also show additional variation due to superimposed polygenic effects. Isoniazid is an example: there is continuous variation within each of the two populations of rapid and slow acetylators (see Fig. 13.1, page 121).

Introduction of New Drugs and Clinical Trials

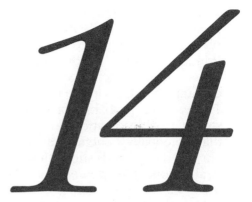

(*with Paul J. Morrison*)

History **132**

UK regulatory system **133**

Codes of practice in the research and development process **133**

The process of drug development **134**

Preclinical studies **135**

Clinical trials **136**

Clinical drug development **139**

Generic drugs **142**

Ethics committees **142**

Globalization **142**

HISTORY

Many years before Christ, man discovered, presumably by trial and error, that certain plant extracts influence the course of disease. Primitive tribes used extracts containing active drugs such as opium, ephedrine, cascara, cocaine, ipecacuanha and digitalis. These were probably often combined with strong psychosomatic therapies and the fact that potentially beneficial agents survived the era of magic and superstition says a great deal about the powers of observation of those early 'researchers'.

Many useless, and sometimes deleterious, treatments also persisted through the centuries but the desperate situation of the sick and their faith in medicine delayed recognition of the harmful effects of drugs. Any deterioration following drug administration was attributed to disease progression rather than adverse drug effects. There were notable exceptions to the faith in medicine and some physicians had a short life expectancy as a consequence!

During the present century there has been an almost exponential growth in the number of drugs introduced into medicine. The 1932 *British Pharmacopoeia* lists only 213 medical products. By 1990 this had increased to almost 3500. Many advances can be attributed to the necessities of war; however, properly controlled clinical trials, which are the cornerstone of new drug development, only became widespread after World War II for which the well-organized vaccine trials of the MRC (Medical Research Council) must take much credit. Some conditions did not require clinical trials, e.g. the early use of penicillin in conditions which had previously been invariably fatal. Many early trials were aided 'ethically' by insufficient drug supplies necessitating a 'non-treatment' group.

Although the necessity of clinical trials became apparent after the war it was not until after the early 1960s that the appalling potential of drug-induced disease was realized worldwide. Thalidomide was first marketed in West Germany in 1956 as a sedative/hypnotic as well as a treatment for morning sickness. The drug was successfully launched in various countries, including Britain in 1958, and was generally accepted as a safe and effective compound with little hangover effect. However, in 1961 it became clear that its use in early pregnancy was causally related to a rare congenital abnormality, phoccomelia, in which the long bones fail to develop. At least 600 such babies were born in England and more than 10 000 afflicted babies were born worldwide.

The thalidomide tragedy stunned the medical profession, pharmaceutical industry and public, precipitating a worldwide revolution in drug development.

In the UK the Committee on the Safety of Drugs was set up in 1963 under the chairmanship of Sir Derrick Dunlop.

Parallel drug evaluation procedures were being implemented worldwide. In the USA thalidomide had not been approved by their drug regulatory body, the Food and Drug Administration (FDA), which was at that time by far the most advanced in the world. The advanced development of the FDA was also attributable to a serious drug toxicity (including several deaths) in the USA in the late 1930s when diethylene glycol (a highly toxic solvent) was used to dissolve one of the then new antimicrobial agents sulfanilamide. As a result the FDA required all new drugs to be submitted to the FDA for approval. Approval of thalidomide was delayed by the FDA, not for its teratogenic potential, which was then unknown, but for another relatively uncommon side effect, of peripheral neuritis. The FDA regulations were, however, extensively tightened following the thalidomide disaster, requiring extensive testing of drugs in animals before testing is permitted in humans.

The current practices of drug development all have their foundations in the responses of society and, consequently, governments to the thalidomide disaster and have as their basic ethos a desire to devise a process which will, as a primary objective, minimize the risks and, secondarily, optimize the benefits to society of new therapeutic agents.

UK REGULATORY SYSTEM

The Medicines Act 1968 provides for the licensing of all medicinal products and controls their sale, supply and advertizing. The Health and Agriculture Ministers are the 'licensing authority'. The Medicines Control Agency (MCA) performs the administrative and secretarial function. The Medicines Commission is an advisory body to the licensing authority and is distinct from the Committee on Safety of Medicines (CSM) which is an independent group of clinicians, clinical pharmacologists, toxicologists, pathologists and others who advise the licensing authority on the safety, quality and efficacy of medicinal products as well as the investigation and monitoring of adverse reactions once a drug has been licensed. In practice it is the CSM which is the regulatory review body for the UK advising when certificates to perform clinical trials [Clinical Trials Certificates (CTC) or Clinical Trials Exemption Certificates (CTX)] should be issued to pharmaceutical companies and advising, following review of all the data from a submission, on the granting of a product license which will allow the company to market the drug.

The UK is also subject to the European Union (EU) Pharmaceutical Directives and at present a regulatory system is evolving to harmonize national and EU regulations.

CODES OF PRACTICE IN THE RESEARCH AND DEVELOPMENT PROCESS

In order to control the standards of research required and the quality of data produced during the drug development process a series of codes of practice has been drawn up by the regulators. All research and development data submitted for review to the regulatory environment are expected, and in some countries legally required, to have been performed under these codes of practice.

The three codes of practice are:

- Good Pharmaceutical Manufacturing Practice (GPMP or GMP).
- Good Laboratory Practice (GLP).
- Good Clinical Research Practice (GCRP or GCP).

These codes were first set out formally in the UK as guidelines by the Association of the British Pharmaceutical Industry (ABPI) and followed in 1991 by an EC Directive. This sets out a comprehensive code of practice for the performance of clinical studies.

*T*HE PROCESS OF DRUG DEVELOPMENT

The process of developing new therapeutic agents is highly regulated. The average cost of taking a new chemical entity (NCE) from the laboratory to the market place in 1990 was more than £150 million and the process took approximately 12 years.

The contemporary process follows well-defined pathways:

1. Discovery/design.
2. Synthesis.
3. Preclinical testing.
4. Clinical testing.
5. Regulatory approval – product license.
6. Postmarketing surveillance.

Drug discovery and design

Although, historically, successes have been obtained using random screening of organic molecules for biological activity, the contemporary drug design process is highly directed. The major advances in molecular biology over the past decade, in particular our understanding of receptors, their structure and the mechanism of the interactions of endogenous substances with them, together with powerful computer technology (computer aided design) means that the drug design process has become a highly specialized branch of pharmaceutical research.

Biotechnology

Some of the most exciting new molecules are coming from the biotechnology revolution.

Our ability to splice (genes (including human genes) into bacterial and yeast chromosomes and to extract from these organisms large quantities of natural human and other proteins has presented a myriad of new challenges: for example, the natural anticoagulant secreted by the leech (hirudin) is now being biotechnologically produced in large quantities and is in advanced clinical trials as a therapeutic anticoagulant.

Some biotechnology products currently in use or development include:

- Calcitonin gene-related peptide.
- Luteinizing hormone-releasing factor.
- Granulocyte colony-stimulating factor.
- Interferons.
- Interleukins.
- Human insulin.
- Growth hormone.
- Hirudin.
- Hemoglobin.
- Factors VIII and IX.
- Epoetin.

Synthesis

Once the moiety to be tested has been identified and its structure established the process for its synthesis must be developed and verified, be it chemical or biotechnological. The manufacture of ethical pharmaceuticals must be performed according to the guidelines of GMP.

*P*RECLINICAL STUDIES

The fundamental tenet of testing drugs in animals is that such information helps to predict the efficacy and toxicity of drugs that are candidates for clinical use. However, although animal testing of potential drugs has been extensive for many years some of the routinely performed studies are of unproven value.

Pharmacology

Compounds must be shown to demonstrate specific pharmacological activity. General pharmacological profiles of compounds are also required (e.g. autonomic, cardiovascular, central nervous system), so-called secondary pharmacology.

Acute toxicity

The estimated lethal dose (LD) is usually evaluated in rodents. There is no need for estimation of the formal LD_{50}, which requires large numbers of animals, except for agents such as vaccines, which may have variable toxicity between batches.

Chronic toxicity

Based on acute toxicity data, three or four dose levels are selected and administered daily for a minimum of 14 days to two species, one rodent (usually rat) and one non-rodent (usually dog). The doses selected are intended to include a 'no effect' dose level (NOEL), low dose, mid dose and a top dose at which fatalities will occur. It is essential to include a placebo dose group. In life, biochemical, hematological and urinalysis profiles are performed as well as physical examinations. Blood samples are also taken for measurement of concentrations of the drug. From these data it may be possible to establish:

1. If the drug is absorbed.
2. An estimate of half-life in the different species and in some cases toxic effects may be correlated not with the dose administered but with the plasma concentration (toxicokinetics). At the end of the study all the animals are killed, *post mortems* performed and a full histopathological examination performed on all organs.

In parallel with these studies more detailed pharmacokinetic and metabolic studies will be performed often using radiolabelled drugs.

DURATION OF CHRONIC STUDIES

If up to three doses of the drug are to be given to humans in the next phase of clinical development, then the results of 14 days' toxicity testing, including gonadal and general histology, should be provided. For repeat dosing of up to 10 days in humans, animal toxicity testing for 28 days with information about gonadal and general histology should be available. Dosing for 6 and, less commonly, 12 months is required by some nations although the value of these studies is uncertain.

MUTAGENICITY

The bacterial mutagenic potential of the compound will be tested, usually in *Salmonella typhi* (the Ames test).

Regulatory bodies now also require at least one mammalian mutagenicity test. If the compound is not extensively metabolized an *in vitro* test (e.g. Chinese hamster ovary cell) is appropriate. There is sound logic in using an *in vivo* model (e.g. mouse micronuclear test) where significant metabolic transformation of the drug occurs. A total of 4 types of test are often performed.

Carcinogenicity testing

Carcinogenicity testing will be required early in the development process if:

1. The structure of the drug or its metabolites in humans suggest similarities to known carcinogens.
2. There are equivocal mutagenicity data.
3. Histopathological findings from toxicity studies are suspicious.
4. The drug, or its metabolites, has an exceptionally long half-life in humans.

Reproductive testing

As most initial studies in humans are performed in males only, most reproductive studies are not usually performed until the drug under development shows efficacy in humans. In general, women of child-bearing potential are not exposed to these compounds until reproductive tests are complete.

The tests cover three distinct areas:

- Segment 1 – fertility.
- Segment 2 – teratology.
- Segment 3 – peri- and postnatal development.

There is increasing pressure for a greater exposure of female subjects to drugs under development and this may lead to an enhancement in the scope of reproductive tests and acceleration of their implementation in the research and development (R & D) cycle.

CLINICAL TRIALS

Physicians read clinical papers, review articles and pharmaceutical advertizements describing clinical trial results. The incompetent and unscrupulous author can hide deficiencies in design and possibly publish misleading data. The major medical journals are well refereed although supplements to many medical journals are less rigorously reviewed for scientific value. An understanding of the essential elements of clinical trial design enables a more informed interpretation.

Assessment of a new treatment by clinical impression is not adequate. Diseases may resolve or relapse spontaneously, coincidental factors may confound any interpretation and the power of placebo and enthusiastic investigators are a major influence on subjective response. In order to minimize these factors and eliminate bias any new treatment should be rigorously assessed by carefully designed, controlled clinical trials.

Objectives

The first step in clinical trial design is to determine which questions need to be answered and then refine these further into the primary objectives which are practical to achieve in the trial. The question may be straightforward, for example does treatment A prolong survival in comparison with treatment B following diagnosis of small cell carcinoma of the lung? Survival is a clear objective parameter. However, other factors such as quality of life must be assessed as objectively as possible so that a fair comparison can be made. Within such a study subgroups of patients may be identified and differences in response determined; for example, treatment A may be found to be most effective in those patients with limited disease at diagnosis whereas treatment B may be most effective in those with widespread disease at diagnosis.

Randomization

Patients who agree to enter such a study must be randomized so that there is an equal chance of receiving treatment A or B. If treatment is not truly randomized then bias will occur; for example, the investigator might consider treatment B to be less well tolerated and thus decide to treat particularly frail patients with treatment A. Multicenter studies are often necessary in order to recruit adequate numbers of patients and it is essential to ensure the treatments are fairly compared. If treatment A is confined to one center/hospital and treatment B to another many factors may affect the outcome of the study due to differences between the centers such as interval between diagnosis and treatment, individual differences in determining entry criteria, facilities for treatment of complications, differing attitude to pain control, ease of transport etc.

Inclusion/exclusion criteria

For any study inclusion/exclusion criteria must be carefully determined before the study commences. Maximizing patient safety and minimizing confounding factors whilst ensuring the criteria are not so strict that the majority of patients with the diagnosis are excluded must be considered. The definition of a healthy elderly subject is a moot point. It is normal once one is over the age of 65 to have a reduced creatinine clearance, to be on some concomitant medication and to have a history of allergy to something. If these are exclusion criteria one is studying a 'superfit' elderly population and not a normal population.

Double-blind design

In addition to true randomization a 'double-blind' design should be employed whenever possible to reduce both subject and observer bias. Unfortunately this is not always possible; for example, if in the comparison of treatment A and treatment B described above, treatment A consists of regular intravenous infusions whilst treatment B consists of oral medication the 'blind' is broken. As 'survival' duration is 'hard' objective data, this should not be influenced markedly, whereas softer endpoints such as state of well-being are more easily confounded.

Withdrawals

The number of patients withdrawn from each treatment and the reason for withdrawal (subjective, objective, logistic) must be taken into account. For example, if in an antihypertensive study comparing two treatments administered for 3 months only the data from those who completed 3 months' therapy with treatment X or Y are analyzed, this may show both treatments were equally effective. If, however, 50% of the patients on treatment X withdrew after 1 week because of adverse effects, that conclusion is erroneous. Hence both an 'intention-to-treat' analysis and a 'treatment received' analysis should be presented.

Placebo

If a placebo control is ethical and practical this often enhances the accurate interpretation of trial data and enables efficacy to be determined. It is well recognized that placebo treatment lowers blood pressure. This is partly due to patient familiarization with study procedures whose effect can be minimized by a placebo 'run-in' phase of 4 weeks. This ideally allows confirmation of diagnosis. To control for placebo effect and allow for the natural course of the disease there should also be a placebo group during the treatment phase.

Trial design

There is no one perfect design for comparing treatments. Studies should be prospective, randomized, double blind and placebo controlled when possible. Parallel group studies are those in which patients are randomized to receive different treatments. Although tempting, using historical data as a control is often misleading and should only be used in exceptional circumstances. Usually one of the treatments is the standard, established treatment of choice, i.e. the control, whilst the other is an alternative, often a new treatment which is a potential advance. In some more chronic diseases and often when investigating pharmacodynamic effects and pharmcokinetics a crossover design where each subject acts as his or her own control can be employed. Intraindividual variability in response is usually much less than interindividual variability. The treatment

sequence must be evenly balanced to avoid order effects and there must be adequate 'washout' to prevent a carryover effect from the first treatment. This design is theoretically more 'economical' in subject numbers but seldom applicable in practice.

Statistics

Research papers often quote P values in determining the value or otherwise of a difference. This is of limited value as a clinically significant difference may be missed if the sample size is too small (type II error). It is possible to calculate the number of patients required to establish a given difference between treatments at a specified level of statistical confidence. For a continuous variable one needs an estimate of the mean and standard deviation which one would expect in the control group. This is usually available from historical data but a pilot study may be necessary. The degree of uncertainty around observed differences should be reported as confidence intervals, usually 95%. Such intervals will diminish as the sample is increased. Confidence intervals are used to determine the 'power' of a study to identify a difference. Confidence intervals reflect the effects of sampling variability on the precision of a procedure and are important to quote when a 'non-significant' result is achieved.

The conventional threshold for a statistically significant result is usually $P < 0.05$, i.e. there is a 1:20 risk of a false positive result (type I error).

If many parameters are analyzed some apparently 'significant' differences will be identified by chance; for example, if 100 parameters are analyzed in a comparison of two treatments one would expect to see a significant difference in five of those parameters. One must also consider the clinical importance of any statistically significant result; for example, a drug may cause a statistically significant decrease in blood pressure in a study, but if it is only 0.2 mmHg it is not of any clinical relevance.

One should discuss the design and sample size of any clinical trial with a statistician at the planning phase. Statistics cannot completely answer the question as to when a randomized controlled trial should be stopped, however, and such trials may occasionally be unethical if one treatment is greatly superior to the other. Clearly it is neither ethically nor economically reasonable to continue with a trial once the result has clearly favored one alternative. A design of a trial which permits timely and efficient termination of a comparison is the sequential design. In this design patients are paired so that the alternative treatments are represented in each pair. For each pair a judgment based upon agreed criteria is made as to the superiority of one of the treatments. This judgment is termed a preference. Pairs for which no preference for any one treatment can be made do not enter the analysis. The results of each preference are plotted on a chart such as that shown in Fig. 14.1. The shape of boundaries in the chart is drawn up using statistical criteria. When the line of preference crosses the upper or lower boundaries of the chart the trial is terminated since at this point a clear difference at a previously decided level of statistical significance has been demonstrated. Pairing of successive entrants to a trial automatically removes variation due to gradual trends in response occurring throughout the trial, for example changes in natural history of the disease, altered standards of assessment of response. The use of sequential trials may rapidly obtain an answer to a problem, but on the other hand

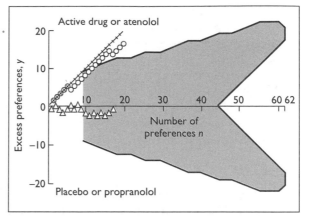

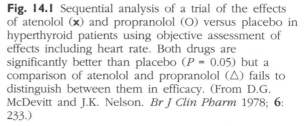

Fig. 14.1 Sequential analysis of a trial of the effects of atenolol (**x**) and propranolol (O) versus placebo in hyperthyroid patients using objective assessment of effects including heart rate. Both drugs are significantly better than placebo ($P = 0.05$) but a comparison of atenolol and propranolol ($\triangle$) fails to distinguish between them in efficacy. (From D.G. McDevitt and J.K. Nelson. *Br J Clin Pharm* 1978; **6**: 233.)

if there is actually no difference, or only a small difference, between treatments the sequential trial requires more patients than non-sequential trials to establish this.

Sequential trials are not always suitable and an ethical dilemma which has not been satisfactorily solved is whether a trial should be stopped by breaking the double blind if the organizers suspect that a proportion of the patients are responding well (or badly) to a new drug.

Any physician conducting a clinical trial must not forget that the prime objective of all studies is to benefit patients. The patients' welfare must be of paramount importance.

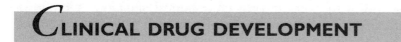

CLINICAL DRUG DEVELOPMENT

For the majority of new drugs the development process in humans, following a satisfactory preclinical safety evaluation, proceeds through four distinct phases. These are summarized below:

Phase I

- Not regulated in the UK unless patients involved; local Ethics Committee approval is required.

- Initial exposure of humans to investigational drug (first in humans).
- Safety evaluation.
- Assessment of pharmacokinetics and pharmacodynamics in healthy subjects.
- Usually healthy male volunteers.
- Usually single site.
- 12–100 subjects/protocol.
- 50–200 subjects in total.

Phase II

- Requires Licensing Authority approval; either a full clinical trials certificate (CTC) or a clinical trials exemption certificate (CTX).
- Initial safety evidence.
- Initial efficacy evidence.
- Identification of dose range for phase III trial.
- Well controlled with narrowly defined patient population.
- Single or multicenter.
- 100–500 patients in total.
- Usually double blind, randomized and often placebo controlled.

Phase III

- Requires Licensing Authority approval; either CTC or CTX.
- Efficacy and safety objective.
- Expanded and controlled.
- Collection of data on a large patient population with indication.
- Provide information on overall benefit/risk.
- Can be placebo or active controls.
- Large multicenter.
- 1000–5000 patients total.
- Usually double blind.

Phase IV

- Postmarketing studies (i.e. after approval).
- Exposure of drug to a wider population.
- Different formulations, dosages, duration of treatment, drug interactions and other drug comparisons studied.
- New age groups, races and other types of patients studied.
- Detection and definition of previously unknown or inadequately quantified adverse events and related risk factors.

Phase I

This initial human exposure is generally to healthy, young men unless toxicity is predictable (e.g. cytotoxic agents, murine monoclonal antibodies). These individuals volunteer to be given the drug under strictly controlled, hospitalized, expert medical supervision.

Prediction of the effects of drugs in humans by extrapolation from animal data is at best of limited value. Consequently very small initial doses, usually some fraction of the no effect dose in the toxicologically most sensitive animal species, is used. Initially single doses are administered to small groups (6–12 subjects) in placebo-controlled, double-blind studies. Following a satisfactory full review of all safety data from an initial group, a higher dose will be evaluated in the next group. Biochemical, hematological and urinalysis testing together with electrocardiographic (ECG) monitoring, blood sampling for plasma levels of drug and adverse event monitoring are the basic requirements for these studies.

This process is repeated until some predefined endpoint such as a particular plasma concentration, a pharmacodynamic effect or maximum tolerated dose is reached. Occasionally other factors may influence the decision to terminate a development program such as unacceptable cost of the drug, the amount to be given, unacceptable bulk of drug to be administered.

Using the pharmacokinetic, safety and pharmacodynamic information from the single rising dose studies, multiple dosing studies are performed under the same, strictly controlled, clinical conditions. These studies will attempt to reflect both the size and frequency of the prescribed dose to be used in the projected clinical situation. A range of doses should be tested with the projected clinical dose included ideally as one of the middle doses. Tolerance, pharmacokinetics and pharmacodynamics are evaluated paying particular attention to evidence of disproportionate accumulation (i.e. non-linearity of the pharmacokinetics).

In modern phase I development it is also desirable, whenever possible, for an evaluation of the pharmacological activity (pharmacodynamics) of the compound to be made at this stage of the development process. This may take a number of forms:

1. Direct, for example sedation, anticoagulation.
2. Indirect, for example QT prolongation of some antidysrhythmics, prolactin secretion with some antipsychotics.
3. Pathology simulation, for example antagonism of the effects of an endotoxin infusion, prevention of ipecac-induced vomiting by 5-hydroxytryptamine ($5HT_3$) receptor antagonists.

Phase II

If the drug satisfactorily completes the phase I program and appears promising the pharmaceutical, pharmacological, toxicological and phase I human (although these are not mandatory in the UK) study reports are submitted to the regulators, together with information on the proposed clinical studies as part of an application for a licence to perform clinical trials with the drug. The granting of either a CTC or a CTX permits authorized protocols to be performed, subject to Ethics Committee approval.

Having established the dose range that is well tolerated by healthy subjects and, in some cases, also identified doses which produce the desired pharmacological effects, the first patient studies are implemented. These first studies in patients are designed to determine the initial safety profile of the drug in patients, to establish clinical efficacy and, thirdly, to define the dose range to be used in the next, more extensive, stage of clinical trials (phase III). Relatively small numbers of tightly defined patient populations are used in well-controlled studies, usually in a small number of expert centers. This is one of the most critical stages of the development process for it is at this stage that the key decisions on the clinical doses to be used are taken.

Phase III

Phase III is the phase of formal clinical trials in which the efficacy of the new drug is usually compared with reference drugs of established efficacy. During this stage the aim is to identify those patient groups who respond more and less well to increased patient exposure in terms of numbers and duration of therapy and to identify less common adverse reactions. During this period the manufacturers will be setting up plant for large-scale manufacture and undertaking further pharmaceutical studies on drug formulation, bioavailability and stability. The medical advisers to the company will, in association with their pharmacological, pharmaceutical and legal colleagues begin gathering together the large amount of data necessary to make formal application to the Licensing Authority via the CSM for a product license. The size of the submission documents may extend to several hundredweights of paper. Marketing approval may be general or granted subject to certain limitations which may include restriction to hospital practice only, restriction in indications for use or a requirement to monitor some particular action or organ function in a specified number of patients. All prescribing doctors are provided with a factual data sheet giving information on each new medicine and the contents of this must be agreed with the CSM. It must provide all the information necessary to make a proper decision as to whether the drug is indicated (i.e. it is not an advertizement) and must also detail all known hazards of the drug. Doctors are also reminded (by means of an inverted triangle symbol beside its entry in the BNF) that this is a recently introduced drug and that any suspected adverse reaction should be reported to the CSM.

It is usual for possible drug interactions between the new compound and commonly prescribed drugs to be investigated at this time. Often these studies will be performed in healthy volunteers (phase IB).

Phase IV

Phase IV studies are prospective trials performed after marketing approval (the granting of a Product License). They may be studies to investigate new formulations, dosage requirements, drug interactions or patient groups and may also help in the detection of previously unrecognized adverse events (chapter 11).

Postmarketing surveillance

The CSM closely monitors newly licensed drugs for adverse events through the yellow card reporting system (chapter 11).

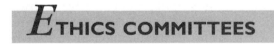

GENERIC DRUGS

Once the patent life of a drug has expired anyone may manufacture and sell their version of that drug. The generic drug producer does not have to perform any of the R & D process other than to demonstrate that their version of the drug is bioequivalent to the standard formulation. This usually means that the plasma concentration–time curves for the generic product must be demonstrated to be sufficiently similar to the standard preparation to be clinically equivalent.

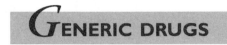

ETHICS COMMITTEES

All protocols for clinical trials must be reviewed and approved by a properly constituted independent ethics committee. The objectives of the ethics committee are:

1. To protect the subjects of research.
2. To preserve the rights of research subjects.

3. To provide public reassurance.

Key issues for ethical review include a genuine humanitarian need for the research, validity of study procedures, informed consent and insurance of subjects.

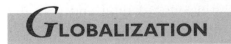

GLOBALIZATION

Today the drug development process is so costly that large markets (i.e. global markets) are necessary to recoup the R & D investment. Consequently, there has been a significant move towards globalization and harmonization of the R & D process culminating in the first International Conference on Harmonization (ICH) in Brussels 1991. The aim of this conference was to produce globally accepted regulations for drug approval. It is hoped that these conferences will lead to a globally accepted system of drug development in the next century without stifling research with excessive bureaucracy and will facilitate the early introduction of valuable new therapies whilst maximizing patient protection.

The Nervous System II

Hypnotics and Anxiolytics

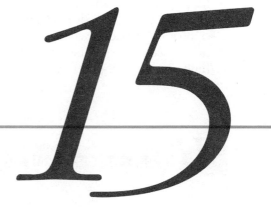

(with Roy G. Spector)

Introduction   **148**

Hypnotics and sleep difficulties   **148**

Anxiolytics and other drugs in the treatment of anxiety   **156**

INTRODUCTION

Hypnotics induce sleep and anxiolytics reduce anxiety. There is considerable overlap between them. Thus drugs that induce sleep, also reduce anxiety when given in subhypnotic doses. Conversely benzodiazepines (which are anxiolytic) while causing less drowsiness than alcohol or the barbiturates in equivalent anxiolytic doses, are nevertheless also hypnotic drugs. Neither hypnotics nor anxiolytics are suitable for the *long-term* management of insomnia or anxiety due to rapid induction of tolerance and dependence.

HYPNOTICS AND SLEEP DIFFICULTIES

Insomnia is common: in one Scottish survey, 45% of women and 15% of men over 45 years regularly took prescribed hypnotics. Not only is such drug treatment relatively ineffective in chronic insomnia, but drugs are also inappropriately prescribed for physiological changes in sleep patterns. For example, in the elderly, total sleep time is reduced and this is accompanied by more frequent wakening. Such phenomena are normal and do not constitute insomnia.

Sleep

Although we spend about one-third of our lives asleep, the function of sleep is not known. Two theories concern somatic and cerebral biochemical recuperation and neurophysiological functions such as consolidation of memory and sorting of sensory data.

Sleep comprises two alternating states: rapid eye movement (REM) sleep and non-REM sleep. During REM sleep there is dreaming. This is accompanied by maintenance of synaptic connections and increased cerebral blood flow. Non-REM sleep includes sleep of different depths – in the most deep of which the electroencephalogram (EEG) shows a slow wave pattern, growth hormone is secreted and protein synthesis occurs.

Drugs produce states that superficially resemble physiological sleep but lack the normal mixture of REM and non-REM phases. Hypnotics usually suppress REM sleep and when discontinued there is an excess of REM (rebound) which is associated with troubled dreams punctuated by repeated wakenings. During this withdrawal state falling from wakefulness to non-REM sleep is also inhibited by feelings of tension and anxiety. The result is that patient and doctor are tempted to restart medication to suppress the withdrawal phenomena.

Management of insomnia

It is important to exclude causes of insomnia that require treating in their own right, for example:

1. Pain, for example due to arthritis or dyspepsia.
2. Dyspnea, for example as a result of left ventricular failure, bronchospasm, cough.
3. Frequency of micturition.

4. Full bladder and/or loaded colon in the elderly.
5. Drugs such as caffeine, or rebound from the effects of alcohol.
6. Depression.
7. Anxiety.

Much chronic insomnia is due to dependence on hypnotic drugs.

Some individuals need very little sleep. Shortened sleep time is common in the elderly. Patients with dementia often have a very disturbed sleep rhythm.

1. Hypnotics should only be considered if insomnia is severe and causing intolerable distress. They should only be used for short periods (at most 2–4 weeks) and, if possible, taken intermittently. On withdrawal the dose and frequency of use should be gradually tailed off.
2. Benzodiazepines are currently the hypnotics of choice, but may fail in the elderly and alternatives such as chlormethiazole can be helpful.
3. Prescribing more than one hypnotic at a time is not recommended.
4. Drugs of other types may be needed when insomnia complicates psychiatric illness. Sleep disturbances accompanying depressive illness usually respond to antidepressives such as amitriptyline. Antipsychotics such as chlorpromazine or thioridazine may help to settle patients suffering from dementia who have nocturnal restlessness.
5. Hypnotics should not be routinely given to hospital patients or in any other situation.
6. Whenever possible non-pharmacological methods such as relaxation techniques, meditation, cognitive therapy, controlled breathing or mantras should be used. Some experience sleepiness after a warm bath and/or sexual activity. A milk-based drink before bed can promote sleep but may cause weight gain. Daytime sleeping should be advised against. Increased daytime exercise improves sleep at night.
7. Alcohol is not recommended because it causes rebound restlessness and sleep disturbance after the initial sedation has worn off. Tolerance and dependence

develop rapidly. It also causes dehydration (*gueule de bois*) and other unpleasant manifestations of hangover.

Drugs used to treat sleep disturbances

BENZODIAZEPINES

These drugs share the same properties and are anxiolytic, anticonvulsant, muscle relaxants and induce sleepiness. It is likely that some relative specificity occurs in individual drugs; for example, clonazepam is more anticonvulsant than other members of the group at equisedating doses.

Use

1. Panic attacks and some other forms of acute agitation.
2. Intravenous benzodiazepines (such as diazepam and midazolam) are powerfully anxiolytic and at appropriate doses cause anterograde amnesia. These properties are useful for procedures such as endoscopy, electrocardioversion and operations under local anesthesia.
3. Relief of spasticity in neurological disease and reduction of muscle spasm due to pain.
4. Intravenous benzodiazepines are rapidly effective in terminating some drug-induced abnormal movements such as acute dystonia caused by metoclopramide.
5. Long-term treatment of some forms of epilepsy and the emergency treatment of status epilepticus.
6. Tetanus.
7. Short-term management of insomnia.

The benzodiazepines are not suitable for the long-term treatment of anxiety or for chronic insomnia.

Long-acting benzodiazepines used as hypnotics include nitrazepam, flunitrazepam and flurazepam. Loprazolam, lormetazepam and temazepam act for a shorter time and therefore cause less hangover and accumulation. Members of the group that are classified as anxiolytics (e.g. diazepam) are as effective as hypnotics as these drugs.

Mechanism of action

Benzodiazepines act by binding the γ-aminobutyric acid (GABA$_A$) receptor–chloride channel complex and facilitate the opening of the channel in the presence of GABA. This increases hyperpolarization-induced neuronal inhibition.

Adverse effects

These mainly involve the nervous system, but other forms of toxicity may be encountered:

1. **Central nervous system**

   (a) Sedation: feelings of fatigue, sleepiness and mental slowing are usually dose dependent. Memory disturbances are common.

   (b) Other consequences of CNS depression: ataxia, dysarthria, motor incoordination, diplopia, blurred vision, weakness, vertigo, increased risk of motor vehicle and other accidents, confusion, apathy.

   (c) States resembling Korsakoff's psychosis and alcoholic intoxication are sometimes produced. Occasionally these drugs precipitate outbreaks of rage and violence, presumably due to the release of anxiety-repressed hostility. Some patients taking triazolam developed severe anxiety, depersonalization, feelings of unreality, paranoia, hyperacusis and restlessness. It remains controversial as to whether this was specific to triazolam or related to use of this drug at effectively higher doses than other benzodiazepines.

   (d) Less common and more unpredictable effects are:

      i. Stimulation instead of sedation, similar to paradoxical excitement in children given barbiturates.

      ii. Antisocial behavior, probably a consequence of alcohol-like intoxication.

      iii. Hypnagogic hallucinations during the induction of sleep. Nitrazepam can cause nightmares that often involve stressful incidents in the patient's past.

      iv. Diazepam has occasionally been associated with depression and suicide.

      v. Patients with organic brain disease may respond adversely to large doses of diazepam and develop tremulousness, crying episodes, impaired concentration, nocturnal confusion and agitation.

      vi. Diazepam inhibits stage 4 (slow wave) sleep and suppresses attacks of night terrors (which arise during this phase of sleep). However, attacks may be displaced to the waking hours.

2. **Allergic reactions** are uncommon. Chlordiazepoxide has produced urticaria, angiodema and maculopapular eruptions. Light sensitivity dermatitis, fixed drug eruptions, non-thrombocytopenic purpura and swelling of the tongue have been described with benzodiazepine treatment. Acute anaphylaxis has also been reported.

3. **Other toxic effects** There is no convincing evidence that these drugs are toxic to hematopoietic tissues, liver or fetus. However, there is one report of a child born with absent first digits and a dislocated head of radius when the mother took diazepam in the first trimester of pregnancy.

4. **Intravenous diazepam**

   (a) Cardiovascular and respiratory depression are uncommon. Patients particularly prone to develop hypotension or apnea are those with serious underlying disease such as respiratory failure in chronic lung disease and those who have been previously given other central depressant drugs.

   (b) Local pain is commonly experienced on repeated intravenous injections of diazepam which can cause phlebitis. The incidence of this complication is reduced by flushing the vein with

150–250 ml isotonic saline. Intra-arterial benzodiazepine can cause arterial spasm and gangrene.

An emulsion of diazepam in intralipid is less irritating to vein and perivenous tissues if leaking occurs. Diazepam emulsion injection is available in 10 mg vials.

Drug dependence and withdrawal syndrome

Benzodiazepine dependence is usually caused by large doses taken for prolonged periods, but withdrawal states have also arisen after limited drug exposure. Fits can occur in the first week after withdrawal. The full withdrawal picture appears after an interval of 3–8 days and includes a cluster of features unusual in anxiety states, although frank anxiety and panic attacks commonly develop as well. Perceptual distortions (such as feelings of being surrounded by cotton wool), visual and auditory hallucinations, paranoia, feelings of unreality, depersonalization, paresthesiae, headaches and other pains, blurring of vision, dyspepsia and influenza-like symptoms are all characteristic. Depression and agoraphobia are also common. The syndrome may persist for many weeks. Withdrawal from benzodiazepines in patients who have become dependent should be gradual. If this proves difficult then an equivalent dose of a long-acting benzodiazepine should be given as a single night-time dose instead of shorter acting drugs. The dose should then be reduced in small fortnightly steps. Psychological support is usually needed. β-blockers or antidepressants should only be used if other measures fail.

Pharmacokinetics

Benzodiazepines are pharmacodynamically similar to one another: the differences between them arise due to their differing pharmacokinetics. Relationships between clinical effects and plasma concentrations of the benzodiazepines are imprecise and weak although in general terms the higher the plasma level the greater the effect. Routine measurement of plasma benzodiazepine concentrations is not useful since no clear therapeutic range has been established.

Benzodiazepines are well absorbed orally. Clorazepate is hydrolyzed in the stomach to an active metabolite, desmethyldiazepam (nordiazepam), the rate of hydrolysis depending upon acidity. The rate but not the extent of total absorption of clorazepate as nordiazepam is reduced by antacids. Absorption of chlordiazepoxide is also slowed by antacid, although the total amount finally absorbed is unaffected, so that steady-state concentration is unaltered during chronic use.

Absorption of most benzodiazepines from intramuscular injections is less rapid and produces lower peak plasma levels than following oral administration. The unreliability of the intramuscular route is important when sedation of uncooperative patients is required, for example in alcohol withdrawal or acute anxiety. However, lorazepam is reliably and rapidly absorbed following intramuscular injection.

Diazepam or midazolam are injected intravenously before procedures such as endoscopy. Early short-lived high peak blood levels are accompanied by amnesia. During the next 30–60 min there is a rapid α-phase decline and then slower (β phase) decline follows (diazepam half-life ($t_{1/2}$) = 20–50 hours; midazolam $t_{1/2}$ = 2 hours). The active desmethyl metabolite of diazepam has a $t_{1/2}$ of 36–200 hours but the α-hydroxy metabolite of midazolam has a $t_{1/2}$ of only 1–1.5 hours.

Sometimes at 6 hours there is a rise in blood concentration and reappearance of sedation, due to reabsorption of drug excreted in the bile (enterohepatic recirculation).

Benzodiazepines are highly protein bound in plasma, for example, at therapeutic concentrations chlordiazepoxide is 87–88% and diazpam is 95% bound.

With the exception of clorazepate the major site of metabolism of benzodiazepines is the liver. There is an interrelated pattern of benzodiazepine metabolites, many of which are pharmacologically active and are used therapeutically. Desmethyldiazepam occupies a central position. This substance has a very long $t_{1/2}$ and at steady state its concentration may exceed that of the parent substance. This explains the common hangover effects of continued administration of diazepam for example. Temazepam, which does not form this metabolite and is largely excreted unchanged as glucuronide, has a shorter $t_{1/2}$ and causes less prolonged sedation. To increase this advantage it is administered as a polyethylene glycol solution in capsules to speed absorption so that elimination of the total dose administered commences within a short time of administration (Fig. 15.1). Flurazepam is completely and rapidly metabolized in humans ($t_{1/2}$ = 2 hours) and flurazepam concentrations in peripheral blood are negligible. It is metabolized by human intestinal mucosa and the metabolites formed then undergo further transformation in the liver with a consequent difference in the pattern of metabolites found in hepatic portal and hepatic vein blood. The main active metabolite, desalkylflurazepam, has a half-life of 40–250 hours.

Because of the long $t_{1/2}$ of most of these drugs a single daily dose is sufficient to produce adequate steady-state levels. Benzodiazepines are only weak microsomal enzyme inducers and are safe to administer with oral anticoagulants (in contrast to barbiturates). Age influences diazepam elimination and the elderly have longer (up to 60%) half-lives for chlordiazepoxide and diazepam than the young. This means that with chronic dosing there is a greater delay in achieving steady state, with a consequent increased risk of failure to recognize adverse effects such as memory impairment as being drug related. The apparent volume of distribution of diazepam (which is lipid soluble) is also increased in old age because of the greater proportion of body fat in the elderly. Since clearance is directly proportional to volume of distribution and inversely proportional to $t_{1/2}$ diazepam clearance is unchanged as the altered $t_{1/2}$ and distribution volume offset one another. Oxazepam elimination does not require demethylation and is unaffected by aging.

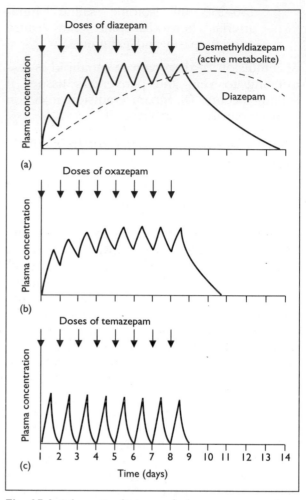

Fig. 15.1 Schematic diagram of plasma concentrations following daily dosage of three benzodiazepines. Note in (a) the accumulation of both diazepam and its active metabolite, and in (b) and (c) the absence of accumulation and active metabolites for oxazepam and temazepam.

Clearance of chlordiazepoxide and diazepam is reduced in patients with cirrhosis of the liver but that of oxazepam is unaffected, and oxazepam is therefore preferred for these patients.

Drug interactions

Pharmacodynamic interactions of benzodiazepines with other centrally acting drugs are common, whereas clinically significant pharmacokinetic interactions are not. Such pharmacodynamic interactions can lead to:

1. **Acute potentiation** of the sedative effects of alcohol, histamine (H_1) antagonists, nabilone (a synthetic cannabinoid used as an antiemetic for nausea and vomiting caused by cytotoxic drugs and unresponsive to conventional antiemetics) and other hypnotics.
2. **Chronic effects** Although benzodiazepines are highly protein bound, clinically significant interactions due to displacement of other protein bound drugs such as oral anticoagulants are not observed.

Pharmacokinetic interactions include:

- Cimetidine inhibition of the metabolism of benzodiazepines.
- Omeprazole inhibition of the metabolism of diazepam.
- Carbamazepine and phenytoin acceleration of the metabolism of clonazepam.
- Erythromycin inhibition of the metabolism of midazolam.

FLUMAZENIL

Flumazenil is a benzodiazepine antagonist. It can be used to assist diagnosis in the management of multiple drug overdose and to reverse benzodiazepine sedation. It is short acting and so sedation may return. Flumazemil can cause nausea, flushing, anxiety and fits.

CHLORMETHIAZOLE

Use

1. Is useful as a hypnotic in the elderly because its short action reduces the risk of severe hangover, ataxia and confusion the next day.
2. Effective in acute withdrawal syndrome in alcoholics but use should be carefully supervised and treatment limited to a maximum of 9 days.
3. Given intravenously to terminate status epilepticus.
4. Sedative during surgery under local anesthesia.

Mechanism of action

Even though the structure of chlormethiazole shares some features with the molecule of thiamine, there is no evidence that its actions have any relevance to this, and its mechanism remains unkown.

Adverse effects

1. Chlormethiazole readily causes dependence and should be used as a hypnotic for short periods only. Its use should be avoided or strictly controlled in patients with a history of drug dependence.
2. Nasal, pharyngeal and conjunctival discomfort and headache are frequently experienced during induction.
3. Gastric irritation is common.
4. High doses cause cardiovascular and respiratory depression. Especially during intravenous therapy the patient must be kept under close observation and the dose adjusted if necessary. Prolonged infusions result in drug accumulation which can lead to fatal respiratory depression.
5. Confusion and paradoxical excitement are uncommon.
6. Intravenous administration can cause thrombophlebitis. Intra-arterial infusion must be avoided because arterial spasm can lead to loss of a limb.
7. Despite its short half-life, drowsiness may be experienced on the following day and driving skills can be impaired.

Contraindications

- Pulmonary insufficiency.
- Hepatocellular failure.
- Alcohol dependence if alcohol is still being consumed.
- Breast feeding.

Pharmacokinetics

Absorption following oral administration is rapid, peak plasma levels being attained at 60 min. The $t_{1/2}$ is 50 min. Sedation and sleep usually occur 30–60 min after taking the drug orally. When given orally, chlormethiazole undergoes extensive first-pass metabolism (85%) which may be dose-dependent and results in low bioavailability by this route. In cirrhosis the oral bioavailability is increased about ten-fold, although its elimination is only slightly retarded. This results from decreased first-pass metabolism by the damaged liver. Chlormethiazole should therefore be given in reduced oral dosage in patients with cirrhosis of the liver.

Drug interactions

- Potentiation of the actions of alcohol and other CNS depressants.
- Cimetidine impairs the metabolism of chlormethiazole and so increases its action.

PROMETHAZINE

This H_1 antihistamine is sometimes used as a hypnotic, particularly for children. It is available without prescription for hypnotic purposes.

Uses

Promethazine is of value in children if itching or allergy is causing sleep disturbance. Otherwise there is nothing to recommend promethazine as a hypnotic.

Mechanism of action

Histamine mediates arousal and wakefulness by acting on receptors in the ventral posterior hypothalamus. Antihistamines produce sedation by inhibition of activity in long caudal tracts arising in this part of the hypothalamus.

Adverse effects

1. Antimuscarinic actions: dry mouth, constipation, reduced sweating, hesitancy of micturition, aggravation of glaucoma; hallucinations, confusion in the elderly, excitement.
2. Convulsions, involuntary movements.
3. Nightmares.
4. Hangover, bad temper.
5. Respiratory and cardiovascular depression; abnormal cardiac rhythms.
6. Dependence and tolerance.

Contraindications

- Because of the antimuscarinic actions, promethazine should not be used in patients with glaucoma, prostatic syndrome and fever.
- Individuals with focal cerebral lesions are more likely to have fits with this drug.
- Liver failure is an absolute contraindication.

Pharmacokinetics

Promethazine is well absorbed from the gastrointestinal tract, but subject to extensive first-pass metabolism. It is highly bound to plasma proteins, but freely passes the placental barrier and can cause sedation in the neonate when given to the mother during labor.

Drug interactions

- Alchohol and other sedatives: enhanced sedation.
- Antidepressants: tricyclics increase antimuscarinic and sedative effects.

ZOPICLONE

Use

Zopiclone is a non-benzodiazepine hypnotic which enhances GABA activity used in the short-term management of insomnia.

Mechanism of action

Zopiclone binds to the GABA–chloride channel complex, probably at the benzodiazepine-binding site. Although zopiclone has no structural similarity to the benzodiazepines, it appears to act in the same way by prolonging GABA-induced opening of the chloride channel. This appears to be the basis of its muscular relaxing, antiepileptic and anxiolytic/sedative actions.

Adverse effects

These are similar to those of the benzodiazepines, but there are some differences:

1. Bitter, metallic taste.
2. Anorexia, nausea, vomiting.
3. Persistent drowsiness, ataxia, uncoordination, confusion and depression the following day.
4. Soon after the first dose, psychological toxic effects may develop: auditory and

visual hallucinations, amnesia, aggression, other behavioral disturbances including agitation.

Contraindications

• Previous psychiatric illness or history of drug abuse.

Pharmacokinetics

Peak blood level occurs 1.5 hours after oral administration, but this is delayed in patients with cirrhosis of the liver. Terminal half-life 3.5 to 6.5 hours. This may be prolonged to over 8 hours in cirrhotic patients. Zopiclone enters breast milk, in which levels are about half that of the plasma.

Drug interactions

• Potentiation of alcohol, benzodiazepines and other central depressants.

CHLORAL AND DERIVATIVES

Use

Chloral is often used in pediatric practice. There is no evidence that chloral derivatives have any advantages over benzodiazepines and they are more prone to cause rashes and gastric irritation. They are not recommended for elderly or debilitated patients.

Mechanism of action

Chloral has a 'type II' hypnotic action (like alcohol and volatile anesthetics). Thus it enters hydrophobic regions of neuronal membranes and causes reversible swelling and disruption of crystalline structure. This inhibits the rapid opening of the sodium channel in neurons.

Adverse effects

1. Gastric irritation (triclofos and dichloralphenazone are less irritating than chloral hydrate).
2. Rashes.
3. Headache, hangover.
4. Ketonuria, disturbance of other urinary tests.
5. Paradoxical excitement; delirium.
6. Tolerance and dependence.
7. Renal damage on prolonged use.
8. Excreted in milk.

Contraindications

• Chronic obstructive lung disease.
• Fever.
• Heart failure.
• Gastritis and peptic ulcer.
• Renal failure (contraindicated if the glomerular filtration rate is less than 50 ml/min).

Pharmacokinetics

Chloral is well absorbed from the gastrointestinal tract and partly metabolized to trichlorethanol (active, $t_{1/2}$ = 7–11 hours) and trichloracetic acid (inactive). Chloral is not an enzyme inducer, but phenazone (in dichloralphenazone) is.

Drug interactions

• Chloral enhances sedation due to alcohol and other CNS depressants. It may transitorily enhance the anticoagulant effects of warfarin.
• Dichloralphenazone can interact with drugs such as warfarin by inducing cytochrome P_{450}.

Special problems and special groups

JET LAG

Jet lag consists of fatigue, sleep disturbances, headache and difficulty in concentrating. It is due to mismatching of the body clock (circadian dysrhythmia) against a new time environment with its own time cues (Zeitgebers). Resetting the internal clock is hastened by conforming to the new time regime: thus one should rest in a dark room at night, even if not tired, and eat, work and socialize during the day. Sufferers should not allow themselves to sleep during the day. Hypnotics at night can make things worse if sleepiness is experienced the next day.

However, sometimes short-acting benzodiazepines may be effective if taken before going to bed for two or three nights.

Melatonin may help sleep patterns and improves daytime well being if taken in the evening. It is not yet generally available.

NIGHT WORK

Night work causes more serious sleep difficulties than jet lag because hypnotics cannot be used for long periods. Also, drug-induced sleep during the day precludes family and other non-work activities. A better strategy is to allow the subject to have a short non-drug-induced sleep during the night shift. This will improve the subject's work efficiency towards the end of the night and also reduce his or her sleep needs during the day.

CHILDREN

The use of hypnotics in children is not recommended apart from unusual situations such as on the night before an anticipated unpleasant procedure in hospital. Hypnotics are sometimes used for night terrors. Children are prone to experience paradoxical excitement with these drugs.

ELDERLY

Hypnotics increase the risk of falls and nocturnal confusion. Even short-acting drugs can lead to ataxia and hangover the next morning.

ANXIOLYTICS AND OTHER DRUGS IN THE TREATMENT OF ANXIETY

Anxiety is fear, and is usually a normal reaction. Pathological anxiety is sufficiently severe fear such that it is disabling. Such a reaction may be a response to a threatening situation (such as having to make a speech) or to a non-threatening event (such as leaving one's front door and going into the street).

General principles and management

1. Distinguish anxiety as a functional disturbance from a manifestation of organic brain disease, or general illness (such as rheumatoid arthritis and tuberculosis).
2. Assess the severity of accompanying depression.
3. Most patients are best treated without drugs, but with cognitive therapy, relaxation techniques and simple psychotherapy.
4. Some patients are improved by taking regular aerobic exercise.
5. In the few selected severely anxious patients who are given anxiolytic drugs, these are only given for a short period (up to 2–4 weeks) because of the risk of dependence.
6 Desensitization can be useful when severe anxiety comes on in well-recognized situations (e.g. agoraphobia, arachnophobia etc.). Anxiolytic drugs are sometimes given intermittently and with a flexible dose scheme in such situations.
7. Benzodiazepines are the usual anxiolytics used in situations 5 and 6 above. Buspirone is equally effective and less hypnotic than the benzodiazepines.

8. β-blockers are sometimes useful in patients with prominent peripheral symptoms such as palpitations or tremor. They do not improve muscular tension, fear and dry mouth.
9. Tricyclic antidepressants may be effective in severe anxiety and in preventing recurrent panic attacks.
10. Monoamine oxidase inhibitors (used only by specialists) can be useful in treating anxiety with depression, phobic anxiety, recurrent panic attacks and obsessive–compulsive disorders.
11. Individual panic attacks usually are terminated by benzodiazepines, which may have to be supplemented with phenothiazines such as chlorpromazine. Such antipsychotic drugs are not used for long-term treatment of anxiety because of the risk of Parkinsonism and tardive dyskinesias.

BUSPIRONE

This belongs to a group of azaspirodecanediones which are relatively anxiolytic without marked hypnotic, anticonvulsant or muscle relaxant properties.

Use

Buspirone is used in anxiety states, but prolonged treatment is avoided as the risks of tolerance and dependence have not been fully evaluated. Response may be delayed up to 2 weeks. Buspirone does not prevent or alleviate benzodiazepine withdrawal symptoms.

Mechanism of action

Buspirone does not bind to benzodiazepine receptors nor potentiates GABA effects. It is a 5-hydroxytryptamine ($5HT_{1A}$) partial agonist and its antianxiety actions are related to this. It also acts on central dopamine receptors.

Adverse effects

1. Nausea, dizziness, headache, nervousness, dysphoria. Drowsiness is uncommon.
2. Rarely palpitations due to tachycardia. Chest pain.
3. Sweating, dry mouth.
4. Confusion and fatigue are uncommon. Driving performance may be impaired.

Contraindications

- Pregnancy, and during lactation.
- Severe hepatic or renal failure.
- Epilepsy.

Drug interactions

Potentiation of the actions of alcohol and other central depressants has not been documented, but it is prudent to avoid taking alcohol with buspirone.

Schizophrenia and Behavioral Emergencies

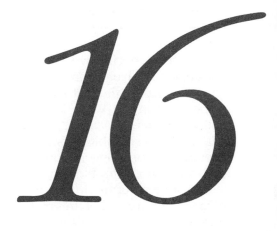

(with Roy G. Spector)

Schizophrenia **160**

Behavioral emergencies **167**

SCHIZOPHRENIA

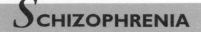

Introduction

Drugs that are effective in acute schizophrenia generally share many of the properties of chlorpromazine, the first member of the group to be used in the West. These include central antidopaminergic actions on the extrapyramidal and mesolimbic systems and on the chemoreceptor trigger zone, antimuscarinic and α-adrenoceptor-blocking properties.

The older terms major tranquilliser and neuroleptic are either misleading or uninformative. At the moment the label antipsychotic seems the most reasonable.

Pathophysiology

Much effort in investigating the mode of action of the antipsychotics has been directed to why they are so effective in schizophrenia. The dopamine theory of schizophrenia postulates that this mental illness arises because of excessive dopamine activity in the mesolimbic system, and that drugs with antipsychotic properties block dopamine D_2 receptors in the brain. There is an impressive correlation between the potencies of antipsychotics in the clinic and their potencies as antagonists of D_2 receptors which extends across several orders of magnitude. However, the relation between dopamine and schizophrenia is unlikely to be one of simple excess, since *post mortem* and neuroimaging techniques have usually failed to show definite increases in dopamine in the central cerebral nuclei of patients. Interpretation of these studies is complicated by prior use of antipsychotic drugs, however. L-Dopa can cause hallucinations in normal individuals but does not produce the full picture of schizophrenia. The closest drug-induced psychosis to naturally occurring schizophrenia is caused by amphetamines. Amphetamine does increase the release of dopamine (as well as other central amines), but the psychosis it produces can outlast drug use by many months, so it seems probable that, as with depressive illness, alterations in slowly adapting receptor-related processes such as up-regulation are involved.

Twenty to thirty per cent of patients with schizophrenia do not respond to the chlorpromazine type of D_2 antagonists. A high proportion of such refractory patients respond to clozapine, another type of antipsychotic drug which is an exception to the rule that antipsychotic potency is related to potency as a D_2 receptor antagonist. Clozapine has only weak D_2-blocking activity, but acts on other receptors, especially muscarinic, 5-hydroxytryptamine receptors ($5HT_2$, $5HT_3$) and D_1. It is thus possible that antipsychotic activity could be due to anti-5HT or non-D_2 dopamine antagonism in such patients. Recent evidence from ligand binding studies in *post mortem* brain tissue strongly suggests that a sub-type of D_2 receptors known as D_4 may be the key receptor to be overexpressed in schizophrenia. Regional dopamine differences may be involved such as low mesocortical activity with high mesolimbic activity.

General principles of management

1. Treatment is started in hospital promptly after diagnosis. Unnecessary delay in treatment has been associated with a poorer prognosis.
2. Social difficulties and other aggravating factors should be attended to.
3. Chlorpromazine is frequently successful on its own in acute psychotic episodes.

4. Once first rank symptoms have been relieved by drugs, the patient should return home and to work on low-dose antipsychotic maintenance treatment.
5. Sometimes maintenance treatment can be withdrawn early with no relapse. Many patients follow a chronic course with few acute episodes, and remain stable on maintenance medication. Some show progressive deterioration punctuated by frequent acute episodes despite continuing drug treatment.
6. Selected patients with refractory illness are treated by specialists with clozapine. (Leukopenia is common with this drug and frequent blood counts are mandatory.)
7. Schizophrenics are poor at taking tablets. Injections of depot antipsychotics (such as fluphenazine decanoate) remove many compliance problems.
8. The type and dose of medication should be reviewed systematically during mainte nance treatment.
9. Anticholinergics are not given routinely with antipsychotics but only if Parkinsonism develops.

Drugs used in treatment

PHENOTHIAZINES

Group 1 (aliphatic side chain): chlorpromazine, methotrimeprazine, promazine. Profoundly sedating, moderately antimuscarinic, moderate extrapyramidal effect.
Group 2 (piperidine side chain): pericyazine, pipothiazine, thioridazine. Moderately sedating, much antimuscarinic action, little extrapyramidal effect.
Group 3 (piperazine side chain); fluphenazine, perphenazine, prochlorperazine, trifluoperazine. Little sedation, little antimuscarinic action, high extrapyramidal effect.

BUTYROPHENONES

Haloperidol, benperidol, droperidol, trifluoperidol. Similar to group 3 phenothiazines.

DIPHENYLBUTYLPIPERIDINES

Fluspirilene, pimozide.

THIOXANTHINES

Flupenthixol, zuclopenthixol.

OXYPERTINE AND LOXAPINE

Similar to phenothiazines in toxicity.

CLOZAPINE

Very little extrapyramidal toxicity. Sedating. Agranulocytosis is common.

SULPIRIDE AND REMOXIPRIDE

Little sedation and extrapyramidal effects.

Mechanism of action

The majority of antipsychotics block dopamine receptors (D_1 and D_2) in the forebrain. D_1 receptors are positively linked to adenylyl cyclase. D_2 receptors inhibit adenylyl cyclase and also act by other mechanisms. Most antipsychotics have an affinity and antagonistic potency at D_2 sites that parallels their clinical efficacy. Their action on D_1 receptors is variable.

Blockade of D_2 receptors induces extrapyramidal effects. Repeated administration causes an increase in D_2 receptor sensitivity due to an increase in abundance of these receptors. This appears to underlie the tardive dyskinesias that are caused by prolonged use of most antipsychotics.

Clozapine has low affinity for D_1 and D_2 receptors but is more active against D_1 than D_2 and has little or no extrapyramidal toxicity. It does not increase the numbers and sensitivity of D_2 receptors in the forebrain, and prevents the supersensitivity to dopamine induced by other antipsychotics. However, clozapine is powerfully antimuscarinic and is also an antagonist of α_1- and

α_2-receptors and of $5HT_1$ and $5HT_2$ receptors. On repeated dosing it increases the sensitivity of α_1-receptors and possibly of muscarinic receptors.

Loxapine has a typical spectrum of antipsychotic activity, including dopamine (D_2) antagonism and muscarinic antagonism. However, it also potentiates 5HT activity by blocking its reuptake into neurons.

PHENOTHIAZINES

The choice of drug is largely determined by the demands of the clinical situation, in particular the degree of sedation needed and the patient's susceptibility to extrapyramidal toxicity and hypotension.

Use

1. Schizophrenia: Antipsychotic drugs are more effective against first rank (positive) symptoms (hallucinations, thought disorder, delusions, feelings of external control) than against negative symptoms (apathy and withdrawal). Piperazine phenothiazines are especially suitable for patients with circumscribed paranoid delusional states (e.g. monosymptomatic delusions).
2. Other excited psychotic states including mania and delirium.
3. Antiemetic and antihiccough.
4. Premedication and in neuroleptanalgesia techniques in surgery.
5. Terminal illness, including potentiating desired actions of opioids while reducing nausea and vomiting.
6. Severe agitation and panic.
7. Aggressive and violent behavior.
8. Movement and mental disorders in Huntington's disease.

Adverse effects

1. Akathisia is the most common movement disturbance caused by antipsychotics and is an important cause of poor compliance. The spectrum of the disturbance includes agitation, insomnia and restlessness. The latter resembles the spontaneous condition of restless legs (Ekbom's syndrome) with aching at rest and the irresistible urge to move. The accompanying emotional changes include anxiety and feelings of inner tension. Acute akathisia starts soon after starting or increasing the dose of antipsychotics, even within an hour or two. It can persist despite dose reduction and sometimes persists after drug withdrawal. Such tardive akathisia may be difficult to distinguish from tardive dyskinesias. The two can coexist.

2. The tardive dyskinesias are several neurological disorders producing persistent, repetitive, dystonic athetoid or choreiform movements of voluntary muscles. Usually the face and mouth are involved causing repetitive sucking, chewing and lip smacking. The tongue may be injured. The movements are usually mild but can be severe and incapacitating. It follows months or years of antipsychotic treatment and typically becomes more severe on stopping the drug for a substantial time or perhaps even permanently.

3. The most common adverse effects are dose-dependent extensions of pharmacological actions:

   (a) Anticholinergic: dry mouth, nasal stuffiness, constipation, urinary retention, blurred vision.
   (b) Postural hypotension due to peripheral α-adrenergic blockade, which is rarely severe unless used in conjunction with other vasoactive drugs (antihypertensives, anesthetics). Gradual build-up of dose improves tolerability.
   (c) Sedation (which may be desirable in agitated patients), drowsiness and confusion. Tolerance usually develops after several weeks on a maintenance dose but can be overcome by an increased dose. Emotional flattening is common but it may be difficult to distinguish this feature from schizophrenia. Depression may develop, particularly following treatment of hypomania and is again hard to distinguish confidently from the natural history of manic depressive disease. Acute confusion is uncommon.

4. Abnormal involuntary movements occur including tremor, seizures, Parkinsonism, dystonia and dyskinesia. All but the last of these are reversible. Acute dystonias can appear within a week of beginning the drug but the other reactions can be delayed for months. There seems to be no relationship between dose and their appearance. Their pathogenesis probably results from blockade of dopamine receptors, although tardive dyskinesias may involve actual structural change.

5. Jaundice occurs in 2–4% of patients taking chlorpromazine, usually during the second to fourth weeks of treatment. It is due to intrahepatic cholestasis and is a hypersensitivity phenomenon associated with eosinophilia. Substitution of another phenothiazine may not reactivate the jaundice.

6. Ocular disorders observed during chronic administration include corneal and lens opacities and pigmentary retinopathy. This may be associated with cutaneous light sensitivity. Recent studies implicate the hydroxylated metabolites of chlorpromazine as the culprit in the ocular disorders.

7. Another type of hypersensitivity reaction involves the skin. Five per cent of patients develop urticarial, maculopapular or petechial rashes. These disappear on withdrawal of the drug and may not recur if the drug is reinstated. Contact dermatitis and light sensitivity are common complications. Abnormal melanin pigmentation may develop in the skin.

8. Chlorpromazine consistently raises serum cholesterol levels. Glucose tolerance may be impaired.

9. Blood dyscrasias are uncommon but may be lethal, particularly leukopenia and thrombocytopenia. These usually develop in the early days or weeks of treatment. The estimated incidence of agranulocytosis is approximately 1 in 10 000 patients receiving chlorpromazine.

10. Sudden cardiac arrhythmia and arrest occurs with phenothiazines in the absence of gross structural damage although mitochondrial abnormalities have been noted in heart muscle. T-wave abnormalities and increased frequency of ventricular premature beats are noted on the ECG.

11. Malignant neuroleptic syndrome is another rare and potentially fatal complication of neuroleptics. Its clinical features are rigidity, hyperpyrexia, stupor or coma, and autonomic disorders. It responds to treatment with dantrolene (an intracellular Ca^{2+} antagonist).

12. Fits can be precipitated, particularly in alcoholics. Pre-existing epilepsy may be aggravated.

13. Impaired temperature control with hypothermia in cold weather and hyperthermia in hot weather.

The Boston Collaborative Survey indicated that adverse reactions are most common in patients receiving high doses and usually occur soon after starting treatment. The most common serious reactions were fits, coma, severe hypotension, leukopenia, thrombocytopenia and cardiac arrest.

Contraindications

- Coma due to cerebral depressants, bone marrow depression, pheochromocytoma, epilepsy, chronic respiratory disease, hepatic impairment, Parkinson's disease.
- *Caution*: elderly – especially in hot or cold weather.
- Pregnancy, lactation.
- Alcoholism.

Pharmacokinetics

The pharmacokinetics of antipsychotic drugs have been little studied. They have multiple metabolites. Their large apparent volumes of distribution (V_d) (e.g. for chlorpromazine $V_d = 22$ l/kg) result in low plasma concentrations presenting technical difficulties in estimation. Most is known about chlorpromazine. When given orally it is incompletely absorbed with a bioavailability of about 30%. This is further decreased by the presence of food or by simultaneous administration of anticholinergic drugs and some antacids.

Animal studies suggest considerable degradation of chlorpromazine in the gut before entering the portal circulation (a prehepatic first-pass effect). Peak plasma levels are reached in 2–3 hours but the $t_{1/2}$ varies between 2 and 24 hours in different individuals. Plasma steady-state concentrations are reached in around 1 week and have been reported as ranging from 10 to 1200 ng/ml in psychotic patients. Changes of dose more often than every 5 days are therefore inadvisable, and daily dosing is adequate in most patients. A single night-time dose will increase compliance and the sedative effects of the drug are maximal when they are most needed. Absorption is unreliable after intramuscular injection, possibly due to local precipitation of drug.

Chlorpromazine is an unstable molecule that rapidly forms an inactive sulfoxide on exposure to light. It has 168 potential metabolites, 70 of which have been identified in humans. The general routes of metabolism are:

1. Demethylation producing nor_1- and nor_2-chlorpromazine, which are sedative and enter the brain.
2. Oxidation producing sulfoxides and N-oxides, which are pharmacologically inactive.
3. Hydroxylation producing 3-hydroxy- and 7-hydroxychlorpromazine. Although 7-hydroxychlorpromazine has been implicated in the production of skin pigmentation, it appears to be an important antipsychotic metabolite and is probably more active than the parent substance.
4. Conjugation with glucuronic acid and sulfate.

Metabolism is primarily by hepatic microsomes although the brain, kidneys, lungs and gut also play a part.

Chlorpromazine is 90–95% bound in plasma, mainly to albumin, and is concentrated in some tissues; for example, brain concentration is four to five times that of plasma.

Following a single dose, a clear relationship has been established between peak plasma concentration and effects such as sedation, pulse rate, pupil size, salivary secretion and orthostatic hypotension, although the threshold for response varies from patient to patient. With chronic administration plasma chlorpromazine concentration may fall while the antipsychotic effect becomes manifest. Possibly this results from increased metabolism due to self-induction or else the anticholinergic effect of chlorpromazine results in delay in absorption and increased gut metabolism. Therapeutic drug monitoring of plasma chlorpromazine concentration is not useful in ordinary clinical practice. The relationship between plasma concentration and therapeutic effect is not well established, but concentrations of 35–350 ng/ml have been associated with clinical improvement and severe toxicity is seen above 600 ng/ml. Quantitation of metabolites may prove useful in future: patients who respond usually have higher ratios of 7-hydroxychlorpromazine + chlorpromazine to chlorpromazine sulfoxide than unresponsive patients.

Thioridazine has been partially investigated but presents most of the same problems as chlorpromazine. The $t_{1/2}$ varies from 10 to 36 hours with a tendency to prolongation in the elderly. A diurnal variation in metabolism (some metabolites are active) has been described, elimination being slowed during sleep.

Drug interactions

- Alcohol and other CNS depressants – enhanced sedation.
- Hypotensive drugs and anesthetics – enhanced hypotension.
- Increased risk of cardiac arrhythmias with drugs that prolong QT interval (e.g. amiodarone, sotalol).
- Tricyclic antidepressants – higher blood concentrations and increased antimuscarinic actions.
- Anticonvulsants – reduced efficacy.
- Desferrioxamine – avoid prochlorperazine.
- Domperidone and metoclopramide – increased extrapyramidal effects and akathisia.
- Antagonism of anti-Parkinsonian dopamine agonists (these are in any event contraindicated in schizophrenia).
- Lithium-increased risk of extrapyramidal effects.

BUTYROPHENONES

Use

Butyrophenones (e.g. haloperidol) are used as for phenothiazines but in addition haloperidol and droperidol are used for rapid control of hyperactive psychotic states. They are used for short periods because of the high incidence of extrapyramidal effects.

Haloperidol used in tics, Gilles de la Tourette syndrome and choreiform disorders.

Benperidol has been used in deviant hypersexual antisocial behavior (value not established).

Trifluoperidol has been used particularly for manic psychosis.

Adverse effects

These are similar to those of phenothiazines but butyrophenones are generally less sedating, less hypotensive, less antimuscarinic and have more extrapyramidal toxicity.

Contraindications

- As with phenothiazines.
- Avoid in basal ganglia disease.

Pharmacokinetics

Haloperidol is well absorbed after oral administration, bioavailability being approximately 60%. The $t_{1/2}$ for elimination is 12–38 hours and so steady-state levels are reached within a week of constant dosing. There is a linear relationship between dose and plateau plasma levels. Haloperidol is oxidized in the liver via oxidative dealkylation and does not form pharmacologically active metabolites. Metabolism may show a diurnal rhythm, being slowed in sleep. The relationship between plasma level and therapeutic effect is not firmly established: and therapeutic drug monitoring is not indicated, although 3–10 ng/ml has been suggested as the therapeutic range.

Drug interactions

As phenothiazines, in addition:

- Fluoxetine increases haloperidol levels.
- Carbamazepine lowers haloperidol levels.
- Lithium increases risk of extrapyramidal and other neurotoxicity of haloperidol.

DIPHENYLBUTYL PIPERIDINES (FLUSPIRILENE AND PIMOZIDE)

Use

Psychiatric uses of phenothiazines but particularly:

1. Monosymptomatic hypochondriacal psychoses.
2. Paranoid psychosis.
3. Mania.
4. Short-term management of excitement and psychomotor agitation.
5. Certain obsessive–compulsive states which have not responded to selective serotonin reuptake inhibitors.
6. Perhaps in apathetic withdrawn schizophrenic patients.

Adverse effects

1. As with phenothiazines, but less sedative than chlorpromazine.
2. Serious cardiac arrhythmias have been associated with administration of pimozide. An ECG must be taken before treatment in all patients, and periodic ECGs taken during treatment if daily doses of 16 mg or more are given.

Contraindications

- Avoid in children.
- Contraindicated if a significant cardiac arrhythmia, history of arrhythmia, pre-existing congenital prolongation of QT interval, concurrent cardioactive drugs, electrolyte disturbance which could affect the heart, in particular hypokalemia.
- Otherwise as with phenothiazines (e.g. avoid in epilepsy).

Pharmacokinetics

Pimozide is long-acting ($t_{1/2}$ = 18 hours) and a single daily dose is given in the maintenance treatment of schizophrenia. Fluspirilene is also long acting and can be injected at intervals of 1–2 weeks in microcrystalline low soluble form.

Drug interactions

- Similar to phenothiazines.
- Can potentiate arrhythmic toxicity of cardioactive drugs.

THIOXANTHENES (FLUPENTHIXOL, ZUCLOPENTHIXOL)

Use

1. As for psychiatric uses of phenothiazines, but not for mania.
2. Also, low doses of flupenthixol may be effective in depression when tricyclics have failed.
3. Intramuscular flupenthixol is given every 2 weeks for chronic schizophrenia especially in apathetic patients. Zuclopenthixol is used in schizophrenia and other psychoses, especially with hostile and aggressive behavior.

Adverse effects

Flupenthixol is less sedating than chlorpromazine but more prone to produce extrapyramidal toxicity.

Contraindications

- Zuclopenthixol should not be used in apathetic or withdrawn states.
- Flupenthixol should not be used in mania and psychomotor hyperactivity.
- These drugs are not used in children and in patients with porphyria.

OXYPERTINE

Use

1. Similar to psychiatric uses of phenothiazines including mania.
2. Violent and impulsive behavior.
3. Short-term adjunctive management of psychomotor agitation.

Adverse effects

1. Like the phenothiazines but less likely to cause extrapyramidal toxicity.
2. Low doses can cause agitation and hyperactivity.
3. High doses cause sedation.

LOXAPINE

Use

1. Similar to psychiatric uses of phenothiazines including acute and chronic psychoses.
2. Perhaps most used in paranoid schizophrenia.

Adverse effects

1. See phenothiazines.
2. Relatively little sedation, but overdose can cause serious cardiac and neurological toxicity, also dermatitis, pruritus, light sensitivity and seborrhea.

Pharmacokinetics

Loxapine is well absorbed via the small intestine, but is subject to presystemic metabolism. There are active metabolites which are excreted by the kidney. Elimination $t_{1/2}$ = 7 hours.

Drug interactions

- See phenothiazines.

CLOZAPINE

Use

1. Clozapine is at least as effective as other antipsychotics in schizophrenia and furthermore is effective in up to 60% of patients who have not responded to other drugs.
2. Unlike D_2 antagonists, clozapine is effective against negative as well as positive symptoms.

Adverse effects

1. Clozapine causes less movement disorders than other antipsychotics: dystonias and tardive dyskinesias are rare. Neutropenia or agranulocytosis develops in up to 3% of patients taking clozapine for a year (cf 0.01–0.1% with other antipsychotics). Because of this only psychiatrists should prescribe clozapine, and blood monitoring is mandatory, including a pretreatment full blood picture.
2. Other adverse effects: fits (3–4% of patients); drowsiness; salivation; dizziness; constipation; nausea; vomiting; weight gain; transient hypertension; hypotension.

Drug interactions

- Lithium increases central nervous system adverse effects of clozapine.

SULPIRIDE AND REMOXIPRIDE

The drugs are chemically different from other antipsychotics and show some selectivity in their activity in schizophrenia with relatively little extrapyramidal toxicity.

Use

1. Sulpiride in high doses controls florid positive schizophrenic symptoms.
2. Lower doses have an alerting effect on apathetic and withdrawn schizophrenics.

Adverse effects

Sulpiride toxicity is similar to that of phenothiazines with the exception of a lack of jaundice or skin reactions. Remoxipride causes little sedation and little extrapyramidal toxicity. It can produce headache, insomnia, difficulty concentrating, aggression, nausea and hypersalivation.

Contraindications

- Remoxipride is contraindicated in depressive illness.
- Both drugs are contraindicated in porphyria.

*B*EHAVIORIAL EMERGENCIES

Mania

Acute attacks are managed with antipsychotics, but the long-term prophylactic treatment of choice is lithium. The control of hypomanic and manic episodes with chlorpromazine is often dramatic. Lithium is also effective in acute episodes but response is delayed for 1–2 weeks.

Acute psychotic episodes

Patients with organic disorders may experience fluctuating confusion, hallucinations and transient paranoid delusions. Violent incidents sometimes complicate schizophrenic illness.

MANAGEMENT

Antipsychotics and benzodiazepines either separately or together are most often used in violent and disturbed behavior. Paraldehyde is an effective and safe parenteral drug, but can cause painful lesions unless given by deep intramuscular injection.

Haloperidol can rapidly terminate violent behavior but hypotension, although uncommon, can be severe, particularly in patients who are already critically ill.

Chlorpromazine is no longer recommended by intramuscular injection because of the formation of painful and irritating crystalline deposits in the tissues. It also causes hypotension.

In treating violent patients large doses of antipsychotics are needed. The result is that extrapyramidal toxicity, in particular acute dystonias, develop in up to a third of patients. Prophylactic anti-Parkinsonian drugs such as procyclidine may be given, especially in patients who are particularly prone to movement disorders.

The combination of lorazepam and haloperidol has been successful in otherwise resistant delirious behavior.

Oral medication, especially in liquid form is the preferred mode of administration, but rectal, intramuscular or intravenous routes may have to be used. Droperidol acts equally rapidly whether given intramuscularly or intravenously.

Antipsychotics, such as chlorpromazine, should not be given in alcohol withdrawal states, in alcoholics and those dependent on benzodiazepines because of the danger of causing fits.

Mood Disorders

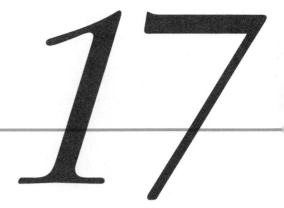

(with Roy G. Spector)

Depressive illnesses and antidepressants   **170**

Lithium and tryptophan   **177**

Special groups   **179**

DEPRESSIVE ILLNESSES AND ANTIDEPRESSANTS

Many forms of depression respond well to drugs. However, a difficulty in finding out which types of illness improve with drug treatment, is that psychiatrists often move the diagnostic goalposts: the definitions of subtypes of depression in the *Diagnostic and Statistical Manual of Mental Disorders* (American Psychiatric Association, Washington) differ in the versions of 1952, 1968, 1980, 1987 and 1992.

From a biochemical point of view there are probably different types of depression (which do not correspond predictably to clinical variants) depending on which neurotransmitter is involved, and which may respond differently to different drugs.

10 days to 3 weeks to alleviate depression. Such a long time course suggests a resetting of postsynaptic or presynaptic receptor sensitivity. For example inhibiting presynpatic receptors could down-regulate reducing feedback inhibition and leading to increased release of monoamine transmitters. There is evidence that long-term antidepressant treatment does down-regulate monoamine receptors (including presynaptic α_2-adrenoceptors). 5-Hydroxytryptamine receptors ($5HT_2$) are also down-regulated by these drugs. It is also likely that the brain stem râphé systems have a built in inertia which slows down mood changes. The pontine and medullary râphé nuclei are the main CNS sites of 5HT 1A receptors.

Pathophysiology

The monoamine theory of mood is mainly based on evidence from the actions of drugs:

1. Reserpine (which depletes neuronal stores of noradrenaline (NA) and 5-hydroxytryptamine (5HT)) and α-methyltyrosine (which inhibits NA synthesis) cause depression.
2. Tricyclic drugs of the amitriptyline type (which raise the synaptic concentration of NA and 5HT) are antidepressant.
3. Monoamine oxidase inhibitors (which increase total brain NA and 5HT) are antidepressant.

From this it was suggested that depression could be due to a cerebral deficiency of monoamines. A difficulty with this theory is that amphetamine and cocaine, which act like tricyclic drugs in raising the synaptic content of NA, are not antidepressive although they do alter mood. Even worse, the tricyclic antidepressants block amine reuptake from synapses within 1 or 2 hours of administration but take

General principles of management

1. Depression is common, but is underdiagnosed. It can be recognized during routine consultations, but additional time may be needed.
2. Patients should talk about their depression symptoms but need encouragment to do this because of feelings of shame, admission of failure and fear that the doctor will not understand (or has no time).
3. Drug treatment is not usually appropriate at the mild end of the severity range. Listening, and simple psychotherapy may be helpful. The possibility of altering social factors should be examined. Regular aerobic exercise often improves mild depression.
4. Drugs are used in more severe depression, especially with melancholic ('endogenous') features. Even if depression is related to interpersonal difficulties or other life stresses (including physical illness) antidepressant drugs may be useful. Drugs

used in the initial treatment of depression include the older tricyclics and related drugs (e.g. amitriptyline; dothiepin); other non-tricyclic amine uptake inhibitors (e.g. mianserin, viloxazine, iprindole); 5HT (serotonin) uptake inhibitors, both mixed (e.g. trazodone; lofepramine) and selective (e.g. fluvoxamine; fluoxetine); monoamine oxidase inhibitors (MAOI; e.g. phenelzine); and thioxanthenes (e.g. flupenthixol, chapter 16).

5. Major depressive episodes usually respond to tricyclic antidepressants such as amitriptyline in adequate dosage (usually 125–150 mg daily). Such drugs should be given as part of a combined therapeutic program. The aims and strategy of the various measures must be agreed with the patient, and the toxic effects of the drugs discussed before treatment is started. The delay of 10 days to 3 weeks before improvement starts should also be stressed.

6. After successful treatment of the acute episode, drug treatment is continued for at least 4–6 months to avoid relapse. The initial effective dose is maintained during this time unless toxic effects necessitate a reduction in dose. The drug is withdrawn gradually to avoid insomnia, panic and other withdrawal symptoms.

7. In refractory depression, other drug treatment or electroconvulsive therapy (ECT) are considered. Alternative drug strategies include (a) adding lithium to a tricyclic to give a lithium blood level of 0.6–0.8 mmol/l, (b) MAOI – usually prescribed only by psychiatrists, (c) MAOI plus a tricyclic – but only in expert psychiatric hands, (d) small doses of flupenthixol (for short-term treatment only).

8. Prophylaxis with lithium or a low-dose tricyclic is considered in recurrent illness as in unipolar or bipolar affective disorders. Patients and their families should be warned about the possibility of relapse and what to do if it happens. Cognitive therapy has a protective effect against relapse.

9. Electroconvulsive therapy is considered when delay for the drug to act in a major depressive episode cannot be tolerated or is hazardous.

10. Chronic mood depression (dysthymia) responds less well to drugs. Major depression can be superimposed on dysthymia (double depression) and successful treatment of the major depression may leave residual dysthymia.

11. Melancholic depression (which used to be called endogenous depression) usually responds well to tricyclics if there was a stable personality before the illness.

12. Atypical depression is used to describe depressed patients without melancholic features who respond positively to favorable life events, but are chronically oversensitive to rejection. These patients do not usually respond well to drugs. There may be a marginally better response to MAOIs than to tricyclics.

13. Major depression with psychotic features (such as delusions) requires specialist treatment. Antidepressants and antipsychotics may be needed in combination. Such patients may respond to ECT.

14. Psychiatric referral is advised if there is no response to treatment – partly because there could be a more severe underlying psychiatric illness or drug/alcohol abuse. Other important reasons for referral to a specialist center are suicide potential, violent behavior, self neglect or other forms of self harm.

15. Many of the newer antidepressants are less toxic in overdose and have different side effects from the amitriptyline type of tricyclic.

SPECIAL SITUATIONS

Tricyclics have antimuscarinic actions and can thus aggravate prostatism, constipation and glaucoma. Less antimuscarinic effects are caused by trazodone, mianserin and maprotiline or by 5HT uptake inhibitors.

Mianserin and tricyclics aggravate epilepsy. 5-Hydroxytryptamine uptake inhibitors and trazodone appear to be less toxic in this respect, but can nevertheless cause fits.

Tricyclics in overdose cause cardiac arrhythmias and mianserin or trazodone are safer in patients with heart disease.

TRICYCLICS AND RELATED ANTIDEPRESSANTS

Use

1. Depressive illnesses, in particular major depressive episodes and melancholic depression.
2. Atypical oral and facial pain.
3. Prophylaxis of panic attacks.
4. Phobic anxiety.
5. Obsessive–compulsive disorders.
6. Imipramine has some efficacy in nocturnal enuresis.

Although these drugs share many properties, their profiles vary in some respects, and this may alter their use in different patients. The more sedative drugs include amitriptyline, dothiepin and doxepin. These are more appropriate in agitated or anxious patients than withdrawn or apathetic patients in whom imipramine or nortriptyline, which are less sedative, are preferred. Protriptyline is usually stimulant.

Imipramine and amitriptyline (tertiary amines) have more powerful anticholinergic and cardiac toxic effects than secondary amines (e.g. nortriptyline).

Mechanism of action

The tricyclics block uptake 1 of monoamines into cerebral (and other) neurons. Thus the concentration of amines in the synaptic cleft rises. Imipramine has equally powerful inhibition of NA and 5HT uptake, whilst amitriptyline has a more powerful effect on 5HT. Nortriptyline acts mainly on NA uptake. In general the tertiary amines have a more powerful action on 5HT uptake than do secondary amines.

Inhibition of uptake 1 is established long before depression is alleviated and so the two events are not directly related. A slow adaptive decrease in presynaptic amine receptor (e.g. α_2) sensitivity may be the physiological basis for clinical benefit by enhancing amine release from the prejunctional neuron.

Adverse effects

1. **Autonomic (anticholinergic)** Dry mouth, constipation, rarely paralytic ileus, tachycardia, paralysis of accommodation, aggravation of narrow-angle glaucoma, postural hypotension, vomiting, retention of urine, dry skin due to loss of sweating.
2. **Central nervous system** Fine tremor, sedation, but also paradoxically sometimes insomnia, decreased rapid eye movement (REM) sleep, twitching, convulsions, dysarthria, paresthesia, ataxia. Uncommonly: confusion, mania, schizophrenic excitement. Anticholinergic and sedating actions are more pronounced with tertiary amine drugs than with secondary amines.

   Increased appetite and weight gain, particularly with the sedative tricyclics, is common. On withdrawal of the drug there may be gastrointestinal symptoms such as nausea and vomiting, headache, giddiness, shivering and insomnia. Sometimes anxiety, agitation and restlessness follow sudden withdrawal.
3. **Cardiovascular** Postural hypotension. Rarely, sudden death due to a cardiac arrhythmia. In overdose a range of tachyarrhythmias and intracardiac blocks may be produced.
4. **Allergic and idiosyncratic** reactions include marrow suppression and jaundice (both rare).

Contraindications

- Epilepsy.
- Recent myocardial infarction, heart block.
- Mania.
- Porphyria.

Pharmacokinetics

Tricyclic antidepressants, being lipid soluble, are readily absorbed from the gastrointestinal tract. Tricyclics may delay their own absorption and that of other drugs, due to their anticholinergic effect in decreasing gastric emptying rate and intestinal peristalsis.

Protein binding of these drugs is high (e.g. imipramine 85%), this and their large apparent volume of distribution (V_d) (e.g. imipramine, 28–61 l/kg body weight; nortriptyline, 25–55 l/kg) make dialysis inappropriate in overdose. These drugs are therefore present in free form in plasma only at very low concentrations after distribution. Tricyclics are extensively metabolized, and there is considerable presystemic hepatic metabolism (e.g. imipramine 53%). Demethylation of the side chain occurs commonly, thus imipramine is metabolized to desipramine and amitriptyline is similarly converted into nortriptyline. These monomethyl derivatives are pharmacologically active. Ring hydroxylation, which abolishes activity, also occurs before conjugation and excretion of polar metabolites in urine.

Studies in twins revealed a five-fold variation in $t_{1/2}$ for nortriptyline (18–93 hours) and a two-fold variation in V_d. No correlation exists between these variables in unrelated subjects, but there is good agreement within monozygotic twins, suggesting that interindividual variability in these parameters is largely genetically determined. The plasma protein binding of nortriptyline varies to give a two-fold range of unbound drug and this may also be under genetic control and so contribute to the two-fold difference in V_d.

Given this degree of variability in pharmacokinetic disposition it is not surprising that there is a wide scatter (5–30-fold) in plasma steady-state levels between individuals on the same dose. Thus patients receiving imipramine, 3.5 mg/kg/day, have steady-state plasma concentrations of 95–1020 ng/ml and nortriptyline given in a dose of 100 mg at night produces steady-state concentrations varying between 120 and 681 ng/ml. Hepatic enzyme induction is also important and lower plasma steady-state levels of tricyclic antidepressants are present in patients who smoke (nicotine and polycyclic hydrocarbons are inducing agents), drink alcohol or take barbiturates.

Only 70% of depressed patients respond adequately to tricyclic antidepressants. One explanation may be the wide variation in individual plasma concentrations of these drugs that is attained with a given dose. However, the relationship between plasma concentration and response is not well defined. A multicenter collaborative study organized by the World Health Organization failed to demonstrate any relationship whatsoever between plasma amitriptyline concentration and clinical effect. Measurement of tricyclic antidepressant concentrations in plasma may be useful in cases of suspected overdose but not as a guide to therapy.

Drug interactions

- Antagonism of antiepileptics.
- Potentiation of sedation with alcohol and other central depressants.
- Antihypertensives and diuretics increase orthostatic hypotension.
- Hypertension and cardiac arrhythmias with adrenaline, noradrenaline or ephedrine.

NON-TRICYCLIC ANTIDEPRESSANTS

This is a mixed group, and includes mianserin, viloxazine, iprindole and maprotiline. Some of these drugs have properties similar to the tricyclics.

Use

1. Maprotiline and mianserin are used in depression when sedation is needed.
2. Mianserin has little anticholinergic and cardiac toxicity and can be used when such actions have to be particularly avoided.
3. Viloxazine may be useful when tricyclics have led to an unacceptable increase in appetite and weight gain.

The efficacy of these drugs in depression is less firmly established than that of the amitriptyline group, but mianserin may be preferred in patients who are judged to be at high suicide risk.

Mechanism of action

Maprotiline is a powerful inhibitor of NA reuptake with some effect on 5HT uptake. Viloxazine has an equally powerful action on NA and 5HT reuptake. Iprindole blocks uptake 1 of NA in the brain but has no such action peripherally.

Mianserin has no effect on uptake 1 but blocks central α_2-receptors thus enhancing NA release.

Adverse effects

1. All drugs in this group can cause fits, but maprotiline especially so. Maprolitine and

viloxazine are significantly anticholinergic and have cardiovascular toxicity, but less than amitriptyline. Mianserin has little anticholinergic and cardiotoxic activity, but causes severe orthostatic hypotension.

2. Viloxazine is not sedating but causes nausea and hypotension.
3. Iprindole is mildly sedating, but mianserin is very sedating. When mianserin is given, a full blood count is needed every 4 weeks during the first 3 months of treatment, because of the risk of agranulocytosis and aplastic anemia, particularly in the elderly. If signs of infection (e.g. mouth ulcers) occur, a blood count should be obtained and mianserin discontinued if there is evidence of bone marrow suppression.

Contraindications

- Epilepsy.
- Recent myocardial infarction, heart block. However, mianserin poses little cardiac risk in such patients.

Pharmacokinetics

Generally similar to the tricyclics, with high lipophilicity and high V_d. Viloxazine is not highly protein bound and has a short half-life (2–5 hours). The half-life of mianserin is 15 hours and that of maprotiline is 48 hours.

Drug interactions

Generally similar to the tricyclics, but mianserin greatly potentiates sedation due to alcohol and other central depressants and greatly increases the severity of orthostatic hypotension with antihypertensives.

5-HYDROXYTRYPTAMINE (SEROTONIN) REUPTAKE INHIBITORS

These include drugs with a mixed action (trazodone and lofepramine) and selective serotonin reuptake inhibitors (SSRI) such as fluvoxamine, fluoxetine, paroxetine and sertraline. These drugs are safer in overdose than the amitriptyline group. Selective serotonin reuptake inhibitors do not stimulate appetite and have much less antimuscarinic side effects than the tricyclics and other catecholamine uptake inhibitors.

Use

1. In depression (but have similar efficacy to tricyclics and are much more expensive).
2. In chronic anxiety and as prophylaxis for panic attacks.

SSRI are also useful in:

3. Obsessive compulsive states.
4. Bulimia nervosa.
5. Seasonal affective disorder, especially accompanied by carbohydrate craving and weight gain.
6. Possibly effective as prophylactic agents in recurrent depression.

Selective serotonin reuptake inhibitors are well tolerated in the elderly.

Mechanism of action

Selective serotonin reuptake inhibitors block neuronal uptake of 5HT and do not primarily influence other neurotransmitter systems. Trazodone has additional direct blocking action on some 5HT receptors and α_2 prejunctional adrenoceptors.

5-Hydroxytryptamine pathways influence mood and behavior and regulate appetite, sleep, aggression and anxiety levels. Selective serotonin reuptake inhibitors augment 5HT activity in depression without unwanted effects on histamine, cholinergic and noradrenergic pathways.

Adverse effects

1. The most common adverse actions of SSRI are nausea, dyspepsia, diarrhea, dry mouth, headache, insomnia and dizziness. These tend to become less severe after 1–2 months of treatment.
2. Selective serotonin reuptake inhibitors have less anticholinergic and cardiotoxic actions than the amitriptyline group. Trazodone has very little anticholinergic and cardiac toxicity. Epilepsy can be precipitated.

3. Trazodone is very sedating; lofepramine is less sedating. Selective serotonin reuptake inhibitors are usually non-sedating but may cause insomnia and do not usually cause orthostatic hypotension.
4. Fluoxetine has been associated with a rare fatal systemic vasculitis of which rash may be the first clinical sign. It has also been said to cause violent and suicidal thoughts, but such thoughts are more likely to be due to the underlying psychiatric illness for which the drug is used.
5. Trazodone, rarely, can cause priapism. Delayed ejaculation affects a substantial minority of men treated with sertraline.

Contraindications
- Hepatic and renal failure.
- Epilepsy.

Pharmacokinetics

Trazodone has a shorter half-life (4 hours) than the tricyclics.

Selective serotonin reuptake inhibitors have similar pharmacokinetic profiles, but differ in their half-lives. The elimination half-lives of fluvoxamine, paroxetine and sertraline range from 15 to 30 hours, while fluoxetine has a half-life of approximately 2 days and its active metabolite, norfluoxetine, a half-life of approximately 7 days.

Drug interactions
- Combinations of SSRI with lithium, tryptophan or MAOI may enhance efficacy, but are currently contraindicated because they increase the severity of 5HT-related toxicity. In the worst reactions, the life-threatening 5HT syndrome develops. This consists of hyperthermia, restlessness, tremor, myoclonus, hyperreflexia, coma and fits. After using MAOI it is recommended that 2 weeks elapse before starting SSRI. Avoid fluoxetine for at least 5 weeks before MAOI.
- The action of warfarin is probably enhanced by fluoxetine and paroxetine.
- Antagonism of anticonvulsants.
- Fluoxetine raises blood concentrations of haloperidol.

MONOAMINE OXIDASE INHIBITORS

These drugs were little used for many years because of their toxicity, in particular potentially lethal food and drug interactions causing hypertensive crises. Non-selective MAOI should only be prescribed by specialists experienced in their use. They can be effective in some forms of refractory depression and anxiety states, for which they are generally reserved. The recent introduction of moclobemide, a reversible selective MAO-A inhibitor, may lead to more widespread use of this therapeutic class.

Tranylcypromine is the most hazardous because of its stimulant activity. The non-selective MAOI of choice are phenelzine and isocarboxazid.

Use
1. Monoamine oxidase inhibitors can be used alone or (with close psychiatric supervision) with a tricyclic antidepressant, in depression which has not responded to tricyclic antidepressants.
2. In phobic anxiety and depression with anxiety.
3. In patients with anxiety who have agoraphobia, panic attacks or multiple somatic symptoms.
4. Hypochondria and hysterical symptoms may respond well.
5. For atypical depression with biological features such as hypersomnia, lethargy and hyperphagia.

Mechanism of action

Phenelzine, isocarboxazid and tranylcypromine irreversibly inhibit both A and B forms of monoamine oxidase. Inhibition of the A form decreases deamination of NA and (to a lesser extent) 5HT. The antidepressant effect is presumably related in some way to the increase in vesicular neuronal stores of NA and 5HT. However, the extent of improvement of patients on MAO varies considerably and may be slow, some patients requiring treatment for 6–8 weeks before showing effect. Clinical efficacy of MAOI does not correspond to their efficacy in MAO inhibition. The stores of adrenaline and NA in the adrenal medulla and NA in peripheral sympathetic nerves also increase. This is part of the basis of the hypertensive crisis due to massive release of these amines when indirectly acting sympathomimetic drugs are given concurrently.

Selective inhibitors of MAO-B preferentially decrease deamination of dopamine. This happens with theraputic doses of selegiline (Chapter 18). Higher doses (such as 30 mg) inhibit both A and B types of MAO and have antidepressant activity.

Adverse effects

1. Common: orthostatic hypotension, weight gain, sexual dysfunction, headache and aggravation of migraine, insomnia, anticholinergic actions, edema.
2. Rare and potentially fatal: hypertensive crisis and 5HT syndrome (see interactions), psychotic reactions, hepatocellular necrosis, peripheral neuropathy, convulsions.
3. Stopping a MAOI is more likely to produce a withdrawal syndrome than with tricyclics. The syndrome includes agitation, restlessness, panic attacks and insomnia.

Contraindiations

- Liver failure.
- Cerebrovascular disease.
- Pheochromocytoma.
- Porphyria.
- Epilepsy.

Pharmacokinetics

Monoamine oxidase inhibitors are generally lipophilic and are well absorbed from the gut. They freely penetrate cell membranes and the blood–brain barrier. The hydrazine MAOI produce irreversible inhibition of monoamine oxidase whilst the inhibition produced by the non-hydrazines is reversible. Thus with many of the MAOI, even after cessation of treatment when the drug can no longer be detected in the body, the effects of treatment persist and dangerous toxicity may arise until new enzyme is synthesized, a process that requires several weeks.

Hydrazine MAOI are partly metabolized by acetylation, and slow acetylators more frequently experience toxicity. Differences in therapeutic responsiveness can be detected between acetylator phenotypes. Blood concentration studies relating to clinical effect are not available but would not be expected to correlate usefully with response in the case of irreversible enzyme inhibitors. In one trial depressed patients treated with phenelzine demonstrating an 80% inhibition of platelet monoamine oxidase were more likely to benefit than those with less enzyme inhibition. The relationship between peripheral and central inhibition of monoamine oxidase is unclear.

It has been suggested that response to MAOI is genetically determined and that efficacy could be predicted in a patient if the response of a first-degree relative to the same drug were known. This possible pharmacogenetic variation could reflect biochemical factors, but more evidence is required before it can be accepted.

Drug interactions

Many important interactions occur with MAOI. A treatment card for patients should be carried at all times. It describes precautions and lists some of the foods to be avoided. The interactions are:

- Hypertensive and hyperthermic reactions sufficient to cause fatal subarachnoid hemorrhage, particularly with tranylcypromine. Such serious reactions are precipitated by amines, including indirectly acting sympathomimetic agents such as tyramine (in cheese), dopamine (in broad bean pods and formed from levodopa), amines formed from any fermentation process (as in yoghurt, beer, wine), phenylephrine (including that administered as nose drops and in cold remedies), ephedrine, amphetamine (all can give hypertensive reactions); other amines: pethidine (excitement, hyperthermia), levodopa (hypertension); tricyclic, tetracyclic and bicyclic antidepressants (excitement, hyperpyrexia). Buspirone should not be used with MAOI. Hypertensive crisis may be treated with α-adrenoceptor blockade analogous to medical treatment of patients with pheochromocytoma (chapter 37). Interactions of this type are much less likely to occur with moclobemide since its MAO inhibition is reversible, competitive and selective for MAO-A. MAO-B is free to deaminate biogenic amines. Although experience with moclobemide is limited its side effect profile is similar to that of placebo, and it appears to be relatively safe in overdose.

- Failure to metabolize drugs that are normally oxidized: opioids, benzodiazepines, alcohol (reactions with alcoholic drinks occur mainly because of their tyramine content). These drugs will have an exaggerated and prolonged effect.
- Enhanced effects of oral hypoglycemic agents, anesthetics, suxamethonium, caffeine, anticholinergics (including benzhexol and similar anti-Parkinsonian drugs).
- Antagonism of antiepileptics.
- Enhanced hypotension with antihypertensives.
- Central nervous system (CNS) excitation and hypertension with oxypertine (an antipsychotic) and tetrabenazine (used for chorea).
- Increased CNS toxicity with sumatriptan.

*L*ITHIUM AND TRYPTOPHAN

LITHIUM

Although lithium is widely used in affective disorders, it has a low toxic to therapeutic ratio and serum concentration monitoring is essential. Serum is used rather than plasma because of possible problems due to lithium heparin which is often used as an anticoagulant. Plasma lithium fluctuates between doses and serum concentrations should be measured at a standard time: 12 hours after the previous dose. This measurement is made frequently until steady state is attained and then every 3 months, unless some intercurrent event occurs that could cause toxicity such as desalination or diuretic therapy.

Use

Lithium is effective in acute mania, but its action is slow (1–2 weeks) so antipsychotic drugs such as haloperidol are preferred in this situation (see chapter 16 on drugs in schizophrenia). Its main use is in prophylaxis in unipolar and bipolar affective illness (therapeutic serum levels 0.4–0.8 mmol/l). Lithium is also used on its own or with another antidepressant in refractory depression to terminate a depressive episode or prevent recurrences and aggressive or self-mutilating behavior.

Patients should avoid major dietary changes that alter sodium intake and maintain an adequate water intake.

Different lithium preparations have different bioavailabilities and so the form should not be changed.

Mechanism of action

Lithium increases 5HT actions in the CNS. It acts as a $5HT_{1A}$ agonist, and is also a $5HT_2$ antagonist. This may be the basis for its antidepressant activity and why it increases the CNS toxicity of selective 5HT uptake inhibitors.

The basic biochemical activity of lithium is not known. It has actions on two second messengers:

1. Hormone stimulation of adenylyl cyclase is inhibited, so that hormone-stimulated cyclic adenosine monophosphate (cAMP) production is reduced; this probably underlies some of the adverse effects of lithium such as goiter and nephrogenic diabetes insipidus since thyroid-stimulating hormone (TSH) and antidiuretic hormone activate

adenylyl cyclase in thyroid and collecting duct cells, respectively. Relevance to therapeutic effect is uncertain.

2. Lithium at a concentration of 1 mM inhibits hydrolysis of myoinositol phosphate in brain so lithium may reduce the cellular content of phosphatidyl inositides so altering the sensitivity of neurons to neurotransmitters that work on receptors linked to phospholipase C (including muscarinic and α-receptors).

From these actions it is clear that lithium can modify a wide range of neurotransmitter effects, but its efficacy in both mania and in depression indicates a subtlety of action that is presently unexplained, but may be related to activation of the brain stem râphé nuclei.

Adverse effects

1. When monitored regularly lithium is reasonably safe in the medium term. However, adverse effects occur even in the therapeutic range: in particular tremor, weight gain, edema, polyuria, nausea and loose bowels.
2. Above the therapeutic range (1.3–3 mmol/l) tremor coarsens, diarrhea becomes more severe and ataxia and dysarthria appear. High levels (3–5 mmol/l) cause gross ataxia, coma, fits, cardiac arrhythmias and death.
3. Goiter, hypothyroidism and exacerbation of psoriasis are less common.
4. Renal tubular damage has been described in association with prolonged use.

Contraindications

- Renal disease.
- Cardiac disease.
- Sodium losing states (e.g. Addison's disease, diarrhea, vomiting).
- Myasthenia gravis.
- During surgical operations.
- Avoid when possible during pregnancy and breast feeding.

Pharmacokinetics

Lithium is readily absorbed after oral administration and injectable preparations are not available. Peak plasma concentrations occur 3–5 hours after dosing. The $t_{1/2}$ varies with age because of the progressive decline in glomerular filtration rate, being 18–20 hours in young adults and up to 36 hours in healthy elderly persons. Sustained release preparations are available, but in view of the long $t_{1/2}$ they are not kinetically justified. The evidence that they produce more even plasma levels is not established. They are erratically absorbed in the upper gut and can cause lower intestinal upset. The long absorption $t_{1/2}$ also means that it takes several days to reach steady state and the first samples for plasma level monitoring should be taken after about a week unless loading doses are given. Lithium elimination is almost entirely renal. Like sodium, lithium does not bind to plasma protein and readily passes into the glomerular filtrate; 70–80% is reabsorbed in the proximal tubules but, unlike sodium, there is no distal tubular reabsorption and its elimination is not *directly* altered by diuretics acting on the distal tubule. However, states such as sodium deficiency and sodium diuresis increase lithium retention (and cause toxicity) by stimulating proximal tubular sodium and lithium reabsorption. An important implication of the renal handling of lithium is that neither loop diuretics, thiazides nor potassium-sparing diuretics can enhance lithium loss in a toxic patient but all do enhance toxicity. Dialysis reduces elevated plasma lithium concentration effectively.

Drug interactions

- Lithium concentration in plasma is increased by diuretics and non-steroidal anti-inflammatory drugs.
- Lithium toxicity is increased by concomitant administration of haloperidol, serotonin uptake inhibitors, calcium antagonists (such as diltiazem) and anticonvulsants (phenytoin and carbamazepine) without change in plasma concentration.
- Lithium increases the incidence of extrapyramidal effects of antipsychotics.

L-TRYPTOPHAN

Tryptophan is the amino acid precursor of 5HT. On its own or with other antidepressants or lithium it sometimes benefits refractory forms of depression. However, L-tryptophan has been withdrawn from general use because of its association with an eosinophilic myalgic syndrome characterized by intense and incapacitating fatigue, myalgia and eosinophilia. Arthralgia, fever, cough, dyspnea and rash may also develop over several weeks. The eosinophil count usually exceeds $2000/\mu l$. A few patients develop myocarditis.

L-Tryptophan remains available on a named patient basis, for those whom no other treatment has helped.

SPECIAL GROUPS

THE ELDERLY

Depression is common in the elderly in whom it tends to be chronic and has a high rate of recurrence. Treatment with drugs is made more difficult because of slow metabolism and sensitivity to anticholinergic effects. Lower doses are therefore needed than in younger patients.

Lack of response may indicate true refractoriness of the depression, sadness due to social isolation or bereavement. The possibility of underlying disease such as hypothyroidism (which increases in incidence with age) should be considered.

Lofepramine and SSRI cause fewer problems in patients with prostatism or glaucoma than do the tricyclic antidepressants because they have less antimuscarinic action. Dizziness and falls due to orthostatic hypotension are less common with nortriptyline than imipramine. Mianserin has fewer anticholinergic actions but blood dyscrasias occur in about 1 in 4000 patients.

EPILEPSY

No currently used antidepressive is entirely safe in epilepsy, but SSRI are less likely to cause fits than the amitriptyline group, mianserin or maprotiline.

SUICIDE

Successful suicide is a less likely outcome with overdoses of mianserin, trazodone and SSRI than with maprotiline and the amitriptyline group.

SEASONAL AFFECTIVE DISORDER

Seasonal affective disorder many respond well to SSRI, as well as to summer sky fluorescent tube lighting.

Movement Disorders

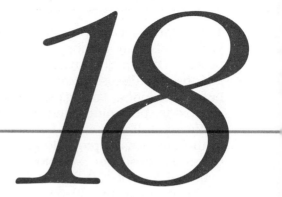

Parkinsonism **182**

Spasticity **188**

Chorea **189**

Dyskinesias **189**

Treatment of other movement disorders **190**

Myasthenia gravis **190**

*P*ARKINSONISM

Pathophysiology

The principal clinical features of Parkinsonism are tremor, rigidity and bradykinesia. The major types are idiopathic Parkinson's disease, toxic (phenothiazines, butyrophenones, manganese and carbon monoxide poisoning) and postencephalitic. Parkinson's disease arises because of cell loss in the nigrostriatal projection and its connections. Parkinsonian symptoms occur after neuronal loss of >70–80% of nerve terminals in the striatum and 50–60% of nerve terminals in the substantia nigra. The nigrostriatal projection consists of very fine nerve fibers travelling from the zona compacta of the substantia nigra to the corpus striatum. This pathway is dopaminergic and inhibitory and the motor projections to the putamen are more affected than both those to the cognitive areas (caudate nucleus and the nucleus accumbens) and to the limbic and hypolimbic regions (Fig. 18.1). Other fibers terminating in the corpus striatum include excitatory cholinergic nerves, noradrenergic and serotoninergic fibers and these are also affected, but to varying extents and the overall effect is a complex imbalance between inhibitory and excitatory influences.

Parkinsonism arises because of deficient transmission at the postsynaptic D_2 receptors, but it appears that stimulation of both D_1 and D_2 is required for optimal response. D_1 receptors activate adenylyl cyclase which

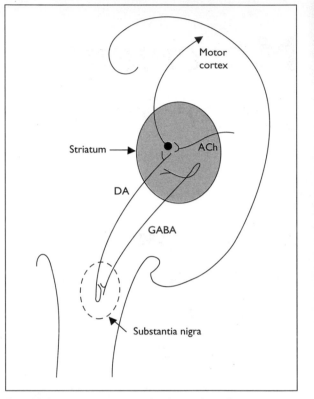

Fig. 18.1 Representation of relationships between cholinergic (ACh), dopaminergic (DA) and GABA-producing neurons in the basal ganglia.

increases intracellular cyclic adenosine monophosphate (cAMP). The antagonistic effects of dopamine and acetylcholine within the striatum have suggested that Parkinsonism results from an imbalance

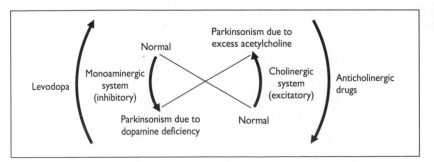

Fig. 18.2 Antagonistic actions of the monoaminergic and cholinergic systems in the production of Parkinsonian symptoms.

between these neurotransmitters (Fig. 18.2). Treatment of Parkinsonism generally involves either a drug that increases dopaminergic activity or reduces the effects of acetylcholine. Ideally, treatment of Parkinsonism should start with removal of the cause; however, in most patients with chronic progressive Parkinsonism this is unknown. Exposure to toxic agents has been considered. 1-Methyl-4-phenyl-1,2,5,6-tetrahydropyridine (MPTP) has been used illicitly on the west coast of the USA as a 'designer drug' and causes severe Parkinsonism. It is converted, in neuronal mitochondria, by the enzyme monoamine oxidase-B (MAO-B) to a toxic free radical metabolite (MPP$^+$). This has led to the hypothesis that idiopathic Parkinsonism may be due to chronic free radical damage to the cells of the substantia nigra. Evidence supporting the hypothesis that excess free radicals are formed in the substantia nigra is (1) mitochondrial glutathione (a free radical scavenger) is low; (2) superoxide dismutase activity is high; (3) the high concentration of monoamine oxidase; and (4) reduced activity of mitochondrial enzyme complex-I in the substantia nigra (this complex is inhibited by MPP$^+$). Free radical scavengers prevent or retard the progression of MPTP-induced extrapyramidal disease in primate models. Selegiline (an anti-Parkinsonian drug that reduces MAO-B activity, thus reducing the formation of free radicals) also has moderate clinical activity in reducing the symptoms and perhaps also the rate of progression of idiopathic Parkinson's disease.

Principles of treatment in Parkinsonism

Drugs producing Parkinsonism, notably the antipsychotics (chapter 16), are withdrawn if possible. Idiopathic Parkinson's disease is a progressive disorder. Treatment consists of using the drugs available to relieve symptoms and if possible reduce the rate of progression

of the disease. Presently there is no consensus as to the best treatment plan to achieve this. In the mildest cases drug treatment may be postponed. However, there is preliminary evidence that selegiline retards the progression of the disease and delays the time until more powerful drugs are required.

In patients with definite disability, treatment should include a levodopa/decarboxylase inhibitor combination, the dose being titrated to produce optimal results. The occurrence of motor fluctuations (on–off phenomena) heralds a more drastic phase of the illness. Initially such fluctuations may be controlled by giving more frequent doses of levodopa (or a sustained release preparation). Addition of a dopamine receptor agonist (e.g. bromocriptine) to the regime may be useful. If on–off phenomena are refractory the dopamine agonist apomorphine will reverse most 'off' periods after 15 min, but its use is complex (see below). Physiotherapy and psychological support are helpful. The experimental approach of implantation of fetal adrenal cells into the substantia nigra of severely affected Parkinsonian patients (perhaps with low-dose immunosuppression) offers an exciting possibility for the future.

Anti-Parkinsonian drugs

MUSCARINIC RECEPTOR ANTAGONISTS

Use

Muscarinic antagonists (e.g. benzhexol, benztropine) are effective in the treatment of Parkinsonian tremor and to a lesser extent rigidity, but produce only slight improvement in bradykinesia. They are usually given in divided doses, which are increased every 2–5 days until optimum benefit is achieved or until toxic effects occur. Their main use is in patients with Parkinsonism caused by antipsychotic drugs in whom these cannot be withdrawn.

Table 18.1 Common muscarinic receptor antagonists.

Drug	Route of administration	Half-life	Metabolism and excretion	Dose (mg)	Special features
Benzhexol	Oral	3–7 hours	Hepatic	1–4 mg tds Maximum 15 mg/day	
Orphenadrine	Oral	13.7–16.1hours	Hepatic-active metabolite	150–400 mg dose ×2/day	Central stimulation
Procylidine	Oral	12.6 hours	Hepatic	2.5 mg tds Maximum 60 mg	

Mechanism of action

These synthetic antimuscarinic drugs block central muscarinic receptors, similar to atropine.

Adverse effects

1. Dry mouth, blurred vision.
2. Possible precipitation of glaucoma and urinary retention; they are therefore contraindicated in some forms of glaucoma and prostatic hypertrophy.
3. Constipation.
4. Confusion and excitement (especially in the elderly).

Pharmacokinetics.

Table 18.1 lists some drugs of this type in common use, with their major pharmacokinetic properties.

Drugs affecting the dopaminergic system

Dopaminergic activity can be enhanced by:

1. Administration of levodopa with a peripheral dopa decarboxylase inhibitor.
2. Release of endogenous dopamine.
3. Stimulation of dopamine receptors.
4. Inhibition of monoamine oxidase type B (MAO-B).

Levodopa and dopa decarboxylase inhibitors

Use

Levodopa (unlike dopamine) can enter nerve terminals in the basal ganglia where it undergoes decarboxylation to form dopamine, partially correcting the nigrostriatal deficiency and improving rigidity and bradykinesia. Levodopa is used in combination with a peripheral (extracerebral) dopa decarboxylase inhibitor (e.g. carbidopa or benserazide). This allows a four- to five-fold reduction in levodopa dose. Clinical benefit appears early (1–2 weeks), and the incidence of vomiting and arrhythmias is reduced. Central adverse effects (e.g. hallucinations) are, however, as common as when large doses of levodopa were given without a dopa decarboxylase inhibitor.

Combined preparations (co-careldopa or co-beneldopa) are available and appropriate. These are given thrice daily starting at a low dose, increased initially after 2 weeks and then reviewed at 6–8 weeks intervals. Without a dopa decarboxylase inhibitor, 95% of levodopa is metabolized outside the brain. In their presence, plasma levodopa concentrations rise (Fig. 18.3), excretion of dopamine and its metabolites falls, and availability of levodopa within the brain for

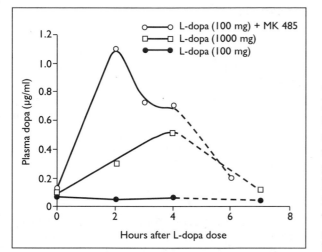

Fig. 18.3 Increased plasma dopa concentrations following combination with a peripheral dopa decarboxylase inhibitor in one patient. (From D.L. Dunner *et al. Clin Pharm Ther* 1971; **12**: 213.)

conversion to dopamine increases. The two available inhibitors are similar.

Adverse effects

1. Nausea and vomiting: this has been reduced with the lower doses of levodopa that are effective when coadministered with a decarboxylase inhibitor.
2. Postural hypotension does not usually persist after the first few weeks, but excessive hypotension may result if antihypertensive treatment is given concurrently.
3. Involuntary movements (dystonic reactions), akathisia (abnormal restlessness and inability to keep still), chorea and jerking of the limbs (myoclonus). Involuntary movements may become worse as treatment is continued and may necessitate drug withrawal.
4. Psychological disturbances: vivid and disturbing dreams; agitation, paranoia, confusion, hallucinations, depression.
5. Cardiac arrhythmias.
6. Endocrine effects of levodopa include stimulation of growth hormone and suppression of prolactin.

Contraindications

- Hypomania and schizophrenia.
- Closed angle glaucoma.

Pharmacokinetics

Levodopa is absorbed from the proximal small intestine and is broken down both by decarboxylases in the intestinal wall and by the gut flora. Oral absorption is therefore somewhat variable. Absorption is improved by coadministration of decarboxylase inhibitors. The plasma $t_{1/2}$ following intravenous infusion is short (30–60 min) and is only moderately prolonged (by about 30%) by decarboxylase blockade. Following oral administration of 15 mg/kg levodopa, peak plasma concentrations occur at 1–2 hours.

Drug interactions

Monoamine oxidase inhibitors can produce hypertensive reactions if given concurrently with levodopa. The hypotensive actions of other drugs are potentiated by levodopa.

Release of endogenous dopamine

AMANTIDINE

Use

Amantidine seldom produces substantial clinical improvement, but approximately 60% of patients experience some benefit. The usual dose is 100 mg twice daily. Severe toxicity is rare.

Mechanism of action

Endogenous dopamine release is stimulated by amantadine, which also inhibits reuptake of dopamine into nerve terminals.

Adverse effects

1. Nightmares, insomnia, dizziness, hallucinations, convulsions.
2. Gastrointestinal upsets and dry mouth.

3. Peripheral edema.
4. Livedo reticularis.
5. Leukopenia (uncommon).

Pharmacokinetics

Amantidine $t_{1/2}$ varies from 10 to 30 hours, so steady-state concentrations are reached after 4–7 days of treatment. It is 95% eliminated by the kidney and should not be used in patients with renal failure.

Dopamine receptor agonists

BROMOCRIPTINE, LYSURIDE, PERGOLIDE AND APOMORPHINE

Use

These are used as adjuncts to levodopa–dopa decarboxylase inhibitor combinations in patients with severe motor fluctuations.

Mechanism of action

Agents in this group are dopaminergic (postsynaptic-D_2) agonists. Pergolide and apomorphine, unlike other drugs in this group, stimulate both D_1 and D_2 receptors.

BROMOCRIPTINE

See also chapter 39.

Use

Bromocriptine is used in conjunction with levodopa–dopa decarboxylase inhibitors, especially in patients showing motor fluctuations (on–off phenomena). There is great individual variation in its efficacy. It is seldom more effective than levodopa and has more marked toxic effects. Its plasma $t_{1/2}$ is 6–8 hours, i.e. longer than that of levodopa. The initial dose is 1 mg at night increased to a total of 10–40 mg in three divided doses. Bromocriptine improves rigidity, tremor and bradykinesia.

LYSURIDE

Use

Use is similar to bromocriptine, and is in addition to stimulating D_2 receptors, an agonist at 5-hydroxytryptamine receptors ($5HT_1$ and $5HT_2$). The starting dose is 200 µg with food at bedtime increasing to a maximum of 5 mg daily in four divided doses.

Adverse effects

These are primarily due to its D_2 agonist activity:

1. Nausea and vomiting, constipation, diarrhea. Nausea can be prevented by pretreatment with the peripheral dopamine receptor antagonist domperidone.
2. Headache, drowsiness, central nervous system (CNS) disturbances.
3. Confusion and orthostatic hypotension (particularly in the elderly).
4. Cardiac arrhythmias – bradycardia.

Pharmacokinetics

Following oral administration absorption is complete, but there is variable first-pass metabolism, yielding a bioavailability of 10–25%. The $t_{1/2}$ is approximately 8 hours and the drug undergoes extensive hepatic metabolism.

PERGOLIDE

Use

This drug is an ergot derivative and best suited to patients with motor fluctuations (on–off phenomena) and with dyskinesias. It is only licensed for use in combination with levodopa, allowing a reduction in levodopa dose. It is best started at a dose of 50 µg at bedtime increasing to 2–5 mg daily in divided doses.

Adverse effects

These are primarily related to its dopaminergic activity and similar to those of lysuride.

Pharmacokinetics

It is rapidly absorbed following oral administration with extensive hepatic metabolism, and a plasma $t_{1/2}$ of 15–42 hours.

Drug interactions

Patients already on selegiline are more prone to psychosis when pergolide is added.

APOMORPHINE

Apomorphine is a powerful dopamine agonist at both D_1 and D_2 receptors and can lead to sustained improvements in patients with refractory motor oscillations (on–off phenomena). It is, however, difficult to use and its use demands specialist input. The problems in its use stem from its pharmacokinetics and side effects, which can only be controlled by coadministration of domperidone. It is extensively hepatically metabolized and is given parenterally. Mean plasma $t_{1/2}$ is only 30 min. Apomorphine treatment is initiated as an inpatient, with pretreatment with domperidone (20–40 mg in divided doses), to control its side effects of nausea, vomiting, postural hypotension and sedation. Initially 0.5 mg is given subcutaneously every 2 hours when an 'off' state is reached. The dose is increased and when the individual dose requirement has been established, administration is changed from intermittent dosing to subcutaneous infusion via a syringe pump.

Monoamine oxidase type B inhibitors

SELEGILINE

Use

One small controlled trial in Parkinson's disease reported that disease progression is slowed in patients treated with selegiline alone, delaying the need to start levodopa. This awaits confirmation. Selegiline is used in conjunction with levodopa and allows a dose reduction of approximately 30% and prolongs the duration of action of levodopa. It is given as a single oral dose of 10 mg in the morning or as two divided doses of 5 mg at breakfast and lunch.

Mechanism of action

There are two forms of monoamine oxidase (MAO): type A (substrates include 5-hydroxytryptamine and tyramine) and type B (substrates include phenylethylamine, benzylamine and tyramine). Pargyline [(an antidepressant monoamine oxidase inhibitor (MAOI)] inhibits both MAO-A and MAO-B. Selegiline selectively and irreversibly inhibits only MAO-B which is mainly localized in neuroglia. Monoamine oxidase type A metabolizes adrenaline, noradrenaline and 5-hydroxytryptamine, while the physiological role of MAO-B is unclear. Both isoenzymes metabolize dopamine. Inhibition of MAO-B could raise brain dopamine levels without affecting other major transmitter amines. Because selegiline selectively inhibits MAO-B, it is much less liable to produce a hypertensive reaction with cheese or other sources of tyramine than non-selective MAOI such as pargyline, iproniazid and phenelzine. It is proposed that any effect of selegiline on retarding the rate of progression of Parkinson's disease is not related to its effect of increasing neuronal dopamine (by MAO-B inhibition and by inhibiting catecholamine reuptake) but to its reducing the activity of MAO-B in producing free radicals and its effect of increasing the activity of superoxide dismutase in the striatum.

Adverse effects

Selegiline is generally well tolerated; side effects are:

1. Agitation and involuntary movements.
2. Confusion, insomnia and hallucinations.
3. Nausea.

Pharmacokinetics

Oral selegiline is well absorbed (100%), but is extensively metabolized by the liver, first to an active metabolite, desmethylselegiline (that also inhibits MAO-B) and then to amphetamine and metamphetamine. Its plasma $t_{1/2}$ is long (with a mean of 39 hours).

Drug interactions

Hypertension occurs at very high doses (60 mg/day: six times the therapeutic dose), MAO-B selectivity is lost and pressor responses to tyramine are potentiated. Hypertensive reactions to tyramine-containing products (e.g. cheese or yeast extract) have been described but are rare. Amantadine and centrally active antimuscarinic agents potentiate the anti-Parkinsonian effects of selegiline.

SPASTICITY

Spasticity is the increase in muscle tone which accompanies decrease in voluntary muscle power due to damage to the cortico-motorneuron pathways in the brain or spinal cord. It can be painful as well as disabling, and is an important problem in patients with upper motor neuron lesions (e.g. following neck injuries to the cord, following stroke, in some patients with multiple sclerosis and in congenital or perinatal spasticity). Treatment is seldom very effective, but physiotherapy or limited surgical release procedures have some place. Drugs that reduce spasticity include diazepam, baclofen and dantrolene, but they have considerable limitations.

Diazepam (chapter 15) facilitates γ-aminobutyric acid (GABA) action. Although spasticity and flexor spasms may be diminished, sedating doses are needed to produce this.

Baclofen also reduces spasticity and flexor spasms by stimulating GABA-β receptors. Effective doses are 5–20 mg 8 hourly. Larger doses cause fits. Less sedation is produced than by equieffective doses of diazepam (15–50 mg daily) but can cause vertigo, nausea and hypotension. Recently there has been interest in administration of low doses of baclofen intrathecally via chronically implanted intrathecal cannulae to maximize efficacy without causing side effects.

DANTROLENE

Use

Dantrolene is less generally useful for symptoms of spasticity than baclofen because muscle power is reduced as spasticity is relieved. It is used intravenously to treat malignant hyperthermia and the neuroleptic malignant syndrome, for both of which it is uniquely effective (chapter 21).

Mechanism of action

Dantrolene acts directly on striated muscle and inhibits excitation–contraction coupling by inhibiting the release of calcium ions from the sarcoplasmic reticulum by blocking calcium channels in the sarcoplasmic reticulum. It is a ryanodine receptor antagonist.

Adverse effects

1. Drowsiness, vertigo, malaise, weakness and fatigue.
2. Diarrhea.
3. Increased serum potassium.

Drug interactions

Calcium channel blockers and intravenous dantrolene cause severe cardiac depression.

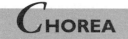HOREA

γ-Aminobutryic acid content in the basal ganglia is reduced in patients with Huntington's chorea. Neuroleptics and tetrabenazine are equally effective in suppressing choreiform movements, but neuroleptics are best avoided in these conditions as they can themselves induce dyskinesias. Tetrabenazine depletes neuronal terminals of dopamine and serotonin, and is given in doses of 25 mg twice daily increasing to 50 mg three or four times a day. It can cause severe dose related depression. Diazepam may be useful.

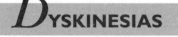YSKINESIAS

Neuroleptic drugs can produce any kind of dyskinesia including (1) drug-induced Parkinsonism; (2) acute dystonic reactions; (3) akathisia; and (4) chronic tardive dyskinesias.

1. Drug-induced Parkinsonism is due to a reduction in dopamine effects in the striatum. Antipsychotic drugs vary in their propensity to produce Parkinsonism because of their varying antimuscarinic activities (high antimuscarinic activity reducing Parkinsonian activity).
2. Acute dystonic reactions can be induced by several antipsychotic drugs or metoclopramide. About 2–10% of patients treated with phenothiazines (especially of the piperazine type), butyrophenones or thioxanthenes develop dystonia. Drug-induced dystonic reactions are caused by an increase in transmitter turnover. This usually occurs in younger patients, and develops rapidly, usually within 48 hours of the start of treatment. There is abrupt onset of torticollis, facial grimacing, dysarthria, labored breathing and involuntary movements. Accompanying these may be scoliosis, lordosis, opisthotonus and dystonic gait. The signs can be abolished by an intravenous injection of 2 mg benztropine, or 5–10 mg procyclidine or l0 mg diazepam.

3. Akathisia is a state of intense restlessness and can be provoked by all the neuroleptic drugs, metoclopramide or by levodopa. There is inability to keep the limbs still or a compulsion to walk or run and an inability to remain seated. Akathisia may begin within days, weeks or months of starting treatment. The pharmacological basis of akathisia is unknown, but is presumably an extrapyramidal disturbance as it may occur with idiopathic Parkinsonism. When drugs have provoked akathisia, it may resolve before or after cessation of drug therapy. Anticholinergic drugs such as benztropine may help.
4. Tardive dyskinesias consist of orofacial chewing and sucking movements, often accompanied by distal limb chorea and dystonia of the trunk. About 15% of patients treated with neuroleptics for over 2 years develop this complication. If treatment is continued, the syndrome persists, but stopping the neuroleptics results in slow improvement in only 40% of patients and sometimes dyskinesia worsens. Tardive dyskinesia is thought to result from the development of 'denervation hypersensitivity' in dopaminergic post-synaptic receptors of the nigrostriatal pathway following chronic receptor blockade by neuroleptics. It is therefore due to a relative preponderance of dopaminergic

effects. This accounts for its exacerbation by drug discontinuation, because of the reduction in receptor blockade, and allows more dopamine to stimulate the sensitized receptors. Administration of increased doses of dopamine antagonists paradoxi-cally initially improves tardive dyskinesia. Use of these drugs in this way can lead to escalating doses, more and more drug being required to suppress the dyskinesia. Neither tetrabenazine nor reserpine cause tardive dyskinesias.

TREATMENT OF OTHER MOVEMENT DISORDERS

Botulinum toxin A

Botulinum toxin A is one of seven distinct neurotoxins produced by *Clostridium botulinum*, which is a glycoprotein. It is available for clinical use as *Clostridium botulinum* toxin A–hemagglutinin complex. It is used by specialists to treat hemifacial spasm, blepharospasm, cervical dystonia (torticollis), jaw closing oromandibular dystonia and adductor laryngeal dysphonia, by local injection into affected muscles, the site of injection being best identified by electromyography. Injection of botulinum toxin A into a muscle weakens it by blocking the release of acetylcholine at the neuromuscular junction. Muscles injected with botulinum toxin A atrophy and become weak over 2–20 days and recover over 2–4 months as new axon terminals sprout and restore transmission. Repeated injections can then be given. Most patients continue to respond to repeated injections over a 5–10 year period. Long-term side effects have presently not been noted, but the best long-term treatment plan is not established. Symptoms are seldom abolished and adjuvant conventional therapy should be given. Adverse effects due to toxin spread causing weakness of nearby muscles and local autonomic dysfunction can occur. In the neck this may cause dysphagia and aspiration into the lungs. Electromyography has detected evidence of systemic spread of the toxin, but generalized weakness does not occur with standard doses. Occasionally a flu-like reaction with brachial neuritis has been reported, suggesting an acute immune response to the bacterial toxin. Neutralizing antibodies to the botulinum toxin A cause loss of efficacy in some cases. Botulinum toxin F does not cross-react with neutralizing antibodies to botulinum toxin A and is effective in patients with torticollis who have botulinum toxin A neutralizing antibodies.

MYASTHENIA GRAVIS

Pathophysiology

Myasthenia gravis is a syndrome of increased fatiguability and weakness of striated muscle and results from an autoimmune process with antibodies to nicotinic acetylcholine receptors. These interact with postsynaptic cholinoceptors at the neuromuscular junction. (Such antibodies may be passively transferred via purified immunoglobulin or across the placenta to produce a myasthenic neonate.)

Antibodies vary from patient to patient and are often directed against sites distinct from the acetylcholine binding site. They none the less interfere with transmission by increasing receptor turnover by complement activation and/or cross-linking of adjacent receptors. Reduction of the number of available receptors results in low-amplitude endplate potentials which in some fibers may be below threshold and so fail to trigger muscle action potentials, thus reducing the power of the whole muscle. Immunologic cross-reactivity exists between antigens in the thymus and the acetylcholine receptor but the stimulus to the production of antibody is unknown.

Diagnosis is aided by the use of edrophonium, a short-acting inhibitor of acetylcholinesterase, which produces a transient increase in muscle power in patients with myasthenia gravis. Edrophonium is also useful in distinguishing a myasthenic crisis from a cholinergic crisis (see below). Therapy of myasthenia is started with oral anticholinesterase drugs, usually neostigmine, 15 mg, 8 hourly and if the disease is progressive or non-responsive then thymectomy or immunosuppressant therapy with glucocorticosteroids and azathioprine are needed. Thymectomy is beneficial in patients with associated thymoma and in patients with generalized disease who can withstand the operation. Thymectomy reduces the number of circulating T lymphocytes capable of assisting B lymphocytes to produce antibody, and a fall in antibody titer occurs after thymectomy, albeit slowly. Corticosteroids and immunosuppressive drugs also reduce circulating T cells. Plasmapheresis is useful in emergencies and reduces the amount of antibody present, producing striking short-term clinical improvement in a few patients.

Anticholinesterase drugs

The defect in neuromuscular transmission may be redressed by cholinesterase inhibitors which inhibit acetylcholine breakdown and increase the concentration of transmitter available to stimulate the receptors.

NEOSTIGMINE

Neostigmine is initially given orally in doses of 15 mg 8 hourly but usually requires more frequent administration (up to 2 hourly) because of a short duration of action (2–6 hours). It is rapidly inactivated in the gut so that the corresponding parenteral dose (1–2 mg) is much smaller. Cholinesterase inhibitors enhance both muscarinic and nicotinic cholinergic effects. The former results in increased bronchial secretions, abdominal colic, diarrhea, miosis, nausea, salivation and lachrymation. Muscarinic effects may be blocked by giving atropine or propantheline, but this increases the risk of overdosage and consequent cholinergic crisis.

PYRIDOSTIGMINE

Pyridostigmine has a more prolonged action than neostigmine and it is seldom necessary to give it more frequently than 4 hourly. The initial dose is 60 mg 8 hourly (equivalent to 15 mg neostigmine) although individual requirements vary and some patients need up to 2000 mg in a day.

Although marked improvement may follow treatment with an anticholinesterase drug most patients must accept some residual disability. Increasing anticholinesterase drug dosage excessively causes increased weakness (cholinergic crisis).

Adjuvant drug therapy

Remissions of myasthenia symptoms are produced by oral administration of prednisolone. Increased weakness may occur at the beginning of treatment which must therefore be instituted in hospital. This effect has been minimized by the use of alternate day therapy starting with 20 mg prednisolone with a gradual increase of dose to 100 mg on alternate days. With such high doses the usual side effects of corticosteroids (chapter 37) are to be expected. The dose is reduced by 5 mg each month for as long as improvement is maintained. Azathioprine, 2.5 mg/kg, (chapter 47) has been successfully used either on its own or combined with glucocorticosteroids for its 'steroid-sparing' effect.

Myasthenic and cholinergic crisis

Severe weakness leading to paralysis may result from either a deficiency (myasthenic crisis) or an excess (cholinergic crisis) of acetylcholine at the neuromuscular junction. Clinically the distinction may be difficult and an injection of the very short-acting anticholinesterase edrophonium with improvement is diagnostic of myasthenic crises.

EDROPHONIUM

Edrophonium, a short-acting cholinesterase inhibitor given as 10 mg intravenously, is a useful aid to diagnosis. This transiently improves a myasthenic crisis and aggravates a cholinergic crisis. Because of its short duration of action any deterioration of a cholinergic crisis is unlikely to have serious consequences, although facilities for artificial ventilation must be available. In this setting it is important that the strength of essential (respiratory or bulbar) muscles be monitored using simple spirometry (forced expiratory volume in 1 second, FEV_1, and forced vital

capacity, FVC) during the test rather than that of non-essential (limb or ocular) muscles.

Myasthenic crises may develop as a spontaneous deterioration in the natural history of the disease, or as a result of infection or surgery. Drugs should not be overlooked as potential precipitants:

1. Aminoglycosides, for example, neomycin, streptomycin.
2. Other antibiotics, including erythromycin and polymyxin.
3. There is enormously increased sensitivity to non-depolarizing neuromuscular-blocking drugs, but reduced sensitivity to suxamethonium.
4. Quinine.
5. Respiratory depressants such as benzodiazepines (these also reduce muscle tone).
6. Antiarrhythmic drugs reduce the excitability of muscle membrane and lignocaine, procainamide and propranolol may increase weakness.

TREATMENT

Myasthenic crisis

Treatment of myasthenic crisis is with neostigmine, 0.5 mg, intramuscularly repeating this every 20 min with frequent edrophonium tests. Artificial ventilation may be needed.

Cholinergic crisis

Treatment of myasthenia with anticholinesterases can be usefully monitored by observation of the pupil (a diameter of 2 mm or less in normal lighting suggests overdose). Overdosage produces a cholinergic crisis and further drug should be withheld.

Anticonvulsants

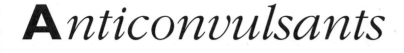

Introduction **194**

Mechanisms of action of anticonvulsants **194**

General principles of treatment of epilepsy **194**

Drug interactions with anticonvulsants **201**

Anticonvulsants and pregnancy **202**

Anticonvulsant osteomalacia **202**

Status epilepticus **202**

Withdrawal of anticonvulsant drugs **202**

Febrile convulsions **203**

INTRODUCTION

Epilepsy is characterized by recurrent seizures. An epileptic seizure is a paroxysmal discharge of cerebral neurones associated with a clinical event apparent to an observer, for example a tonic clonic (*grand mal*) seizure, or as an abnormal sensation perceived by the patient, for example a distortion of consciousness in temporal lobe epilepsy which may not be apparent to an observer.

A 'funny turn', black out or apparent seizure may be secondary to many events such as hypoglycemia, a vasovagal episode, cardiac arrhythmias, drug withdrawal, migraine and transient ischemic attacks. Precise differentiation is essential not only to avoid the damaging social and practical stigma associated with epilepsy but also to ensure appropriate medical treatment. Febrile seizures are a distinct problem and are discussed at the end of this chapter.

MECHANISMS OF ACTION OF ANTICONVULSANTS

The pathophysiology of epilepsy and the mode of action of antiepileptic drugs are poorly understood. These agents are not all sedative, but selectively block repetitive discharges at concentrations below those that block normal impulse conduction. Carbamazepine and phenytoin prolong the inactivated state of the sodium channel and reduce the likelihood of repetitive action potentials. Consequently normal cerebral activity, which is associated with relatively low action potential frequencies, is unaffected whilst epileptic discharges are suppressed.

γ-Aminobutyric acid (GABA), acts as an inhibitory neurotransmitter by opening receptor-operated chloride channels that lead to hyperpolarization and suppression of epileptic discharges. In addition to the receptor site for GABA the GABA receptor/channel complex includes benzodiazepine and barbiturate recognition sites which can potentiate GABA antiepileptic activity. Vigabatrin (γ-vinyl-γ-amino butyric acid) irreversibly inhibits GABA transaminase, the enzyme that inactivates GABA. The resulting increase in synaptic GABA probably explains its antiepileptic activity.

Glutamate is an excitatory neurotransmitter. A glutamate receptor, the N-methyl-D-aspartate (NMDA) receptor, is important in the genesis and propagation of high frequency discharges. Lamotrigine inhibits glutamate release and has anticonvulsant activity.

GENERAL PRINCIPLES OF TREATMENT OF EPILEPSY

Before treatment is prescribed the following questions should be asked:

1. Are the fits truly epileptic and not due to some other disorder (e.g. syncope, cardiac arrhythmia)?

2. Is the epilepsy caused by a condition that requires treatment in its own right (e.g. brain tumor, brain abscess, alcohol withdrawal)?

3. Are there remediable or reversible factors that aggravate the epilepsy or precipitate individual attacks?

4. Is there a clinically important risk if the patient is left untreated?
5. What type of epilepsy is present?

The ideal anticonvulsant would completely suppress all clinical and electroencephalographic evidence of the patient's epilepsy while producing no immediate or delayed side effects. This ideal does not exist (in the UK at least 16 anticonvulsant preparations are available) and the choice of drug depends on the balance between efficacy and toxicity and the type of epilepsy being treated. Table 19.1 summarizes the commonest forms of epilepsy and their drug treatment.

Control should initially be attempted using a single drug, chosen on the basis of the type of epilepsy. The dose is increased until either the seizures cease or the blood drug concentration (chapter 8) is in the toxic range and/or signs of toxicity appear. It should be stressed that some patients have epilepsy which is controlled at drug blood concentrations below the usual therapeutic range and others do not manifest toxicity above the therapeutic range. Thus estimation of drug plasma concentration is to be regarded as a guide but not an absolute arbiter. The availability of plasma concentration monitoring of antiepileptic drugs has allowed the more efficient use of individual drugs and is a crude guide to compliance. In a recent study of phenytoin monotherapy

for *grand mal* and focal epilepsy only 10% of new patients required the addition of a second drug whereas over half would have done so if concentrations had not been measured. If a drug proves to be ineffective it should not be suddenly withdrawn since this may provoke status epilepticus. Another drug should be introduced in increasing dosage whilst the first is gradually withdrawn.

Few studies have investigated combined drug therapy although empirically this is sometimes necessary. In most, but not all cases, effects are additive. Combinations of three or more drugs probably do more harm than good by increasing the chances of adverse drug reaction without improving seizure control. Many antiepileptic drugs are enzyme inducers so pharmacokinetic reactions are common; for example, carbamazepine reduces plasma concentrations of phenytoin.

Individual antiepileptic drugs

ETHOSUXIMIDE

Use

Ethosuximide is one of a group of succinimide drugs and is effective in *petit mal* absences. It is continued into adolescence and then gradually withdrawn over several months. If a drug for *grand mal* is being given concurrently, this is continued for a further 3 years. The daily dose usually lies between 0.5 and 2 g by mouth.

Adverse effects

Apart from dizziness, nausea and epigastric discomfort, side effects are rare and there are few doubts about its safety. *Grand mal* and *petit mal* may coexist in the same child, and a drug such as phenytoin may need to be added since ethosuximide is not effective against *grand mal*.

Table 19.1 Choice of drug in various forms of seizure.

Form of epilepsy	First choice	Other drugs
Tonic clonic (*grand mal*)	Carbamazepine Phenytoin Valproate	Phenobarbitone Primidone Vigabatrin Lamotrigine
Partial (focal) seizures	Valproate	Clonazepam Phenytoin Carbamazepine Lamotrigine
Absence seizures (*petit mal*)	Ethosuximide Valproate	Clonazepam
Myoclonic jerks	Valproate	Clonazepam

Pharmacokinetics

Ethosuximide is well absorbed following oral administration. Plasma half-life is 70 hours in adults but only 30 hours in children. Thus ethosuximide need be given only once daily and steady-state values are attained within 7 days.

Plasma concentration estimations are not usually required, but effective concentrations lie in the range 40–120 mg/l; the average dose which will attain this is 20 mg/kg/day. In practice 500 mg is given as the initial dose and this is increased by 250 mg every week until attacks are prevented. Extensive hepatic metabolism produces two major metabolites which are inactive. No significant plasma protein binding occurs and the cerebrospinal fluid (CSF) drug concentration is similar to that in plasma.

PHENYTOIN

Use

Phenytoin is one of the drugs of choice in the treatment of tonic clonic (*grand mal*) and partial (focal) seizures, including psychomotor attacks. For adults the usual dose is approximately 300 mg/day given as a single dose, but individualization is essential. Plasma concentration is measured after 2 weeks. According to clinical response and plasma concentration, adjustments should be small (e.g. 50 mg at a time) and no more frequent than every 4–6 weeks. Phenytoin illustrates the usefulness of therapeutic drug monitoring (chapter 8), but not all patients require a plasma phenytoin concentration within the therapeutic range of 10–20 mg/l for optimum control of their seizures.

Adverse effects

1. **Nervous system** High concentrations produce a cerebellar syndrome (ataxia, nystagmus, intention tremor, dysarthria), involuntary movements and sedation. Seizures may paradoxically increase with phenytoin intoxication. High concentrations cause psychological disturbances.
2. '**Allergic**' Rashes, drug fever and hepatitis may occur. Predisposition to these associated severe but rare effects (and also to lymphadenopathy, see below) is probably genetically predetermined by an abnormality in phenytoin metabolism. Oddly, but importantly, such patients can show cross-sensitivity to carbamazepine.
3. **Skin and collagen changes** Coarse facial features, gum hypertrophy, acne, hirsutism may appear.
4. **Hematological** Macrocytic anemia which responds to folate is common; rarely aplastic anemia; lymphadenopathy ('pseudolymphoma' which rarely progresses to true lymphoma).
5. **Effects on fetus** (difficult to distinguish from effects of epilepsy). There is increased perinatal mortality, raised frequency of cleft palate, hare lip, microcephaly and congenital heart disease.

Pharmacokinetics

Intestinal absorption is variable. There is wide variation in the handling of phenytoin, and in patients taking the same dose there is a 50-fold variation in steady-state plasma concentrations. The following factors contribute to the variation:

1. Age: Phenytoin clearance increases with age and this is correlated with lower protein binding and plasma albumin levels in the elderly. Young children metabolize phenytoin faster than adults.
2. Body weight: This influences volume of distribution (0.6 l/kg).
3. Sex: This makes a small contribution, steady-state levels being lower in females.
4. Metabolism: This is under polygenic control and varies widely between patients accounting for most of the interindividual variation in steady-state plasma concentration.

Phenytoin is extensively metabolized by the liver and less than 5% is excreted unchanged. The enzyme responsible for elimination becomes saturated at concentrations within the therapeutic range and phenytoin exhibits dose-dependent kinetics which, because of its low therapeutic index, makes clinical use of phenytoin difficult. Successive equal dose increments result in a disproportionate

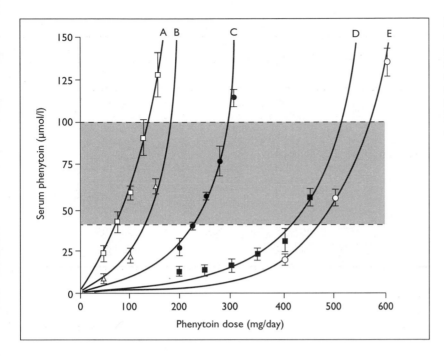

Fig. 19.1 Relationship between daily dose of phenytoin and resulting steady-state serum level in five patients on several different doses of drug. The curves were fitted by computer assuming Michaelis–Menten kinetics. (From A. Richens and A. Dunlop. *Lancet* 1975; ii: 247.)

increase in plasma concentration (Fig. 19.1) as drug metabolism approaches saturation. The clinical implications are:

1. Dosage increments should be 50 mg or less once the plasma level is within the therapeutic range.
2. Fluctuations above and below the therapeutic range occur relatively easily due to changes in the amount of drug absorbed or by forgetting to take a tablet. This behavior also magnifies bioavailability differences and clinical intoxication resulted on one occasion from alteration of the excipient in phenytoin capsules from calcium sulfate to lactose (see chapter 4).
3. Drug interactions are common since administration of a second drug such as isoniazid (which inhibits phenytoin metabolism), or carbamazepine (which enhances it), results in clinically important effects on steady-state plasma concentrations.

The saturation kinetics of phenytoin make it invalid to calculate $t_{1/2}$ since the rate of elimination depends upon the plasma level and enzyme saturation. After a single dose of phenytoin the $t_{1/2}$ is around 10–17 hours, but in patients on continuous phenytoin therapy the $t_{1/2}$ of an isotopically labeled tracer dose of phenytoin may be as long as 140 hours. Practically, this means that the time to reach a plateau plasma concentration is longer than is predicted from the $t_{1/2}$ of a single dose of the drug. Hence if necessary (e.g. in patients with status epilepticus) a loading dose (800–1000 mg) is used. Eight hourly dosing is unnecessary and single daily dosage is effective and helps compliance.

Phenytoin is extremely insoluble and crystallizes out in intramuscular injection sites and this route should never be used. For the rapid attainment of therapeutic plasma concentrations intravenous injection is needed. To improve solubility the parenteral preparation has a pH of 10 and precipitation of the free acid occurs if the injection is added to intravenous infusion fluids. The high pH is irritant to veins and tissues. Phenytoin should not be given at rates of greater than 50 mg/min because at higher rates of administration cardiovascular collapse, respiratory arrest and seizures may occur. Electrocardiographic monitoring with measurement of blood pressure every minute during administration is essential. If

Table 19.2 Metabolic interactions of anticonvulsants.

Enzyme-inducing effects of antiepilepetic drugs		Drugs that inhibit the metabolism of anticonvulsants	
Antiepileptic drug	Drugs whose metabolism is enhanced	Inhibitor	Anticonvulsant
Carbamazepine	Warfarin	Amiodarone	Phenytoin
Phenobarbitone	Oral contraceptives	Fluoxetine	Phenytoin, carbamazepine
Phenytoin	Theophylline	Diltiazem, nifedipine	Phenytoin
Primidone	Cyclosporin	Chloramphenicol	Phenytoin
	Some tricyclic antidepressants	Disulfiram	Phenytoin
	Doxycycline	Erythromycin & clarithromycin	Carbamazepine
	Corticosteroids	Cimetidine	Phenytoin
	Anticonvulsants	Isoniazid	Carbamazepine, ethosuximide, phenytoin
		Metronidazole	Phenytoin
		Miconazole, fluconazole	Phenytoin
		Valproate	Lamotrigine

blood pressure falls, administration is temporarily stopped until blood pressure rises satisfactorily.

At therapeutic concentrations 90% is bound to albumin and to two α-globulins which also bind thyroxine. In uremia, displacement of phenytoin from plasma protein binding results in lower total plasma concentration, and a lower therapeutic range. If this is not appreciated and the dose increased, toxicity will result. Sodium valproate also increases the ratio of free to total phenytoin by this mechanism.

Other important interactions occur via alterations in the hepatic metabolism of phenytoin. Drugs that impair or induce metabolism are summarized in Table 19.2.

Phenytoin elimination is impaired in liver disease. Chronic renal disease may result in unusually low levels because of hypoalbuminemia in patients with nephrotic syndrome or displacement of protein-bound phenytoin by accumulated endogenous metabolites in patients with renal failure.

PHENOBARBITONE

Phenobarbitone is an effective drug for tonic and partial seizures but is sedative in adults and causes behavioral disturbances and hyperkinesia in children. It may be tried as a second-line drug for atypical absence, atonic and tonic seizures. Rebound seizures may occur on withdrawal. Monitoring plasma concentrations is less useful than with phenytoin because tolerance occurs and the relationship between plasma concentrations and therapeutic and adverse effects are less predictable than is the case with phenytoin.

Other adverse effects include rashes, anaphylaxis, folate deficiency, aplastic anemia and congenital abnormalities.

CARBAMAZEPINE

Use

Carbamazepine is structurally related to the tricyclic antidepressants. In addition to its effectiveness in all forms of epilepsy except absence seizures, it is effective in trigeminal neuralgia and in the prophylaxis of mood swings in manic-depressive illness (chapter 17). Carbamazepine is a drug of choice for tonic clonic epilepsy. A dose of 100–200 mg is given twice daily followed by a slow increase in dose until seizures are controlled. At higher doses the daily dose may have to be divided into a three or four times daily regime to reduce side effects. A dose of 1200 mg daily is sometimes required. Assays of serum concentration are a useful guide to compliance, rapid metabolism, or drug failure if seizures continue. The therapeutic range is 4–12 mg/l.

Pharmacokinetics

Carbamazepine is slowly but well absorbed following oral administration. Plasma levels fluctuate widely during absorption. Plasma $t_{1/2}$ after a single dose is 25–60 hours but on chronic dosing this falls to 10 hours, possibly due to enzyme induction. A controlled release preparation reduces the peak plasma concentration and fluctuations in carbamazepine concentration during treatment. It is indicated in patients whose adverse effects (dizziness, diplopia and drowsiness) correlate with peak drug concentrations and for patients who have difficulty in complying with three or more doses per day.

At therapeutic concentrations carbamazepine is 75% bound to plasma protein and it is feasible to use salivary carbamazepine concentrations (which reflect unbound drug in the plasma) as an alternative to blood analysis.

Adverse effects

Adverse effects are common but seldom severe. They are particularly troublesome early in treatment. Sedation, ataxia, giddiness, nystagmus, diplopia and slurred speech occur in 50% of patients with plasma levels over 8.5 mg/l. Carbamazepine can cause hyponatremia and water intoxication due to an antidiuretic action. Carbamazepine is contraindicated in patients with atrioventricular (AV) conduction abnormalities and a history of bone marrow depression or porphyria. Use in pregnancy has been associated with fetal neural tube defects and hypossadias.

Drug interactions

Carbamazepine should not be combined with monoamine oxidase inhibitors.

BENZODIAZEPINES

See chapter 15.

Use

Benzodiazepines (e.g. diazepam, nitrazepam, clobazepam and clonazepam) have anticonvulsant properties in addition to their anxiolytic and other actions. Unfortunately on prolonged usage tolerance to their antiepileptic properties tends to develop. Clonazepam was introduced specifically as an anticonvulsant: its chief uses are as maintenance therapy and in status epilepticus in which diazepam or clonazepam given intravenously is the treatment of choice. Clonazepam has a wide spectrum of activity, having a place in the management of the motor seizures of childhood, particularly absences and infantile spasms. It is also useful in psychomotor and myoclonic epilepsy in patients not adequately controlled by phenytoin or carbamazepine.

Clonazepam is given in divided doses of 4–8 mg/day in adults. The intravenous dose is 0.5–2 mg. Intravenous diazepam is indicated in status epilepticus. Rectal diazepam is a useful alternative in children.

Adverse effects

Adverse effects are frequent and about 50% of patients experience lethargy, somnolence and dizziness with clonazepam. This is minimized by starting with a low dose then gradually increasing it. In many cases sedation disappears on chronic treatment. More serious effects are muscular incoordination, ataxia, dysphoria, hypotonia and muscle relaxation, increased salivary secretion and hyperactivity with aggressive behavior.

Pharmacokinetics

Clonazepam is well absorbed orally and the $t_{1/2}$ is about 30 hours. Neither therapeutic nor adverse effects appear to be closely related to plasma concentrations. Control of most types of epilepsy occurs within the range 30–60 ng/ml. Clonazepam is extensively metabolized to inactive metabolites

SODIUM VALPROATE

Use

Sodium valproate (dipropylacetate) is effective against several forms of epilepsy: tonic clonic, absence, psychomotor epilepsy, and myoclonic epilepsy. Dosage starts at 600 mg daily in divided (8 hourly) doses after meals and is increased every 3 days by 200 mg/day, until control is achieved. This is generally in the range 1000–2000 mg/day but may be up to 2500 mg/day. The onset of effect is slow and may take several days.

Adverse effects

Adverse effects most commonly involve the alimentary system. Toxic effects include:

1. Nausea, vomiting, abdominal pain (may be reduced by enteric-coated tablets).
2. Enhancement of sedatives (including alcohol).
3. Thrombocytopenia (usually associated with high dosage). Platelet count should be checked before surgery and if any abnormal bruising occurs.
4. Temporary hair loss.
5. False positive ketone test in urine which may cause confusion in the management of diabetes has been reported.
6. Teratogenic effects (neural tube defects and hypossadias) have been reported.
7. Rarely hepatic necrosis has developed particularly in children taking high doses and suffering from congenital metabolic disorders.
8. Acute pancreatitis is another rare complication.

Pharmacokinetics

Valproate is well absorbed when given orally (95–100% bioavailability). Like other fatty acids it is highly bound (approximately 90%) to plasma protein, showing a two-fold inter-individual variation in the amount of free drug. Like phenytoin, there is reduced binding in uremia and the unbound drug shows good correlation with serum creatinine. The plasma $t_{1/2}$ is 7–10 hours. Little progress has been made in identification of metabolites. Possibly the presence of active metabolites explains the relatively slow onset and long time course of action. The brain to plasma ratio is low (0.3) and a large dose (1–2 g/day) is necessary. There is substantial interindividual variation in the handling of the drug. A therapeutic range of 40–80 mg/l has been suggested.

CHLORMETHIAZOLE

Chlormethiazole (chapter 15) is a powerful anticonvulsant which can be given intravenously in the treatment of status epilepticus. When given orally it has a short half-life (1 hour) and is therefore not convenient to use in the day-to-day treatment of epilepsy. It can cause respiratory depression and if given by intravenous infusion careful monitoring of respiratory function is mandatory. In addition if the infusion is prolonged accumulation can occur.

VIGABATRIN

Use

Vigabatrin, a structural analog of GABA, increases brain concentration of GABA (an inhibitory neurotransmitter) through irreversible inhibition of GABA transaminase. It is reserved for the treatment of epilepsy unsatisfactorily controlled by more established drugs. The initial dose is 2 g daily in single or two divided doses then increased or decreased according to response in steps of 0.5–1 g. The usual maximum daily dose is 4 g. Lower doses should be used in the elderly and those with impaired renal function. Vigabatrin should be avoided in those with a psychiatric history.

Adverse effects

1. The commonest reported adverse event (up to 30% of patients) is drowsiness.
2. Fatigue, irritability, dizziness, confusion and weight gain have all been reported.
3. Psychotic reactions occur, including hallucinations and paranoia.

Pharmacokinetics

Absorption is not influenced by food and peak plasma concentrations occur within 2 hours of an oral dose. In contrast to most other anticonvulsants it is not metabolized in the liver but is excreted unchanged via the kidney and has a plasma half-life of about 5 hours. Its efficacy does not correlate with the plasma concentration and its duration of action is prolonged due to irreversible binding to GABA transaminase.

LAMOTRIGINE

Lamotrigine inhibits glutamate, a fast cerebral excitatory transmitter. It is a new drug and is indicated as an adjunctive treatment of partial seizures and generalized tonic clonic seizures not satisfactorily controlled with other drugs. It is contraindicated in hepatic and renal impairment. Side effects include rashes (rarely angioedema and Steven–Johnson syndrome), visual disturbances, dizziness, drowsiness, gastrointestinal disturbances and aggression. The patient must be closely monitored if rash, fever, influenza-like symptoms, drowsiness or worsening of seizure control develops, particularly in the first month of treatment as this may herald rapidly progressive multi-organ failure and status epilepticus.

GABAPENTIN

Gabapentin has recently been licensed as an 'add on' therapy in the treatment of partial seizures. It is a GABA analog but its mechanism of action is uncertain. Initial studies suggest it is generally well tolerated with somnolence being most frequently reported. It is well absorbed after oral administration and is eliminated by renal excretion; the half-life averages 5–6 hours. It does not interfere with the metabolism or protein binding of other anticonvulsants.

*D*RUG INTERACTIONS WITH ANTICONVULSANTS

Clinically important interactions with other drugs occur with several antiepileptics. The therapeutic ratio of antiepileptics is often small, and changes in plasma concentrations can seriously effect both efficacy and toxicity. In addition, antiepileptics are prescribed over long periods so that there is a considerable chance of them being sooner or later combined with another drug.

Several mechanisms are involved:

1. Enzyme induction, so that the hepatic metabolism of the antiepileptic is enhanced, plasma concentration lowered and efficacy reduced.
2. Enzyme inhibition, so that the metabolism of the antiepileptic is impaired with the development of higher blood concentrations and toxicity.
3. Displacement of the antiepileptic from plasma binding sites so that more free drug is available. For example, sodium valproate displaces phenytoin, altering its therapeutic range.

In addition to this several antiepileptics (e.g. phenytoin, phenobarbitone, carbamazepine) are themselves powerful enzyme inducers and may alter the metabolism of other drugs. Table 19.2 shows the effect of some drugs on the metabolism of widely used antiepileptics and the effect of antiepileptics on the metabolism of other drugs.

Antiepileptics and the oral contraceptive

Phenytoin, phenobarbitone and carbamazepine induce the metabolism of estrogen and can lead to unwanted pregnancies. Patients taking antiepileptics and wishing to take an oral contraceptive should use one containing at least 50 μg estrogen.

ANTICONVULSANTS AND PREGNANCY

The benefit of treatment outweighs the risk to the fetus. The risk of teratogenicity is greater if more than one drug is used (chapter 9).

ANTICONVULSANT OSTEOMALACIA

Enzyme induction reduces serum 25-hydroxy-cholecalciferol. Subclinical or symptomatic rickets or osteomalacia can develop due to deficient vitamin D. The deficit is increased by the poor diet and lack of sunlight which is the lot of many institutionalized epileptics. Associated hypocalcemia rarely causes fits. Good diet should be encouraged in epileptics and vitamin D supplement prescribed if necessary.

STATUS EPILEPTICUS

Status epilepticus is a medical emergency with a mortality of about 10% with neurological and psychiatric sequelae possible in the survivors. Rapid suppression of seizure activity is essential and can usually be achieved with intravenous benzodiazepines (e.g. diazepam, formulated as an emulsion, 10 mg i.v.). The rectal route is useful in children and if venous access is difficult (chapter 10). False teeth should be removed, an airway established and oxygen administered as soon as possible. The dose of diazepam is repeated if fitting continues. Transient respiratory depression and hypotension may occur. Relapse may be prevented with intravenous phenytoin and/or early recommencement of regular anticonvulsants. Identification of any precipitating factors, such as hypoglycemia, alcohol, drug overdose, low anticonvulsant plasma concentrations and non-compliance may influence the immediate and subsequent management. If intravenous benzodiazepines and phenytoin fail to control the fits, removal to an intensive care unit and assistance from an anesthetist are essential. Chlormethiazole or thiopentone are commonly used in this situation.

WITHDRAWAL OF ANTICONVULSANT DRUGS

All anticonvulsants are associated with adverse effects. It has been estimated that up to 70% of patients eventually enter a prolonged remission and do not require medication; however, it is difficult to know if a prolonged seizure-free interval is due to efficacy of the antiepileptic drug treatment or true remission. Those with a history of adult onset epilepsy of long duration which has been difficult to control, partial seizures and/or underlying cerebral disorder have a less favorable prognosis. Drug withdrawal itself may precipitate seizures and the possible medical and social consequences of recurrent seizures (e.g. loss of driving licence) must be carefully discussed with the patient. If drugs are to be withdrawn, the dose should be reduced gradually, for example over 6 months with strict instructions to the patient to report any seizure activity.

FEBRILE CONVULSIONS

Febrile seizures are the most common seizures of childhood. A febrile convulsion is defined as a convulsion that occurs in a child aged between 3 months and 5 years with a fever but without any other evident cause, such as an intracranial infection or previous non-febrile convulsions. Approximately 3% of children have at least one febrile convulsion of whom about one-third will have one or more recurrences and 3% develop epilepsy in later life.

In spite of the usually insignificant medical consequences a febrile convulsion is a terrifying experience to parents. Most children are admitted to hospital following their first febrile convulsion. If prolonged the convulsion can be terminated with either rectal or intravenous diazepam. If the child is under 18 months old, pyogenic meningitis should be excluded. It is usual to reduce fever using paracetamol, removal of clothing, tepid sponging and fanning. Fever is usually due to viral infection but if a bacterial cause is found this should be treated.

Uncomplicated febrile seizures have an excellent prognosis so the parents can be confidently reassured. They should be advised how to reduce fever and how to deal with a subsequent fit should it occur. Although phenobarbitone and sodium valproate have been used as long-term regular prophylaxis in children to reduce the occurrence of febrile convulsions there is no evidence that this reduces the likelihood of developing epilepsy in later life and their benefits are outweighed by the sedation and behavioral disturbances caused by phenobarbitone and the small risk of hepatic necrosis associated with sodium valproate. Rectal diazepam may be administered by parents as prophylaxis during a febrile illness or to stop a prolonged convulsion.

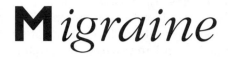

Migraine

Pathophysiology **206**

Drugs used for the acute attack **207**

Drugs used for prophylaxis **209**

PATHOPHYSIOLOGY

Migraine is a common condition, yet its precise pathophysiogical mechanism is poorly understood. The early aura is associated with intracranial vasoconstriction and localized cerebral ischemia and dysfunction have been demonstrated by angiographic and isotopic blood-flow studies. Shortly after this phase the extracranial vessels dilate and pulsate, changes that are associated with local tenderness and the classical headache, which begins unilaterally in the territory of one or other carotid artery.

Serotonin (5-hydroxytryptamine, 5HT) may be the initial stimulus to vasoconstriction but this long-standing hypothesis remains controversial; noradrenaline has also been suggested as a possible mediator of this effect. Serotonin is a potent vasoconstrictor of extracranial vessels in humans, and it has been postulated that serotonin released from platelets in migraine causes vasoconstriction. This summates with effects of kinins and histamine (produced as a response to ischemia) to cause pain in the affected arteries. Enhanced platelet aggregation has been demonstrated in migraine and this could enhance the effects of vasoconstriction in producing the aura. Uptake and metabolism of 5HT by blood vessels reduces circulating 5HT concentration and removes this counterbalance to vasodilator substances such as kinins, prostaglandins and histamine. These then act on the unstable vasculature to produce inappropriate vasodilatation and pain. The initial stimulus to platelet 5HT release is unknown. One hypothesis is that migraineurs have inherently unstable cerebral vasculature prone to excessive contraction and dilatation when stimulated by factors that in normal subjects produce only minor effects (Fig. 20.1)

Ingestion of vasoactive amines in food by a migraine sufferer may cause inappropriate responses of intra- and extracranial vessels. Several other precipitating factors are recognized anecdotally, although in some cases, for example precipitation by chocolate, they are not easily demonstrated scientifically. These include physical trauma; local pain from sinuses; cervical spondylosis; sleep (too

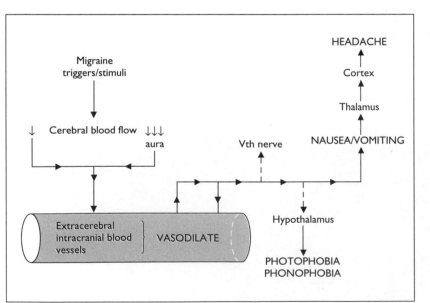

Fig. 20.1 Pathophysiology of migraine.

much or too little); ingestion of tyramine-containing foods such as cheese; allergy, for example to wheat, eggs, fish; stress; hormonal changes, for example menstrual cycle; fasting and hypoglycemia.

Some of the most effective prophylactic drugs against migraine inhibit 5HT reuptake by platelets and other cells, thus maintaining plasma 5HT levels and so preventing vasodi-latation. Several such drugs have additional antihistamine and anti-5HT activity which blocks the permeability-increasing actions of these transmitters.

The assessment of drug efficacy in migraine is bedevilled by the fact that migraine is paroxysmal and variable in intensity and severity and no stimulus exists that will reproducibly initiate an attack.

DRUGS USED FOR THE ACUTE ATTACK

In the majority of patients with migraine the combination of a mild analgesic with an antiemetic and if possible a period of rest aborts the acute attack. Until recently the small proportion of migraine sufferers in whom this treatment was inadequate were given ergotamine. The introduction of sumatriptan has increased the therapeutic armamentarium appreciably. This is an expensive drug, but has an important role in disabling migraine resistant to simple therapy.

SIMPLE ANALGESICS

Aspirin, 900 mg, or paracetamol, 1 g, are useful in treatment of the headache. They are cheap and are effective in about three-quarters of patients. During a migraine attack gastric stasis occurs and this impairs drug absorption. It is therefore suggested that a soluble aspirin preparation be employed and this may be usefully coupled with metoclopramide (which acts both as an antiemetic – useful if nausea is a prominent symptom – and enhances gastric emptying) if necessary. Combination preparations of metoclopramide, 5 mg, and aspirin, 325 mg, or with paracetamol, 500 mg, are available. They should be avoided if possible in adolescents and women in their twenties because of the risk of spasmodic torticollis and dystonia.

ANTIEMETICS

Antiemetics are useful in their own right if gastrointestinal symptoms are troublesome. Although no controlled studies comparing their efficacy have been performed it is reasonable to avoid antiemetics with sedative properties (e.g. antihistamines, phenothiazines) and on this account metoclopramide – a dopamine and weak $5HT_3$ antagonist (chapter 31) – or domperidone (chapters 18 and 31) are appropriate choices.

SUMATRIPTAN

Use

Sumatriptan, 6 mg, is injected subcutaneously. Prepacked dosage vials are available for self injection and the maximum recommended dose is 12 mg/24 hours, a second injection being administered at least 1 hour after the first. Orally sumatriptan is taken as 100 mg tablets. The maximum recommended dose is 300 mg/24 hours. It can be taken at any time during a migraine attack but is most effective if taken early on. It is used to treat acute migraine or acute cluster headaches, and relieves headache and nausea in 65–85% of attacks. It is more effective than ergotamine, but has a short half-life so headache recurs after a single dose in 30–40% of patients.

Mechanism of action

Sumatriptan is a selective agonist of $5HT_{1D}$ receptors which are found predominantly in the cranial circulation. Sumatriptan causes carotid vasoconstriction in a dose-dependent manner. There is a small amount of vasoconstriction in other vascular beds, notably the coronary and pulmonary vasculature, and sumatriptan causes a significant but transient systemic pressor response.

Adverse effects

1. Transient pain at the injection site.
2. Flushing, dizziness, weakness.
3. Paresthesiae.
4. Pressure or tightness in any part of the body, particularly the chest. Chest pain is particularly worrying as it is possible that it could be due to coronary artery vasoconstriction, although there is no conclusive evidence to support this view.
5. Nausea and vomiting after oral administration.

Pharmacokinetics

Sumatriptan is rapidly absorbed after both oral and subcutaneous administration, with a T_{max} of 45 and 15 min, respectively. The drug is approximately 100% bioavailable after subcutaneous injection, in comparison to 14% bioavailability after oral administration; food does not affect oral absorption. Sumatriptan undergoes substantial presystemic hepatic metabolism to an inactive indole acetic acid metabolite. Eight per cent is metabolized and 20% is excreted unchanged via the kidney. The $t_{1/2}$ is 2 hours, protein binding is low and because of its lipid solubility it has a large volume of distribution.

Contraindications

Sumatriptan should not be used in patients with ischemic heart disease or Prinzmetal angina, or severe hypertension.

Drug interactions

Sumatriptan should not be combined with ergotamine, MAOI, lithium, or 5HT reuptake inhibitors.

ERGOTAMINE

Use

Ergotamine is only used in acute migraine; it is advisable to start oral, rectal or inhalation ergotamine treatment at a dose of 1 mg only (e.g. half a cafergot suppository or three puffs of an ergotamine medihaler). The corresponding intramuscular dose is 0.25 mg.

Mechanism of action

Ergotamine has partial α-adrenergic agonist (vasoconstrictor) actions. Structurally the lysergic acid moiety of the molecule resembles both 5HT and noradrenaline and it blocks 5HT uptake by platelets and blood vessels thus allowing 5HT to activate vasoconstrictor receptors. It is believed to act by vasoconstriction.

Adverse effects

1. Nausea and vomiting, due to too high a dose, may be misinterpreted as due to undertreatment, a potentially disastrous error.
2. Peripheral vascular system: coldness of extremities, Raynaud's phenomenon, intermittent claudication, paresthesiae and digital gangrene (treatment of ergot-induced vasospasm is by means of a vasodilator such as nitroprusside or an organic nitrate).
3. Rebound headaches which may persist for several days following discontinuation of the drug if used excessively.

Contraindications

Ergotamine should not be used in pregnancy, and only in exceptional circumstances in patients with cardiac and peripheral vascular disease.

Pharmacokinetics

Ergotamine shows marked interindividual variations in absorption when administered orally, undergoing extensive hepatic metabolism. Less than 5% is excreted unchanged.

DRUGS USED FOR PROPHYLAXIS

Prophylactic therapy is not used unless two or more attacks occur each month. Due to the relapsing/remitting natural history of migraine, prophylactic therapy should be given for 4–6 months and then withdrawn.

PIZOTIFEN

Use

Pizotifen is often the first choice in migraine prophylaxis. It is related to the tricyclic antidepressants. The initial dose is 0.5 mg (given at night as it causes drowsiness) and this can be increased up to 3 mg if necessary.

Mechanism of action

Pizotifen is a $5HT_2$ antagonist. It also has mild antimuscarinic and antihistamine activity.

Adverse effects

1. Drowsiness.
2. Appetite stimulation and weight gain.
3. Dizziness.
4. Muscle pain.

Pharmacokinetics

Pizotifen is well absorbed (80%) and undergoes extensive hepatic metabolism. Only 1% of a dose is excreted unchanged in the urine. The $t_{1/2}$ is 26 hours and it has a large volume of distribution.

Drug interactions

Pizotifen should not be used with monoamine oxidase inhibitors, and potentiates the drowsiness and sedation of sedatives, tranquillizers and antidepressants.

PROPRANOLOL AND OTHER β-ADRENORECEPTOR BLOCKERS

β-Adrenoreceptor antagonists have prophylactic efficacy compared to placebo. Their mechanism in this regard is uncertain but they may act by opposing dilatation of extracranial vessels. Atenolol or metoprolol are effective and easy to use (chapters 25 and 26). β-Blockers potentiate the peripheral vasoconstriction caused by ergotamine and these drugs should not be given concurrently.

METHYSERGIDE

Use

Methysergide should only be used under specialist hospital supervision because of its severe toxicity. It is highly effective as prophylaxis (up to 80% of patients) in a dose of 1–2 mg two or three times daily with meals. Initially 1 mg is given at night and the dose is slowly increased up to 2 mg 6 hourly. After 6 months it is stopped for at least 1 month. Its use is indicated only in patients who, despite other attempts at control, experience such severe and frequent migraine as substantially to interfere with their work or social activities. The smallest dose that suppresses about 75% of the headaches is used because of toxicity.

Mechanism of action

Methysergide has powerful $5HT_2$ blocking activity with partial agonist activity on $5HT_1$ receptors and also some anti-inflammatory and vasoconstrictor effects.

Adverse effects

1. Gastrointestinal disturbances: nausea, vomiting, diarrhea and abdominal pain.
2. Neurological disturbances: mild euphoria, dissociation, experiences of unreality, hyperesthesia.
3. Weight gain and edema.
4. Reversible vasoconstriction: angina, intermittent claudication, abdominal angina.
5. Fibrosis in the peritoneum and thorax: retroperitoneal fibrosis is not clearly dose related but is related to prolonged use.

Symptoms may be minimal and progression to end-stage renal failure may occur insidiously.

CALCIUM CHANNEL BLOCKERS

Flunarizine, 10 mg daily, is the most effective of this class of drugs in migraine prophylaxis. These drugs are useful in terminating the aura in patients who have aura without headache.

Verapamil, 40 mg tds, is commonly used as prophylaxis against cluster headaches.

TRICYCLIC ANTIDEPRESSANTS

These (chapter 17) are effective in preventing attacks in some patients independent of their mood. The probable mechanism is via 5HT and noradrenaline reuptake blockade. Amitryptyline in low dose (e.g. 10–25 mg at night) is often adequate.

Anesthetics and Muscle Relaxants

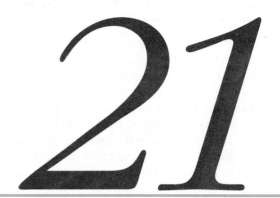

(*with Mark Edwards*)

General anesthetics   **212**

Inhalational anesthetics   **212**

Intravenous anesthetics   **216**

Neuroleptanalgesia   **219**

Sedation in the intensive care unit   **220**

Premedication for anesthesia   **220**

Muscle relaxants   **221**

Malignant hyperthermia   **223**

Local anesthetics   **224**

GENERAL ANESTHETICS

Mechanism of action

The mode of action of anesthetics is still debated. All general anesthetics act on the mid-brain reticular activating system and cerebral cortex to produce complete but reversible loss of consciousness. The principal site of action is probably the neuronal lipid bilayer plasma membrane or hydrophobic domains of membrane proteins buried within it. Here the drugs block sodium and potassium channels inhibiting nerve impulse transmission. Support for this theory includes the observations that the anesthetic potency of drugs is highly correlated with their lipid solubility and the fact that high atmospheric pressures (applied experimentally in animal experiments) can lead to reversal of anesthesia, presumably as a result of physical changes in cell membranes.

General anesthetics are usually considered in two groups:

1. Inhalational anesthetics.
2. Intravenous anesthetics.

INHALATIONAL ANESTHETICS

Uptake and distribution

Several physical properties influence the performance of anesthetic agents. The saturated vapor pressure (SVP) determines the maximum proportion of atmospheric pressure that can be occupied by a saturated vapor of the substance and thus gives an indication of how readily a high concentration can be achieved at atmospheric pressure. For halothane the SVP is 243 mmHg at 20°C which translates into a maximum attainable concentration of 33%, the usual maintenance concentration of halothane being 0.5–2%. The minimum alveolar concentration (MAC) indicates the minimum alveolar concentration of an agent required to prevent reflex response to surgical stimulation; for example, the minimum required to prevent reflex response to surgical stimulation in 50% of the population is the MAC 50. Once an adequate quantity of anesthetic agent has built up in the alveoli further uptake depends on its passage into the circulation. This is governed by the following factors:

1. The concentration gradient across the alveolar membrane between the alveolar air and pulmonary capillary blood. Pulmonary capillary blood concentration is dependent on tissue uptake.
2. Relative solubility in blood. This is expressed as the blood–gas solubility coefficient. A high value indicates a high solubility in blood and a low value a low solubility. The alveolar concentration of an agent with a low blood solubility rises rapidly as little drug is taken up into the circulation. The alveolar concentration determines the arterial tension of an agent and therefore the concentration gradients to other tissues especially the brain. It follows that agents with low blood solubility rapidly produce high arterial tensions and therefore large concentration gradients between the blood and brain. This leads to rapid induction and, on discontinuing

administration, rapid recovery. Conversely agents that have a high blood solubility only build up an adequate arterial (and therefore brain) tension gradually making induction slow and recovery prolonged.

3. Pulmonary blood flow. This normally equates to cardiac output. As pulmonary flow increases more agent is removed from the alveoli thereby delaying the rise in arterial tension and making induction longer. Conversely, a fall in pulmonary blood flow, for example in shock, hastens induction.

4. Pulmonary ventilation. Changes in ventilation have little influence on induction with insoluble agents as the alveolar concentration is always high. However, soluble agents show marked rises of alveolar concentration with increased ventilation.

Commonly used inhalational anesthetic agents include:

- Halothane.
- Enflurane.
- Isoflurane.
- Nitrous oxide.

HALOTHANE

Use

Halothane is 2-bromo-2-chloro-1,1,1-trifluoro-ethane. It is a potent inhalational anesthetic. The boiling point is 50°C and the saturated vapor pressure at 20°C is 243 mmHg. It is decomposed by light and is stored in amber-colored bottles, stabilized by 0.01% thymol. It does not react with soda lime and is non-inflammable. It has a blood–gas partition coefficient of 2.5 and an MAC in oxygen of 0.75%. The vapor has a sweet odor, is non-irritant and not unpleasant to smell. For induction of anesthesia 2–4% vapor is administered and for maintenance 0.5–2% is used. It is a poor analgesic, but with nitrous oxide and oxygen it is very useful for many purposes. Whilst apparently simple to use its therapeutic index is relatively low and overdosage is easily produced. Warning signs are bradycardia, hypotension and tachypnea.

Particular aspects of the use of halothane relate to the following:

1. Moderate muscular relaxation is produced, but is rarely sufficient for major abdominal surgery. As with other volatile anesthetics the actions of most non-depolarizing muscle relaxants are augmented.
2. Heat loss is accelerated and may aid hypothermic techniques.
3. It is useful:
   (a) When quiet spontaneous respiration is required.
   (b) In bronchitic and asthmatic patients.
   (c) For gaseous induction of children.

Adverse effects

1. **Cardiovascular system**
   (a) Increased myocardial excitability, ventricular extrasystoles, ventricular tachycardia and ventricular fibrillation may occur. Predisposing factors include carbon dioxide retention, adrenaline administration, atropine and sensory stimulation during light anesthesia. Ventricular extrasystoles can be controlled by intravenous β-adrenoceptor blockers.
   (b) Bradycardia mediated by the vagus and hypotension. This may be treated with a slow intravenous injection of atropine. Deaths have occurred from myocardial failure.
   (c) Blood pressure usually falls during halothane anesthesia. This is probably due to central vasomotor depression and myocardial depression.
   (d) Cerebral blood flow is increased which contraindicates its use where reduction of intracranial pressure is desired (e.g. head injury, intracranial tumors).

2. **Respiratory system** Respiratory depression commonly occurs resulting in decreased alveolar ventilation. Respiratory center depression usually precedes myocardial depression and is dose dependent. Although the depth of respiration is decreased there is tachypnea.

3. **Central nervous system** Despite generalized central nervous system (CNS)

depression, the drug is not a good analgesic and also may lead to convulsions. Psychological changes may persist for over a week after administration.

4. **Liver** Halothane can produce massive hepatic necrosis or subclinical hepatitis following anesthesia. However, the incidence of massive necrosis due to halothane is very low. Patients most at risk are middle-aged, obese women who have previously (within 28 days) had halothane anesthesia. The basic lesion appears to be a hypersensitivity type of hepatitis which is independent of halothane dose.

5. **Uterus** Halothane can cause uterine atony and *postpartum* hemorrhage.

Pharmacokinetics

Twenty per cent of administered dose is metabolized in the liver, the balance being lost in exhaled air. Metabolites are slowly cleared from the body and can be detected in the urine for up to 3 weeks.

ENFLURANE

Use

Enflurane is 2-chloro-1,1,2-trifluoroethyl, difluoromethyl ether. It is a volatile liquid with an ethereal smell (boiling point 56.5°C). It has a blood–gas coefficient of 1.8 and an MAC of 1.68 % in oxygen. For induction an initial inspired concentration of 1% is gradually increased to 4–5% in oxygen or a nitrous oxide–oxygen mixture. For maintenance 1–3% concentration is used. Enflurane is a potent general anesthetic which has the potential advantage of producing direct muscle relaxation and reversible potentiation of muscle relaxants. It is commonly used in anesthetic practice, particularly if multiple anesthetics are necessary (as liver dysfunction is rare), or rapid recovery is important.

Adverse effects

1. **Cardiovascular system** Enflurane depresses myocardial contractility more than halothane, but sensitizes the myocardium to catecholamines less than halothane.

2. **Respiratory system** Respiratory depression is common, but is only a problem if spontaneous ventilation is required during deep anesthesia.

3. **Central nervous system** High concentrations can produce spike and wave activity in the electroencephalogram (EEG), particularly in children. In the presence of hypocapnia this may lead to *grand mal* fits.

4. **Uterus** Uterine tone is reduced increasing the risk of *postpartum* hemorrhage.

5. **Kidney** Transient loss of renal concentrating ability leading to polyuria has been reported following prolonged enflurane anesthesia. This may be related to accumulation of fluoride ion or another separate metabolite of enflurane producing a mild degree of reversible nephrotoxicity.

Pharmacokinetics

Enflurane is relatively insoluble, so only a small fraction (approximately 2.5%) is metabolized. However, free fluoride ion is released by this process and during prolonged anesthesia this may lead to nephrotoxicity in susceptible patients.

ISOFLURANE

Use

Isoflurane is 1-chloro-2,2,2-trifluoroethyl difluoromethyl ether (boiling point 48.5°C). It has a blood–gas partition coefficient of 1.4 and an MAC of 1.15% in oxygen. Isoflurane is a less soluble isomer of enflurane, and is widely used. It potentiates the action of muscle relaxants. It produces dose-dependent peripheral vasodilatation and therefore hypotension but with less depression of the myocardium than halothane or enflurane. This makes it the agent of choice for use in hypotensive anesthesia as cardiac output is well maintained. The relative cardiostability of isoflurane also makes it popular for use in patients with cardiac disease. Cerebral blood flow is little affected by isoflurane anesthesia which makes it an agent of choice during neurosurgery. Uterine tone is well maintained compared with halothane or enflurane thereby reducing the likelihood of anesthetic associated *postpartum* hemorrhage.

Adverse effects

1. **Cardiovascular system** Hypotension from peripheral vasodilatation. High concentrations (greater than 2 MAC) may theoretically worsen ischemia in patients with ischemic heart disease due to a 'coronary steal' syndrome where blood flow is increased along the normal vessels at the expense of the already ischemic areas, these being supplied by stressed rigid vessels. Normal clinical use of isoflurane is not associated with this problem.
2. **Respiratory system** Respiratory depression is common and dose dependent. The vapor is also irritant which makes gas induction more difficult than with halothane.

Pharmacokinetics

Because of its low solubility isoflurane is even less metabolized than enflurane (approximately 0.2%), so fluoride accumulation is rare and only seen after prolonged administration (e.g. when used for sedation in intensive care).

NITROUS OXIDE

Use

Nitrous oxide is stable and unaffected by soda lime. It is not irritant. It is a powerful analgesic but a weak anesthetic, with a MAC of 104%. It has a blood–gas partition coefficient of 0.47, which means that anesthesia is induced rapidly. Unconsciousness is not usually attained unless the concentration of inhaled gas is above 70%, but use of less than 30% inhaled oxygen may result in a PaO_2 below 80 mmHg (10.5 kPa), severely limiting its use as a sole agent. Uses include:

1. General anesthesia after premedication, intravenous induction with a volatile or intravenous supplement. There is poor muscle relaxation, not adequate for abdominal surgery.
2. Premixed nitrous oxide and oxygen in equal volumes can be administered on a demand system and it is useful as an analgesic in labor, during postoperative physiotherapy, changing of surgical dressings, removal of drainage tubes and other painful procedures.
3. Concomitant administration of nitrous oxide with one of the volatile anesthetics reduces the MAC value of the volatile agent by up to 75%.

Adverse effects

1. Nitrous oxide on its own, like nitrogen, produces progressive hypoxia and can result in death or permanent neurological sequelae. With adequate (20% or more) oxygen, nitrous oxide does not depress respiration but does potentiate respiratory depression due to barbiturates and narcotic analgesics.
2. Nitrous oxide in the alveolar gas equilibrates with the pulmonary capillary blood, tissues and gas-containing spaces, whilst nitrogen is removed and passes into the alveoli. Because of the large difference in their blood–gas partition coefficients, much less nitrogen will leave the circulation compared with the nitrous oxide entering. Thus pressure can increase in the gut, lungs, middle ear and sinuses. Ear complications and pneumothorax may occur.

   After cessation of administration of nitrous oxide, the rapid outflow into the alveoli can result in diffusion hypoxia, i.e. the gas diffuses out very quickly and can account for up to 10% of the expired volume; this displaces alveolar air so that the patient is left a hypoxic mixture to breathe.
3. Prolonged administration (as in tetanus treatment) has resulted in megaloblastic anemia due to interference with the action of vitamin B_{12}, and agranulocytosis.

Pharmacokinetics

Nitrous oxide is eliminated unchanged from the body, mostly via the lungs. Despite its high solubility in fat most is eliminated within minutes of stopping administration.

New agents

Two potentially important inhalational anesthetic agents (sevoflurane and desflurane) are being developed. Sevoflurane, being non-irritant, promises to be the best agent for smooth, rapid gaseous induction of anesthesia, affords cardiovascular stability and allows for rapid recovery. It has the potential disadvantage of being metabolized to the same extent as enflurane. Desflurane is the most cardio-stable agent yet developed and also affords rapid induction and recovery. Metabolism is of the order of only 0.02%. Problems with its use are (1) its extreme pungency, and (2) being highly volatile at room temperature, it requires a special vaporizer.

Occupational hazards of inhalational anesthetics

Apart from the obvious risks to patients, the effects of prolonged exposure to inhalational agents on anesthetists and other theatre personnel have to be considered. Among postulated hazards are abortion, low birth-weight infants, congenital disorders and cancer in adults. Although much of the evidence is controversial, evidence is accumulating that such exposure may be hazardous and that all possible precautions to ensure efficient removal of anesthetic gases from the environment must be taken.

INTRAVENOUS ANESTHETICS

Uptake and distribution

Uptake depends on a number of factors including the concentration of agent, the site, rate and volume of injection, and circulation time – a low cardiac output resulting in a longer induction time. Redistribution rather than metabolism is the main factor influencing waking time following a single bolus dose of an intravenous anesthetic. The anesthetic action depends on administration of a large enough bolus to produce a high blood–brain concentration gradient. Plasma concentration falls rapidly due to dilution in the bloodstream followed by distribution to other body tissues. Metabolism then follows at a rate of approximately 10–20% per hour of the total dose.

SODIUM THIOPENTONE

Use and pharmacokinetics

Sodium thiopentone is used to induce general anesthesia (and also in status epilepticus,

chapter 19). It dissolves in water and a 5% solution has a pH of 10.8. Sodium carbonate, 1.6%, is added to the powder to prevent formation of free acid on exposure to atmospheric carbon dioxide. It is therefore an extremely irritant solution. Its safe use depends critically on understanding its pharmacokinetics. A dose of 4–5 mg/kg intravenously produces loss of consciousness within 10 s and general anesthesia for about 5 min. The plasma half-life of the drug is 6 hours but the rapid course of action is explained by its high lipid solubility coupled with the rich cerebral blood flow which ensures rapid penetration into the brain. The short-lived anesthesia results from the rapid fall (α phase, chapter 3) of the blood concentration, which occurs due to distribution of drug into the tissues. Drug is then transferred rapidly back out of the brain into blood to maintain equilibrium. Following the initial uptake of thiopentone into brain the main early transfer is into muscle. In the hypovolemia and vasoconstriction occurring in shock, this transfer is reduced and sustained high concentrations develop in brain and heart, producing prolonged and sometimes fatal depression of these organs. These facts were unknown during the early use of the drug. The mortality from thiopentone use in trauma, for example after the Pearl Harbor attack, was consequently a staggering 1 in 80, and thiopentone is now used only for induction and not for maintenance of anesthesia. Metabolism, mainly side chain oxidation, is almost complete and occurs in the liver, muscles and kidneys. The metabolites are excreted via the kidneys. Reduced doses are used in the presence of impaired liver or renal function.

Adverse effects

1. **Central nervous system** There is depression of many central functions including respiratory and cardiovascular centers. Subanesthetic doses are not analgesic and indeed produce hyperalgesia. Cerebral blood flow and metabolism are reduced (this is turned to advantage when thiopentone is used in neuroanesthesia).

2. **Cardiovascular system** The force of cardiac contraction and therefore cardiac output is reduced. Cardiac arrest can occur in patients with pre-existing heart disease. There is dilatation of peripheral capacitance vessels with a fall in blood pressure and reduction in renal blood flow.

3. **Respiratory system** In addition to centrally mediated respiratory depression, there is an increased tendency to laryngo- and bronchospasm.

4. **Allergy and other adverse effects** These can manifest as urticaria or anaphylactic shock due to histamine release. Necrosis of tissue and peripheral nerve injury can occur due to accidental extravascular administration and arterial spasm following accidental injection into an artery. Postoperative restlessness and nausea are common.

5. **Thiopentone** should be avoided or the dose reduced in patients with shock, anemia, uremia, cardiac disease and in immature infants. Acute porphyria can be precipitated in susceptible patients.

PROPOFOL

Use

Propofol is the newest of the commonly used anesthetic induction agents. Owing to its short duration of action and the rapid clear-headed recovery that ensues from its use, it has superseded thiopentone as an intravenous induction agent in many centers. It is formulated as an emulsion in egg phosphatide/soya bean oil at a concentration of 10 mg/ml. Its main advantage over other agents is that it is rapidly metabolized and has no active metabolites. After a single dose patients recover after approximately 5 min with a clear head and no hangover. It may have amnesic and antiemetic actions. Uses include:

1. Intravenous induction. A dose of 2–2.5 mg/kg depending on patient response will provide generally smooth induction of anesthesia lasting for approximately 5 min, making it especially useful for short procedures and day case surgery. Special caution is, however, needed following day case surgery because delayed recovery can occur, and delayed convulsions have also been reported.

2. Maintenance of anesthesia. Total intravenous anesthesia (TIVA) using propofol in doses of 6–12 mg/kg/h in conjunction with oxygen or oxygen-enriched air ± nitrous oxide, opioids and muscle relaxants relies on the short half-life of propofol. It is 'environmentally friendly', avoiding the need for volatile fluorocarbons that have been implicated in damaging the ozone layer. In addition, propofol has little effect on cerebral blood flow (unlike nitrous oxide and volatile agents), making TIVA with propofol a useful technique in neuroanesthesia.

3. Sedation. Doses of 2–3 mg/kg/h can be used where sedation is required, for example in intensive care or during investigative procedures.

Adverse effects

1. **Cardiovascular system** Propofol produces greater cardiovascular depression than other intravenous agents and should be

avoided in patients with cardiac disease or where hypovolemia exists.

3. **Respiratory system** Apnea following injection is generally more marked than with thiopentone and may require assisted ventilation. Laryngeal reflexes are obtunded to a greater degree than with other intravenous induction agents. Histamine release can occur and bronchospasm has been reported occasionally in susceptible patients.

3. **Nutrition** Long-term sedation in intensive care using propofol can lead to a substantial extra calorie load (in the form of lipid) which should be accounted for if the patient is receiving parenteral nutrition.

KETAMINE

Use

Ketamine is used as a parenteral anesthetic, but has adverse effects (see below). Because of its ease of administration and safety, its use is widespread in countries where there are few skilled anesthetists. Its safety relates to the fact that, unlike other injectable anesthetics, it is a respiratory and cardiac stimulant (rather than depressant). The altered state of consciousness that it produces differs from conventional anesthesia in that there is profound sedation and analgesia, but there may be 'dreaming' and muscle tone is increased. It has been used for management of mass casualties or for anesthesia of trapped patients to carry out amputations etc.

Adverse effects

1. **Ketamine** was developed from phencyclidine (now used only as an animal tranquillizer and drug of abuse because of its ability to cause psychosis). Ketamine can cause similar, though less severe hallucinatory experiences consisting of vivid, unpleasant, brightly colored dreams of a hallucinatory character occurring in some 15% of patients during recovery and often accompanied by delirium. 'Flashbacks' can occur over many months. This can occur in children, and it is unfortunate that

ketamine has been used widely for procedures in this age group.

2. **Intracranial pressure** is increased by ketamine and its safety in patients with raised intracranial pressure has been questioned.

3. **Cardiovascular system** Blood pressure is raised by 25–30 mmHg and pulse by 10–15 beats/min, which may be dangerous in hypertensive patients or in those with heart failure or a history of cerebrovascular accident.

4. **Respiratory system** Respiration is mildly stimulated and salivation is increased, producing a risk of fluid aspiration into the lungs.

Pharmacokinetics

Plasma $t_{1/2}$ is 2.5–4 hours. Ketamine is 5–10 times more lipid soluble than thiopentone and rapidly passes the blood–brain barrier. An intravenous dose of 2 mg/kg produces anesthesia within 30 s which lasts for 5–10 min. Unconsciousness is probably terminated by redistribution of drug from the brain to other tissues as with thiopentone, but some of its metabolites have pharmacological activity which may be responsible for postanesthetic hallucinations.

BENZODIAZEPINES

See chapters 15 and 19.

Use

Diazepam has been used for induction and to supplement nitrous oxide anesthesia. Despite good amnesia and less cardiorespiratory depression than the other short-acting intravenous agents, it is not popular for induction. It is slow to act, can cause pain during injection and ensuing thrombophlebitis. Unpredictable cardiovascular depression may occur and a full recovery is prolonged. Despite these drawbacks, it is used as a psychosedative for minor procedures such as dentistry, endoscopy and cardioversion. The incidence of thrombophlebitis with intravenous diazepam has been substantially reduced by using a preparation made up as an emulsion in soya bean oil.

Midazolam is a benzodiazepine with a short plasma half-life (approximately 2.5 hours). It rarely produces thrombophlebitis and onset of hypnosis is more rapid than with diazepam. Recovery times after single doses of diazepam and midazolam are similar but midazolam produces more amnesia which is useful for procedures such as endoscopy or bone marrow trephine. It should not be used in repeated doses as accumulation occurs. The use of benzodiazepines for induction of anesthesia is usually confined to the slow induction of poor-risk patients.

A specific benzodiazepine antagonist **flumazenil** allows for rapid reversal of benzodiazepine sedation/anesthesia. However, it has a short half-life of less than 1 hour which often leads to resedation if given as a single bolus dose. This characteristically occurs when the patient has been returned to the ward where observation is less intense than in the recovery area. Respiratory depression and hence hypoxia may therefore be missed. Routine use of flumazenil after benzodiazepine sedation/anesthesia is not recommended.

OPIOIDS

High-dose opioids (chapter 22) such as fentanyl have been used to induce anesthesia in poor-risk cardiac patients as they afford cardiostability, as well as helping to reduce markedly the stress response to cardiac surgery. In this context fentanyl has been used in doses of up to 50 µg/kg (compare this with a normal single bolus dose of fentanyl of 50–150 µg). It is important to realize that even with these massive doses awareness under anesthesia has occurred and such procedures should be accompanied either with a small dose of a volatile agent or with concomitant administration of benzodiazepines to produce amnesia. High-dose opioids can also cause marked muscle rigidity making assisted ventilation difficult. This can be abolished by the use of muscle relaxants. Opioids are also used in neuroleptanalgesia.

Neuroleptanalgesia

Neuroleptanalgesia is a state of inactivity and reduced response to external stimuli. Symptoms of psychomotor agitation disappear and the patient is in a state of analgesia and sedation although able to understand and answer simple questions and obey commands. This state can be useful in complex diagnostic procedures, or nitrous oxide may be added to induce unconsciousness. Neuroleptanalgesia is commonly produced by a combination of droperidol (a butyrophenone 'tranquillizer') and an opioid (fentanyl or phenoperidine).

DROPERIDOL

Droperidol is a butyrophenone and so produces extrapyramidal effects. It is also a potent α-adrenoceptor antagonist and has quinidine-like properties. It has a short distribution phase half-life. It is usually given as an intramuscular or intravenous injection. The rapid distribution results in a rapid onset of action. The plasma elimination $t_{1/2}$ is 2–3 hours but droperidol has a depressant effect on behavior for up to 48 hours when given in usual doses (10 mg). About 10% of the drug is excreted unchanged, the rest undergoes hepatic metabolism to inactive products.

FENTANYL

Fentanyl is the opioid most commonly employed with droperidol to produce analgesia (alfentanyl or phenoperidine are alternatives). It is exceptionally potent having approximately 100 times the analgesic activity of morphine. It is also used to depress respiration in patients requiring prolonged assisted ventilation. It distributes rapidly into tissues following injection accounting for its rapid action. The $t_{1/2}$ is 2–4 hours. Fentanyl is rapidly and extensively metabolized but the short duration of action (the peak effect lasts only 20–30 min) is probably due to redistribution of drug from brain to tissues, like thiopentone. Particular care should therefore be taken after multiple injections where accumulation of the drug may occur because of saturation of tissue stores. As with other opioids respiratory depression can be reversed by naloxone. Bradycardia can be antagonized by atropine and muscular rigidity can be relieved by muscle relaxants.

SEDATION IN THE INTENSIVE CARE UNIT

Both ventilated and spontaneously breathing patients in intensive care frequently require sedative/analgesic drugs, both for humanitarian reasons and to reduce responses to stress, for example hypertension, tachycardia, tachypnea, that are undesirable in patients with compromised cardiac function or neurological disease. The choice of agent(s) used is tailored to meet the needs of the individual patient and regularly reviewed. This is particularly important where long-acting opioids or benzodiazepines are being used whose action may be prolonged due to accumulation of drug and active metabolites. Similarly ultra-short-acting drugs like propofol may not be the most suitable agents to use if ventilation is potentially destined to be used for several weeks as in tetanus. Most sedative drugs are given by continuous intravenous infusion both for convenience of administration and controllability, and include opioids, benzodiazepines (e.g. diazepam or midazolam) and anesthetics (e.g. propofol). Propofol is increasingly used where short-term sedation is required because its lack of accumulation results in rapid recovery.

PREMEDICATION FOR ANESTHESIA

Premedication was originally introduced to facilitate induction of anesthesia with agents such as chloroform and ether that are irritant and produce copious amounts of secretions. Modern induction methods are simple and not unpleasant and the chief aim of premedication is now to allay anxiety in the patient awaiting surgery. Inadequate premedication may lead to the administration of larger doses of anesthetic than would otherwise have been required thereby resulting in delayed recovery. Agents used include sedatives (e.g. benzodiazepines), opioids (e.g. papaveretum), phenothiazines, and muscarinic receptor antagonists (e.g. atropine).

*M*USCLE RELAXANTS

Muscle relaxants are reversible muscle paralyzers. They are grouped as:

1. Non-depolarizing agents (competitive blockers), such as vecuronium and atracurium. These bind reversibly to the motor endplate nicotinic cholinoceptor competing with acetylcholine and thereby preventing endplate depolarization and blocking neuromuscular transmission.
2. Depolarizing agents, such as suxamethonium which bind acetylcholine receptors at the neuromuscular junction, but act as agonists. The motor endplate is prevented from responding normally to acetylcholine by maintaining it in a constant state of depolarization. These drugs also exert a non-depolarizing action after the initial phase of depolarization which may relate to receptor desensitization.

All muscle relaxants are highly charged molecules and do not readily pass through plasma membranes into cells. They are usually administered intravenously and are distributed by blood flow and diffusion throughout the body. Changes in muscle blood flow or cardiac output can thus alter the speed of onset of neuromuscular blockade.

Non-depolarizing agents

TUBOCURARINE

Use

Curare, an arrow poison used by South American Indians, is derived from the plant *Chondrodendron tomentosum*. The active alkaloid, tubocurarine, is an isoquinoline derivative which has neither analgesic nor anesthetic properties but can release histamine and is a weak ganglion blocker. A dose of 0.5 mg/kg intravenously is used to produce muscle relaxation sufficient for intubation and controlled ventilation. At the end of the procedure the effect of tubocurarine can be reversed by the injection of an anticholinesterase such as neostigmine, 2.5–5 mg, which increases the amount of acetylcholine at the endplate by preventing its breakdown by acetylcholinesterase. Neostigmine is preceded by atropine, 1.2 mg, or glycopyrrolate, 0.5 mg, to prevent the parasympathetic effects of acetylcholine by blocking muscarinic receptors.

Pharmacokinetics

Curare is not absorbed when taken orally: hence Indians could safely eat the animals they killed with poisoned arrows. The half-life is about 100 min. The duration of paralysis is determined by drug elimination Some tubocurarine is metabolized but 30% is excreted unchanged in the urine. Renal excretion is by glomerular filtration and no secretion or reabsorption takes place via tubular epithelium because of the high degree of ionization of the drug. Biliary excretion occurs in dogs but has not been demonstrated in humans. After intravenous administration, the effect comes on rapidly, reaches a maximum at 3 min and persists for approximately 40–50 min, although following repeated administration a more prolonged effect results. The action is prolonged in acidotic patients and shortened in alkalosis. Volatile anesthetics intensify and prolong the action of tubocurarine. There is poor penetration of the placental barrier and usual doses do not affect the fetus or cross the blood–brain barrier.

Adverse effects

1. Hypotension due to autonomic ganglion blockade.
2. Occasional bradycardia.
3. Histamine release can cause flushing of the face and upper chest and very rarely bronchospasm and circulatory collapse.

4. In the presence of respiratory acidosis, myasthenic syndromes, concurrent administration of β-receptor blockers, aminoglycosides, frusemide and some tetracyclines prolongation of neuromuscular blockade may occur.

PANCURONIUM

Use

Pancuronium is a non-depolarizing muscle relaxant with a rapid onset of action, a peak effect at 2–3 min and duration of action of 60–90 min. It is about five times more potent than D-tubocurarine.

Pharmacokinetics

The $t_{1/2}$ of pancuronium is similar to D-tubocurarine (100 min). It is partly metabolized by hepatic microsomes, but a large fraction is eliminated by the kidneys so patients with reduced renal function show reduced elimination and prolonged neuromuscular blockade. Pancuronium, like tubocurarine, does not pass the blood–brain or placental barriers.

VECURONIUM

Use

Vecuronium is a relatively new non-depolarizing agent with an onset of action similar to pancuronium but a duration of action of approximately 30 min. A full intubating dose of vecuronium, 0.1 mg/kg, can usually be reversed successfully by anticholinesterases after only 15–20 min. It has minimal effect on heart rate or blood pressure and does not release histamine.

ATRACURIUM

Use

Atracurium is a non-depolarizing muscle relaxant with a rapid onset of action similar to vecuronium and a duration of 20–30 min. The intubating dose is 0.5 mg/kg. Flushing of the face and chest, hypotension or rarely bronchospasm may result from histamine release. Continuous infusion of atracurium is

popular in intensive care to facilitate intermittent positive pressure ventilation (IPPV) and during long surgical cases it can provide stable and readily reversible muscle relaxation as it does not accumulate. It is unique in that it is inactivated spontaneously in plasma by Hoffman elimination, a chemical process that requires neither hepatic metabolism nor renal excretion. This makes it the agent of choice for use in patients with significant hepatic and renal impairment. One metabolite, laudanosine, rarely causes epileptic fits.

NEW AGENTS

New non-depolarizing agents have been developed that are claimed to approach the speed of onset of suxamethonium whilst retaining ease of reversibility. Mivacurium and rocuronium are two such agents but as yet neither is in common use.

Depolarizing agents

SUXAMETHONIUM

Use

Suxamethonium is the dicholine ester of succinic acid and thus structurally resembles a dimer of acetylcholine. Solutions of suxamethonium are unstable at room temperature and must be stored at 4°C. They lose activity if mixed with thiopentone with which they are incompatible. Suxamethonium is used to obtain short duration muscle relaxation as needed for tracheal intubation, during bronchoscopy, orthopedic manipulation and electroconvulsive therapy. Because of the muscarinic effects of suxamethonium, atropine or glycopyrrolate is usually given before its use. A single adult dose of 1 mg/kg intravenously produces paralysis for 2–4 min. Apnea lasting more than 15 min is considered abnormal.

Adverse reactions

1. Prolonged apnea can occur. In about 1 in 2800 of the population a genetically

determined abnormal plasma pseudo-cholinesterase is present which has poor catalytic activity (chapter 13). Slow hydrolysis of suxamethonium in these patients produces prolonged apnea, sometimes lasting several hours. Acquired deficiency of cholinesterase may be caused by malnutrition, dehydration, electrolyte disturbances, anemia, liver disease (parenchymatous and obstructive), carcinomatosis, radiation, poisoning (e.g. organophosphorus). However, even very low blood cholinesterase levels acquired due to these diseases only prolong suxamethonium apnea by several minutes.

2. Muscle fasciculations are often produced several seconds after injection of suxamethonium and are associated with muscular pains after anesthesia.

3. Occasionally hypertonicity develops for 3–5 min and is then replaced by hypotonicity. Rarely this hypertonicity may develop into malignant hyperpyrexia (see below).

4. Owing to its muscarinic action repeated doses of suxamethonium without prior administration of atropine or glycopyrrolate can cause bradycardia or asystole.

5. Suxamethonium may cause an increase in salivary and gastric secretion and is contraindicated in severe glaucoma because it increases intraocular pressure.

6. It can precipitate ventricular fibrillation due to potassium release from striated muscle in hyperkalemic patients. For this reason it is contraindicated in patients with neuropathies, myopathies or severe burns.

7. Suxamethonium can produce anaphylactic reactions.

8. Neostigmine prolongs its action by increasing endogenous acetylcholine.

Pharmacokinetics

The action of suxamethonium is terminated by metabolism by plasma enzymes that are subject to genetic variation (chapter 13): pseudocholinesterase first converts it into succinyl monocholine. This is also a depolarizing muscle blocker but has only 1/20 of the potency of the parent compound. Succinyl monocholine is further hydrolyzed to choline and succinic acid. The plasma $t_{1/2}$ of succinylcholine is 2–4 min. In the absence of any enzyme activity non-enzymic hydrolysis continues at a rate of 5% per hour.

MALIGNANT HYPERTHERMIA

This is a rare but potentially lethal complication of anesthesia. All the volatile anesthetic agents and suxamethonium have been implicated in its causation. It consists of a rapid increase in body temperature accompanied by tachycardia and generalized muscle spasm. Severe acidosis and hyperkalemia can lead to serious arrhythmias.

Treatment

Treatment includes the following:

1. Discontinue the anesthetic and administer 100% oxygen via a vapor-free breathing system.

2. Administer dantrolene sodium intravenously: this inhibits excitation–contraction coupling in striated muscle by interfering with intracellular calcium mobilization, thus relieving muscle spasm. Intravenous boluses of 1 mg/kg are given as required at 5–10 min intervals to a maximum of 10 mg/kg.

3. Correction of acidosis and prompt treatment of serious arrhythmias.

4. Administration of 50% glucose and insulin to correct hyperkalemia.

5. Cooling.

LOCAL ANESTHETICS

Introduction

Many surgical procedures can be performed as well under local or regional anesthesia as with general anesthesia. A local anesthetic may well be considered the method of choice for patients with severe cardiorespiratory disease as the 'risk of general anesthesia is avoided and in many cases there is potential for good quality postoperative analgesia (epidural), and avoidance of systemic narcotic analgesics. Alternatively a local anesthetic nerve block is often useful as an adjunct to general anesthesia.

LIGNOCAINE

Use

Lignocaine is the most widely used local anesthetic in the UK (its use as an antiarrhythmic drug is discussed in chapter 29). For procedures such as lumbar puncture or bone marrow trephine it is used to anesthetize the skin and deeper pain-sensitive membranes such as the periosteum, and may be infiltrated locally, or applied topically as a gel or drops to mucous membranes. Lignocaine is chemically stable and like most local anesthetics is a weak base with a pK_a of 7.86. The unionized form is lipid soluble and spreads through tissues penetrating cell membranes. This necessary conversion to the unionized form explains why local anesthetics are less active (or inactive) if injected into an inflamed area due to low pH from local tissue acidosis. Local anesthetics act on the plasma membranes of excitable cells. The resting transmembrane potential is unaffected but the rapid inflow of sodium ions which is the ionic basis of the upstroke of the action potential is prevented. Like other local anesthetics small unmyelinated fibers are depressed first and larger myelinated fibers last. The order of loss of function is therefore: pain, temperature, touch, proprioception and motor function. Lignocaine does not affect vascular smooth muscle, but is available in combination with adrenaline which causes vasoconstriction and hence prolongs its effect.

Adverse effects

Toxicity (chapter 29) is uncommon after lignocaine is used as a local anesthetic but cardiovascular and central nervous complications can occur. A rough guide for maximum local administration is 7 mg/kg with adrenaline and 3 mg/kg without adrenaline. Toxicity can readily result from accidental intravenous administration of lignocaine. Absorption following topical application can be very rapid (e.g. from the larynx, bronchi or urethra) and levels in plasma may be reached similar to those after intravenous injection. Preparations containing adrenaline must not be injected into the digits (to produce a 'ring' block) because of the risk of vasospasm in digital end arteries and consequent ischemia. Systemic allergy is uncommon.

BUPIVACAINE

Bupivacaine is a commonly used long-acting amide local anesthetic especially for epidural/spinal anesthesia. Peripheral nerve and plexus blockade with bupivacaine 0.5% can have a duration of action of 5–12 hours. Epidural blockade is much shorter at about 2 hours but is still longer than for lignocaine. Relatively short duration of epidural block is related to the high vascularity of the epidural space and consequent rapid uptake of anesthetic into the bloodstream. Bupivacaine is the agent of choice for continuous epidural blockade in obstetrics as the rise in maternal (and therefore fetal) plasma concentration occurs less rapidly than with lignocaine. Bupivacaine has a mild vasodilator action that makes the addition of adrenaline less effective than with lignocaine. The maximum recommended doses are 2 mg/kg plain and 3 mg/kg with adrenaline added. Toxicity is more marked than with lignocaine. The first sign of toxicity can be cardiac arrest from ventricular fibrillation, which is often resistant to defibrillation.

PRILOCAINE

Prilocaine is similar in structure and actions to lignocaine, but is claimed to be less toxic. It is most useful when a high concentration or large total amount of local anesthetic is needed, for example for injection into vascular areas such as the perineum or for use in intravenous regional anesthesia (e.g. Biers' block). For topical analgesia a 4% solution is used. Adrenaline has a smaller effect in prolonging the duration of analgesia with prilocaine than with lignocaine, and in dental procedures prilocaine is often used with the peptide vasoconstrictor felypressin. Excessive doses can lead to systemic toxicity, dependent on plasma concentration, and the maximum safe dose is approximately 8 mg/kg.

Pharmacokinetics

Prilocaine is metabolized by amidases in the liver, kidney and lungs. The rapid production of oxidation products, particularly o-toluidine and nitrosotoluidine, may give rise to methemoglobinemia which is, however, of clinical importance only if there is severe anemia or circulatory failure.

COCAINE

Cocaine (see also chapter 49) is the major local anesthetic alkaloid in the leaves of the South American coca plant. It is used topically in nasal operations and other ear, nose and throat (ENT) procedures. A reasonable dose for surface analgesia is 3 mg/kg with a maximum total of 200 mg. Because of its inhibitory effects on amine uptake, cocaine potentiates adrenaline so the addition of a vasoconstrictor is unnecessary. Acute intoxication can occur, consisting of restlessness, anxiety, confusion, tachycardia, angina, cardiovascular collapse, convulsions, coma and death. In the central nervous system (CNS), initial stimulation gives rise to excitement and raised blood pressure followed by vomiting. This may be followed by fits and CNS depression. Small doses produce central respiratory stimulation; larger doses depress respiration.

BENZOCAINE

Benzocaine is a surface anesthetic which is comparatively non-irritant and has low toxicity. Compound benzocaine lozenges (containing 100 mg benzocaine) are used to prevent nausea and vomiting during the taking of dental impressions and for the passage of bronchoscopes and esophagoscopes in the conscious patient. They can also be used to alleviate the pain of local oral lesions such as aphthous ulcers, acute pharyngitis, lacerations and carcinoma of the mouth.

Analgesics and the Control of Pain

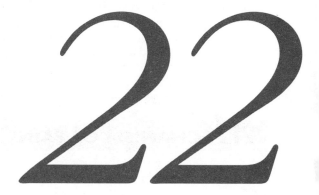

Introduction **228**

Mechanism of pain **228**

Potential sites of action of analgesics **229**

Analgesics in terminal disease **229**

Management of postoperative pain **230**

Drugs used to treat mild or moderate pain **231**

Drugs for severe pain **236**

Opioid antagonists **242**

INTRODUCTION

Pain is a common symptom and is important as it both signals 'disease' (in the broadest sense) and aids diagnosis. However, by definition it is a wretched sensation and its relief is one of the most important duties of a doctor. Fortunately, pain relief was one of the earliest triumphs of pharmacology, although less happily physicians and nurses are only recently beginning to use the drugs available adequately and rationally.

MECHANISM OF PAIN

Pain is usually triggered by a potentially harmful peripheral stimulus. The perception of such stimuli is termed nociception, and is not quite the same as the subjective experience of pain which contains a strong central and emotional component. Consequently the intensity of pain is often poorly correlated with the intensity of the nociceptive stimulus, and many clinical states associated with pain are due to a derangement of the central processing of afferent information such that a stimulus that should be regarded as innocuous is perceived as painful. Trigeminal neuralgia is an extreme example where a minimal mechanical stimulus to the face can trigger excruciating pain. An effect of the context in which pain occurs on the intensity of what is experienced is a general phenomenon. Postoperative pain provides a striking demonstration of the importance of higher functions in the perception of pain: when patients are provided with devices that enable them to control their own analgesia they report superior pain relief but use less analgesic medication than when this is administered by nursing staff.

The afferent nerve fibers involved in nociception are slowly conducting unmyelinated C fibers that are activated by stimuli of various kinds (mechanical, thermal and chemical) and fine myelinated ($A\delta$) fibers that conduct more rapidly but respond to similar stimuli. These afferents synapse in the dorsal horn of gray matter in the spinal cord in laminae I, V and II (the substantia gelatinosa). The cells in laminae I and V cross over and project to the contralateral thalamus, whereas cells in the substantia gelatinosa have short projections to laminae I and V and function as a 'gate', inhibiting transmission of impulses from the primary afferent fibers. The gate provided by the substantia gelatinosa can also be activated centrally by descending pathways. There is evidence of a similar gate mechanism in the thalamus. Descending inhibitory controls are very important, a key component being the small region of gray matter in the mid-brain known as the periaqueductal gray area. Stimulation of this area causes profound analgesia. The main pathway from this area runs to the nucleus raphe magnus in the medulla, and thence back to the dorsal horn of the cord connecting with the interneurons involved in nociception.

Stimulation of nociceptive endings in the periphery is predominantly chemically mediated. Bradykinin, prostaglandins and various neurotransmitters (e.g. 5-hydroxytryptamine, 5HT) and metabolites (e.g. lactate) or ions (e.g. K^+) released from damaged tissue have been implicated. Capsaicin, the active principle of red peppers, potently stimulates and then desensitizes nociceptors. The neurotransmitters of the primary nociceptor fibers include fast neurotransmitters [including glutamate and probably adenosine triphosphate (ATP)] and various neuropeptides including substance P and calcitonin gene-related peptide (CGRP) whose function is uncertain. Neurotransmitters that are known to play a part in modulating the nociceptive pathway include opioid peptides (metenkephalin and β-endorphin) that are present in the substantia gelatinosa, the periaqueductal gray area and the nucleus raphe magnus; 5HT, which is the transmitter of the axons running from the nucleus raphe magnus to the dorsal horn; and noradrenaline which is the transmitter of inhibitory fibers running from the locus ceruleus to the dorsal horn.

POTENTIAL SITES OF ACTION OF ANALGESICS

1. At the site of injury, by interfering with the chemical mediators involved in nociception. This is responsible for analgesic actions of the non-steroidal anti-inflammatory drugs (NSAID).
2. By blocking transmission in peripheral nerves as with local anesthetics.
3. By modifying transmission at the dorsal horn. This explains some of the actions of opioids and of nefopam and some of the antidepressants that inhibit axonal reuptake of 5HT and noradrenaline. This is also believed to account for the effect of vibromassage, transcutaneous electrical nerve stimulation (TENS) and perhaps acupuncture.
4. By interfering with the central appreciation of pain or by inhibiting its emotional concomitants. This is an important mode of action of the opioids and may also contribute to the analgesic action of antidepressants.

ANALGESICS IN TERMINAL DISEASE

The relief of pain in terminal disease, usually cancer, requires careful use of analgesic drugs:

1. It is important to use a large enough dose to relieve the pain completely. There is an extraordinarily wide range (about 1000-fold differences) in dose needed to suppress pain in different individuals, but very few patients need very high doses, and most need 200 mg/day or less of oral morphine.
2. Drug dependence is not a problem in this type of patient.
3. It is much easier to keep the patient free from pain than to relieve pain and its attendant anxiety when it has fully developed. Therefore in chronic pain and terminal illness regular administration is necessary. Ordinary preparations of morphine or diamorphine (used to establish pain relief, see below) usually have to be given at least four times daily. Strict adherence to 4 or 6 hourly injection regimes when the patient is requesting 3 hourly relief is inhumane and unnecessary.
4. If possible use oral medication, and once pain control is established change to a slow release morphine preparation. In addition to convenience this produces a smoother control of pain without peaks and troughs of analgesia.
5. Tolerance is not a problem in this setting, the dose being increased until pain relief is obtained.

A variety of analgesic drugs may be used depending on the severity of the pain and the preference of the patient. The World Health Organization (WHO) has endorsed a simple stepwise approach of moving from non-opioid to weak opioid to strong opioid. For mild pain paracetamol, aspirin or codeine (a weak opioid) or a combined preparation (e.g. coproxamol) is usually satisfactory.

Bone pain is often most effectively relieved by local radiotherapy rather than by drugs, but non-steroidal anti-inflammatory drugs are useful in some patients in whom such pain is partly prostaglandin mediated, and reduce opioid requirements in such patients. Bisphosphonates (see chapter 36) can also be extremely effective for bone pain in this setting. Buprenorphine, dissolved under the tongue, is useful for more severe pain and it has the advantage of a rather longer action than most powerful analgesics, but should not be combined with other opioids because it is a partial agonist (see below).

For short-term analgesia to cover dressings etc., dextromoramide orally or by injection is effective for 2–3 hours. For severe pain morphine or diamorphine are the drugs of choice. Their use is described in the sections on these drugs below. Doses are adjusted so that the patient is kept pain-free. Rarely, because of vomiting or the severity of the pain, morphine requires to be given by injection but such nausea and vomiting often resolve after a few days. Chlorpromazine or prochlorperazine can be used to reduce nausea and vomiting and may increase analgesia. Narcotic drugs are constipating and suppress appetite which is often very poor: despite hydration and as much fiber as is tolerated in the form of fruit and vegetables most patients require a stimulant laxative such as senna, or glycerine suppositories. Spinal administration of opioids is not routinely available but is sometimes useful for those few patients with opioid-responsive pain that have intolerable systemic side effects when morphine is given orally. Perhaps around one-quarter of patients with terminal cancer have some degree of endogenous depression. A trial of an antidepressant is worthwhile if this is suspected, but patients on opioids should be started on a low dose (e.g. imipramine, 25 mg) which is increased as required.

*M*ANAGEMENT OF POSTOPERATIVE PAIN

Unfortunately, postoperative pain has traditionally been managed by analgesics prescribed by the most inexperienced surgical staff and administered at the discretion of nursing staff untrained in the humane use of analgesia. Recently anesthetists have become more involved in management of postoperative pain, and in some hospitals specific pain teams have been set up with some notable improvements. There are several general principles:

1. Surgery results in pain as the anesthetic wears off. This causes fear in the patient, reinforcing anxieties about his or her illness and about the hospital environment thus making the pain worse. This vicious circle can be avoided by time spent preoperatively explaining the procedure, and giving reassurance that pain is expected, will be transient and will be controlled.

2. Analgesics are always more effective in preventing the development of pain than in treating it when it has developed. Regular use of mild analgesics can be highly effective. Non-steroidal anti-inflammatory drugs (e.g. ketorolac, which can be given parenterally) can have comparable efficacy to opioids when used in this way. They are particularly useful after orthopedic surgery.

3. Parenteral administration is usually only necessary for a short time postoperatively, after which analgesics can be given orally.

Where suitable devices are available the best way to give parenteral opioid analgesia is often by intravenous or subcutaneous infusion under control of the patient ('patient controlled analgesia,' PCA). Opioids are particularly effective in visceral pain and are especially valuable after abdominal surgery. Some operations (e.g. cardiothoracic surgery) cause both visceral and somatic pain and regular prescription of both an opioid and non-opioid analgesic is appropriate. Once drugs can be taken by mouth slow release morphine, meptazinol or buprenorphine prescribed on a regular basis are effective. Breakthrough pain can be treated by additional oral or parenteral doses of morphine.

4. Pethidine does not cause bronchoconstriction, and is therefore better for asthmatics than morphine which causes bronchoconstriction via liberation of histamine. It must still be used with great care in such patients because of its respiratory depressant action. Nefopam is useful when respiratory depression is an especial concern.

5. Antiemetics (e.g. metoclopramide, prochlorperazine) should be routinely prescribed on an 'as needed' basis. They are only required by a minority of patients, but should be available without delay when needed. The rectal route of administration is often appropriate.

6. Nitrous oxide/oxygen mixture (50/50) can be self administered and is useful during painful procedures such as dressing changes or physiotherapy, and in obstetrics.

DRUGS USED TO TREAT MILD OR MODERATE PAIN

PARACETAMOL

Uses

Paracetamol is an antipyretic and mild analgesic with little, if any, anti-inflammatory properties and no antiplatelet action. It has no irritant effect on the gastric mucosa and can be used in place of aspirin in individuals who are intolerant of aspirin. It is useful in pediatrics since, unlike aspirin, it has not been associated with Reye's syndrome and can be formulated as a stable suspension. The usual adult dose is 0.5–1 g repeated at 4–6 hour intervals if needed.

Mechanism of action

Paracetamol inhibits prostaglandin biosynthesis, but by a different mechanism from that of aspirin and the other NSAIDs. Prostaglandin biosynthesis requires the presence of peroxides as cofactors for the action of cyclo-oxygenase, and paracetamol reduces peroxide tone. This effectively prevents prostaglandin biosynthesis in tissues where peroxide concentration is low (such as brain), but not where this is high (as at sites of inflammation, especially in the presence of pus).

Adverse effects

Rashes and blood dyscrasias have been reported but are rare. There is no evidence of nephrotoxicity following short-term therapeutic use. The most important toxic effect is hepatic necrosis leading to liver failure after overdose, but renal failure in the absence of liver failure has also been reported after overdose. There is no convincing evidence that paracetamol causes chronic liver disease when used regularly in therapeutic doses, earlier reports probably being attributable to concomitant alcohol abuse. Paracetamol is structurally closely related to phenacetin, raising the issue of whether its long-term abuse causes analgesic nephropathy. It has been claimed that this does not occur, but some epidemiological evidence (from the USA) failed to exonerate it. Long-term use of large doses is, in any event, to be discouraged.

Pharmacokinetics, metabolism and interactions

Absorption of paracetamol following oral administration is increased by concomitant administration of metoclopramide and there is a significant relationship between gastric emptying and absorption. Paracetamol is rapidly metabolized in the liver and has a plasma half-life ($t_{1/2}$) of 75–180 min. The major metabolites are sulfate and glucuronide products, which are excreted in the urine (approximately 25% and 75% of the dose, respectively) accompanied by 1–4% unchanged drug. When paracetamol is taken in overdose the capacity of these conjugating mechanisms is exceeded, plasma $t_{1/2}$ of paracetamol is increased and a reactive metabolite, N-acetyl benzoquinone imine (NABQI), is formed by a cytochrome P_{450}-dependent metabolic pathway. N-acetyl benzoquinone imine is extremely toxic and causes hepatocellular damage unless inactivated by conjugation with reduced glutathione. This is the reason for giving acetylcysteine to such patients, as this repletes the supply of reduced glutathione in the liver.

ASPIRIN

Use

Antiplatelet uses of aspirin are described in chapters 26 and 27. As an antipyretic and mild analgesic it has similar efficacy to paracetamol while being less well tolerated. Unlike paracetamol it has anti-inflammatory properties especially when used in high doses (3.6 g daily or more), and is for this reason particularly useful in disorders (including rheumatic fever) where there is an inflammatory component. The dose of aspirin varies, depending on the type of pain being treated. For minor pains the usual dose for an adult is 600 mg repeated 4–6 hourly if required, taken after food. Various preparations are available, including regular as well as buffered, soluble and enteric-coated forms. Enteric coating is intended to reduce local gastric irritation, but these preparations have variable bioavailability, and much of the gastric toxicity of aspirin is due to inhibition of prostaglandin biosynthesis (see below), rather than direct gastric irritation. Consequently their use does not obviate the adverse effects of aspirin on the gastric mucosa. The same applies to benorylate, a prodrug ester of aspirin with paracetamol.

Mechanism of action

Salicylates produce their major analgesic and anti-inflammatory effects by inhibition of prostaglandin E_2 and prostacyclin biosynthesis at the site of pain production. Whether they have some additional central analgesic action is unclear. Their antipyretic effect is due to inhibition of the synthesis of prostaglandins E_2 and D_2 in the hypothalamus, which is the site of temperature regulation. Aspirin inhibits cyclo-oxygenase irreversibly by acetylating a serine residue in the active site and hence preventing access of substrate (arachidonic acid) to the active site. Salicylic acid (to which aspirin is metabolized) and other salicylates inhibit the enzyme reversibly but much less potently than does aspirin. In overdose salicylates increase respiration by a direct stimulant action on the respiratory centre and also uncouple oxidative phosphorylation leading to inefficient cellular respiration, lactic acidosis and fever.

Adverse effects and contraindications

1. Salicylism: high therapeutic or excessive doses of salicylates cause tinnitus, deafness, nausea, vomiting and occasionally abdominal pain and flushing.
2. Regular use of aspirin, even in low dose, frequently causes dyspepsia, and this is even more common when anti-inflammatory doses are used. Blood loss from the stomach can be life threatening. With prolonged treatment chronic low-grade gastrointestinal blood loss may be sufficient to cause iron deficiency anemia. The mechanism of the gastrotoxicity of aspirin is inhibition of gastric prostaglandin E_2 biosynthesis. Prostaglandin E_2 is the main prostaglandin made by the human stomach, and is involved in protecting the stomach in several ways: it inhibits acid secretion,

protects the mucosa by stimulating mucus secretion and perhaps at the cellular level also, and increases the clearance of acid that has diffused into the submucosa by causing local vasodilatation. Aspirin and other NSAIDs damage the stomach by impairing these protective mechanisms, and perhaps also by damaging the mucosal barrier directly by chemical irritation. Aspirin should not be given to patients with active peptic ulceration. It should not be given at the same time as anticoagulants and preferably should be taken with or after meals. Buffered aspirin reduces the risk of bleeding but this can still occur.

3. Wheezing, sometimes accompanied by urticaria and rhinorrhea, occurs in aspirin-sensitive asthmatics (approximately 2% of asthmatics). This is associated with the presence of nasal polyps and similar reactions to other NSAID and tartrazine (a yellow food dye). The mechanism of this adverse effect is evidently connected with the pharmacological action of aspirin rather than an allergic reaction to the drug. An individual who is aspirin sensitive is predictably sensitive to structurally un-related NSAIDs that share its pharmacological effect on cyclo-oxygenase. It is probably related to an alteration in the proportions of cyclo-oxygenase products (prostaglandins) to lipoxygenase products (leukotrienes) in the lung. Lipoxygenase is not inhibited by NSAIDs and acts on the same substrate as cyclo-oxygenase (arachidonic acid) to produce leukotrienes. These may be involved in the pathophysiology of asthma in some individuals: leukotriene B_4 is a dihydroxy fatty acid that plays a role in inflammation by causing chemotaxis, and sulfidopeptide leukotrienes (mainly C_4 and D_4) comprise the biological activity that used to be called slow-reacting substance of anaphylaxis (SRS-A) and cause bronchoconstriction.

4. Salicylates may provoke gout due to reduced uric acid excretion due to inhibition of tubular urate secretion. (Conversely high doses of salicylates are uricosuric because of inhibition of tubular urate reabsorption, but this is not clinically useful.)

5. Aspirin can cause hepatitis especially in patients with systemic lupus erythematosus and other connective tissue disorders. This effect is dose dependent and usually requires a plasma concentration of more than 250 µg/ml. The main changes are elevation of the serum enzymes. Histological change is minimal and liver function tests revert to normal on stopping the drug.

6. Reye's syndrome, a rare disease of children with high mortality, is characterized by hepatic failure and encephalopathy often occurring in the setting of a viral illness. It occurs frequently, although not invariably, after ingestion of aspirin. The cause of this epidemiological association is not known.

Pharmacokinetics

The gastrointestinal absorption of salicylates is rapid, with an apparent absorption half-life of soluble aspirin of 5–15 min. Aspirin is subject to considerable presystemic metabolism to salicylate, so plasma concentration of aspirin is much lower than of salicylate following an oral dose (Fig. 22.1).

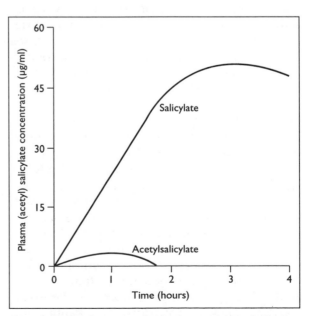

Fig. 22.1 Plasma levels of salicylate and acetylsalicylate following 650 mg aspirin given orally demonstrating rapid conversion of acetylsalicylate to salicylate.

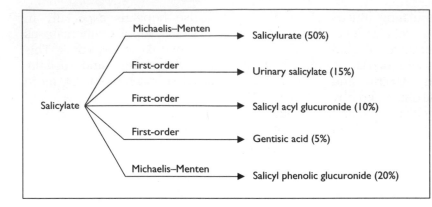

Fig. 22.2 The main pathways of salicylate metabolism.

Some of the selectivity of aspirin for platelet cyclo-oxygenase is probably due to exposure of platelets to high concentrations of aspirin in portal blood, whereas tissues are exposed to the lower concentrations present in the systemic circulation. Salicylates are extensively bound (80–85%) to plasma albumin. Salicylate is metabolized in the liver by five main parallel pathways, two of which are saturable, and is also excreted unchanged in the urine by a first-order process. This is summarized in Fig. 22.2. The formation of salicylurate is of interest since it is one of the relatively few drug metabolism processes that occur in mitochondria and is easily saturable. Consequently salicylate has dose-dependent (non-linear) kinetics: for doses lower than 4 mg/kg the plasma disappearance of salicylate follows approximately first-order kinetics with an apparent $t_{1/2}$ of 2–4 hours but for higher doses elimination is non-linear and $t_{1/2}$ may be as long as 15–30 hours. Clinically this means that for example doubling the daily dose from 2 to 4 g raises the amount of salicylate in the body at steady state disproportionately from 1.3 to 5.3 g. It also requires a longer time to reach steady state using a larger daily dose. Urinary elimination of salicylate is influenced by pH, being more rapid in alkaline urine which favors the charged (polar) anionic form which is not reabsorbed rather than the free acid. This property is utilized in the treatment of salicylate overdose by alkalinization of the urine by administration of sodium bicarbonate.

Drug interactions

The pharmacodynamic interaction of misoprostol, a prostaglandin E analog or of H_2 antagonists with aspirin (and other NSAIDs) is potentially useful. It may permit aspirin to be tolerated by individuals who otherwise experience unacceptable dyspepsia, and reduces the risk of hemorrhage, albeit at considerable expense, and the risk of toxicity and side effects from the second drug. Consequently, the routine use of such drugs in patients who do not experience dyspepsia is not recommended. Salicylates potentiate gastric irritation by alcohol and potentiate the effects of some oral hypoglycemic agents. They increase the risk of bleeding in patients receiving oral anticoagulants by their effects on platelets, their gastrotoxicity and, in large doses, by a hypoprothrombinemic effect. Aspirin should not be given to neonates with hyperbilirubinemia because of the risk of kernicterus as a result of displacement of bilirubin from its binding site on plasma albumin.

IBUPROFEN

Ibuprofen has a similar analgesic potency to paracetamol and in addition has useful anti-inflammatory activity, so it is an alternative to aspirin for painful conditions with an inflammatory component such as sprains and minor soft tissue injury. It is also useful in dysmenorrhea. It is a reversible cyclo-oxygenase inhibitor, but causes rather less gastric irritation than aspirin and other NSAIDs, and is available in the UK over the counter. The usual dose is 400–800 mg three times a day after food. A suspension is available for use in children. It is also less potent than the other NSAIDs and is therefore not recommended in the more severe inflammatory disorders such as gout, where one of the stronger prescription only NSAIDs such as indomethacin is appropriate. It can cause other adverse reactions common to the NSAIDs including causing reversible renal impairment in patients with cirrhosis, nephrotic syndrome or heart failure, and it reduces the efficacy of antihypertensive medication and of diuretics by a non-specific pharmacodynamic interaction.

TOPICAL NON-STEROIDAL ANTI-INFLAMMATORY DRUGS

Several NSAIDs (incuding benzydamine, ibuprofen, felbinac and piroxicam) are available as topical preparations. Systemic absorption occurs but is modest. There is some evidence that these are effective in soft tissue injuries and other localized inflammatory conditions, but the effect is small and of uncertain clinical importance. They occasionally cause local irritation of the skin, but adverse effects are otherwise uncommon.

NEFOPAM

Use

Nefopam is chemically and pharmacologically unrelated to other analgesics, being a cyclized analog of orphenadrine. It is used for moderately severe pain, being intermediate in potency between aspirin and morphine. Unlike the NSAIDs it does not injure the gastric mucosa, and it is less of a respiratory depressant than the opioids, and does not cause dependence. It is used in postoperative or acute pain, and in the relief of cancer pain, and is particularly useful in patients in whom the respiratory depression caused by opioids is unacceptable. It is more expensive than opioids or NSAIDs. The usual dose is in the range 30–90 mg by mouth three times a day, adjusted according to response. The usual intramuscular dose is 20 mg every 8 hours.

Mechanism of action

Nefopam is a potent inhibitor of uptake of 5HT, noradrenaline and dopamine by nerve terminals, and it potentiates descending 5HT and other aminergic pathways that operate the gate mechanism for pain described above. Given intravenously it has mild positive chronotropic and inotropic effects due to potentiation of endogenous catecholamines. It has activity in some animal models that suggests that it may have antidepressant activity, in common with other 5HT reuptake inhibitors that are marketed for this indication (such as sertraline). In higher concentrations it has antimuscarinic activity, which accounts for some of its adverse effects.

Adverse effects and contraindications

Nefopam has few severe (life-threatening) effects, although convulsions, cerebral edema and fatality can result from massive overdose. It is contraindicated in patients with a history of epilepsy. It is also contraindicated in patients receiving monoamine oxidase inhibitors (see below). Similarly, its cardiac effects are such that it should not be used in acute myocardial infarction since it increases myocardial oxygen demand and may also be pro-arrhythmogenic. In contrast to the relative paucity of severe adverse effects, nefopam causes a high incidence of minor adverse effects, especially after parenteral use. These include sweating, nausea, headache, dry mouth, insomnia, dizziness and anorexia. Nefopam is contraindicated in glaucoma, and can cause urinary retention in men with prostatic hypertrophy. Neither tolerance nor drug dependence has been demonstrated.

Pharmacokinetics

Nefopam is rapidly absorbed (15–30 min) following oral administration. The plasma $t_{1/2}$ is 4–8 hours. It is extensively metabolized by the liver to inactive compounds excreted in the urine. Presystemic metabolism is substantial.

Drug interactions

Nefopam can cause potentially fatal hypertension with monoamine oxidase inhibitors (MAOI), and potentiates the arrhythmogenic effect of halothane.

COMBINED ANALGESIC TABLETS

A large number of fixed combinations of analgesics are marketed. There are a number of problems with these and their use is seldom justified. For example, coproxamol is a combination of dextropropoxyphene with paracetamol. Dextropropoxyphene is similar structurally to methadone but it is a weaker analgesic. Its elimination half-life is 12–24 hours and the half-life of its active metabolite norpropoxyphene is 24–48 hours. Although the combination is very widely used there is no clear evidence that it is superior to other mild analgesics given alone. The disparity in half-lives of the two components is a disadvantage when single doses are used but with repeated doses a higher steady-state blood concentration is reached which may account for its apparent efficacy when taken regularly. Overdose can be fatal (due to respiratory depression or atrioventricular (AV) block) particularly if alcohol is taken in addition: large doses of naloxone are required to displace dextropropoxyphene from opioid receptors, and treatment for paracetamol toxicity as described above will also be required. High doses of dextropropoxyphene produce euphoria and consequently abuse and dependence occur.

DRUGS FOR SEVERE PAIN

Opioids

Opium is derived from the dried milky juice exuded by incised seed capsules of a species of poppy *Papaver somniferum* that is grown in Turkey, India and South East Asia. Its medicinal properties were recognized as long ago as the third century BC. Homer refers to it in the Odyssey as 'nepenthes', a drug given to Odysseus and his followers 'to banish grief or trouble of the mind'. Sydenham introduced laudanum (tincture of opium) into English medicine in the 17th century and wrote that 'few would be willing to practice medicine without opium'. Osler referred to it as 'God's own medicine'. Opium had social as well as medical uses, and was not originally regulated. Several literary figures were 'opium eaters', including Scott and Coleridge as well as de Quincey. A number of notably discreditable events including the opium wars and the mistreatment of Chinese laborers on the Panama canal ensued from the commercial, social, moral and political interests involved in its worldwide trade and use. Opium is a complex mixture of alkaloids, the principal components being morphine, codeine and papaverine. The main analgesic action of opium is due to morphine. Papaverine is a vasodilator and is used for local injection into the corpora cavernosa of the penis in the treatment of erectile impotence (chapter 38).

Until 1868 opium could be purchased without prescription from grocers' shops in the UK. During the last 100 years it has been realized that opium was not without disadvantages, particularly the development of dependence. Much work has gone into synthesizing morphine analogs in the hope of producing a drug with the therapeutic actions of morphine but without its disadvantages. However, the analgesic actions of opioids are closely related to their potential for abuse and the history of this field has not been encouraging in that morphine was introduced as a non-addictive alternative to opium and this in turn was superseded by diamorphine which was believed to be non-addicting. Synthetic drugs such as pethidine, dextropropoxyphene and pentazocine were originally thought to lack abuse potential, but are now known to cause dependence and abuse.

Morphine is active when given by mouth, a more rapid effect can be obtained if it is administered intramuscularly or intravenously, but the potential for abuse is much increased. Some anesthetists give opioids such as fentanyl by the epidural route, especially during obstetrical surgery such as Cesarian section.

OPIOID RECEPTORS

Stereospecific receptors with a high affinity for opioid analgesics are present in neuronal membranes. They are found in high concentrations in the periaqueductal gray matter, the limbic system, the pulvina of the thalamus, the hypothalamus, medulla oblongata and the substantia gelatinosa of the spinal cord. Narcotic antagonists (e.g. naloxone) and certain analgesic peptides also bind to these receptors. These peptides are widely distributed throughout the nervous system. They can be divided into three groups:

1. Encephalins, leu-encephalin and met-encephalin, pentapeptides differing in only one amino acid.
2. Dynorphins which are extended forms of the above and are more potent in binding to opioid receptors and more powerful analgesics.
3. Endorphins (e.g. β-endorphin).

These peptides are derived from larger precursors (pro-opiomelanocortin, pro-encephalin and pro-dynorphin) and may act as neurotransmitters or as longer acting neurohormones.

There are three types of opioid receptor: μ, δ and κ; a fourth category, the σ-receptors are now generally not classified as opioid receptors because they bind non-opioid psychotomimetic drugs such as phencyclidine and the only opioids that bind appreciably to them are the benzomorphans (e.g. pentazocine) that have psychotomimetic properties.

Blocking opioid receptors with naloxone has little effect in normal individuals but in patients suffering from chronic pain it produces hyperalgesia. This suggests that a pre-existing stimulus is required to activate the pain-inhibiting function of the opioid system. Physical and emotional stress can produce analgesia which is reversed by naloxone. Electrical stimulation of areas of the brain rich in encephalins and opioid receptors (such as the periaqueductal gray matter), elicits analgesia which is abolished by naloxone implying that it is caused by liberation of endogenous opioids. Pain relief by acupuncture may also be mediated by encephalin release, because it is antagonized by naloxone.

Narcotic analgesics are believed to exert their effects by entering the brain and binding to opioid receptors. The resulting pattern of pharmacological activity depends on their affinity for the various receptors and whether they are full or partial agonists. The affinity of narcotic analgesics for μ receptors parallels their analgesic potency. In addition to their involvement in brain function the opioid peptides may well play a neuroendocrine role. Administration in humans suppresses the pituitary–gonadal and pituitary–adrenal axis and stimulates the release of prolactin, thyroid-stimulating hormone (TSH) and growth hormone. High concentrations of opioid peptides are present in sympathetic ganglia and adrenal medulla. Their function at these sites has not been elucidated but they may play an inhibitory role in the sympathetic system.

Following repeated administration of an exogenous opioid, the sensitivity of the receptors decreases, necessitating an increased dose to produce a constant effect ('tolerance'). On withdrawal of the drug, endogenous opioids are not sufficient to stimulate the insensitive receptors resulting in a withdrawal state characterized by autonomic disturbances including pallor, sweating and piloerection ('cold turkey').

MORPHINE

Use

1. The most important use of morphine is for pain relief. For acute pain following injury

an average adult requires 10 mg subcutaneously or intramuscularly repeated at 4–6 hour intervals. A large patient suffering severe pain may need 15–20 mg. Conversely, the elderly or debilitated and individuals with renal or hepatic insufficiency will require less than the usual dose (one-quarter to one-half). Previous analgesic requirements (if known) should be taken into account in selecting a dose.

2. Morphine may be given as an intravenous bolus if rapid relief is required (e.g. during myocardial infarction) and the usual dose is 5 mg. Intermittent subcutaneous injections can safely be self administered by preloaded devices in suitably selected patients postoperatively. Such devices can only deliver a fixed maximum dose in any period to avoid accidental overdose. Furthermore, morphine in large doses causes sleep (Morpheus was the god of sleep) before respiratory arrest, so otherwise healthy postoperative patients who overdose fall asleep and therefore stop activating the device before coming to harm.

3. Alternatively, morphine can be given continuously by an infusion pump (e.g. postoperatively), either intravenously or subcutaneously. This is very effective and relatively small doses are required.

4. Morphine is effective orally although rather larger doses may be needed owing to presystemic metabolism. Single doses of oral morphine are not very effective, but repeated oral doses produce a smoother and more prolonged analgesic action than intermittent bolus injections and this is particularly useful in terminal malignant disease. Morphine is given by mouth initially regularly 4 hourly as an elixir, giving additional doses as needed between the regular doses as a 'top-up', the daily dose being reviewed daily and titrated upward depending on the need for additional doses and by asking the patient about the severity of the pain. Once the dose requirement is established, sustained release morphine 12 hourly is substituted. If nausea is a problem an antiemetic (e.g. chlorpromazine) is useful. Constipation is anticipated and consumption of dietary fiber and fluid encouraged together with a stimulant laxative (e.g. senna) or glycerine suppositories. Morphine is used as premedication before anesthesia.

5. Spinal (epidural or intrathecal) administration of morphine is effective at much lower doses than when given by other routes and therefore causes fewer systemic side effects. It is useful in those few patients with opioid-responsive pain who experience intolerable side effects when morphine is given by other routes. A short trial (3 days) using a simple percutaneous catheter precedes implantation of a more elaborate system, and this requires considerable back up.

6. Continuous subcutaneous infusions by pump can be useful in the terminally ill, but there is an advantage in using diamorphine rather than morphine for this purpose since its greater solubility permits smaller volumes of more concentrated solution to be used.

7. Morphine is very effective in the relief of acute left ventricular failure. How this is achieved is unknown, but probably involves depression of pulmonary reflexes and dilatation of capacitance vessels (pulmonary vessels and great veins) thus reducing cardiac preload. The usual dose is 5–10 mg intravenously.

8. Morphine depresses the cough center and has been used in small doses to treat cough. Codeine is preferred for this indication. Cough suppression does not involve endorphin receptors and this property of opiates is not stereospecific, so that D-isomers, such as dextromethorphan, are effective antitussives.

9. Morphine has also been used in the symptomatic relief of diarrhea but codeine is preferred for this indication.

Mechanism of action

Morphine relieves both the perception of pain and the emotional response to it, as a result of its action as a full agonist on opioid receptors (especially μ, but also δ and κ) in the brain and spinal cord. These receptors are localized at several sites that have been implicated in nociception including the periaqueductal gray matter and substantia gelatinosa. In addition to these important central actions it has recently been shown that activation of peripheral opioid receptors on primary afferent terminals involved in nociception also causes analgesia, probably by modulating the adenylyl cyclase second messenger system that is activated by prostaglandins and other peripheral mediators that sensitize peripheral nociceptors. (The evidence for this comes from the analgesic effect of low doses of intra-articular morphine after arthroscopic knee surgery.) Morphine causes pupillary constriction by stimulating μ/δ-receptors in the Edinger–Westphal nucleus in the mid-brain. This action is not of therapeutic importance but provides a useful diagnostic sign in narcotic overdosage or chronic abuse. Morphine dilates capacitance and resistance vessels by both neurally and locally mediated mechanisms. The former results from withdrawal of efferent sympathetic vasoconstrictor discharge causing attenuation of the tonic α-adrenergic stimulation of the peripheral circulation. Morphine also causes peripheral histamine release and thus vasodilatation and, in some patients, bronchoconstriction. In some patients it may also cause bradycardia due to stimulation of the vagal center in the medulla. If such bradycardia is poorly tolerated (as may occur immediately following myocardial infarction), it can be corrected by atropine.

Adverse effects

Certain types of patient are particularly sensitive to the pharmacological actions of morphine. These include the very young, the elderly, those with chronic lung disease, myxedema, chronic liver disease and chronic renal failure. Overdose leads to coma. Morphine depresses the sensitivity of the respiratory center to carbon dioxide, thus causing a progressively decreased respiratory rate. Patients with decreased respiratory reserve from asthma, bronchitis, emphysema or hypoxemia of any cause are more sensitive to the respiratory depressant effect of opioids. Bronchoconstriction occurs via

histamine release, but is usually mild and clinically important only in asthmatics, in whom morphine is best avoided. Morphine causes vomiting in 10–15% of patients by stimulation of the chemoreceptor trigger zone. This action is mediated by dopamine receptors rather than opioid receptors, and can be antagonized by dopamine receptor antagonists (e.g. chlorpromazine). Morphine increases smooth muscle tone throughout the gastrointestinal tract, which is combined with decreased peristalsis, due to an action on μ/δ receptors in the ganglion plexus in the gut wall. The result is constipation with a hard dry stool. The increase in muscle tone also involves the sphincter of Oddi and morphine causes a rise in intrabiliary pressure which lasts for 2–3 hours. Dependence (both physical and psychological) is particularly liable to occur if the drug is used for the pleasurable feeling it produces rather than in a therapeutic context. Nightmares occur in about 1% of patients and can be helped by haloperidol 2–4 mg at night. Patients with prostatic hypertrophy may suffer acute retention of urine as morphine increases the tone in the sphincter of the bladder neck. Allergic phenomena are rare but rashes and even acute anaphylaxis have been described.

Pharmacokinetics

Like other organic bases opioids are well absorbed and morphine can be given orally or by subcutaneous, intramuscular or intravenous injection. After intramuscular injection the peak therapeutic effect is achieved in about 1 hour and it lasts for 3–4 hours. Morphine is metabolized largely by combination with glucuronic acid but also by N-dealkylation and oxidation, about 10% being excreted in the urine as morphine and 60–70% as the glucuronide. Metabolism occurs in the liver and gut wall and the oral bioavailability of morphine is 16–64%. The dose/plasma relationship for morphine and its main metabolite is linear over a wide range of oral dosage. Morphine-6-glucuronide has analgesic properties, and may account for a considerable part of the analgesic action of morphine. Only low concentrations of this active metabolite appear in the blood after a single oral dose which may explain why single doses of oral morphine are not very effective. With repeated dosing the concentration of morphine-6-glucuronide increases correlating with the high efficacy of repeated dose oral morphine. Morphine-6-glucuronide is eliminated in the urine, and the reason why patients with renal impairment can experience severe and prolonged respiratory depression when treated with morphine is accumulation of this active metabolite rather than of morphine itself. (Early reports of morphine accumulation in patients with renal impairment relied on assays that failed to distinguish morphine from morphine-6-glucuronide.) The birth of opiate-dependent babies born to addicted mothers demonstrates the ability of morphine to cross the placenta. The plasma protein binding of morphine is unusual in that it appears to be largely to an immunoglobulin (rather than to albumin). Unlike diamorphine morphine does not cross the blood–brain barrier rapidly and its potent central effects reflect very high receptor affinity and sensitivity.

Drug interactions

- Useful pharmacodynamic interactions with antiemetics (e.g. prochlorperazine, haloperidol) and laxatives (e.g. senna) have been mentioned above.
- Morphine augments other central depressants, and should not be combined with MAOI.
- Antagonists (e.g. naloxone) are used in overdose and sometimes (e.g. naltrexone) in managing addicts after withdrawal.

DIAMORPHINE

Use

Diamorphine is diacetylmorphine. Its actions are similar to those of morphine although it is more potent as an analgesic when given by injection (7.5 mg morphine is equivalent to 5 mg diamorphine). There has been a clinical impression that side effects including vomiting are less common with diamorphine than with morphine and that it has a greater euphoric effect. This is not supported by objective evidence and the drugs are very similar. Diamorphine is also said by some to have greater addictive potential than morphine and it is banned from use in the USA for this reason. Again this is unsupported by firm evidence, although the more rapid central effect of intravenous diamorphine than of morphine (faster 'buzz'), due to rapid penetration of the blood–brain barrier, makes it plausible. Diamorphine is used for the same purposes as morphine. It can be given intravenously, the usual dose being 2.5–5 mg. It is more soluble than morphine and this may be an advantage if large doses are being given by injection (e.g. as continuous subcutaneous infusion).

Adverse effects

The adverse effects of diamorphine are as for morphine.

Pharmacokinetics

After injection diamorphine is hydrolyzed (deacetylated) to form 6-acetylmorphine (which is pharmacologically active) and morphine. Both diamorphine and 6-acetylmorphine are metabolized very rapidly, the half-life of diamorphine after intravenous injection being about 3 min. This occurs in the liver and other organs including the brain. Diamorphine and 6-acetylmorphine enter the brain more rapidly and in greater amounts than morphine, accounting for the more rapid clinical effect of diamorphine than morphine. Fifty to seventy per cent of the injected dose can be recovered from urine, mostly as conjugated metabolites. After oral administration of diamorphine, only morphine appears in the blood, presumably due to the considerable presystemic metabolic conversion of both diamorphine and 6-acetylmorphine to morphine. The amount of circulating morphine after oral diamorphine is about 20% less than that from the same dose of oral morphine, suggesting that giving oral diamorphine is merely an inefficient way of giving morphine.

PETHIDINE

Use

The actions of pethidine are similar to those of morphine, but it is less potent, even in high doses and pupillary constriction is not a consistent finding. It causes similar respiratory depression, vomiting and gastrointestinal smooth muscle contraction as morphine but does not constrict the pupil, release histamine or suppress cough. It produces little euphoria but causes dependence. Pethidine is widely used in obstetrics as it does not reduce the activity of the pregnant uterus and is relatively short acting. The usual dose is 25–100 mg parenterally or 50–150 mg orally.

Pharmacokinetics

Hepatic metabolism is the main elimination route, less than 50% being excreted unchanged in the urine. The major metabolites are an N-demethylated product, norpethidine, and a hydrolysis product, pethidinic acid, and its conjugates. Norpethidine, which only appears in blood after multiple doses, is about half as active as an analgesic as pethidine but has twice its convulsant activity. The $t_{1/2}$ of pethidine is 3–4 hours in healthy individuals, but this is approximately doubled in patients with cirrhosis or hepatitis. Higher plasma pethidine concentrations also occur in elderly patients in whom the initial parenteral dose should not exceed 25 mg. Pethidine crosses the placenta, and placental blood may contain a higher concentration than maternal blood. Pethidine or its metabolites may be responsible for respiratory depression of the neonate and this is exacerbated by the prolonged elimination $t_{1/2}$ in neonates of about 22 hours (seven times longer than in healthy adults).

Drug interactions

- Monoamine oxidase inhibitors: a syndrome characterized by rigidity, hyperpyrexia, excitement, hypotension and coma has occurred when these drugs are given together. Its mechanism is unknown.
- Pethidine, like other opiates, delays gastric emptying, thus interfering with the absorption of coadministered drugs. Delayed gastric emptying is particularly of concern in obstetrics, since Mendelson's syndrome is a leading cause of maternal mortality.

METHADONE

Use

Methadone has very similar actions to morphine, but it is less sedating and longer acting. Its main use is by mouth to replace morphine or diamorphine when these drugs are being withdrawn in the treatment of drug dependence. A single oral dose of methadone given once daily under supervision may be less damaging than leaving addicts to seek diamorphine illicitly. Many of the adverse effects of opioid abuse are related to parenteral administration with its attendant risks of infection, for example endocarditis, human immunodeficiency virus (HIV) or hepatitis. The intention is to reduce craving by occupying opioid receptors, simultaneously reducing the 'buzz' from any additional dose taken. The slower onset following oral administration reduces the reward and reinforcement of dependence. The relatively long half-life reduces the intensity of withdrawal and permits once daily dosing under supervision.

Pharmacokinetics

After oral dosage, the peak blood concentration is achieved in about 4 hours. Methadone is 40% protein bound to albumin and the plasma $t_{1/2}$ is approximately 7 hours following a single intramuscular dose. The metabolism of methadone seems rather variable, particularly with repeated doses, so that with prolonged administration accumulation can occur.

CODEINE

Use

This is the methyl ether of morphine but has only about one-tenth of its analgesic potency. (Dihydrocodeine is a commonly prescribed alternative.) Although codeine is converted to morphine it produces little euphoria and is of low addiction potential. As a result it has been used for many years as an analgesic for moderate pain (15–60 mg 4 hourly), as a cough suppressant (codeine linctus BPC contains 15 mg/5 ml) and for symptomatic relief of diarrhea.

Adverse effects

Constipation and nausea are the most commonly encountered problems.

Pharmacokinetics

Codeine has a plasma $t_{1/2}$ of 3.2 hours, but free morphine also appears in plasma following codeine administration, and it has been suggested that codeine acts as a prodrug producing a low but sustained concentration of morphine. Sufficient morphine may enter the brain to produce analgesia without causing a high risk of abuse. Some individuals are poor metabolizers of codeine with the result that they produce little morphine and experience less if any analgesic effect.

PENTAZOCINE

Pentazocine is a partial agonist on opioid receptors (especially κ-receptors with additional actions on σ-receptors which result in hallucinations and thought disturbances. It also increases pulmonary artery pressure. Its use is not recommended.

BUPRENORPHINE

Use

Buprenorphine is a partial agonist. It can be given sublingually in doses of 0.2–0.4 mg and given this way is useful in controlling chronic pain of various types. In common with other partial agonists buprenorphine occupies a much larger fraction of the receptors to produce its analgesic effect than does a full agonist. Consequently it can precipitate pain and cause withdrawal symptoms in patients who have received other opioids, and much larger doses of naloxone are required to displace it from the receptors in the treatment of overdose than are needed to treat overdosage with a full agonist.

Pharmacokinetics

Like other opiates buprenorphine is subject to considerable hepatic first-pass metabolism if administered orally, but this can be circumvented by absorpion through the buccal mucosa when it is administered sublingually. It is metabolized by dealkylation and glucuronidation before excretion predominantly in bile. The duration of pain relief is a little longer than morphine.

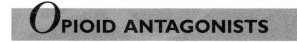

OPIOID ANTAGONISTS

Minor alterations in the chemical structure of opioids result in drugs that are competitive antagonists.

NALOXONE

Naloxone is derived from oxymorphone. It is a pure competitive antagonist of opioid agonists at μ-receptors. It is given intravenously, the usual dose being 0.8–2.0 mg for the treatment of poisoning with full agonists (e.g. morphine), higher doses (up to ten times the recommended dose, depending on clinical

response) being needed for overdosage with partial agonists (e.g. dextropropoxyphene, buprenorphine). Its effect is rapid and if a satisfactory response has not been obtained in 3 min the dose may be repeated. If the patient does not respond, the diagnosis of opioid overdose should be reconsidered. The action of many opioids outlasts that of naloxone which has a $t_{1/2}$ of 1 hour and a constant rate infusion of naloxone (e.g. up to 5 mg/hour) may be needed. It can also be used to reverse the effects of morphine postoperatively, or in the management of the apneic infant after birth when the mother has received an opioid during labor. Naloxone precipitates acute withdrawal symptoms in opiate-dependent patients.

NALTREXONE

Naltrexone hydrochloride is an orally active opioid antagonist at μ and other opioid receptors that is used in specialized clinics as adjunctive treatment to reduce the risk of relapse in former opioid addicts who have been detoxified. Such patients receiving naltrexone in addition to supportive therapy are less likely to resume illicit opiate use (detected by urine measurements) than those receiving placebo plus supportive therapy. Drop-out rate is, however, high due to non-compliance. Naltrexone has weak agonist activity but this is not clinically important, and withdrawal symptoms do not follow abrupt cessation of treatment. The usual dose is 25 mg increasing to 50 mg daily, and it should not be started until the addict has been opioid free for at least 7 days for short-acting drugs such as diamorphine or morphine or 10 days for longer acting drugs such as methadone because it can precipitate a severe and prolonged abstinence syndrome. Naltrexone has not been extensively studied in non-addicts, and most of the symptoms that have been attributed to it are those that arise from opioid withdrawal. In addition one reversible case of idiopathic thrombocytopenic purpura and several of other rashes have been reported. It has a number of neuroendocrine effects including increased plasma concentrations of β-endorphin, cortisol and luteinizing hormone (LH) (indeed it has been used experimentally to induce ovulation in women with amenorrhea secondary to hypothalamic disease, although it is not licensed for such use in the UK). Evidence of reversible hepatocellular damage is inconclusive but it is recommended that liver enzymes are determined before and at intervals during treatment. It is completely absorbed following oral administration, but is rapidly and variably metabolized ($t_{1/2}$ = 1–10 hours); the main metabolite is 6β-naltrexol which is much less potent than the parent drug but may none the less have important biological activity by virtue of its slower elimination.

The Musculoskeletal System

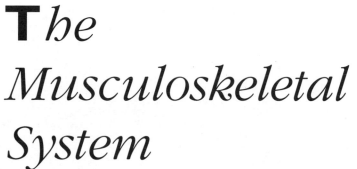
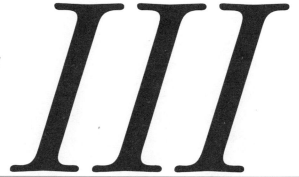

Anti-inflammatory Drugs and the Treatment of Arthritis

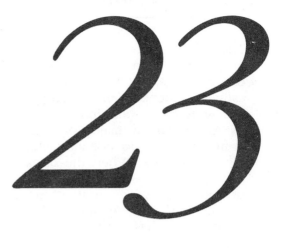

Rheumatoid and other chronic arthritides **248**

Drugs that suppress the rheumatoid process **253**

Hyperuricemia and gout **257**

*R*HEUMATOID AND OTHER CHRONIC ARTHRITIDES

Introduction

The cause of rheumatoid arthritis is unknown and current treatment entails the use of drugs that have been found empirically to influence some aspect of the disease. Non-steroidal anti-inflammatory drugs (NSAIDs) play a major part in controlling symptoms, but do not alter the underlying disease process. When the disease is resistant and progressive in spite of NSAIDs, one of the suppressive group of drugs can be added to the therapeutic regime, although their efficacy has been hard to establish and their toxicities make close monitoring mandatory. Patients should not, however, be allowed to become permanently disabled without a trial of such agents being at least considered. The place of glucocorticoids in treatment has changed over the years. There is no doubt that they suppress the inflammatory process and produce rapid and dramatic relief. However, with prolonged use side effects become more and more prominent and glucocorticoids are now only used when other measures have failed or sometimes in an elderly patient in whom a rapid therapeutic response is required to prevent them becoming permanently bedridden.

Non-steroidal anti-inflammatory drugs

USE

This group of drugs is widely used in the treatment of rheumatoid and seronegative arthritides including ankylosing spondylitis, psoriatic arthropathy and gout, and for cases of osteoarthrosis with a marked inflammatory component. They are valuable in suppressing inflammation in these miserable and chronic conditions, but are not believed to influence the course of the disease favorably in terms of progression to disability and deformity. Differences in anti-inflammatory activity between different NSAIDs are small, but there is considerable interpatient variation in clinical response. About two-thirds of patients respond to any NSAID, but among the remaining third, individuals may well respond to one drug having failed to respond to another. Consequently, if no response is obtained after 3 weeks, a drug of a chemically distinct class should be substituted on an empirical basis. Some NSAIDs are also used as general purpose analgesics for other types of pain (e.g. dysmenorrhea, muscular sprains and other soft tissue injuries), as described in chapter 22 on analgesia.

CYCLO-OXYGENASE INHIBITION: EFFECTS, ADVERSE EFFECTS AND INTERACTIONS COMMON TO NON-STEROIDAL ANTI-INFLAMMATORY DRUGS

All NSAIDs inhibit the enzyme cyclo-oxygenase and this is the basis of most of their therapeutic as well as their undesired actions. Aspirin is unique in inhibiting the enzyme irreversibly, and has a unique place as an antiplatelet drug. Aspirin is not, however, especially potent as an anti-inflammatory drug and the doses needed to achieve an adequate anti-inflammatory effect are associated with considerable toxicity. More potent reversible cyclo-oxygenase inhibitors are therefore preferred for this indication. Cyclo-oxygenase is a key enzyme in the synthesis of prostaglandins and thromboxanes. Two isoforms of the enzyme occur, a constitutive form (cox-1) present in platelets and other tissues and an inducible form (cox-2) formed in inflamed tissues as a result of stimulation by cytokines. There is currently great interest in the development of inhibitors specific for cox-2. Cyclo-oxygenase products are important mediators of the erythema, edema, pain and fever of inflammation, both by direct actions on the microvasculature, on nociceptive afferent C and Aδ fibers and on the hypothalamus, and by synergizing with other inflammatory mediators such as bradykinin, histamine, activated complement components (C5a) and platelet-activating factor. Both inflammation and pain are reduced as a result of inhibition of prostaglandin synthesis. Some NSAIDs have additional anti-inflammatory actions, including reduced superoxide and hydroxyl anion radicals and inhibition of leukocyte migration.

The NSAIDs share several adverse effects in common as a result of inhibition of cyclo-oxygenase, although not all members of the group cause these effects to an equal extent. Inhibition of prostaglandin E_2 biosynthesis is associated with increased leukotriene B_4 biosynthesis and leukocyte adhesion in microvasculature in the stomach and predisposes to gastric damage and peptic ulceration. Dyspepsia is common with all NSAIDs and hematemesis is their most frequent life-threatening adverse effect. Ibuprofen (which is available over the counter in the UK) is less potent than other NSAIDs, and gastric toxicity is correspondingly less common.

Non-steroidal anti-inflammatory drugs cause wheezing in a subgroup of aspirin-sensitive asthmatics (who sometimes also have a history of nasal polyps and urticaria), probably as a result of disturbing the balance of cyclo-oxygenase to lipoxygenase products (see chapter 22). All NSAIDs are likely to cause wheezing in aspirin-sensitive individuals.

The main prostaglandins made in human kidneys are prostacyclin (PGI_2) and prostaglandin E_2. Non-steroidal anti-inflammatory drugs predictably cause functional renal impairment in patients with pre-existing glomerular disease (e.g. lupus nephritis) or with systemic diseases in which renal blood flow is dependent on the kidneys' ability to synthesize vasodilator prostaglandins. These include heart failure, salt and water depletion, cirrhosis and nephrotic syndrome. The elderly, with their reduced glomerular filtration rate and reduced capacity to eliminate NSAIDs, are especially prone to this problem. Renal impairment manifests as a progressive increase in serum creatinine that is rapidly reversible if the NSAID is stopped promptly. All NSAIDs can cause this effect, but it is seldom seen with aspirin (which is a weak inhibitor of renal cyclo-oxygenase) or low doses of sulindac. This is because sulindac is a prodrug that acts through an active sulfide metabolite; the kidney converts the sulfide back into the inactive sulfone. Sulindac therefore is relatively 'renal sparing', although at higher doses, renal impairment does occur. For the same reason (inhibition of renal prostaglandin biosynthesis) NSAIDs all interact non-specifically with antihypertensive medication, and concurrent use of NSAID is a common cause of loss of control of blood pressure in treated patients. Again, and for the same reasons, aspirin and sulindac are less likely to cause this interaction. Both PGE_2 and PGI_2 are natriuretic as well as being vasodilators, and NSAIDs consequently cause salt and water retention, antagonize the effects of diuretics and exacerbate heart failure. As well as reducing sodium reabsorption, NSAIDs can also reduce lithium clearance, and lithium levels should be more closely monitored in patients on maintenance doses of lithium in whom treatment with an NSAID is initiated. Non-steroidal anti-inflammatory drugs can also increase plasma potassium, especially in patients with diabetes who may have underlying hyporeninemic hypoaldosteronism, and in patients with renal impairment or who are receiving drugs that elevate potassium (potassium supplements, potassium-sparing diuretics or converting enzyme inhibitors). Finally, NSAIDs are a well-recognized cause of acute interstitial nephritis, sometimes presenting as a nephrotic syndrome that is slowly reversible on withdrawing the drug.

CLASSIFICATION OF NON-STEROIDAL ANTI-INFLAMMATORY DRUGS BY CHEMICAL STRUCTURE

1. Salicylates and related substances.
2. Indoleacetic acids.
3. Propionic acids.
4. Anthranilic acids.
5. Phenylacetic acids.
6. Oxicams.
7. Pyrazolones.

Indoleacetic acids

These include indomethacin and sulindac.

INDOMETHACIN

Use

Indomethacin has a powerful anti-inflammatory action but only weak analgesic action. It is used in treating rheumatoid arthritis and associated disorders, ankylosing spondylitis and gout. Adverse effects are rather common so in chronic disorders it is best to start treatment with a single dose of 25 mg daily and increase this gradually up to 25 mg three times daily. Further increase in dosage is unlikely to increase effectiveness. In acute gout the initial dose is 50 mg orally repeated after 4 hours and then 6 hourly for a few days. It can be given as a suppository (100 mg) at night to relieve morning stiffness in rheumatoid arthritis and slow release preparations are available.

Adverse effects

Indomethacin produces side effects in at least 25% of patients. The most common are headaches and occasionally other central nervous symptoms such as light-headedness, confusion or hallucination. Gastric intolerance is common and renal and pulmonary toxicites occur as with other NSAIDs (see above).

Pharmacokinetics

Indomethacin is readily absorbed by mouth or from suppositories. Indomethacin undergoes extensive hepatic metabolism and both parent compound and metabolites take part in enterohepatic circulation. Mean half-life ($t_{1/2}$) is 7–10 hours, but hepatic elimination is prolonged in patients with biliary obstruction. Indomethacin and inactive metabolites are also excreted in urine.

Drug interactions

Anticoagulants worsen hemorrhage should peptic ulceration or gastritis occur during treatment with indomethacin. Actions of antihypertensive drugs and diuretics are opposed by indomethacin. Triamterene (as commonly prescribed in the combination product 'Dyazide™') should especially be avoided, as its addition to maintenance doses of indomethacin resulted in reversible renal failure in two of four previously healthy volunteers.

SULINDAC

Use

Sulindac is used in rheumatic conditions of all types including gout. The dose is 100–200 mg twice daily. Its relative lack of effect on renal cyclo-oxygenase (see above) is useful when low doses are used in patients with hypertension or with diseases where renal blood flow is dependent on prostaglandin biosynthesis (e.g. cirrhosis, heart failure, nephrotic syndrome), although its selectivity is not absolute and careful monitoring is mandatory in such patients.

Adverse effects

Sulindac is generally well tolerated, the main adverse effects being gastrointestinal disturbance, rashes and central nervous system effects such as sweating and vertigo.

Pharmacokinetics

Sulindac undergoes conversion to an inactive sulfone and a reversible conversion to an active sulfide. The sulfide metabolite is approximately as potent as indomethacin and has a $t_{1/2}$ of 18 hours. Enterohepatic recycling of sulindac followed by conversion back to sulfide contributes to the maintenance of high plasma concentrations of active compound. The kidney converts the sulfide back to inactive prodrug, accounting for the relative lack of cyclo-oxygenase inhibition in the kidney.

Propionic acids

This group is among the most generally useful, with a relatively low incidence of side effects. Ibuprofen is commonly used as an over-the-counter analgesic and is described in chapter 22 on analgesics. Naproxen is a more potent member of the group and has emerged as one of the first choices in treatment of inflammatory arthritis as it combines efficacy with a low occurrence of adverse effects.

NAPROXEN

Use

Naproxen is used in rheumatic and muscu-loskeletal diseases. It is useful in dysmenor-rhea and in the prophylaxis and treatment of migraine. The usual dose is 250–500 mg twice daily.

Mechanism of action

Naproxen is approximately 20 times as potent an inhibitor of cyclo-oxygenase as aspirin. An additional property of note is inhibition of leukocyte migration, with a potency similar to that of colchicine.

Adverse effects and drug interactions

Adverse effects and interactions of naproxen are generally mild, although effects common to NSAIDs occur.

Anthranilic acids

MEFENAMIC ACID

Use

Mefanamic acid is used for mild to moderate pain in rheumatoid arthritis and related conditions and dysmenorrhea. It has weak anti-inflammatory effects. The usual dose is 500 mg three times daily. Blood tests are required if it is to be used chronically (see below).

Adverse effects

Mefanamic acid causes adverse effects common to NSAIDs, of which renal failure in the elderly is especially noteworthy. It also causes several distinctive adverse effects: diarrhea, drowsiness, neutopenia and autoim-mune hemolytic anemia in which antibody is directed against normal red cells (for this reason it can interfere with blood cross-matching). Thrombocytopenia and severe rashes can occur, and overdose causes convulsions.

Pharmacokinetics

Mefanamic acid is absorbed slowly after oral administration, peak concentration occurring at 2–3 hours. It is 98.5% bound to plasma proteins and is converted to inactive metabo-lites by the liver.

Phenylacetic acids

This group (e.g. diclofenac) is similar to the propionic acids. Diclofenac has an action and adverse effects similar to those of naproxen. It is available as a slow-release preparation (75–100 mg once daily with food) and as suppositories. Intramuscular injection (75 mg once or twice daily deep into the buttock) is useful for short periods (1–2 days at most) for controlling postoperative pain, especially after orthopedic or dental surgery, and for renal colic.

Oxicams

PIROXICAM

The use and side effects of piroxicam are similar to those of other NSAIDs. It is extensively metabolized and has a long half-life (35–60 hours) so a once daily dose (20 mg) is used.

Pyrazolone compounds

PHENYLBUTAZONE

Use

Phenylbutazone is a powerful anti-inflammatory agent, but a weak analgesic with some uricosuric action. Serious side effects (see below) are frequent and in the UK its use is restricted to hospital practise where it still has some place in the treatment of ankylosing spondylitis. The initial dose is 400 mg daily in divided doses with meals and this is reduced to the minimum dose that will control symptoms, usually 100–200 mg daily. Suppositories, 250 mg, are available.

Adverse effects

Phenylbutazone has a number of unpleasant side effects which affect about 10–20% of patients.

1. Depression of the bone marrow (especially neutropenia) which is usually, but not always, reversible on stopping the drug.
2. Peptic ulceration.
3. Rashes.
4. Salt and water retention which may cause edema, hypertension and heart failure in patients with impaired cardiac function.
5. Hepatitis.

Pharmacokinetics

Phenylbutazone is well absorbed, extensively bound to plasma protein and metabolized in the liver. Oxyphenbutazone is an active metabolite with similar properties to phenylbutazone. Inactivation is to the glucuronide, which is excreted in urine. Slow elimination is a concern in view of its toxicity: mean $t_{1/2}$ is 72 hours (very considerably longer in some individuals).

Drug interactions

Phenylbutazone stereospecifically inhibits breakdown of the active S(−) enantiomer of warfarin, thereby causing its accumulation and increasing the risk of hemorrhage. It also inhibits metabolism of tolbutamide, enhancing its hypoglycemic effect. It inhibits secretion of methotrexate into the urine, while simultaneously displacing it from plasma protein.

Glucocorticoids

Glucocorticoids are discussed in chapters 37 and 47. Despite their rapid and often profound effect on the inflammatory component of rheumatoid arthritis and several other inflammatory arthropathies they have such severe long-term effects if used systemically in pharmacological doses that their use is now highly circumscribed. Prednisolone is generally preferred for systemic use when a glucocorticoid is specifically indicated, for example, for giant cell arteritis (for which high-dose daily steroid treatment saves sight); in lower dose for polymyalgia rheumatica; for selected patients with systemic lupus erythematosus with ongoing inflammatory problems (especially in renal glomeruli or brain), active polyarteritis nodosa, myositis or dermatomyositis. A brief course of high-dose prednisolone is usually given to suppress the disease, followed if possible by dose reduction to a maintenance dose of 7.5 mg or less given as a single dose first thing in the morning when endogenous glucocorticoids are at their peak. A marker of disease activity (e.g. the erythrocyte sedimentation rate in patients with polymyalgia or giant cell arteritis) is followed as a guide to dose reduction. An important use of glucocorticoids in rheumatoid arthritis and inflammatory osteoarthritis is by intra-articular injection to reduce pain and deformity in a joint. Glucocorticoids can be given locally into soft tissues (avoiding direct injection into a tendon as this can lead to rupture) to relieve periarticular pain, and when injected into the subacromial bursa is more effective in the treatment of painful shoulder than is naproxen. It is essential to rule out infection before injecting a steroid preparation into a joint, and meticulous aseptic technique is needed to avoid introducing infection. A suspension of a poorly soluble drug such as triamcinolone acetonide (a potent halogenated synthetic steroid also used topically to treat a variety of skin diseases) is used to give a long-lasting effect. The patient is warned to avoid excessive weight bearing or over use of the joint should the hoped for improvement materialize, since this predisposes to joint destruction. Multiple injections over a period of time also cause joint destruction and bone necrosis, and are to be avoided for this reason. Steroid induced myopathy is a particular problem with the fluorinated derivatives, and triamcinolone is to be avoided in patients with a history of steroid myopathy for this reason.

DRUGS THAT SUPPRESS THE RHEUMATOID PROCESS

Several drugs are not analgesic and do not inhibit cyclo-oxygenase but do suppress the inflammatory process in rheumatoid arthritis and some of the seronegative arthritides, perhaps by inhibiting excessive cytokine liberation. They only have a part to play in management of patients with progressive disease. They are sometimes rather optimistically labeled 'disease-modifying' agents; in fact it is very difficult to prove or disprove some effect on the natural history of a relapsing/remitting and unpredictably progressing disease such as rheumatoid arthritis. Because of their toxicity, they are reserved for patients with progressive disease, although there is a tendency among rheumatologists to use them earlier than in the past (despite the lack of regulatory body approval for such use in most cases), with close monitoring for toxicity and the patient fully informed as to their toxic as well as their desired effects.

GOLD SALTS

Use

Gold was originally introduced to treat tuberculosis. Although ineffective it was found serendipitously to have antirheumatic properties, and has been used to treat patients with rheumatoid arthritis since the 1920s. Sodium aurothiomalate is administered weekly by deep intramuscular injection: week 1, 10 mg; week 2, 20 mg; week 3, 50 mg; and thereafter 50 mg weekly until a total of 1.0 g has been given followed by maintenance treatment of 50 mg monthly. Benefit is not anticipated until 300–600 mg has been administered. About 75% of patients improve with reduction in joint swelling, disappearance of rheumatoid nodules and a fall in erythrocyte sedimentation rate (ESR). Urine must be tested for protein and full blood count (with platelet count and differential white cell count) performed before each injection. Auranofin is an oral gold preparation with less toxicity and similar (although probably slightly less) efficacy as sodium aurothiomalate. The usual starting dose is 3 mg twice daily, changing to 6 mg as a single daily dose if tolerated. If the response is inadequate after 6 months the dose is increased to 3 mg three times a day. If there is no response after a further 3 months the drug is stopped. Monitoring of blood counts and urine is performed monthly.

Mechanism of action

The precise mechanism of the therapeutic action of gold salts is unknown. Several effects could contribute to their efficacy in rheumatoid arthritis: gold–albumin complexes are phagocytosed by macrophages and polymorphonuclear leukocytes and concentrated in their lysosomes where gold inhibits lysosomal enzymes that have been implicated in causing damage to joints. Furthermore, gold binds to sulfydryl groups and inhibits sulfydryl–disulfide interchange in immunoglobulin and complement which could influence progression of autoimmune processes.

Adverse effects

Adverse effects from gold are often troublesome and sometimes dangerous: some adverse effect occurs in up to half of all treated patients, in half of whom they are severe.

1. Rashes are an indication to stop treatment as they can progress to exfoliation.
2. Photosensitive eruptions, urticaria and erythematous reactions to gold are often preceded by itching.
3. Glomerular injury can be severe, resulting in nephrotic syndrome, so treatment must be withheld if more than a trace of proteinuria is present and not resumed until the urine is protein free.
4. Blood dyscrasias can develop rapidly and consequently become established despite frequent routine blood counts.
5. Stomatitis can be troublesome, and suggests the possibility of neutropenia.
6. Diarrhea is common, and can often be improved by a bulk laxative such as bran.

Unusually an exacerbation of symptoms occurs shortly after each injection. Auranofin is generally better tolerated than injections of aurothiomalate, although similar toxicities occur.

Pharmacokinetics

The plasma half-life of gold increases with repeated administration and may vary from 1 day to several weeks. It is bound to plasma proteins and is concentrated in inflamed areas. It is excreted in urine and a small amount lost in the feces. Total elimination from the body takes a long time and gold continues to be excreted in urine for up to 1 year after a course of treatment.

PENICILLAMINE

Use

Penicillamine is a breakdown product of penicillin. It is effective in Wilson's disease and in cystinuria and more recently has found a place in the management of rheumatoid arthritis. It is given orally between meals (ideally an hour before food). The initial dose is 125 mg daily for 1 month, then 250 mg daily for a further month, increasing by 125–250 mg per month until a response is achieved. Clinical improvement is anticipated only after 6–12 weeks. When improvement is well established, the dose is gradually reduced (by 125–250 mg every 6 weeks) to the minimum effective maintenance dose. This is usually 500–750 mg daily, but as high as 1.5 g is sometimes used. Results are similar to those obtained with gold. Weekly blood and urine tests (including platelet and differential and absolute white cell counts and urine protein) are carried out initially, and then monthly during maintenance treatment. Treatment should be discontinued if there is no improvement within a year.

Mechanism of action

Penicillamine has several mechanisms of action including metal ion chelation via its sulfydryl group, and dissociation of macroglobulins. It also inhibits release of lysosomal enzymes in inflamed connective tissue.

Adverse effects

Adverse effects of penicillamine are common and can be dangerous. They are commoner in patients with poor sulfoxidation phenotype.

1. Bone marrow hypoplasia, thrombocytopenia and leukopenia occur and can be fatal: they are indications to stop treatment.

2. Immune complex glomerulonephritis is common and causes mild proteinuria in 30% of patients. The drug should be stopped until it resolves and then treatment resumed at a lower dose. Heavy proteinuria, with or without edema, is an indication to stop the drug permanently.
3. Other symptoms include hypersensitivity reactions with urticaria, nausea (minimized by taking the drug on an empty stomach), anorexia, taste loss (usually transient), systemic lupus erythematosus-like syndrome, and myasthenia gravis.

The toxicity of penicillamine is such that it should only be used by clinicians with experience of the drug and meticulous patient monitoring.

Contraindications

Penicillamine is contraindicated in systemic lupus erythematosus, and should be used with caution, if at all, in patients with renal or hepatic impairment.

Pharmacokinetics

Penicillamine is well absorbed from the gut in the fasting state. A number of hepatic metabolites are formed and rapidly excreted following acute dosing. Some of the active substance is tightly bound to plasma proteins and tissues and is slowly excreted over several months during and after chronic dosing.

Drug interactions

Absorption of penicillamine is prevented by antacids, iron or zinc (which bind to its sulfydryl group). It should not be used with concurrent gold, chloroquine or immunosuppressive treatment, because of increased toxicity.

CHLOROQUINE AND HYDROXYCHLOROQUINE

Use

Chloroquine, an antimalarial 4-aminoquinoline, and hydroxychloroquine have an effect in rheumatoid arthritis comparable with that of gold. They are also used in systemic lupus erythematosus, but are contraindicated in psoriatic arthritis because they worsen psoriatic skin disease. They are better tolerated than gold or penicillamine, but cause severe ocular toxicity if the recommended dose is exceeded. Eye examination is performed before starting treatment to establish a baseline and the patient advised to stop taking the drug and seek immediate advice if vision changes. Toxicity is rare if the dose of chloroquine is less than 4 mg/kg body weight daily or of hydroxychloroquine sulfate less than 6.5 mg/kg body weight daily. The usual adult dose of chloroquine for this indication is 200 mg, administered after food. Remission of symptoms in rheumatoid arthritis usually occurs after 2–3 months of treatment.

Mechanism of action

Chloroquine is not an analgesic or anti-inflammatory drug. It is concentrated in lysosomes, altering the pH and interfering with lysosomal enzyme function and with antigen processing by macrophages.

Adverse effects

1. Chloroquine retinopathy is heralded by bilateral central visual field defects with normal fundal appearances; in late retinopathy concentric rings of pigmentation are deposited around the macula, the so-called 'bull's eye' macula. Choroquine is concentrated in melanin in the eye and may cause damage by binding to retinal DNA. Corneal deposition also occurs, but is less serious.
2. Common adverse effects include nausea, vomiting, diarrhea, dizziness, headache, abdominal pain and rashes.
3. Pigmentation of the hard palate occurs in about one-quarter of patients on long-term treatment, and reversible bleaching of the hair also occurs.

Pharmacokinetics

Chloroquine accumulates slowly and while plasma concentrations are very variable and often low, progressive tissue binding occurs and it is this tissue binding with nucleoprotein and melanin that probably produces many of its toxic effects. About 50% of chloroquine is excreted unchanged in urine, the remaining 50% being metabolized in the liver.

SULFASALAZINE

Use

Sulfasalazine was originally introduced for the treatment of rheumatoid arthritis, and only subsequently found to be effective in maintaining remission in inflammatory bowel disease. Its efficacy in rheumatoid arthritis has recently been confirmed. It is given as enteric-coated tablets, initially 500 mg daily, increasing by 500 mg at weekly intervals to a maximum of 2–3 g daily in divided doses. Blood counts and liver function tests are checked monthly for the first 6 months and 3 monthly thereafter. Improvement usually starts within 2–3 months in patients who respond favorably, and sulfasalazine may be continued for several years if effective. Clinicians believe that it is probably rather less effective than gold or penicillamine but less toxic and better tolerated, although direct comparative trials are lacking.

Mechanism of action

The mechanism of action of sulfasalazine in rheumatoid arthritis is unknown.

Adverse effects

1. Life-threatening blood dyscrasias caused by sulfasalazine are rare, although less so than in patients with inflammatory bowel disease.
2. Common side effects include nausea, vomiting, headache, dizziness, rashes (rarely Stevens–Johnson syndrome), rarely hepatitis and pancreatitis.
3. Sulfasalazine colors urine orange and can stain soft contact lenses.

Pharmacokinetics

Sulfasalazine is poorly absorbed from the small intestine and is split into sulfapyridine and 5-aminosalicylic acid in the colon, both moieties probably being important for its action in rheumatoid arthritis.

Immunosuppressants

Immunosuppressants have similar activity to gold, penicillamine or chloroquine and are useful in patients who have failed to respond to these drugs.

AZATHIOPRINE

Use

Azathiaprine (see also chapter 47) is used to prevent rejection following organ transplantation. It is a cytotoxic immunosuppressant and has also proved effective in various conditions that involve derangement of the immune system including rheumatoid arthritis and systemic lupus erythematosus, Crohn's disease, chronic active hepatitis and autoimmune hemolytic anemia. It is useful in psoriatic arthropathy. The usual adult dose is 1.5–2.5 mg/kg body weight daily in divided doses with food. Blood counts are done monthly and if neutropenia or thrombocytopenia occurs the dose is reduced.

Mechanism of action

The precise mechanism whereby azathioprine produces immunosuppressant effects is unknown. It impairs B cell function with reduced immunoglobulin synthesis, inhibits the cellular component of the inflammatory response, and depresses cellular proliferation via its active metabolite 6-mercaptopurine. The mechanism of 6-mercaptopurine is itself not fully understood: it probably exerts its cytotoxic effects by a combination of incorporation into DNA, inhibition of purine biosynthesis and inhibition of DNA synthesis and repair.

Adverse effects

1. Bone marrow depression is the most common severe side effect of azathioprine.
2. Severe pancytopenia occurs in about 1% of patients treated with more than 2.5 mg/kg daily.
3. It is carcinogenic with a small increase in the risk of lymphomas, mesenchymal tumors and other malignancies.

4. Opportunistic infections may occur.
5. Alopecia is common.
6. Nausea and vomiting which is reduced by taking the drug with food are also common.
7. Dose-related cholestatic hepatitis and drug fever with myalgia and rashes are less common.

Pharmacokinetics

Oral absorption is high. Mean $t_{1/2}$ is 3–5 hours, but azathioprine is rapidly metabolized to 6-mercaptopurine which is pharmacologically active. 6-Mercaptopurine is itself rapidly metobolized and has a mean $t_{1/2}$ of 1–1.5 hours.

Drug interactions

Allopurinol inhibits breakdown of 6-mercaptopurine by xanthine oxidase and necessitates a 75% reduction in the dose of azathioprine. Azathioprine should not be used concurrently with penicillamine.

METHOTREXATE

Use

Methotrexate is an antimetabolite. It is a folic acid analog and is used in cancer chemotherapy as well as in immunosuppression. It is effective in rheumatoid arthritis and in psoriatic arthritis, in which it improves skin as well as joint manifestations. It is also effective in Wegener's granulomatosis. The initial dose for arthritis is 2.5 mg by mouth once a week, increasing slowly to a maximum of 15 mg weekly. Full blood count and liver function tests are carried out weekly to begin with and then monthly.

Mechanism of action

Methotrexate inhibits dihydrofolate reductase. How this accounts for its effects on the immune system is not known.

Adverse effects

Severe adverse effects of methotrexate include bone marrow suppression, gastrointestinal mucositis and cirrhosis (acute elevations of liver enzymes are however common and usually return to normal within 1–2 weeks). Minor effects include nausea and vomiting.

Pharmacokinetics

Methotrexate is 25–50% absorbed following oral dosing, and has a mean $t_{1/2}$ of 8–10 hours. It is approximately 60% protein bound in plasma. It is eliminated partly by hepatic metabolism but also importantly as unchanged drug in the urine by secretion into the proximal tubule. It must therefore not be used (or used with great caution) in patients with renal impairment.

Drug interactions

Other acidic drugs that are secreted into urine by the proximal tubular transport mechanism (chapter 6) reduce the clearance of methotrexate, and can be expected to increase its toxicity, especially if they also compete with it for protein binding. These include probenecid, aspirin and probably other NSAIDs and uricosuric drugs.

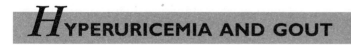

HYPERURICEMIA AND GOUT

Uric acid is the end product of purine (adenine and guanine) metabolism in humans, and gives rise to problems because of its limited solubility. Crystals of uric acid evoke a severe inflammatory response in patients with gout, cause chalky deposits (tophi) in cool extremities (e.g. pinna of ear, toes) and cause renal stones and/or renal tubular obstruction. The final stages in the production of uric acid are shown in Fig. 23.1. Two of these stages are dependent on xanthine oxidase. In most mammals uricase converts uric acid into allantoin which is rapidly eliminated by the kidneys, but

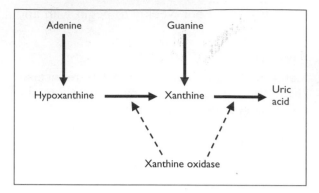

Fig. 23.1 The final stages of the production of uric acid.

humans (as well as higher apes and Dalmatian dogs) lack uricase so the less soluble uric acid must be excreted. Uric acid is filtered by the glomerulus but 98% is reabsorbed in the proximal tubule with subsequent secretion into the distal tubule. It is more soluble in an alkaline urine (which favors the charged anionic urate rather than free uric acid) and one factor in the development of uric acid stones is impairment of the ability to excrete alkaline urine. It is possible to lower the plasma uric acid concentration by increasing renal excretion of uric acid or by inhibiting its synthesis.

Hyperuricemia may arise:

1. As a result of a genetically determined defect of metabolism causing overproduction of uric acid, as occurs in primary gout.
2. As a result of increased breakdown of nuclear material which is seen in leukemia and similar disorders, particularly when treated by cytotoxic drugs.
3. When excretion is decreased, as occurs in renal failure or when tubular excretion of uric acid is diminished by diuretics or by low doses of salicylates, pyrazinamide or clofibrate.

Acute gout

The acute attack is treated by anti-inflammatory analgesic agents (e.g. indomethacin, 50 mg, three times a day, naproxen, piroxicam,

ketoprofen or diclofenac). Aspirin is contraindicated because of its effect on urate excetion. Colchicine, which is relatively specific in relieving the symptoms of acute gout, is an alternative to an NSAID but commonly causes diarrhea.

COLCHICINE

Use

Colchicine is derived from the autumn crocus. It is a useful alternative to NSAIDs in patients with gout in whom NSAIDs are contraindicated, for example patients with heart failure. Its efficacy is similar to indomethacin. It is also used in patients with other forms of crystal arthropathy (e.g. pseudogout) and with familial Mediterranean fever and certain forms of Behçet's disease that are associated with excessive polymorphonuclear leukocyte migration into sites of tissue injury. It does not interact with warfarin. For acute attacks it is given in doses of 1 mg initially followed by 0.5 mg orally every 2–3 hours until pain is relieved or diarrhea occurs, up to a maximum of 10 mg. The course should not be repeated within 72 hours. Colchicine can also be used prophylactically in doses of 0.5 mg two or three times daily. It is relatively contraindicated in old or feeble patients and in those with renal or gastrointestinal disease.

Mechanism of action

The primary action of colchicine is to bind to microtubular proteins. The most important results of this are:

1. Toxic concentrations cause arrest of cell division at metaphase. (This phenomenon is exploited in making chromosome preparations *ex vivo*.)
2. Inhibition of leukocyte migration and hence reduced inflammation.

Adverse effects

1. The most important adverse effects of colchicine are nausea, vomiting and diarrhea, probably due to a direct effect on intestinal mucosa and some patients cannot tolerate colchicine.

2. Excessive doses cause gastrointestinal hemorrhage, rashes and renal failure.
3. Peripheral neuropathy (probably related to the role of microtubular proteins in axonal transport), alopecia and blood dyscrasias occur with prolonged use.

Pharmacokinetics

Colchicine is rapidly absorbed from the gastrointestinal tract. The mean $t_{1/2}$ is 30 min. It is partly metabolized and a major portion is excreted via bile and undergoes entero-hepatic circulation, contributing to its gastrointestinal toxicity.

Chronic treatment for recurrent gout

ALLOPURINOL

Use

Allopurinol is used as long-term medication to treat patients with recurrent gout, especially those with severe tophaceous gout, urate renal stones, gout with renal failure, acute urate nephropathy and as prophylaxis to prevent this complication in patients about to undergo treatment of leukemias and lymphomas with cytotoxic drugs. Plasma uric acid concentration should be kept below 0.42 mmol/l. The initial dose is 100 mg daily after food, increased gradually if necessary to a maximum of 600 mg daily. Allopurinol is of no use for the treatment of acute gout and its use may provoke acute gout during the first few weeks of treatment. Concurrent indomethacin or colchicine is therefore given during the first month of treatment.

Mechanism of action

Allopurinol is a xanthine oxidase inhibitor and decreases production of uric acid. Precipitation into joints or elsewhere is therefore much less likely and uric acid is mobilized from tophaceous deposits which slowly disappear.

Adverse effects

The theoretical risk of forming xanthine stones has not proved to be a practical problem although crystals of xanthine, hypoxanthine and oxypurinol (which appear to be harmless) are found in the muscles of allopurinol-treated patients. Mild dose-related rashes and more serious hypersensitivity reactions (including Stevens–Johnson syndrome) occur, especially in patients with renal failure and are presumably due to accumulation of metabolites. Malaise, nausea, vertigo, alopecia and hepatotoxicity are uncommon.

Pharmacokinetics

Allopurinol is well absorbed from the intestine. The mean plasma $t_{1/2}$ is about 3 hours. Hepatic metabolism yields oxypurinol which is itself a weak xanthine oxidase inhibitor.

Drug interactions

- Allopurinol decreases the rate of breakdown of 6-mercaptopurine (the active metabolite of azathioprine). If these drugs are used concomitantly the dose of 6-mercaptopurine or azathioprine should be reduced.
- Inactivation of oral anticoagulants is impaired by allopurinol, and the frequency of monitoring INR must be increased in patients on long-term warfarin treatment in whom allopurinol is started, with dose adjustment if necessary.

URICOSURIC DRUGS

Use

These drugs (e.g. sulfinpyrazone, probenecid) have largely been rendered obsolete by allopurinol, but continue to be useful in the few patients needing prophylactic therapy who have severe adverse reactions to allopurinol. Uricosuric drugs inhibit active transport of organic acids by renal tubules. Their main effect on the handling of uric acid by the kidney is to prevent the reabsorption of filtered uric acid by the proximal tubule, thus greatly increasing excretion. After a week the initial dose (250 mg daily for probenecid, 100 mg daily for sulfinpyrazone) is increased until a satisfactory plasma concentration of uric acid is obtained. An acute attack of gout may be precipitated if treatment is started with a large dose. Concurrent treatment with an anti-inflammatory drug while initiating treatment with probenecid reduces this risk, but at the expense of increased risk of NSAID toxicity since these drugs are also eliminated by the organic acid secretory mechanism (chapter 6). Sulfinpyrazone is a weak NSAID in its own right, and a flare of gout is less likely when using it. The patient should drink enough water to have a urine output of 2 litres/day during the first month of treatment and sodium bicarbonate or potassium citrate mixture given to keep urinary pH above 7.0. Other adverse effects include rashes and gastrointestinal upsets.

The Cardiovascular System IV

Prevention of Atheroma: Lowering Plasma Cholesterol and Other Approaches

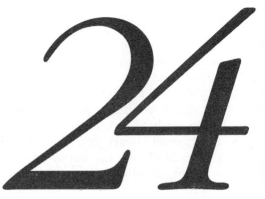

Introduction **264**

Pathophysiology **264**

Prevention of atheroma **267**

Screening **269**

Approach to therapy **269**

Drugs used to treat hyperlipidemia **272**

Treatment of hyperlipidemia at extremes of age and during pregnancy **277**

*I*NTRODUCTION

Atheroma is the commonest cause of ischemic heart disease, stroke and peripheral vascular disease in western countries. Since these are the major causes of morbidity and mortality among adults in industrialized societies, its prevention is of great importance. A family history of myocardial infarction in a first degree relative, especially at an early age, confers an increased risk of ischemic heart disease, and genetic factors are likely to be important in the development of atheroma. Epidemiological observations including the rapid change in incidence of coronary disease in Japanese migrants from Japan (low risk) through Hawaii (intermediate risk) to the west coast of the USA (high risk), and the recent substantial decline in coronary risk in the USA, indicate that environmental factors are of paramount importance in the pathogenesis of atheroma. Such observations further suggest that if environmental risk factors are altered this results quite rapidly in an altered incidence of disease.

*P*ATHOPHYSIOLOGY

Atheromatous plaques are *focal* lesions of large and medium-sized arteries. They start as fatty streaks in the intima, and progress to proliferative fibro-fatty growths that protrude into the vascular lumen and limit blood flow. These plaques are rich in both extracellular and intracellular cholesterol. During their development they do not initially give rise to symptoms, but as they progress they may cause angina pectoris, intermittent claudication, or other symptoms according to their anatomical location. They may rupture or ulcerate, in which event the subintima acts as a focus for thrombosis: platelet–fibrin thrombi propagate and can occlude the artery causing myocardial infarction or stroke.

Epidemiological observations from the Framingham study have shown that there is a strong positive relationship between the concentration of circulating cholesterol, specifically of the low density lipoprotein (LDL) fraction, and the risk of atheroma. This relationship is non-linear and depends strongly on the presence or absence of other risk factors including male sex, arterial hypertension, cigarette smoking, diabetes mellitus, positive family or personal history of premature ischemic heart disease, electrocardiographic or echocardiographic abnormalities (Fig. 24.1).

Figure 24.2 shows an outline of the metabolic pathways involved in lipid tranport. Approximately two-thirds of cholesterol circulating in the blood is made in the liver. Hepatocytes synthesize cholesterol and bile acids from acetate, and secrete them in bile into the intestine where they are involved in fat absorption. The rate-limiting enzyme in cholesterol biosynthesis is called 3-hydroxyl 3-methylglutaryl coenzyme A reductase (HMGCoA reductase). Fat is absorbed in the form of triglyceride-rich chylomicra. Free fatty acid is cleaved from triglyceride in these particles by lipoprotein lipase, an ectoenzyme on the surface of endothelial cells. Free fatty acids are used as an energy source by striated muscle, or stored as fat in adipose tissue. Chylomicron remnants are taken up by hepatocytes to complete the exogenous cycle. The endogenous cycle consists of the secretion of triglyceride-rich (and hence very low density) lipoprotein particles (VLDL) that also contain cholesterol by the

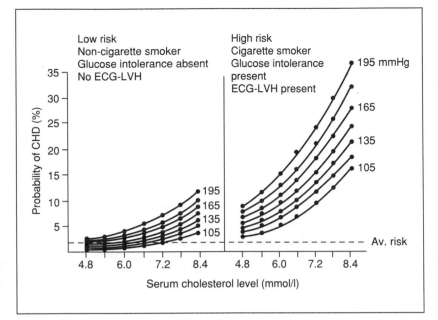

Fig. 24.1 Probability of developing coronary heart disease in 6 years: 40-year-old men in the Framingham Study during 16 years of follow-up. The numbers to the right of the curves show the systolic blood pressure (mmHg).

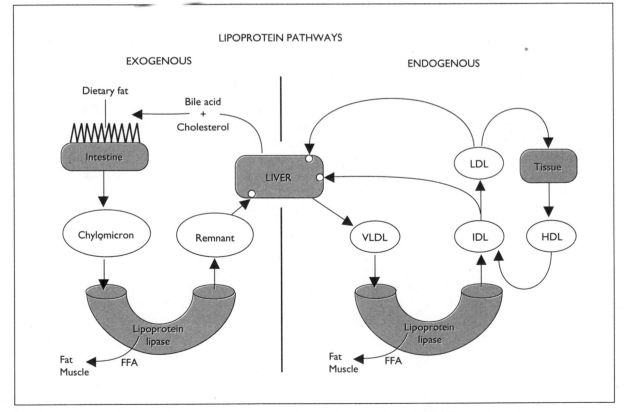

Fig. 24.2 Lipoprotein transport. FFA = free fatty acids. VLDL = very low density lipoprotein. IDL = intermediate density lipoprotein. LDL = low density lipoprotein. HDL = high density lipoprotein.

liver into the blood, followed by removal of free fatty acid by lipoprotein lipase in the capillaries. This results in progressive enrichment of the particles with cholesterol with an increase in their density through intermediate density to low density lipoprotein (LDL). It is circulating LDL that is especially atherogenic. Low density lipoprotein particles bind to receptors (LDL receptors) located in coated pits on the surface of hepatocytes, so the plasma concentration of LDL is determined by a balance between LDL synthesis and hepatic uptake. Low density lipoprotein that enters arterial walls at sites of endothelial damage can be remobilized in the form of high density lipoprotein (HDL); however, it may become oxidized and taken up by macrophages.

There have been no good subprimate animal models of atheroma until recently, but the advent of transgenic mice deficient in specific key enzymes and receptors in lipoprotein metabolism is rapidly transforming this fast moving field. None the less, most of our understanding of atheroma comes from human pathology (dating from the classical studies of Rokitanski, Duguid and of Florey) and from experimental studies in primates (especially those of Ross). Intimal injury is believed to initiate the atheromatous process. Rheological factors (e.g. turbulence) are believed to be responsible for the striking predilection for certain sites (e.g. at the low shear side of the origin of arteries branching from the aorta). The injury may initially be undetectable morphologically, but results in focal endothelial cell dysfunction. Blood monocytes adhere to receptors expressed by injured endothelium, and migrate into the vessel wall where they become macrophages. These possess receptors for oxidized (but not for native) LDL, which they ingest to become 'foam cells'.

Lesions become infiltrated with extracellular as well as intracellular cholesterol. Platelets also adhere to the injured intima. Macrophages and platelets both secrete growth factors, including platelet and macrophage-derived growth factors and transforming growth factor β, which cause migration, proliferation and differentiation of vascular smooth muscle cells and fibroblasts from the underlying media and adventitia. These processes result in the formation of fibro-fatty plaques.

Atheromatous lesions are not necessarily irreversible, and there is indirect evidence from autopsies of people dying of starvation in World War II that implies that severe starvation can probably cause regression. There is currently considerable interest in the possibility that the combination of acceptable dietary restraint with drugs causes regression of atheroma, and evidence to support this. Cholesterol is mobilized from tissues in the form of HDL particles. These are *not* atherogenic: indeed epidemiological studies have identified HDL as being strongly *negatively* correlated with risk of coronary heart disease. There is great interest in the connection between hyperlipidemia and thrombosis, and it has been found that there is a close relationship between one of the apolipoproteins and plasminogen. Apo(a) is present in a lipoprotein called Lp(a) which was first identified as a blood group variant responsible for occasional transfusion reactions. The plasma concentration of Lp(a) varies over a 100-fold range and is strongly genetically determined. Apo(a) is very large and contains multiple repeats of one of the kringles of plasminogen (a kringle is a doughnut-shaped loop of amino acids held together by three internal disulfide bonds). It is likely that this homology leads to interference by Lp(a) with the function of plasminogen, which is the precursor of the endogenous fibrinolytic plasmin, and hence to a predisposition to thrombosis on atheromatous plaques.

PREVENTION OF ATHEROMA

Smoking

Modifiable risk factors for the genesis of atheromatous plaque are potentially susceptible to therapeutic intervention. Cigarette smoking (chapter 49) is a strong risk factor for vascular disease. It causes vasoconstriction via activation of the sympathetic nervous system and platelet activation with a consequent increase in thromboxane A_2 biosynthesis, although the precise mechanism whereby smoking promotes atheroma is unknown. Stopping smoking is of substantial and rapid benefit. Smoking causes considerable physical and psychological dependence, and attempts to give up are often unsuccessful. Much of the dependence is due to the pharmacological effects of nicotine, and nicotine chewing gum or 'patches' for transdermal administration (which are available in the UK as over-the-counter products, chapter 4) are sometimes helpful. They reduce the dysphoria during the first few weeks of stopping smoking, and approximately double the number of people who succeed in remaining off the habit, although the proportion who relapse is still depressingly high. Individuals must not smoke while using nicotine patches, and these should not be used in pregnancy or within 6 weeks of a myocardial infarction or stroke. They should not be used for longer than 3 months since it is not clear how many of the long-term adverse effects of smoking on vascular disease are in fact mediated by nicotine.

Diet and habits

Obesity is extremely common in the UK and is a strong risk factor for atheromatous disease, especially in individuals with a predominantly abdominal distribution of excess fat (high waist:hip ratio). The influence of obesity on cardiovascular risk is partly accounted for by its association with other risk factors such as hypertension and hypercholesterolemia (that is, it may not be an 'independent' risk factor, although recent evidence suggests that it is). This in no way reduces the importance of attaining ideal body weight. Weight reduction in obese individuals restores their life expectancy toward normal. It also has additional benefits in terms of prevention of osteoarthrosis, gout (although acute gout can be precipitated by dieting), diabetes and hiatus hernia.

Treatment of obesity (see also chapter 31, p. 422) is notoriously difficult, and the list of grotesquely inappropriate therapies that have been employed is a testament to human folly. One is reminded of Barnum's dictum that 'there is a sucker born every minute, and one born to take him'. Surgical treatments including wiring the jaws, stapling the stomach and 'apronectomies' have little place. There are good reasons to take regular exercise independent of any effect this may have on body weight, but the effect of increased exercise on body weight is small unless combined with energy restriction. Bulk agents such as methylcellulose have been used in an attempt to produce feelings of satiety, but there is little evidence that they are effective; they cause bloating, flatulence and, rarely, esophageal or intestinal obstruction. They are less palatable than high fiber foods such as jacket potatoes. Centrally acting appetite suppressants have been used, but there is no evidence that they improve the long-term outlook and their history is not reassuring: amphetamines cause dependence as well as a range of neuropsychiatric (e.g. euphoria, nervousness, irritibility, drowsiness, insomnia, tiredness, dizziness, hallucinations, paranoia and depression), gastrointestinal (e.g. dry mouth, nausea, vomiting, constipation or diarrhea) and cardiovascular (e.g. palpitations, arrhythmias) side effects, and use of amphetamine-like drugs (e.g. diethylpropion) is not justified. Fenfluramine is structurally related to amphetamine but has a sedative rather than a stimulant effect. Abuse has occurred, and depression sometimes develops when it is abruptly discontinued. It should not be used in patients with epilepsy or a history of psychiatric illness or drug abuse. Some physicians use fenfluramine or dexfenfluramine (the active dextro isomer) as adjunctive treatment in severe obesity. These drugs should not be used in patients who are only mildly or moderately overweight, and should not be used for longer than 3 months. Increasing basal metabolic rate by treatment with thyroxine is justified only in patients with hypothyroidism. Selective β_3-agonists that exert an action on thermogenesis have been developed that increase energy expenditure and cause weight loss during short-term treatment. There is no evidence of long-term efficacy and they cause muscle tremor in a large fraction of patients, although more selective drugs of this class appear promising.

The desirable range of weight for height in adults is defined by body mass index (BMI):

$$BMI = Weight\ in\ kg/(Height\ in\ m)^2$$

The BMI should be between 20 and 25. Each kilogram of excess weight represents approximately 7000 kcal of stored energy. Dietary restriction of energy intake to create a negative energy balance is the only practicable way to use up the excess stores. Lifelong alteration of dietary habits is needed to maintain ideal body weight, so advice regarding a suitable and acceptable diet is essential. Patients need to be given a target weight and advised as to a realistic rate of weight loss that they should attempt to achieve. Very low calorie and formula diets cause an excessive loss of non-fat body mass, do nothing to improve eating habits in the long term and are not recommended. Instead, advice should center on the importance of small regular meals, reduced fat and increased fiber, with a total energy of 800 kcal or more. An energy deficit of 1000 kcal/day will result in a loss of about 1 kg body weight per week which is the maximum useful rate of weight loss.

Behavioral modification is essential and psychological support (e.g. from groups such as weight watchers) can be valuable.

Diet is important in ways other than weight alone. Saturated fats, as opposed to mono- or polyunsaturated fatty acids are important determinants of plasma cholesterol (see below). Among polyunsaturated fatty acids there may be important differences (e.g. between natural *cis* isomers and potentially atherogenic *trans* isomers present in some margerines). There is epidemiological evidence that eating modest amounts of fish regularly reduces cardiovascular risk independent of providing natural polyunsaturated fatty acids. There is also accumulating evidence that eating food rich in natural antioxidants such as salads (vitamin C) and nuts (vitamin E) reduces cardiovascular risk and is certainly less likely to cause adverse effects than are drugs such as probucol which also has some antioxidant effect but which lowers HDL and has marked toxic effects in animals.

Sedentary habits are a risk factor for atheromatous disease, and regular exercise improves cardiovascular risk. This appears to be independent of any effect on obesity, but perhaps relates to favorable effects on systolic blood pressure, on HDL (which is increased by exercise) and fibrinolysis. Exercise also improves sense of well being, and reduces stress. Other methods of achieving this include meditation and relaxation therapy.

Dyslipidemia

Reducing total plasma cholesterol concentration reduces the risk of coronary heart disease, and can cause regression of atheroma. The potential benefit of lowering plasma cholesterol can be viewed from either an individual or a public health perspective. Individuals with the highest plasma cholesterol concentrations have most to gain from cholesterol lowering measures, especially if they also have other risk factors. However, to achieve maximum impact on the prevalence of coronary artery disease in a country such as the UK it is essential to reduce the average plasma cholesterol concentration of the whole community, not just those at highest individual risk. This is because most vascular events occur in individuals without marked elevations in plasma cholesterol, because the total number of such people is so much greater than the few with very high values. Consequently a shift of the population distri-bution curve toward lower values with a quite modest reduction in the average value would have a very substantial effect on the prevalence of coronary artery disease. These two perspectives are not mutually exclusive, and general dietary advice directed at the population as a whole should be combined with opportunistic screening of individuals, especially those with additional risk factors for vascular disease.

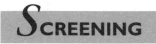

SCREENING

The most cost-effective method of screening for general practitioners and hospital physi-cians is to determine serum cholesterol opportunistically when the occasion offers, provided the patient is not suffering from an acute illness such as influenza or myocardial infarction (since this transiently but profoundly lowers the circulating cholesterol concentration), or from a chronic disease (e.g. dementia, malignant disease or cor pulmonale) that would render treatment inappropriate. The presence of additional risk factors for coronary disease or, even more strongly, of a personal history of vascular disease (e.g. angina, previous myocardial infarction), renders such screen-ing even more appropriate. Physical signs of vascular disease or of hyperlipidemia (e.g. tendon, eruptive or palmar xanthomas; early arcus, xanthelasma) occasionally alert the physician to the possibility of hypercholes-terolemia.

APPROACH TO THERAPY

See Fig. 24.3.

1. Measure height and weight, and determine ideal body weight. Advice regarding healthy eating habits, particularly as regards attaining ideal body weight and avoidance of excessive intake of saturated fats, as well as general advice regarding smoking and regular exercise, should be given to everyone.
2. Since risk of coronary disease rises smoothly with cholesterol concentration recommendations regarding actions that are justified at specified concentrations are arbitrary. As with arterial blood pressure 'lower is better', but, again as for hyper-tension, in practice physicians need an arbitrary framework (such as that recom-mended by the European Atherosclerosis Society) within which to make individual clinical judgments. If the screening choles-terol is < 5.2 mM, dietary advice should be reinforced, but blood sampling need not be repeated unless there are multiple coexistent risk factors, and then probably not for a year or more.
3. A further blood sample should be obtained in the fasted state from individuals with

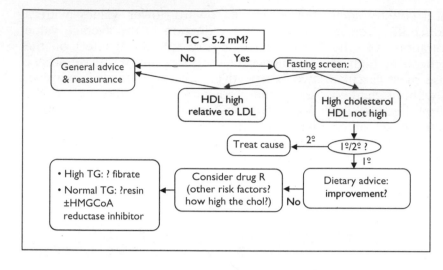

Fig. 24.3 Approach to dyslipidemia. TC = total cholesterol. HDL = high density lipoprotein. TG = triglyceride. 1° = primary dyslipidemia. 2° = secondary dyslipidemia. HMGCoA = β-hydroxy-β-methylglutaryl coenzyme A.

total cholesterol > 5.2 mM on the initial screen. This is sent to the laboratory for determination of total cholesterol (TC), triglycerides (TG) and HDL. (Total cholesterol is little influenced by whether or not blood is sampled during fasting, but triglyceride concentration is grossly elevated during absorption of food due to the presence of chylomicra.) From these values, LDL can be calculated using the Friedwald equation:

$$LDL = TC - (HDL + TG/2.2) \text{ mM}$$

This second sample reduces the chance of acting on a value that was elevated due to laboratory variation. It also identifies individuals (often women) with total cholesterol > 5.2 mM but with relatively high levels of HDL and LDL < 3.8 mM, who are *not* at increased risk of coronary disease and can be reassured.

4. The possibility of secondary hypercholesterolemia (Table 24.1) is considered in

individuals with total cholesterol > 5.2 mM and LDL > 3.8 mM. It is especially important to consider the possibility of hypothyroidism which can be asymptomatic and commonly causes hypercholesterolemia. Hypertriglyceridemia raises the possibility of excessive alcohol consumption, and further history and laboratory evidence such as elevated γ-glutamyl transpeptidase activity or raised mean corpuscular volume may be informative. If present, such underlying disorders are treated.

5. A detailed dietary history is obtained, and more intense dietary advice given to individuals with total cholesterol > 5.2 mM. This should include advice to reduce intake of egg yolks (which are rich in cholesterol), and items high in saturated fat including red meat, sausages, bacon, offal, butter, full cream milk and fried foods together with advice to trim fat from food before cooking, use of grilling, poaching or microwave, and a relative increase (through substitution) of vegetables, fish, chicken and corn or olive (mono-unsaturated) oil. Blanket recommendations are not very likely to be successful; what is usually recommended is total fat < 30% of calories, ratio of unsaturated to saturated fat >1.0 (>1.4 if more severe), cholesterol <300 mg daily (<200 mg if more severe) and calories to achieve/maintain ideal body weight. It is

Table 24.1 Secondary dyslipidemia.

Disorder	Main lipid disturbance
Diabetes	Mixed
Hypothyroidism	Cholesterol
Alcohol excess	Triglyceride
Nephrotic syndrome	Cholesterol
Renal failure	Mixed
Primary biliary cirrhosis	Cholesterol

important to try to give advice that will be acceptable to each individual for the long term. Effects of diet vary depending on the enthusiasm and time spent by physician and dietitian and on motivation and cultural background of the patient. A recent overview of the effect of dietary intervention concluded that milder measures had little effect, but there is considerable individual variation and the important thing is to determine response to diet by measuring total serum cholesterol after 4–8 weeks, with further encouragement and follow-up as needed.

6. Drug treatment is considered for individuals in whom total cholesterol fails to fall below 5.2 mM despite dietary advice. The higher the cholesterol the greater the potential benefit from such treatment; however, the decision to start drug treatment also needs to take account of the presence or otherwise of additional risk factors. The gradient of the function relating coronary risk to plasma cholesterol concentration is smooth, the slope of the line being determined by the presence or absence of other risk factors (Fig. 24.1), and lipid lowering drugs are not without adverse effects. Decisions as to the concentration of cholesterol at which the benefit of treatment outweighs the risks, inconvenience and expense are still contentious; what follows is based on our current practice. A personal history of coronary artery disease (i.e. secondary as opposed to primary prevention) or of familial hypercholesterolemia are the strongest indications for drug intervention, and we generally recommend treating such patients with drugs in order to lower total cholesterol to <5.2 mM, although there are as yet only small studies to justify this aggressive approach. (These include several studies that have demonstrated regression of coronary atheroma on repeat angiography as a result of hypolipidemic therapy.) The presence of two or more other risk factors generally prompts us to initiate drug treatment at concentrations of serum cholesterol of >6.5 mM. In the absence of other risk factors we initiate drug treatment only if the total cholesterol is persistently >7.5 mM despite adherence to dietary advice, and then only in selected patients.

7. Choice of drug. Resins reduce plasma cholesterol concentration and reduce the risk of coronary artery disease but the magnitude of their effect is modest and there is a high incidence of gastrointestinal side effects. They are useful as single agents in patients with mild disease and, in combination with HMGCoA reductase inhibitors, in patients with very severe disease. Since they are not absorbed and have been used extensively they are also a rational choice in children with severe familial hyperlipidemias in whom they may prevent disease progression and buy time while the safety and efficacy of some of the newer agents and strategies such as HMGCoA reductase inhibitors and gene therapy are explored. Resins increase plasma triglyceride, so they should not be used in patients with hypercholesterolemia and coincident marked hypertriglyceridemia. If triglycerides are elevated as well as cholesterol the possibility of excessive alcohol intake is reviewed, and appropriate advice given if necessary. If the patient is obese, calorie restriction is intensified. Fibrates and nicotinic acid derivatives are effective at lowering cholesterol in patients with high cholesterol together with markedly elevated triglycerides. Fish oil is also effective at lowering triglycerides, but has little effect on cholesterol and so is only indicated as a pharmacological intervention in rare patients suffering recurrent pancreatitis or eruptive xanthomas as a result of severe hypertriglyceridemia.

DRUGS USED TO TREAT HYPERLIPIDEMIA

ANION EXCHANGE RESINS

Use

Cholestyramine or colestipol are used to treat patients with hypercholesterolemia. The American lipid research clinics trial of middle-aged men with primary hypercholesterolemia showed that addition of such a resin to dietary treatment resulted in approximately a 13% fall in plasma cholesterol concentration and that this was associated with a 20–25% reduction in coronary heart disease over a 7.5 year follow-up period. Cholestyramine and colestipol are similar in their safety and efficacy, but cholestyramine consists of much coarser particles and individual patients may prefer one or other for this reason. Resins are taken as a suspension, and are more palatable if dispersed in fruit juice than in water.

Some patients prefer to make up the following day's supply the night before and leave it in the refrigerator. This results in a soft suspension rather than a gritty one. The dose of cholestyramine is 8–24 g daily given as a single' dose or divided 8 hourly immediately before meals. Other uses of these resins include:

- Diarrhea due to ileal resection or Crohn's disease.
- Diarrhea after vagotomy or in diabetic autonomic neuropathy.
- Pruritus in incomplete biliary obstruction.

Mechanism of action

Bile acid binding resins (Fig. 24.4) are not absorbed from the intestine and bind bile acids in the gut lumen, disrupting micelles

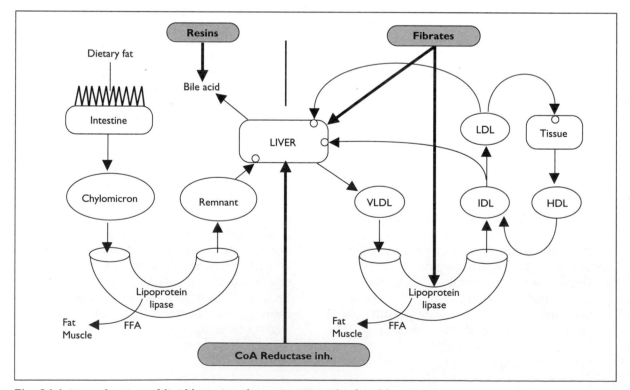

Fig. 24.4 Sites of action of lipid-lowering drugs. See Fig. 24.2 for abbreviations.

and thereby inhibiting reabsorption of bile salts and cholesterol so that their fecal excretion is increased. This lowers plasma cholesterol in two ways:

1. A larger proportion of cholesterol synthesized by the liver is converted into bile salts and less enters the circulation as cholesterol and its esters.
2. Bile acids inhibit the rate-limiting 7-hydroxylation step in cholesterol oxidation so the resins increase cholesterol breakdown.

However, cytoplasmic cholesterol exerts negative feedback inhibition on HMGCoA reductase which is rate limiting in cholesterol *synthesis*. Lowering plasma cholesterol by means of a resin removes this inhibition and accelerates cholesterol production. Accelerated cholesterol synthesis therefore limits the magnitude of the effect of resins on plasma cholesterol. This accounts for the marked synergy between resins and HMGCoA reductase inhibitors which block cholesterol synthesis.

Adverse effects and contraindications

Since resins are not absorbed the major side effects relate to the gut and consist of bloating, wind, abdominal discomfort and distension, constipation or diarrhea, and anorexia. These affect around one-third of patients. Constipation can usually be controlled with a stool softener such as dioctyl sodium sulfosuccinate. Absorption of vitamins D, K and folic acid is reduced and supplements may be needed especially in children, pregnant women and nursing mothers. If uncorrected, prolonged use can predispose to hemorrhage due to reduced synthesis of vitamin K-dependent coagulation factors. Resins are contraindicated in patients with complete biliary obstruction.

Drug interactions

Bile acid binding resins give rise to several clinically important interactions due to interfering with absorption of other drugs such as thiazides, antibiotics, warfarin, thyroxine and digoxin. All other drugs should be taken at least 1 hour before or 4–6 hours after a dose of resin. The potentially useful interaction between resins and HMGCoA reductase inhibitors has been described above.

FIBRATES

Use

Several fibrates including bezafibrate and gemfibrozil are in common clinical use. Fenofibrate has similar actions, but in addition has a uricosuric effect; hyperuricemia and gout commonly coexist with hypertriglyceridemia so this is of some clinical utility in such patients. Clofibrate (which was used in a World Health Organization, WHO, trial) is less used because it increases biliary cholesterol secretion and therefore predisposes to gallstones. Its use is therefore limited to patients who have had a cholecystectomy. Further, while it reduced the number of myocardial infarctions in the WHO trial, this was offset by an increased number of cancers of various kinds. The meaning of this has been extensively debated, but remains obscure. If it is a real effect rather than a statistical accident it does not appear to be a class effect, since there is no excess of cancers in patients treated with gemfibrozil in other trials (e.g. the Helsinki Heart Study). These have shown that fibrates have a marked effect in lowering plasma triglyceride, with a modest (around 10%) reduction in LDL and similar increase in HDL. Coronary heart disease was reduced by about one-third. The Helsinki Heart Study was not designed to detect a change in overall mortality, which would require a very large number of patients. Nevertheless, concern has been expressed over the apparent lack of effect on longevity, and in particular the possibility that fibrates predispose to accidents or other violent deaths has been widely if inconclusively aired. The dose of gemfibrozil is 600 mg twice daily. Bezafibrate is available in a slow-release preparation that is administered as a single night time dose of 400 mg.

Mechanism of action

The mechanism of the fibrates (Fig. 24.4) is incompletely understood. They stimulate lipoprotein lipase (hence their marked effect on triglyceride concentrations) and also increase LDL uptake by the liver. In addition to their effects on plasma lipids the fibrates lower fibrinogen and improve glucose tolerance, although it is unknown if these potentially advantageous changes are clinically important.

Adverse effects

Fibrates can all cause myositis, especially in alcoholics (in whom they should not be used) and in patients with impaired renal function in whom elimination is prolonged and protein binding reduced. They can also further reduce renal function in such patients. In addition they cause a variety of gastrointestinal side effects including nausea, and abdominal discomfort. Headache, impotence and urticaria have also been reported.

Contraindication

They should be used with caution if at all in patients with renal or hepatic impairment. They should not be used in patients with gallbladder disease or with hypoalbuminemia (e.g. from nephrotic syndrome). They are contraindicated in pregnancy and in alcoholics (this is particularly important because alcohol excess causes hypertriglyceridemia, Table 24.1).

Pharmacokinetics

Both bezafibrate and gemfibrozil are completely absorbed when given by mouth, highly protein bound and excreted mainly by the kidneys.

Drug interactions

Fibrates potentiate oral anticoagulants, and bezafibrate (though not gemfibrozil) potentiates the hypoglycemic effect of the sulfonylureas. Concurrent use with an HMGCoA reductase inhibitor increases the risk of myositis.

HMGCoA REDUCTASE INHIBITORS

Use

Simvastatin and pravastatin are available in the UK, and many similar drugs are being developed. They are generally similar, although simvastatin is more widely distributed in the body since it is less polar than pravastatin which is distributed selectively to the liver (which is its site of action) by virtue of a specific uptake mechanism. Both drugs are highly effective in lowering LDL cholesterol, especially in patients with heterozygous familial hypercholesterolemia in whom they are particularly useful. Outcome studies have yet to be reported, so their effect on cardiac morbidity and mortality can only be inferred from their effect on the surrogate endpoint of LDL cholesterol, which they lower by approximately 30–35%. This could translate into a substantial effect on cardiac disease (perhaps as much as a 60–70% reduction), but many physicians have reasonably adopted a wait-and-see strategy in relatively low-risk patients with mixed common forms of hyperlipidemia until the results of large-scale phase III clinical trials looking at clinical endpoints are available and more is known about long-term safety. HMGCoA reductase inhibitors are given by mouth as a single dose of 10–40 mg at bed time. The dose is adjusted on the basis of repeat plasma lipid determinations.

Mechanism of action

HMGCoA reductase is the rate-limiting step in cholesterol biosynthesis from acetate. Inhibition of this enzyme results in reduced cytoplasmic cholesterol in hepatocytes, which respond by increasing the synthesis of LDL receptors that are expressed on their surface membranes. This in turn increases hepatic LDL uptake from plasma, reducing plasma LDL concentration. HMGCoA reductase inhibitors have little effect on plasma concentrations of triglycerides or of HDL.

Adverse effects and contraindications

HMGCoA reductase inhibitors are generally very well tolerated. Mild and infrequent side effects include nausea, constipation, diarrhea, flatulence, fatigue, insomnia and rash. More serious adverse events are rare but include rhabdomyolysis, hepatitis and angioedema.

Liver function tests should be obtained before starting treatment and at intervals thereafter, and patients warned to stop the drug and report at once for determination of creatine kinase if they develop muscle aches. HMGCoA reductase inhibitors should not be used in alcoholics or patients with active liver disease, nor during pregnancy. In contrast to their great usefulness in patients with heterozygous familial hypercholesterolemia HMGCoA reductase inhibitors are completely ineffective in rare patients with *homozygous* familial hypercholesterolemia (since such individuals are unable to make LDL receptors).

Pharmacokinetics

Simvastatin and pravastatin are well absorbed from the intestine, extracted by the liver (their site of action) and are each subject to extensive presystemic metabolism. Simvastatin is an inactive lactone prodrug which is metabolized in the liver to its active form, the corresponding β-hydroxy fatty acid.

Drug interactions

- The potential for rhabdomyolysis and consequent acute renal failure may be increased by concurrent use of an HMGCoA reductase inhibitor with a fibrate, and close monitoring is mandatory if such a combination is employed.
- The efficacy of HMGCoA reductase inhibitors is substantially increased by concurrent use of a bile acid binding resin, and this may prove useful in treating severely affected individuals, especially those with established disease.

NICOTINIC ACID DERIVATIVES

Use

Nicotinic acid in pharmacological (as opposed to vitamin) doses lowers plasma triglyceride by 30–50% and cholesterol by 10–20%, and increases HDL. Its use is limited by side effects, especially flushing. There is evidence from the coronary drug project that it reduces the rate of reinfarction as well as the surrogate endpoints of plasma lipid concentrations. Reductions in lipid concentrations occur in all types of hyperlipoproteinemia apart from type I. Nicotinic acid is still used in the treatment of heterozygous familial hypercholesterolemia when optimum dietary and resin therapy have not restored plasma lipids to normal, although it has partly been replaced by the HMGCoA reductase inhibitors in this context. Nicotinic acid is started in a low dose (100 mg) and built up slowly to minimize side effects. At least 3 g daily is usually needed for a worthwhile effect. It is given three times daily in divided doses, but many patients prefer to take it as a single dose with their evening meal when they are at home and can cope better with the flushing reaction. The flushing is prostaglandin mediated and may be attenuated by taking aspirin (300 mg) 15–30 min before the dose. Acipimox is a derivative of nicotinic acid with fewer side effects. The dose is 500–750 mg daily in divided doses.

Mechanism of action

Nicotinic acid inhibits secretion of VLDL by the liver into the circulation, thereby reducing plasma triglyceride concentration. Low density lipoprotein particles are derived from VLDL so LDL and cholesterol concentrations are also reduced. Unlike resins, fibrates and statins, nicotinic acid reduces Lp(a), but the mechanism and significance of this effect is unknown. The mechanism of flushing induced by nicotinamide is stimulation of biosynthesis of a vasodilator prostaglandin, prostaglandin D_2, the cellular origin of which is unknown, but is *not* mast cells in this instance.

Adverse effects

Adverse effects of nicotinic acid and its derivatives include flushing, postural hypotension, pruritus, headache, nausea, vomiting, diarrhea, epigastric pain and rashes. Other adverse effects include hepatic dysfunction, exacerbation of peptic ulcer, hyperuricemia, gout and an increase in blood glucose.

Drug interactions

Nicotinic acid may be combined with a bile acid binding resin or with an HMGCoA reductase inhibitor in severe and refractory cases. Its vasodilator effect increases the hypotensive action of antihypertensive drugs.

PROBUCOL

Use

Probucol lowers plasma cholesterol without affecting triglycerides. A trial on regression of atheroma (PQRST) is being undertaken in Sweden but there are no large studies published of its effect on clinical outcome. This is a pity because its actions are distinctive. It produces a modest decline in LDL cholesterol of approximately 8–17%, but also reduces HDL by about 22%, including the HDL2 subfraction that appears particularly beneficial from epidemiological studies. However, it also has potentially advantageous effects notably as an antioxidant. Probucol causes regression of tendon xanthomata of patients with familial hypercholesterolemia, and of fatty deposits in the arteries of Watanabe hereditary hyperlipidemic rabbits. However, until clinical studies are available, reasonable indications for using probucol are extremely limited. Unlike the HMGCoA reductase inhibitors probucol does lower LDL in patients with homozygous familial hypercholesterolemia, since it stimulates non-receptor-mediated LDL catabolism. The usual dose is 500 mg twice daily with food.

Mechanism of action

Probucol stimulates non-receptor-mediated LDL catabolism. It is a powerful antioxidant and is incorporated into LDL. If LDL from a normal or hypercholesterolemic subject is incubated with endothelial cells *in vitro* it undergoes oxidation and is then readily taken up by macrophages that possess receptors for oxidized LDL. However, if LDL from a patient taking probucol is incubated in this way it resists oxidation and is not taken up by macrophages. Foam cells (i.e. macrophages that have ingested oxidized LDL) are important in the progression of atheroma. The effect of probucol on HDL is believed to be due to stimulation of a cholesterol ester transfer protein that transfers cholesterol from HDL to VLDL.

Adverse effects and contraindications

Probucol is well tolerated. Mild and transient diarrhea occurs in a minority of patients on starting treatment. The only potentially life-threatening effect is prolongation of the QT interval, which occurs in about 50% of patients. Interestingly, while probucol is almost completely free of toxicological effects in normal experimental animals, in severely hypercholesterolemic monkeys and dogs high doses of probucol produce QT prolongation and fatal cardiac arrhythmias. A case report of a patient with Ward–Romano syndrome (congenital QT prolongation) who developed *torsades de pointes* while on probucol which reversed on discontinuing the drug, suggests that this effect occurs in humans. For this reason probucol should be avoided in patients with prolonged QT interval or ventricular arrhythmias. It should not be used in pregnancy or by nursing mothers, and, because of its long half-life in the body, should be discontinued 6 months before pregnancy.

Pharmacokinetics

Probucol is very lipophilic, but despite this is poorly absorbed (<10% of the oral dose). Absorption is improved if it is taken with food. It accumulates in fat and is present in fat for up to 6 months. It is bound to LDL but not to plasma albumin. Metabolism is negligible, and elimination is by excretion of unchanged drug in bile with elimination in feces.

Drug interactions

Harmful interactions have not been described, but should be anticipated with drugs that also prolong the QT interval, notably amiodarone, sotolol and antihistamines including astemizole and terfenadine.

FISH OIL

Use

Omega-3 marine triglycerides are effective in reducing plasma triglyceride concentrations, but have no effect on cholesterol concentration (or even increase it). They are used in severe hypertriglyceridemia and may prevent pancreatitis. The recommended dose is 5 g twice daily with food, but many of the clinical studies that have demonstrated effects on plasma lipids used much higher doses. Ordinary cod liver oil cannot be used safely at the required high doses because of the risk of causing vitamin A and/or D toxicity. Isolated hypertriglyceridemia is at most weakly associated with coronary artery disease, and using pharmacological doses of fish oil in the hopes of preventing such disease is of unproven benefit. In contrast eating fish regularly reduces ischemic heart disease.

Mechanism of action

The mechanism whereby marine triglycerides lower plasma triglyceride concentration is unknown. Fish oils have other potentially important effects including inhibition of platelet function and prolongation of bleeding time, anti-inflammatory effects and reduction of circulating fibrinogen. Fish oil is rich in highly unsaturated fatty acids including eicosapentanoic and docosahexanoic acids.

Eicosapentanoic acid substitutes for arachidonic acid and gives rise to 3-series prostaglandins and thromboxanes (i.e. prostanoids with three double bonds in their side chain rather than the usual two), and 5-series leukotrienes. This probably explains their effects on hemostasis since thromboxane A_3 is much less active as a platelet aggregating agent than is thromboxane A_2, whereas prostaglandin I_3 is similar in potency as an inhibitor of platelet function as is prostaglandin I_2 (prostacyclin). Similarly, the alteration in leukotriene biosynthesis probably underlies the anti-inflammatory effects of fish oil, which may be of some clinical benefit in patients with rheumatoid arthritis or with psoriasis.

Adverse effects and contraindications

Side effects include occasional nausea and belching with a fishy after-taste. Fish oil is contraindicated in patients with familial hypercholesterolemia (type IIa hyperlipoproteinemia) in whom it increases total circulating LDL cholesterol.

TREATMENT OF HYPERLIPIDEMIA AT EXTREMES OF AGE AND DURING PREGNANCY

The elderly

The value of drug treatment of hyperlipidemia in the elderly has not been established, and there are no universally accepted guidelines. We treat otherwise healthy individuals with established atheromatous disease aggressively but do not currently recommend screening asymptomatic healthy individuals over the age of 65. In individuals who reach this age while on drug treatment we review the initial indication for treatment. Patients with evidence of established atheromatous disease we continue on current effective treatment. In individuals who have moderately elevated cholesterol and no additional cardiovascular risk factors we consider a trial of 'stepping down' to diet alone, with continued monitoring of plasma lipids.

The young

Children with evidence of familial hyperlipidemia represent a difficult management problem, and specialist advice should be sought. Experience of long-term safety of the most effective class of drug for treating heterozygous familial hypercholesterolemia – the HMGCoA reductase inhibitors – has not been established, and there is a case for dietary modification combined with treatment with an anion exchange resin as a temporizing measure in such children while experience of these drugs accumulates and other promising therapeutic modalities (notably replacement of the gene encoding the LDL receptor) are evaluated.

In pregnancy

The safety of hypolipidemic drugs during pregnancy has not been established, and drugs that are eliminated from the body very slowly should not generally be given to young women for this reason. As with children, a combination of diet with a resin if necessary seems the most reasonable approach in the small number of severely affected individuals.

Hypertension

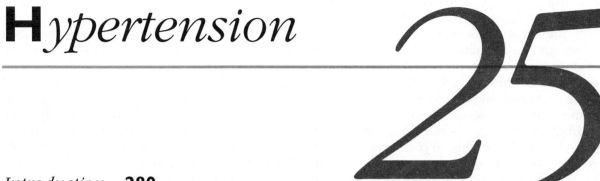

Introduction   **280**

Pathophysiology   **281**

General principles of management   **282**

Drugs used to treat hypertension   **285**

Special situations   **301**

INTRODUCTION

Hypertension is the strongest known modifiable risk factor for ischemic heart disease. It is also responsible for considerable potentially preventable disability from stroke, renal failure and heart failure. Despite this, hypertension continues to be underdiagnosed and undertreated in the UK. This is probably partly because hypertension is difficult to define: arterial pressure has a continuous distribution in the population, and it is arbitrary to divide this into discrete 'hypertensive' and 'normotensive' groups. Additionally, doctors frequently underestimate the magnitude of the excess risk attributable to hypertension over a timescale that is long in relation to clinical trials but relevant to the individual patient, and are sometimes unduly pessimistic about the benefit that treatment confers. To put this in perspective, Beevers and MacGregor (1987) estimate that a 35-year-old man with a blood pressure of 150/100 has an odds on chance of dying before the age of 60 unless active steps are taken to reduce his blood pressure: insurance companies pay close attention to blood pressure for good reason!

Figure 25.1 shows the relationship between usual mean diastolic blood pressure and the risks of coronary heart disease and of stroke redrawn from an overview by an Oxford group of epidemiologists. Over this range of blood pressure the lower the diastolic pressure, the lower the risk of each complication, the relationships being approximately linear. The same group performed a meta-analysis of published trials of antihypertensive drug treatment, and showed that the reduction in diastolic blood pressure achieved by drug treatment reduced the risk of stroke by the full extent predicted, and reduced the risk of coronary disease by about 50% of the maximum predicted, within approximately 2.5 years. These effects are impressive, and form a secure scientific basis for the clinical value of diagnosing and treating hypertension.

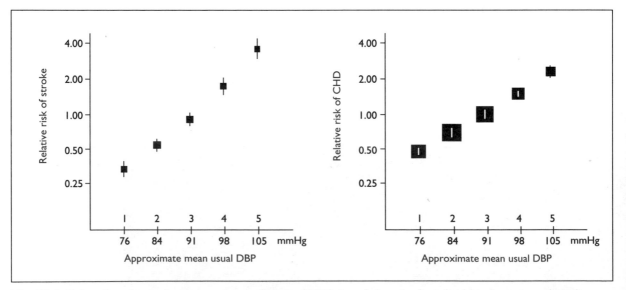

Fig. 25.1 Risks of stroke and coronary heart disease (CHD) in relation to diastolic blood pressure (DBD). (Redrawn from MacMahon *et al. Lancet* 1990; **335**: 765–74.)

*P*ATHOPHYSIOLOGY

Hypertension is occasionally secondary to some distinct disease (Table 25.1). However, most patients with persistent arterial hypertension have essential hypertension.

Arterial blood pressure is determined by (1) cardiac output, and (2) peripheral vascular resistance. Peripheral resistance is determined by the caliber and total cross-sectional area of the resistance vessels (small arteries and arterioles) in the various tissues (Fig. 25.2). One or more of a 'mosaic' of interconnected predisposing factors (including positive family history, obesity, insulin resistance and stress among others) are commonly present in patients with essential hypertension. The importance of intrauterine factors has recently been emphasized by the finding that hypertension in adult life is strongly associated with low birth weight.

Cardiac output may be increased in children or young adults during the earliest stages of essential hypertension. However, by the time hypertension is established the predominant hemodynamic abnormality is usually elevated peripheral resistance. Peripheral resistance is determined by the number and luminal diameters of the resistance vessels. Structural alterations such as reduction of vessel numbers ('pruning') or vessel wall hypertrophy with consequent encroachment on the lumen, as well as functional abnormalities (e.g. increased vasoconstriction or reduced vasodilatation), are believed to be important in determining the increased peripheral resistance in patients with essential hypertension. The genesis of such changes is poorly understood.

The kidney plays a key role in the control of blood pressure and in the pathogenesis of hypertension. Excretion of salt and water controls intravascular volume, which influences the force of contraction of the heart by the Starling mechanism. Secretion of renin influences vascular tone and electrolyte balance. Renal disease (vascular, parenchymal or obstructive) is a cause of arterial hypertension (Table 25.1). Conversely, severe

Table 25.1 Secondary hypertension.

Coarctation of aorta
Renal artery stenosis
Renal disease (parenchymal or obstructive)
Conn's syndrome
Cushing's syndrome
Pheochromocytoma

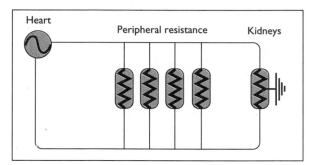

Fig. 25.2 Arterial blood pressure is controlled by the force of contraction of the heart and the peripheral resistance (resistances in parallel through various vascular beds). The fullness of the circulation is controlled by the kidneys, which play a critical part in essential hypertension.

hypertension of any kind causes glomerular sclerosis, manifested clinically by proteinuria and reduced glomerular filtration, leading to a vicious circle of worsening blood pressure and progressive renal impairment. Renal cross-transplantation experiments in several animal models of hypertension, as well as observations following therapeutic renal transplantation in humans, point to the importance of the kidney in the pathogenesis of hypertension.

Non-renal mechanisms are also important in the control of the circulation and in the pathogenesis of hypertension. These include neuronal mechanisms, especially the sympathetic nervous system, and endocrine and autocrine/paracrine mechanisms. The blood pressure of an individual varies widely at different times and this can cause a diagnostic problem. The activity of the sympathetic nervous system causes a continual background of vasoconstrictor tone that varies rapidly to adjust for changes in cardiovascular demand with alterations in posture and physical activity. It is also activated by emotional states such as anxiety and this can result in 'white coat' hypertension.

There has been considerable debate throughout this century as to the possible importance of tonically active vasodilator mechanisms in opposing sympathetically mediated vasocostriction. There is little evidence for tonically active vasodilator *nerves*, except in a few highly specialized vascular beds, nor for tonically active blood-borne vasodilator hormones. However, recent evidence points to a tonically active *paracrine* vasodilator mechanism. Vallance and colleagues recently discovered that inhibition of biosynthesis of nitric oxide (now believed to be the endothelium-derived relaxing factor described by Furchgott) in the human forearm causes marked vasoconstriction. This implies that basal release of nitric oxide by endothelial cells provides a background vasodilator tone in this vascular bed.

Clinically important consequences of hypertension ('end-organ damage') include damage both to large and small blood vessels as well as left ventricular hypertrophy. It is easy to understand how increased arterial pressure causes an increased risk of arterial rupture and bleeding from a weak spot in the arterial wall (e.g. from a Charcot–Bouchard aneurysm, causing a cerebral hemorrhage). The close link between hypertension and atherogenesis is less well understood, but may be related to vascular injury (believed to initiate atherogenesis, chapter 24). Damage to small vessels occurs most floridly in the vasculitis (fibrinoid necrosis) that is the hallmark of accelerated or malignant hypertension, and also underlies the glomerular sclerosis and consequent proteinuria and progressive renal impairment that complicate severe essential hypertension.

GENERAL PRINCIPLES OF MANAGEMENT

1. Make sure you measure the blood pressure accurately, using an appropriately sized cuff and recording Korotkov sounds 1 (systolic) and, where possible, 5 (diastolic). Where Korotkov 5 is unclear record Korotkov 4, making clear in the patient's notes that this was the phase used. Repeat the reading at the end of the examination, especially if the patient is agitated or anxious with tachycardia and pallor or cold extremities.

2. Consider the possibility of an underlying cause: many forms of secondary hypertension including coarctation of the aorta and endocrine tumors are best managed surgically. Renal artery stenosis merits consideration of angioplasty.

3. Seek evidence of end-organ damage. Cotton wool spots, retinal hemorrhages, papilloedema and/or microscopic hematuria in the setting of severe hypertension suggest accelerated or malignant hypertension which is a medical emergency requiring immediate admission to hospital (see below). Such evidence of microvascular damage is rare in modern practice, and in its absence the appropriate tempo of evaluation and treatment is much less precipitate. However, other evidence of end-organ damage including symptoms or signs of atheromatous disease, cardiac hypertrophy (with or without a fourth heart sound), cardiac failure, or evidence of renal impairment also indicate the need for treatment. The most sensitive measure of ventricular hypertrophy is provided by two-dimensional echocardiography; if this is unavailable an electrocardiogram should be obtained, but this is less sensitive. It is important to appreciate that the

absence of evidence of end-organ damage does *not* indicate that treatment is unnecessary.

4. Confirm (or refute) the persistence of clinically significant hypertension by establishing a number of accurate readings on separate occasions. Blood pressure varies in everyone, and it is probably the average of several readings of pressure that is important. Automated ambulatory and/or home readings are sometimes helpful in deciding on the need for treatment in borderline cases, especially in patients with marked sympathetic activation when confronted with doctors ('white-coat' hypertension).

5. Consider the possibility that hypertension is caused by alcohol withdrawal, or by some other drug. Heavy drinkers develop marked hypertension after drinking, even when they are not otherwise obviously in an acute state of alcohol withdrawal. Withdrawal from narcotics also causes hypertension, but the cause is usually obvious. Oral contraceptives can cause hypertension that usually settles when the drug is stopped. Vasoconstrictors including ergotamine and ephedrine as well as amphetamines and related drugs of abuse (e.g. 'ecstasy') can cause acute hypertension, as can ingestion of fermented foods or drink containing tyramine in patients receiving monoamine oxidase inhibitors (chapters 12 and 17). Mineralocorticoids (including carbenoxolone and rare cases of liqorice intoxication) can cause hypertension.

6. Evaluate the patient for other cardiovascular risk factors including serum cholesterol, smoking habits, glucose intolerance, obesity and lack of exercise. Attend to these if present. Risk factors interact positively and are usually supra-additive with hypertension in determining the risk of cardiovascular disease (Fig. 24.1, page 265). Knowledge of these factors should therefore inform the decision whether or not to initiate drug treatment in any individual patient: a usual blood pressure of 150/100 has very different significance in, say, a 35-year-old smoking man with a bad family history of ischemic heart disease and total serum cholesterol concentration of 7.6 mM than in a 70-year-old woman who is of long-lived stock, a life-long non-smoker and with a cholesterol of 5.6 mM.

7. Dietary factors: apart from avoiding excessive alcohol it is important to treat obesity and avoid excessive salt consumption. Some individuals are very sensitive to salt restriction, whereas unfortunately others are not. Statistically, Afro-Caribbean people are more likely to be salt sensitive than white people, at least in the West Indies and USA. Individuals with the highest initial pressures tend to have the greatest falls in pressure in response to a salt-restricted diet, whereas, disappointingly, mild hypertensives who might avoid the need for drug treatment entirely if their pressure were reduced by a similar amount have on average much more modest responses. There is, however, considerable individual variation in response, and English physicians often pay less attention than they should to this harmless intervention, perhaps because it is time consuming to educate patients effectively to achieve a worthwhile reduction in salt intake.

8. Consider other forms of non-drug treatment, for example relaxation techniques, in patients with mild elevations in pressure and stressed lives. These may usefully be combined with other dietary and 'life-style' advice during a run-in phase of repeated observation over several months or more, depending on the pressure.

9. If, taking age, sex and other risk factors into account, it is evident that the patient would derive more benefit than harm from drug treatment, explain this and seek the patient's agreement to long-term treatment, explaining the importance of compliance and the need for regular monitoring. It is important to stress that hypertension is not an illness but a risk factor for illness, and that the object of treatment is not to feel better here and now but rather to stay healthy.

(Antimalarial prophylaxis when visiting the tropics is a useful analogy.)

10. Before starting drug treatment review the possibility of coexisting disease that would limit the choice of drug: a history of gout is a relative contraindication to the use of a diuretic, non-insulin-dependent diabetes will be exacerbated by a thiazide, symptoms of hypoglycemia may be masked by β-blockers in insulin-treated diabetics, and obstructive airways disease, cardiac failure or conduction abnormalities and peripheral vascular disease similarly contraindicate β-blockers.

11. Whenever possible choose a class of drug that has been proved effective in terms of clinical endpoints such as stroke reduction. At present this means a thiazide diuretic or β-blocker. These drugs are relatively inexpensive and their adverse effects are well known and reversible on stopping treatment. Of the two we recommend a thiazide if other things are equal, especially if the patient is Afro-Caribbean. Some authorities prefer to initiate treatment with a converting enzyme inhibitor or calcium channel blocker, but in the absence of data from large clinical trials as to the benefits or otherwise of these drugs in patients with mild or moderate hypertension this is hard to justify as universal policy.

12. Start with a low dose and, except in emergency situations, titrate this up gradually. Almost every category of antihypertensive drug that has been introduced into clinical practice has been used initially in too high a dose, with resultant toxicity: hydralazine, thiazide diuretics, propranolol and captopril all exemplify this. One reason is that physicians are impatient to see a rapid reduction in pressure that is elevated as a result of slow processes that initially probably took many months to assert themselves and may require at least as long to regress. The converse is that if antihypertensive medication is discontinued, perhaps because it was initiated before adequate demonstration of persistent hypertension, the hypertension may reassert itself only after several months of normal blood pressure. Close and continued monitoring in such circumstances is therefore mandatory.

13. If control is not established by a single agent consider the possibility of non-compliance. If this is excluded, consider either substitution of a drug of a different category, or addition of a second drug. There is no hard and fast rule about this, but if a drug has had minimal or no effect on its own it may be more reasonable to substitute a different agent, whereas if it has had a real but insufficient effect it is more reasonable to add a second drug with a complementary mechanism of action. In this regard thiazides and β-blockers combine well, as do diuretics and converting enzyme inhibitors, β-blockers and calcium channel blockers, α-blockers with converting enzyme inhibitors and a number of other rational combinations. In patients with severe hypertension, three and occasionally four drugs may be needed. Try to keep such regimes as simple as possible, using once a day or twice a day dosing when possible.

14. Loss of control. If blood pressure control, having been well established, is lost, there are several possibilities. Consider:

(a) Non-compliance: This is the most common cause of loss of control. It is conceptually the simplest but in practice often the hardest to pin down. Hospital admission may be warranted, and if the problem is faced frankly but non-confrontationally the outcome is often surprisingly good.

(b) Drug interaction: The commonest cause with modern antihypertensive treatment is concurrent use of non-steroidal anti-inflammatory drugs (NSAIDs). The NSAIDs all cause increased blood pressure in hypertensive patients receiving antihypertensive drugs, irrespective of the particular category of drug used. The cause is that NSAIDs inhibit the renal biosynthesis of vasodilator/natriuretic prosta-glandins (including prostaglandin E_2 and prostacyclin). All NSAIDs possess this property to some extent, but sulin-dac (which has *relatively* little effect on renal prostaglandin synthesis) is less potent than other NSAIDs in this regard, as is aspirin. Paracetamol and opiates such as codeine do not exhibit this pharmacodynamic interaction, and may be useful in patients with severe hypertension coexisting with painful osteoarthrosis.

(c) Intercurrent event: Patients with hypertension frequently have athero-matous disease. If a plaque in a renal artery progresses to cause hemody-namically significant stenosis, hyper-reninemia may cause a rapid increase in arterial pressure, and even precipitate malignant hyperten-sion. Other possible intercurrent events include renal infarction, and progressive obstructive uropathy in an aging man with prostatic hyper-trophy.

DRUGS USED TO TREAT HYPERTENSION

DIURETICS

Use

Diurctics remain the logical first choice for treating patients with mild hypertension, unless contraindicated by some coexistent disease, and are also valuable in treating more severe cases when they are often combined with another drug or drugs. Diuretics have been shown to reduce the risk of stroke in several large clinical trials, and indeed in the Medical Research Council (MRC) trial they did so significantly more effectively than did β-blockade, although this may have been a statistical quirk. The dose–response curve of diuretics on blood pressure is remarkably flat. The adverse metabolic effects described below are, however, dose related. Thiazides (e.g. bendrofluazide, hydrochlorothiazide) are preferable to loop diuretics for the treatment of uncomplicated hypertension, and are given by mouth as a single morning dose. They begin to act within 1–2 hours and work for 12–24 hours. Treatment should be started using a low dose (e.g. bendrofluazide, 2.5 mg, each morning) and the daily dose may be increased if necessary to 5 mg. Loop diuretics are useful in hypertensive patients with moderate or severe renal impairment, or in patients with hypertensive heart failure.

Mechanism of action

Thiazide diuretics inhibit reabsorption of sodium and chloride ions in the early part of the distal convoluted tubule. Excessive salt intake or a low glomerular filtration rate interferes with their antihypertensive effect, and thiazides are ineffective in anephric patients. Natriuresis is therefore probably important in determining their hypotensive action. However, it is not the whole story, since although plasma volume falls when treatment is started it returns to normal with continued treatment despite a persistent effect on blood pressure, suggesting an additional mode of action. During chronic treatment total peripheral resistance, which is raised initially, slowly falls, suggesting an action on resistance vessels. This could be an autoregulatory change in response to the altered blood volume, or could be due to an effect of the drug in reducing arteriolar tone. Such an effect might be indirect, perhaps involving release of a vasodilator mediator from the kidneys in view of the obligatory requirement of functioning kidneys for thiazide diuretics to be able to exert their hypotensive effect. Vascular responses to pressor agents including angiotensin II and noradrenaline are reduced during chronic treatment with thiazides, which may also influence cation pump activities.

Adverse effects

1. **Impotence** Analysis of the reasons for withdrawal from randomized blind treatment with thiazide from the MRC trial showed a higher rate of impotence than in placebo-treated or β-blocker-treated patients. This may have been exaggerated by the unnecessarily high dose of bendrofluazide (10 mg) used in that study.
2. **Idiosyncratic reactions** Such reactions to diuretics include rashes (which may be photosensitive) and purpura, which may be thrombocytopenic or non-thrombocytopenic.
3. **Increased plasma renin** The contraction of plasma volume caused acutely by diuretics causes increased plasma renin which limits the magnitude of their effect on blood pressure.
4. **Metabolic and electrolyte changes** Thiazide diuretics have several metabolic effects of uncertain clinical significance:

    (a) *Hyponatremia* This is sometimes severe.
    (b) *Hypokalemia* Thiazides are kaliuretic as well as natriuretic, an inevitable consequence of increased sodium ion delivery to the distal nephron where sodium and potassium ions are exchanged. This results in mild hypokalemia in many subjects. Despite this, total body potassium may be little affected during chronic treatment and as long as plasma potassium remains 3.0 mmol/l or greater there is little reason to add potassium supplements (which are unlikely to be effective at tolerable doses) or potassium-sparing diuretics (which have toxicities of their own).
    (c) *Hypomagnesemia* This has been reported, but is seldom of clinical significance in this context.
    (d) *Hyperuricemia* Most diuretics reduce urate clearance. They therefore increase plasma urate concentration and can precipitate gout in predisposed individuals. (There are exceptions to this, e.g. drugs like ticrynafen that combine diuretic and uricosuric actions, but at present none is marketed in the UK because of concerns about toxicity.)
    (e) *Hyperglycemia* Thiazides reduce glucose tolerance, and can cause hyperglycemia in non-insulin-dependent diabetics.
    (f) *Hypercalcemia* Thiazides reduce urinary calcium ion clearance (unlike loop diuretics which increase it), and can therefore precipitate clinically significant hypercalcemia in hypertensive patients with hyperparathyroidism.
    (g) *Hypercholesterolemia* Thiazide diuretics cause a small increase in plasma cholesterol concentration, which may not persist during prolonged treatment. This is of uncertain significance, and does not account quantitatively for the failure of clinical trials to show as big an effect of treatment of hypertension on coronary disease as on stroke. To put it in perspective, MRC trial patients randomized to bendrofluazide (in the high dose – by current standards – of 10 mg daily) actually experienced a *fall* in total cholesterol concentration during treatment, albeit of significantly smaller magnitude than those randomized to placebo. The possible importance of this modest metabolic effect has been overemphasized by sales forces eager to promote newer, relatively expensive, drugs. Provided the dose of diuretic is kept low, adverse metabolic effects are minimal.

Contraindications

The effects of thiazide diuretics described above contraindicate their use in patients with severe renal impairment, in whom they are unlikely to be effective; in patients with non-insulin-dependent diabetes; in patients with a history of gout; and suggest caution in using these drugs in patients with mild hypertension but severe hypercholesterolemia. They should not be used in pre-eclampsia, which is associated with a contracted intravascular volume, unless complicated by left ventricular failure. Diuretics should be avoided in men with prostatic symptoms. It is prudent to discontinue diuretics temporarily in patients who develop intercurrent diarrhea and/or vomiting, to avoid exacerbating fluid depletion.

Drug interactions

In addition to the non-specific adverse interaction with NSAIDs mentioned above, all diuretics interact with lithium. Li$^+$ is similar to Na$^+$ in many respects, and is reabsorbed mainly in the proximal convoluted tubule (chapter 17). Diuretics increase lithium reabsorption in the proximal tubule indirectly by causing volume contraction. This results in increased plasma concentration of Li$^+$, and hence increased likelihood of toxicity. Diuretic-induced hypokalemia and hypomagnesemia can increase toxicity of digoxin (chapters 28 and 29). Combinations of a thiazide with a potassium-sparing diuretic such as amiloride (co-amilozide) or triamterene are widely prescribed but seldom necessary in patients with uncomplicated hypertension, although they are useful in patients who require simultaneous treatment with digoxin, sotolol or other drug that prolongs the electrocardigraphic QT interval.

Potentially useful interactions with other antihypertensive drugs abound: in general, low doses of two or even three drugs may be more effective and better tolerated than larger doses of single drugs. Useful interactions include thiazide/β-blocker, thiazide/angiotensin-converting enzyme inhibitor and thiazide/α-blocker. An unexpected exception to this is provided by most calcium channel blockers whose hypotensive actions are *not* enhanced, and may even be attenuated, by concurrent use of diuretics. This is particularly disappointing as one of the most troublesome adverse effects of dihydropyridine calcium channel blockers is ankle swelling, which is *not* however reduced by diuretics.

β-ADRENOCEPTOR ANTAGONISTS

Use (see also chapter 29 for use in arrhythmias)

Atenolol and metoprolol are currently the β-blocking drugs most widely used to treat hypertension in the UK. β-Blockers lower blood pressure, and have been shown to reduce the risk of stroke in patients with mild essential hypertension, although there is a suggestion from the MRC trial that they may be slightly less effective than diuretics. They reduce the risk of myocardial infarction in hypertensive patients, although there is no evidence that they are better than thiazide diuretics in this regard. They seldom cause postural hypotension. Statistically they are less effective in Afro-Caribbean patients (at least from the USA and Caribbean) than in white people. Chinese people by contrast are usually more sensitive to the effects of β-blocking drugs than are Whites. Treatment is started with a small dose (e.g. atenolol 25 mg, metoprolol 50 mg) and the daily dose increased gradually measuring blood pressure, pulse and, especially in the case of partial agonists (see below), pulse following exercise. Doses of atenolol greater than 100 mg or of metoprolol greater than 200 mg daily are seldom needed, so dose titration is simpler than with propranolol.

β-Blockers are usually well tolerated and although more expensive than thiazide diuretics are much less expensive than calcium channel blockers, converting enzyme inhibitors or modern α-blockers. Unless contraindicated (see below) they are appropriate first-line drugs for patients with essential hypertension who do not tolerate thiazides or as an additional drug in patients whose response to thiazides is inadequate. They are particularly useful in hypertensive patients who have angina pectoris or who have survived myocardial infarction. β-Blockers have been used in women with pregnancy associated hypertension, and lower blood pressure without evidence of adversely affecting pregnancy outcome. The negative inotropic effect of β-blocking drugs may be particularly useful in stabilizing patients with dissecting aneurysms of the thoracic aorta, in whom it is desirable to lower not only the mean pressure but also to reduce the rate of rise of the arterial pressure wave.

Classification of β-adrenoceptor antagonists

Adrenoceptors are classified α or β, based on the effects of different agonists and antagonists. A further subdivision has been made into β_1-receptors, mainly in the heart, and β_2-receptors in blood vessels, bronchioles and other cells and tissues. Non-selective β-adrenoceptor antagonists (e.g. propranolol) compete with agonists at β_1- and β_2-adrenoceptors.

Cardioselective β-blockers (e.g. atenolol, metoprolol) inhibit β_1-receptors but exert little influence on bronchial and vascular β_2-receptors when employed in low doses in experiments on isolated tissues *in vitro*. However, such selectivity is relative rather than absolute, and in clinical practice cardioselectivity is of little relevance: even cardioselective β_1 antagonists (at least those currently available) are hazardous for patients with asthma or obstructive airways disease. Metabolic differences between selective and non-selective β-blockers also appear to be of only marginal importance in clinical practice. The metabolic response to insulin-induced hypoglycemia depends upon hepatic glycogen breakdown (mediated via α-adrenoceptors) and gluconeogenesis (mediated by β_2-adrenoceptors). Thus a β_1-selective blocker should be less likely to blunt the metabolic response of a diabetic who has received excess insulin, but in practice β-blockers are generally best avoided in insulin-requiring diabetics, and there are usually acceptable alternatives available. The popularity of drugs such as atenolol and metoprolol among clinicians rests largely on their convenience for the patient rather than on their selectivity for the β_1-receptor subtype. This convenience relates to their favorable pharmacokinetic properties which enable them to be administered once daily over a small dose range compared to the large range necessitated by the high presystemic metabolism of propranolol.

Some β-blockers (e.g. oxprenolol, pindolol) are partial agonists and possess intrinsic sympathomimetic activity. Partial agonists antagonize full agonists, because they occupy a substantial fraction of the receptors to produce their modest effect, and therefore compete successfully with the more efficacious full agonists which occupy only a small fraction of the receptors to produce a maximal effect. Pure antagonists like atenolol often cause mild bradycardia (heart rate typically around 60/min) because of unopposed vagal activity. By contrast, partial agonists like oxprenolol cause some β-adrenoceptor stimulation and the resting heart rate is often around 80/min. During increased sympathetic activity (e.g. on exercising), the usual tachycardia is, however, blunted by the partial agonist as it is by the pure antagonist. Theoretically drugs with intrinsic sympathomimetic activity might be less liable to induce cardiac failure, peripheral vasoconstriction, depressed atrioventricular conduction or marked bradycardia. This does not generally seem important in practice, but partial agonists are sometimes tolerated by patients with symptomatic peripheral vascular disease who experience unacceptable increased claudication with pure β-antagonists, and partial agonists are also occasionally useful when bradycardia with full antagonists is a problem. β-Blockers have a small effect on serum lipid concentrations: they increase triglyceride concentrations and may decrease high density lipoprotein, although this remains controversial and of uncertain clinical relevance in this context. Pindolol does not have this theoretically detrimental effect.

Since β_2-receptors on resistance vessels increase cytoplasmic cyclic adenosine monophosphate (AMP) thereby causing vasodilatation, β-blocking drugs usually cause a small degree of vasoconstriction. However, some β-blockers have additional actions that cause vasodilatation, theoretically an advantage in treating patients with hypertension. The mechanisms of these so-called vasodilating β-blockers vary: some (e.g. labetolol) have additional α-blocking activity, although the potency of labetalol in blocking α-receptors is much less than on β-receptors. Celiprolol is a relatively selective β_1-antagonist which has additional *agonist* activity at β_2-receptors. Nebivolol causes vasodilatation *in vitro* by releasing endothelium-derived relaxing factor in addition to its β-blocking action, and improves diastolic function *in vivo*. The clinical importance of these actions (if any) has still to be demonstrated.

Mechanism of action

Despite their undoubted efficacy in lowering blood pressure, the mechanism by which β-blocking drugs achieve this is by no means obvious. As explained above, they actually *increase* peripheral vascular resistance in acute dose studies, although this effect is transient and is offset by the fall in cardiac output. They reduce renin secretion by the kidney, and statistically are more likely to be effective in patients with high circulating renin, and less effective in low renin groups (e.g. Afro-Caribbean patients). However, this distinction is of statistical rather than clinical importance, and β-adrenoceptor antagonists are effective in some patients with low plasma renin as well those with high renin hypertension, and their effects are additive with those of converting enzyme inhibitors, so inhibition of renin secretion is unlikely to be the full explanation of their hypotensive action. Propranolol has central effects and reduces sympathetic output from the central nervous system, but again this appears inadequate as an explanation since more polar β-blockers such as atenolol which penetrate the blood–brain barrier much less readily than does propranolol are as effective as propranolol in lowering blood pressure. The hypotensive action of these drugs is therefore attributed, somewhat unsatisfactorily, to their negative inotropic action on the heart. Patients on long-term β_1-antagonists do not usually have a low cardiac output, and it seems likely that additional mechanisms, perhaps involving baroreceptors or other homeostatic adaptations, must also be involved. Possible mechanisms include: (1) β-adrenoceptors located on sympathetic nerve terminals can promote noradrenaline release, and this is prevented by β-receptor antagonists, and (2) local generation of angiotensin II within vascular tissues is stimulated by β_2-agonists.

Adverse effects and contraindications

1. **Intolerance** β-Adrenoceptor antagonists cause a variety of symptoms in apparently healthy individuals, some of whom may not tolerate them in consequence. Of these fatigue, cold extremities, sexual dysfunction and loss of motivation and *joie de vivre* are common. Less often β-adrenoceptor antagonists (especially, but not invariably, non-polar ones like propranolol that cross the blood–brain barrier readily) cause hallucinations or vivid and sometimes horrible dreams.

2. **Airways obstruction** β-Adrenoceptor antagonists, whether non-selective or cardioselective, can cause catastrophic airways obstruction in patients with pre-existing obstructive airways disease, especially asthma, but also emphysema and chronic bronchitis, and are contraindicated in these conditions. Patients with asthma sometimes tolerate a small dose of a selective drug when first prescribed, only to suffer an exceptionally severe attack subsequently, and such drugs should ideally be avoided altogether in asthmatics.

3. **Heart failure** The negative inotropic action of β-adrenoceptor antagonists renders them dangerous in patients with heart failure.

4. **Peripheral vascular disease and vasospasm** β-Adrenoceptor antagonists predictably worsen symptoms of claudication in patients with symptomatic atheromatous peripheral vascular disease. Patients with peripheral vasospasm should also not be prescribed β-blockers which worsen Raynaud's phenomenon. The rather small number of patients with angina in whom coronary artery vasospasm contributes significantly to their 'variant' or 'Printzmetal' angina may also experience a 'paradoxical' worsening of their symptoms if prescribed β-blockers.

5. **Hypoglycemia** The propensity of β-adrenoceptor antagonists to mask symptoms of hypoglycemia (which, apart from sweating which is largely cholinergically mediated, are caused mainly by adrenergic pathways) render them hazardous in patients with insulin-requiring diabetes mellitus. Not only are symptoms of hypoglycemia masked but the rate of recovery from hypoglycemia is slowed, especially by non-selective β-blockers, because adrenaline stimulates gluconeogenesis in striated muscle via β_2-adrenoceptors.

6. **Heart block** β-Adrenoceptor antagonists are contraindicated in patients with minor degrees of heart block, because of the risk of precipitating complete block.

7. **Metabolic disturbance** β-Adrenoceptor antagonists cause several subtle biochemical or metabolic changes of uncertain clinical significance. As mentioned above, they cause a small increase in serum triglyceride concentration and possibly also a small fall in serum high density lipoprotein; it is not, however, clear that these biochemical effects translate into adverse effects on atheroma formation in this context. They cause a small rise in serum potassium because of inhibition of renin release (and hence reduction of aldosterone release) in some individuals, but this is not usually clinically important. Their effect, if any, on glucose tolerance in non-insulin-dependent diabetics is controversial, with some studies finding no effect and others documenting deterioration in glycemic control which may be additive with the effect on blood glucose of thiazide diuretics in such patients.

Pharmacokinetics

β-Adrenoceptor antagonists are well absorbed when administered orally, and are only given intravenously to control blood pressure in rare emergency situations (e.g. dissecting aortic aneurysm) or, occasionally, perioperatively. (They are sometimes also used in treating supraventricular arrhythmias, chapter 29.) Esmolol is a relatively cardioselective β-adrenoceptor antagonist with a very short duration of action which is given by intravenous infusion for these indications, usually in the dose range 50–200 μg/kg/min.

Polarity is an important determinant of the pharmacokinetics of different β-blocking drugs. Propranolol, oxprenolol and metoprolol are among the least, and atenolol and sotolol among the most, polar. The less polar (and more lipophilic) a drug the more extensive and rapid is absorption from the gut but the higher is presystemic metabolism in the gut wall and liver. The dose of propranolol required to cause β-blockade when given intravenously is therefore only a small fraction of that needed when it is given orally (approximately 1 mg compared with 40 mg or more).

Propranolol has an active metabolite (4-hydroxypropranolol), and metoprolol is metabolized by the enzyme that hydroxylates debrisoquine, the activity of which varies between individuals as a balanced polymorphism in the British population. These potentially complicating facts have little bearing on the dose requirements for these drugs in ordinary clinical practice however. Lipophilic β-blockers enter the brain more readily than do polar drugs such as atenolol. Central nervous system side effects such as nightmares and hallucinations occur more commonly with non-polar β-blockers, but can also occur with atenolol. Polar (water-soluble) β-blockers tend to be excreted by the kidneys without metabolism, to have longer half-lives and to accumulate in renal failure.

Non-polar (lipophilic) β-blockers are usually highly protein bound; for example, propranolol is 85–95% bound largely to α_1-acidic glycoprotein (which carries 75% at therapeutic plasma concentrations) and also albumin and lipoproteins. Polar (hydrophilic) β-blockers have low protein binding; for example, atenolol is less than 5% bound. Increased plasma concentrations of acute phase proteins, evidenced by a raised erythrocyte sedimentation rate, cause increased plasma concentrations of highly protein bound β-blockers (e.g. metoprolol, propranolol), but not of drugs like atenolol.

Although age in itself has little effect on β-blocker kinetics, in the population of symptomatic elderly patients seen by doctors, higher plasma levels of oxprenolol and propranolol result despite using lower doses than in the young. This is probably because such patients have high acute phase proteins and raised erythrocyte sedimentation rates. β-Receptor density is however reduced in the elderly thus decreasing tissue sensitivity, so dose reduction is not usually needed as patients age.

Antihypertensive effects of β-blockers outlast plasma levels, and atenolol and metoprolol are each given once daily despite having plasma half-lives of less than 24 hours. Slow release preparations are sometimes employed to optimize control over 24 hours with a single daily dose.

Drug interactions

- **Pharmacokinetic interactions** β-Adrenoceptor antagonists inhibit drug metabolism indirectly by decreasing hepatic blood flow secondary to decreased cardiac output. This causes accumulation of drugs such as lignocaine that have so high a hepatic extraction ratio that their clearance reflects hepatic blood flow, if given concurrently with β-blocking drugs. Conversely, cimetidine increases the effectiveness of propranolol, and may precipitate cardiac failure or other evidence of toxicity, by inhibiting its metabolism by hepatic cytochrome P_{450}-related oxidation.
- **Pharmacodynamic interactions** Increased negative inotropic and atrioventricular (AV) nodal effects occur with verapamil (giving both intravenously can be fatal), lignocaine and other negative inotropes. Exaggerated hypoglycemia with insulin and oral hypoglycemic drugs may be caused by β-antagonists. The antihypertensive effect of β-blockers is antagonized by non-steroidal anti-inflammatory drugs.

DIURETIC/β-BLOCKER COMBINATIONS FOR HYPERTENSION

Most of the β-blockers marketed in the UK are available as combined preparations with a diuretic. These may be useful for improving compliance if the appropriate dosage ratio of diuretic and β-blocker is available. They are also cheaper for the patient, although not for the national health service. Dose inflexibility limits their use. They should never be used as first-line therapy nor should their dose be titrated up to obtain a large dose of β-blocker.

ANGIOTENSIN-CONVERTING ENZYME INHIBITORS

Use

Enalapril, quinapril and a number of other angiotensin-converting enzyme (ACE) inhibitors are effective in lowering blood pressure when taken once daily. Captopril (the first ACE inhibitor in clinical use) needs to be taken twice daily. The ACE inhibitors are a useful addition to a diuretic in patients with moderate or severe hypertension not controlled by diuretic alone. Several ACE inhibitors are also licensed for use as a single agent in patients with mild essential hypertension, although so far there have been no controlled clinical trials to demonstrate that they reduce the risk of stroke or other clinically important events in such patients. Large-scale comparative studies with thiazide diuretics and β-blockers are sorely needed, since there are theoretical reasons to think that converting enzyme inhibitors might perform either worse or better than these proven therapies.

The ACE inhibitors are more expensive than thiazide diuretics or β-blockers, but are well tolerated by most patients and make a useful alternative in patients in whom thiazide diuretics and β-blockers are contraindicated, or who do not tolerate them. Their beneficial effect in patients with heart failure (chapter 28) make an ACE inhibitor particularly useful in hypertensive patients with this complication. A case has been made that ACE inhibitors have a distinctive and favorable effect on the progression of diabetic nephropathy over and above their effect in lowering blood pressure: larger controlled studies are needed to confirm this and determine whether it is clinically important.

Treatment is initiated using a small dose (e.g. enalapril 2.5 mg) given last thing before going to bed, because of the possibility of first dose hypotension. If possible diuretics should be withheld for a day or two before the first dose for the same reason. First dose hypotension is much less problematic, however, than when starting treatment with a converting enzyme inhibitor in patients with heart failure (chapter 28) in whom blood pressure is usually lower, circulating plasma renin activity often higher and diuretic therapy less safe to withhold. The dose is subsequently usually given in the morning and increased in stages to up to 20 mg (enalapril) or 40 mg (quinapril), monitoring blood pressure response.

Mechanism of action

Angiotensin-converting enzyme (also known as kininase 2) catalyzes the cleavage of a pair of amino acids from the carboxy terminus of short peptides, thereby 'converting' the inactive decapeptide angiotensin I to the potent vasoconstrictor angiotensin II. As well as *activating* the vasoconstrictor angiotensin in this way, it also *inactivates* bradykinin and some other vasodilator peptides. Converting enzyme is widely distributed in the body. It is an ectoenzyme, and is present on the luminal surface of vascular endothelial cells. The enzyme has a short tail anchoring it inside the cytoplasm, a transmembrane domain and a large portion which extends extracellularly, where it encounters angiotensin I and other potential substrates in the circulating plasma. This portion contains two active sites, each with a zinc atom. The lung is rich in ACE because of its huge surface area of endothelial cells, and was the first organ identified as containing the enzyme, but other tissues including heart, kidney, striated muscle and brain also contain high activities of ACE both on endothelial cells and elsewhere.

Converting enzyme inhibitors lower blood pressure by reducing angiotensin II, and perhaps also by increasing vasodilator peptides such as bradykinin. The relative contributions to the lowering of blood pressure of inhibition of the circulating renin–angiotensin system and of local renin–angiotensin systems in individual vascular beds have not been worked out: both are almost certainly important in different physiological circumstances. Angiotensin II increases noradrenaline release from sympathetic nerve terminals, so ACE inhibitors reduce sympathetic activity. This probably explains why their use is not associated with reflex tachycardia despite causing arteriolar and venous dilatation. Angiotensin II causes aldosterone secretion from the zona glomerulosa of the adrenal cortex, and inhibition of this contributes to the antihypertensive effect of converting enzyme inhibitors. Angiotensin II is a growth factor for vascular smooth muscle and some other cells, and in some but not all animal models of hypertension converting enzyme inhibitors influence the arteriolar and left ventricular remodelling that are believed to be important in the pathogenesis of human essential hypertension.

Metabolic effects

The ACE inhibitors do not have detectable effects on concentrations of plasma cholesterol or triglycerides. They cause a mild increase in plasma potassium concentration which may be either desirable or problematic depending on renal function and other drugs being used (see adverse effects and drug interactions below).

Adverse effects and contraindications

Converting enzyme inhibitors are generally well tolerated. Captopril has fared especially well when evaluated formally by 'quality of life' questionnaires. Adverse effects include:

1. **First dose hypotension** Steps to minimize this are described above in the section on use.
2. **Dry cough** This is the most frequent (5–30%) symptom during chronic dosing. It is often but not always mild. The cause is unknown but it may be due to kinins accumulating and stimulating cough afferents, perhaps via stimulation of

prostaglandin production. This latter possibility was raised by a study that showed that ACE inhibitor cough could be reduced by treatment with sulindac, which inhibits prostaglandin biosynthesis. Losartan (an angiotensin II receptor antagonist) does not potentiate bradykinin and does not cause cough.

3. **Urticaria and angioneurotic edema** Increased kinin concentrations have been invoked to explain the urticarial reactions and angioneurotic edema sometimes caused by converting enzyme inhibitors, although evidence is incomplete.

4. **Functional renal failure** This occurs predictably in patients with hemodynamically significant bilateral renal artery stenosis, and in patients with renal artery stenosis in the vessel supplying a single functional kidney. Converting enzyme inhibitors are therefore contraindicated in such patients. Plasma creatinine and potassium should be monitored before and during the early weeks of therapy with ACE inhibitors and the possibility of such renal artery stenosis considered in patients in whom there is a marked rise in creatinine. Provided the drug is stopped promptly, such renal impairment is reversible. The explanation of acute reduction in renal function in this setting is that glomerular filtration in these patients is critically dependent on angiotensin II-mediated efferent arteriolar vasoconstriction, and when angiotensin II synthesis is prevented by a converting enzyme inhibitor glomerular capillary pressure falls and glomerular filtration ceases. This possibility should especially be borne in mind in aging patients with atheromatous disease which often involves one or both renal arteries.

5. **Fetal injury** Renal failure occurs in the fetus if converting enzyme is inhibited, resulting in oligohydramnios in addition to other problems including craniofacial malformations. Converting enzyme inhibitors are therefore contraindicated in pregnancy and other drugs are preferred in women of child-bearing potential with essential hypertension.

6. **Hyperkalemia** Converting enzyme inhibitors cause a modest increase in plasma potassium as a result of reduced aldosterone secretion. This may usefully counter the small reduction in potassium ion concentration caused by thiazide diuretics. Increased plasma potassium is, however, potentially hazardous in patients with renal impairment, and great caution must be exercised in this setting. This is even more important when such patients are also prescribed potassium supplements and/or potassium-sparing diuretics including those marketed for hypertension as fixed dose combinations with a thiazide (e.g. co-amilozide) in patients receiving converting enzyme inhibitors.

7. **–SH group-related effects** When first introduced into clinical use captopril was found to cause a cluster of adverse effects including heavy proteinuria, neutropenia, rash and taste disturbance, that were identified as being related to its sulfhydryl group. Similar effects occur with penicillamine, another drug that contains a sulfhydryl group (chapter 23). These dose-related effects seldom occur with the maximum doses of captopril that are now regarded as being useful in treating hypertension (i.e. usually no more than 50 mg twice daily).

Pharmacokinetics

Currently available converting enzyme inhibitors are all active when administered orally, but are highly polar and are eliminated in the urine. Some (e.g. fosinopril) are also metabolized by the liver. Some (e.g. captopril, lisinopril) are active *per se*, while others (e.g. enalapril, quinapril) are prodrugs, and require metabolic conversion to active metabolites (e.g. enalaprilat, quinaprilat). In practice this is of little or no importance. None of the currently available ACE inhibitors penetrates the central nervous system particularly well, and none penetrates to inhibit the testicular enzyme. Enalapril, quinapril and lisinopril are all given once daily, while captopril is administered twice daily. However, ACE inhibitors are effective in many patients with low renin as well as those with high renin hypertension and there is only a poor correlation between inhibition of plasma converting enzyme and chronic hypotensive effect, possibly because of the importance of converting enzyme in various key tissues rather than in the plasma.

Drug interactions

The useful interaction with diuretics has already been alluded to: diuretic treatment increases plasma renin activity, and the consequent activation of angiotensin II and aldosterone limits their efficacy. Converting enzyme inhibitors interrupt this loop and so enhance the hypotensive efficacy of diuretics, as well as reducing thiazide-induced hypokalemia. Conversely, ACE inhibitors have a potentially adverse interaction with potassium-sparing diuretics and potassium supplements, leading to hyperkalemia especially in patients with renal impairment, as mentioned above. As with other antihypertensive drugs, non-steroidal anti-inflammatory drugs increase blood pressure in patients treated with converting enzyme inhibitors.

CALCIUM CHANNEL BLOCKERS

Use

Dihydropyridine calcium channel blockers lower blood pressure and are a useful addition to a β-adrenoceptor antagonist in patients with moderate or severe hypertension who are not adequately controlled by a β-blocker alone. Some of these drugs (e.g. nifedipine, nicardipine, amlodipine) are also licensed for use alone in patients with mild essential hypertension, although so far there have been no controlled clinical trials to demonstrate that they reduce the risk of stroke or other clinically important events in such patients. As with the converting enzyme inhibitors, large-scale comparative studies with thiazide diuretics and β-blockers are sorely needed, since there are theoretical reasons to think that calcium channel blockers might perform either worse or better than these proven therapies. They are particularly useful in patients with angina in addition to hypertension, because of their prophylactic effect in reducing the frequency of this symptom (chapter 26), especially those in whom β-adrenoceptor antagonists (which are also useful prophylactically in patients with angina) are contraindicated. Nifedipine worsens angina in occasional patients, because of reflex tachycardia, and such patients may benefit from diltiazem (which has little effect on heart rate) or verapamil (which slows heart rate via its effect on cardiac conducting tissue).

Calcium channel blockers are more expensive than thiazide diuretics or β-blockers, and similar in cost to converting enzyme inhibitors. They make a useful alternative in patients in whom thiazide diuretics and β-blockers are contraindicated, or who do not tolerate them, although they have several distinct side effects of their own, and are not invariably well tolerated. Amlodipine has a long half-life, and is taken once daily; nifedipine and nicardipine are taken more frequently, although in the case of nifedipine the need for this is minimized by the use of a slow release or of an osmotically powered sustained release formulation. Because of its long half-life the daily dose of amlodipine should not be increased too rapidly. It has in any event a relatively small useful dose range of 5–10 mg.

There has been a vogue in the UK for the use of nifedipine sublingually for the treatment of hypertensive emergencies. A capsule is bitten into and the liquid allowed to remain in the mouth. Used in this way it has been shown that most of the absorbed nifedipine is in fact swallowed, and that this method causes unpredictable and sometimes catastrophic hypotension with consequent watershed infarction of the brain. The drug is not licensed for use in this way, and advice to do so (sometimes given in anonymous editorials) is to be deplored.

Mechanism of action

Calcium channel blockers inhibit the influx of Ca^{2+} through voltage dependent L-type calcium channels. Calcium entry through such channels in vascular smooth muscle controls the contractile state of actomyosin. Calcium channel blockers therefore relax arteriolar smooth muscle, reduce peripheral vascular resistance and lower arterial blood pressure.

Their ability to relax vascular smooth muscle also underlies their use in coronary artery spasm, cerebral vasospasm following subarachnoid hemorrhage (where nimodipine is used) and Raynaud's phenomenon. Calcium channel blockers are negatively inotropic because they inhibit Ca^{2+} entry in cardiac tissue.

Not all chemical classes of calcium channel blockers have the same selectivity for calcium channels in vascular smooth muscle and cardiac tissues, dihydropyridines (e.g. nifedipine, nicardipine, amlodipine) being relatively selective for vascular smooth muscle. Verapamil (a phenylalkylamine calcium channel blocker) is used mainly as an antiarrhythmic drug (chapter 29) because of its effects on the voltage-dependent channels in cardiac conducting tissue; it also blocks Ca^{2+} entry in gastrointestinal smooth muscle, and consequently causes constipation. An attempt to capitalize on the effect of calcium channel blockers on gastrointestinal muscle has been made in treating patients with lower esophageal spasm with nifedipine. Selectivities are only relative: dihydropyridines are negatively inotropic and verapamil causes vasodilatation and is indeed sometimes used to treat hypertension. Diltiazem, a benzothiazepine calcium channel blocker, is often used to treat patients who have recovered from subendocardial myocardial infarction and patients with angina, because it causes less reflex tachycardia than nifedipine.

It has been argued that calcium channel blockers may cause regression of atheroma, and some evidence for this has been provided by a study called INTACT. Measurements of atheromatous plaque at different time points is, however, difficult especially as Ca^{2+} blockers relax healthy coronary artery adjacent to the plaque thereby influencing the apparent tightness of the stenosis. Larger studies are needed to confirm these interesting findings, and determine whether or not they are of clinical relevance.

Metabolic effects

Calcium channel blockers do not affect concentrations of plasma cholesterol or triglycerides or extracellular calcium homeostasis.

Adverse effects

Calcium channel blocking drugs are usually reasonably well tolerated.

1. The commonest adverse effects of the dihydropyridines are flushing and headache which are directly related to arteriolar vasodilatation. These effects are worst when treatment is started and are related to peak plasma concentration. Consequently they are most marked with short-acting drugs such as nifedipine, less marked with slow release formulations and least marked with a long half-life drug such as amlodipine, with which the frequency of these complaints in double blind trials is similar to placebo.

2. Ankle swelling is common with all the dihydropyridines, and often takes some time to become manifest. The reason for the particular propensity of dihydropyridines (as distinct from other calcium channel blockers and most other vasodilators) to cause this side effect is not completely understood: it has been suggested that dihydropyridines preferentially relax arteriolar smooth muscle, thereby exposing the capillaries in the feet to unphysiologically high pressures causing exudation of fluid by the Starling mechanism.

3. The negative inotropic effect of the calcium channel blockers can exacerbate cardiac failure. This propensity is most marked with verapamil and least manifest in the case of the dihydropyridines because of their relative selectivity for vascular smooth muscle, and the tendency for the reduction in cardiac afterload caused by arteriolar dilatation to offset the direct negative inotropic effect of the heart. Indeed these drugs can usefully be combined with β-blockers (which are themselves negatively inotropic) in patients with good cardiac function who do not achieve adequate reduction in blood pressure with a β-blocking drug as a single agent. Caution is however needed in treating patients with even mild degrees of heart failure with a calcium channel blocking drug. It is claimed that nicardipine has less direct

negative inotropic action than other dihydropyridines.

4. Constipation is an undesired effect of phenylalkylamines such as verapamil on gastrointestinal smooth muscle.

Pharmacokinetics

Calcium channel antagonists are absorbed when given by mouth. Parenteral preparations of some dihydropyridines (e.g. nicardipine) are available but are seldom needed for hypertension, in contrast to verapamil which is used intravenously to treat supraventricular arrhythmias (chapter 29). Nifedipine has a short half-life and many of its adverse effects (e.g. flushing, headache) relate to the peak plasma concentration. Slow release preparations improve its performance in this regard, but are limited by the transit time of the bowel. Amlodipine has a half-life of 2–3 days and produces a smooth effect, as well as requiring only once daily administration. Nifedipine is preferred in urgent situations as it permits more rapid dose titration: the useful dose range of the retard formulation is 10–40 mg twice daily. Amlodipine can be phased in subsequently when blood pressure control has been achieved.

Drug interactions

The favorable interaction of calcium channel blocking drugs with β-adrenoceptor antagonists when used orally to treat patients with moderately severe hypertension uncomplicated by cardiac failure has already been discussed. It contrasts with the potentially catastrophic interaction of intravenous verapamil or other calcium channel antagonists when used intravenously to treat patients with tachyarrhythmias.

α-ADRENOCEPTOR ANTAGONISTS

Use

Non-specific α-blockade causes profound postural hypotension and reflex tachycardia. Use of such drugs is limited and specialized: phenoxybenzamine is distinctive in irreversibly alkylating the receptors. It is still uniquely valuable in preparing patients with pheochromocytoma for surgery but has no place in the management of essential hypertension. Prazosin is a selective reversible post- junctional α$_1$-blocker. Unlike phenoxybenzamine, it does not block presynaptic α$_2$-receptors that are normally stimulated by released noradrenaline and which inhibit further transmitter release. Thus there is no interference with this negative feedback pathway, and consequently relatively little tachycardia or increased cardiac output occurs during prazosin therapy compared to phenoxybenzamine. Furthermore α-blockers reduce plasma low density lipoprotein (LDL) cholesterol and increase high density lipoprotein (HDL) cholesterol, effects that could be of value especially in treating patients with coexisting dyslipidemia. Usage of prazosin is, however, limited by the occurrence of severe hypotension and collapse especially following the first dose. Prazosin has a short plasma half-life and is given at least twice daily. Because of these problems α-blockers were not especially widely used. This situation has changed recently with the introduction of doxazosin and terazocin. These drugs are structurally closely related to prazosin. They possess similar α$_1$-selectivity as prazosin but have substantially longer plasma half-lives, permitting once daily use and fewer problems with first dose hypotension.

Long-acting α$_1$-adrenoceptor antagonists are useful additions to diuretics, β-adrenoceptor antagonists, Ca^{2+} antagonists or converting enzyme inhibitors in patients with moderate hypertension who are partially but not adequately controlled on one of these drugs used on its own. Doxazosin is also licensed for use as a single agent in patients with mild essential hypertension, although so far there have been no controlled clinical trials to demonstrate that α$_1$-adrenoceptor antagonists reduce the risk of stroke or other clinically important events in such patients. As with converting enzyme inhibitors and calcium channel blockers large-scale comparative studies with thiazide diuretics and/or β-blockers are needed, since there are theoretical reasons to think that α$_1$-blockers might perform either worse or better (e.g. because of their effects on plasma lipids) than these proven therapies.

It is prudent to start treatment with a long-acting α_1-blocker with a small dose (e.g. 1 mg terazosin) given before going to bed, and to warn patients of the possibility of postural hypotension if they get up during the night. Nevertheless, postural hypotension is less of a problem than with prazosin. The dose may be titrated to up to 16 mg (doxazosin) or 20 mg (terazosin) if necessary. Despite the 10–12 hour plasma half-life the daily dose should not be escalated too rapidly, and the effect on erect as well as supine blood pressure should be monitored. Since α_1-antagonists reduce cardiac afterload and, unlike β-antagonists and calcium channel antagonists, have no direct negative inotropic effect, they are particularly useful as an addition to a converting enzyme inhibitor or diuretic in hypertensive patients with cardiac failure. They also reduce symptoms of bladder outflow tract obstruction, and are useful in men with mild symptoms from benign prostatic hypertrophy who do not desire surgery but who do not tolerate thiazide diuretics because of urinary urgency or nocturia.

Mechanism of action

The sympathetic nervous system is tonically active, and noradrenaline released from postganglionic nerve terminals activates α_1-receptors on vascular smooth muscle causing tonic vasoconstriction via release of Ca^{2+} from intracellular stores by inositol trisphosphate and by influx of Ca^{2+} through receptor-operated as well as voltage-dependent channels. (Voltage-dependent channels are opened indirectly via depolarization of the smooth muscle membrane.) α_1-Blockers cause vasodilatation by antagonizing this tonic action of noradrenaline.

Adverse effects

1. First dose hypotension and postural hypotension have been mentioned above.
2. Other effects including nasal stuffiness, headache, dizziness, dry mouth, impotence

and pruritus have also been reported but are relatively infrequent.
3. α-Blockers can cause urinary incontinence, especially in women with pre-existing pelvic pathology. This is uncommon but it is important to be aware of this possibility since the effect is reversible on stopping the drug.

Metabolic effects

α_1-Adrenoceptor antagonists have a mild favorable effect on plasma lipids, with an increase in HDL and reduction in LDL cholesterol. Whether these desirable biochemical effects translate into a clinically useful reduction in ischemic heart disease is unknown.

Pharmacokinetics

Mean plasma half-life of prazosin is approximately 3 hours; doxazosin and terazosin have plasma half-lives of approximately 10–12 hours and provide acceptably smooth 24 hour control if used once daily.

MINOXIDIL AND POTASSIUM CHANNEL ACTIVATORS

Several vasodilators including cromokalim (and its active stereoisomer lemakalim) and pinacidil have been intensively studied and shown to work by opening K^+ channels. Ironically it has subsequently transpired that several older selective arteriolar vasodilators including minoxidil and diazoxide which had previously been dubbed 'direct acting' also have this mechanism of action. Vascular smooth muscle cells contain high conductance K^+ channels that are controlled by intracellular adenosine triphosphate (ATP). When the ATP concentration is high, these channels are closed but when ATP falls these K^+ channels open. This causes hyperpolarization of the cell membrane which switches off the voltage-dependent Ca^{2+} channels and hence relaxes the contractile apparatus. This probably represents an important link between the metabolic and contractile state of the cell. K^+ channel activators antagonize the action of ATP. This causes the channels to open even when the intracellular ATP concentration is high, with resulting hyperpolarization, relaxation and vasodilatation.

Use

Minoxidil is valuable as a drug of last resort in very severely hypertensive patients. It is added as a third drug to β-blocker and diuretic, and cannot be used on its own since it causes marked reflex tachycardia which necessitates β-blockade and marked fluid retention necessitating use of a loop diuretic. Extraordinarily large doses of loop diuretic (e.g. several hundred milligrams daily of frusemide) are sometimes needed to prevent fluid retention. The side effects of minoxidil render its use unacceptable in any but the most severely affected individuals. Minoxidil is usually given by mouth twice daily, and the dose is titrated from 5 mg daily to up to 40 mg daily, with close attention to body weight: increased weight and other evidence of fluid overload should be countered by increasing the dose of loop diuretic rather than the dose of minoxidil.

Diazoxide is a thiazide analog but is a powerful vasodilator and causes salt and water retention. When used chronically it almost invariably caused significant glucose intolerance (cf. the much milder glucose intolerance sometimes caused by thiazide diuretics). Indeed this effect is now exploited in what is the only remaining indication for diazoxide, namely to prevent hypoglycemia in patients with inoperable insulinoma. This effect on glucose tolerance is due to reduced insulin secretion. It is caused by hyperpolarization of pancreatic islet cells and consequent reduction of insulin secretion secondary to potassium channel activation. Diazoxide was used as an intravenous drug to control blood pressure acutely in patients with malignant hypertension, but safer and more predictable alternatives have superseded it.

Adverse effects

In addition to the reflex activation of the sympathetic nervous system and fluid retention mentioned above minoxidil causes hirsuitism (almost invariably), coarsening of the facial features and, rarely, effusions (pericardial, pleural or ascitic: usually in patients with renal impairment), rash, gastrointestinal intolerance and breast tenderness. Hirsuitism is particularly unacceptable in women. An alcoholic solution of minoxidil sulfate is marketed for topical application, and stimulates hair growth in a few patients with male pattern baldness, but only for as long as it is used.

Pharmacokinetics

Oral absorption of minoxidil is complete. Mean plasma half-life is 3–4 hours, but plasma concentration is not correlated with effect because it works via an active sulfate metabolite. It is eliminated by glucuronide formation followed by renal excretion.

SODIUM NITROPRUSSIDE

Use

Sodium nitroprusside is uniquely valuable in the management of hypertensive encephalopathy and other hypertensive emergencies. It is also used in the management of shock, tissue hypoperfusion and/or cardiac dysfunction (e.g. following cardiopulmonary bypass) when it is combined with a positive inotrope. It is administered by intravenous infusion, the initial dose being 0.5–1.5 µg/kg/min. Constant monitoring of blood pressure in an intensive care unit is required. The dose is adjusted to individual requirements, which are variable: usually within the range 0.5–8 µg/kg/min. A maximum dose limit of 800 µg/min is recommended to avoid cyanide intoxication. Its unique value in treating hypertensive emergencies is due to its very short half-life. Consequently, blood pressure can be titrated precisely by varying the infusion rate. Control can therefore be achieved within minutes and any tendency to an excessive fall in pressure (potentially catastrophic) can be countered within minutes by reducing or discontinuing the infusion. Tachyphylaxis is not generally a problem (in contrast to organic nitrates, chapter 26), but prolonged administration is undesirable because of the possibility of cyanide toxicity. It is not usually necessary to use sodium nitroprusside for longer than 24 hours. When administration for longer than 24 hours is needed plasma concentrations of thiocyanate and of bicarbonate, lactate and pyruvate should be monitored.

Degradation of nitroprusside occurs in the presence of light or acid yielding sodium ferrocyanide and cyanide. This changes the colour of the solution from the normal brownish-pink to blue or dark brown. The stock solution should be diluted only in 5% dextrose: other diluents may produce toxic products. The infusion bottle should be covered with foil to prevent photodeactivation.

Mechanism of action

Nitroprusside liberates nitric oxide under physiological conditions. Nitric oxide diffuses into vascular smooth muscle cells where it combines with a heme group in soluble guanylyl cyclase, hence activating this enzyme and increasing the synthesis of cyclic guanosine monophosphate (cGMP). This cyclic nucleotide reduces the concentration of cytoplasmic Ca^{2+} by causing Ca^{2+} sequestration in the endoplasmic reticulum. This results in relaxation of both arterioles and venous capacitance vessels, lowering peripheral vascular resistance and reducing cardiac pre- as well as afterload. Nitric oxide also inhibits platelet function, but it is not known whether this has consequences of clinical importance.

Adverse effects

Side effects of nitroprusside are usually due to a too rapid reduction in blood pressure because of excessive dose and inadequate monitoring, and disappear with slowing of the infusion rate. Other effects include nausea, palpitation, dizziness, apprehension and muscle twitching, but generally its use is associated with a low incidence of toxicity. Prolonged or excessive dosage has resulted in deaths due to cyanide accumulation. There is a theoretical risk of worsening hypothyroidism because of the inhibitory effect of thiocyanate on iodine uptake and binding by the thyroid. Similarly prolonged nitroprusside infusion could worsen vitamin B_{12} deficiency in patients with pernicious anemia or tobacco amblyopia.

Pharmacokinetics

Each nitroprusside ion liberates five cyanide ions by a non-enzymic reaction with hemoglobin. One cyanide ion is absorbed by reacting with the resultant methemoglobin and the remainder are metabolized by rhodanase, a mitochondrial enzyme system in liver and kidney which is a sulfydryl transferase, converting cyanide to thiocyanate. Vitamin B_{12} is a rhodanase cofactor. Although the half-life of nitroprusside is of the order of seconds, thiocyanate has a half-life of about a week and is excreted largely unchanged.

HYDRALAZINE

Use

Hydralazine was used extensively in severely hypertensive patients whose blood pressure remained unacceptably elevated despite treatment with a β-blocker and diuretic. (The sequence diuretic, diuretic + β-blocker, diuretic + β-blocker + hydralazine was referred to in the USA as 'stepped care'). The introduction of converting enzyme inhibitors and calcium channel antagonists has reduced the need for hydralazine considerably, but it remains useful in occasional patients. In particular there is considerably greater experience with hydralazine than with other vasodilators in treating women with pregnancy hypertension, a situation in which a conservative approach is appropriate. It is usually added to methyldopa or to a β-blocker in women with severe hypertension during pregnancy. It is usually given by mouth twice daily in doses up to 200 mg/day, but in urgent situations (e.g. in pregnant women with severe pre-eclampsia) it can be given as an intravenous infusion.

Mechanism of action

Hydralazine reduces arteriolar resistance by direct relaxation of arteriolar smooth muscle by an unknown mechanism. The resulting reduction in peripheral vascular resistance causes the arterial blood pressure to fall. Its effect is limited by reflex sympathetic activation (evidenced by tachycardia), and by salt and water retention.

Adverse effects

1. Related to direct or reflex-mediated **hemodynamic actions**: flushing, headache, palpitations, edema, angina and nasal congestion. These effects are reduced by coadministration of a β-blocker and diuretic.
2. Drug-induced **systemic lupus erythematosus** (SLE) syndrome: this is almost always reversible when hydralazine is stopped, although months may be required for complete disappearance of the reaction. The incidence is dose dependent and higher in women and slow acetylators (chapter 13). It is not related to the human leukocyte antigen (HLA) types associated with increased incidence of the idiopathic form of SLE.
3. **Peripheral neuropathy**: this is dose related and possibly due to pyridoxine deficiency due to formation of a pyridoxine–hydralazine complex which inactivates the coenzyme. The neuropathy is corrected by pyridoxine supplements.
4. **Blood dyscrasias**: anemia, agranulocytosis and leukopenia have been described but are uncommon with doses of less than 200 mg daily.

Pharmacokinetics

Hydralazine is rapidly and fairly completely absorbed after oral administration, peak levels being reached within 1 hour of dosing. Tissue binding also occurs, particularly in the walls of muscular arteries. This presumably explains why, despite a short plasma half-life the half-offset time of the hypotensive effect is greater than 24 hours following discontinuation of treatment. It is therefore unlikely that a simple relationship exists between plasma hydralazine concentration and the circulatory effects of the drug. Metabolism occurs by hepatic acetylation, the rate of which is genetically determined (chapter 13). Fast acetylators have lower steady-state plasma concentrations, less reduction in blood pressure and a reduced incidence of adverse effects.

GANGLION BLOCKERS

Use

The few remaining indications for ganglion-blocking drugs are in the initial treatment of acute thoracic aortic dissection and in the diagnosis of pheochromocytoma. Trimetaphan is used as an intravenous infusion in patients with acute dissection. It has a swift onset of action and is given as an intravenous infusion at 3–4 mg/min. It not only reduces blood pressure but, unlike other vasodilators such as sodium nitroprusside, it also reduces the rate of rise of the aortic pressure wave (dP/dt). Its hypotensive effect is strongly influenced by posture (because of the 'use dependent' nature of its blocking action, see below), and patients may be managed in a bed adjusted to provide a head-up tilt. Prolonged use is not appropriate, and may be complicated by paralytic ileus. Trimetaphan is best used as a temporizing measure in such patients while the anatomy of their dissection is studied and the tear stabilized while surgery is planned.

Pentolinium is used in a suppression test to differentiate elevated plasma catecholamines due to pheochromocytoma from elevation due to other causes of increased sympathetic outflow such as anxiety: pentolinium does not suppress autonomous catecholamine secretion by pheochromocytomas, but does suppress plasma catecholamine concentrations in patients with increased sympathetic nerve traffic due to anxiety or cardiovascular reflex activation.

Mechanism of action

These drugs block autonomic ganglia (both sympathetic and parasympathetic) by blocking ion channels that are linked to nicotinic cholinergic receptors. The block is thus non-competitive. Ganglion-blocking drugs block ion channels in the open state, so the block is 'use dependent': i.e. if nerve traffic occurs at high frequency the synapse will be blocked more than if synaptic transmission is less frequent. This explains why ganglion blockers are so much more dependent on posture than are α_1-blockers that interrupt the same pathway more distally.

The non-selective effect on autonomic ganglia results in parasympathetic blockade and adverse effects that make these drugs unacceptable for general use.

CENTRALLY ACTING DRUGS

Use

Methyldopa and, to a lesser extent, clonidine continue to have a limited use in the treatment of hypertension. Methyldopa is used in women with hypertension during pregnancy since there is more experience with this drug than with many newer agents in pregnant women, in whom a conservative approach is appropriate. Methyldopa is given by mouth (there is a parenteral formulation, but this is seldom indicated), starting at doses of 250 mg twice daily and increasing if necessary to doses of 3–4 g daily. Methyldopa causes symptoms of drowsiness and fatigue that are intolerable to many adult patients in long-term use, and is seldom used any longer to treat essential hypertension. It was used as an additional treatment in elderly patients inadequately controlled with diuretic alone in the European Working Party on Hypertension in the Elderly study (EWPHE) and, perhaps surprisingly, was well tolerated by this age group, many of whom remained alert and symptom free while taking methyldopa. Clonidine is potent but poorly tolerated. Rebound hypertension, if it is discontinued abruptly, is an uncommon but severe problem and with newer and better tolerated drugs now available clonidine is currently seldom needed, although it is still sometimes used to treat drug addicts during opiate withdrawal to minimize withdrawal symptoms.

Mechanism of action

The central nervous system plays an important role in the regulation of the circulation. Stimulation of α_2-adrenoceptors in the brainstem pontomedullary area decreases sympathetic nervous outflow to the periphery which produces a fall in blood pressure. Clonidine is an α_2-agonist as is α-methylnoradrenaline, a false transmitter synthesized from α-methyldopa and released instead of noradrenaline from the nerve terminals. The hypotensive actions of methyldopa and clonidine are attributed to their central α_2-agonist actions.

Adverse effects

Adverse effects to centrally acting drugs are both common and diverse. They include:

1. Drowsiness, depression, nightmares and, with methyldopa, rarely extrapyramidal features. With clonidine nasal stuffiness is prominent and anticholinergic symptoms of dry mouth and constipation may be troublesome.
2. Sexual dysfunction.
3. Hepatitis (with methyldopa).
4. Coombs' test positive hemolytic anemia (with methyldopa). Reversible leukopenia and thrombocytopenia may also occur.
5. Salt and water retention.
6. Drug fever (with methyldopa).
7. Hypertensive rebound associated with anxiety, sweating, tachycardia and extrasystoles, and rarely hypertensive crisis may be provoked by drug withdrawal (especially from clonidine). Such patients are extremely agitated and present with a clinical syndrome of sympathetic overactivity that is reminiscent of opiate or alcohol withdrawal in addicted patients.

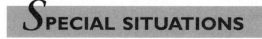

SPECIAL SITUATIONS

ELDERLY

Most vascular events occur in elderly persons who therefore particularly benefit from antihypertensive treatment provided they are otherwise in good health. Evidence for this view comes from several controlled trials including the EWPHE study and the systolic hypertension in the elderly (SHEP) study, which demonstrated significant reductions in myocardial infarction with treatment in this age group. Elderly persons are, however, also at greatest risk of adverse effects and treatment should be mild and dose titration gradual. There are no hard rules about choice of drug. Diuretics (e.g. Dyazide™ which was used in the EWPHE study) are often successful, but should be avoided in men with symptoms of prostatism or women with incontinence; they may need to be temporarily withheld in the event of intercurrent desalinating illness (e.g. with fever, vomiting and diarrhea). β-Adrenoceptor antagonists are also sometimes effective and well tolerated; it is important to obtain an electrocardiogram and make sure there is no evidence of heart block or suggestion of sick sinus syndrome. Converting enzyme inhibitors are usually well tolerated by elderly persons, as are calcium channel antagonists. α-Adrenoceptor antagonists are best avoided because even healthy elderly persons often experience some degree of postural hypotension, and lack the homeostatic mechanisms to compensate for additional causes of postural hypotension. Centrally acting drugs (e.g. methyldopa) were used as add-on treatment in the EWPHE trial.

PREGNANCY

Management of eclampsia/pre-eclampsia

Eclampsia is a leading cause of fetal and maternal mortality. Pre-eclampsia (its forerunner) occurs from the twentieth week of pregnancy and consists of hypertension, proteinuria and edema, often with elevation of plasma urate and liver enzymes and thrombocytopenia and other evidence of consumptive coagulopathy. It can progress rapidly to eclampsia, which is characterized by convulsions. Women with pre-eclampsia should be admitted to hospital. Pre-eclampsia resolves rapidly (usually within a few days) after delivery, although occasionally late *postpartum* eclampsia develops up to 10 days after delivery. Near term the baby

should therefore be delivered promptly. Earlier in gestation attempts to prolong the pregnancy by treating blood pressure and giving anticonvulsants may be worthwhile, although they seldom do more than buy a little extra time and the risks of eclampsia are considerable: if headache or epigastric pain, hyperreflexia, deterioration of renal function or development of consumptive coagulopathy develop, or if the fetus is in jeopardy, delivery should be undertaken promptly whatever the gestational age. Glucocorticoids are something given to accelerate maturation of the fetal lung, and reduce the risk of respiratory disease in the newborn baby.

From this it is evident that drugs have only a secondary part to play in the management of established pre-eclampsia/eclampsia. In women with mildly elevated blood pressure it is appropriate to begin treatment with methyldopa given by mouth. The starting dose is 250 or 500 mg two or three times daily, and the dose can be increased rapidly if necessary to a maximum of 3–4 g daily in divided doses. If this fails to control the blood pressure hydralazine can be added in doses up to 200 mg daily by mouth. In more urgent situations (i.e. when the clinical picture suggests that eclampsia is imminent) blood pressure should be controlled by intravenous hydralazine, given ideally as a constant rate infusion, or, if an infusion pump is not available, as a series of small intravenous boluses, starting with a 5 mg dose followed by 5–10 mg every 20–30 min as needed with continuous monitoring of blood pressure.

Evidence as to the best drug to prevent and treat seizures in this context is incomplete. The largest published experience is that of the Parkland Hospital in Dallas, and this suggests that magnesium administered intravenously to achieve a plasma concentration of 2–3 mmol/l is highly effective, although this has never been formally proved in clinical trial. Use of magnesium is appropriate in women in whom hyperreflexia or other features of imminent eclampsia develop, provided renal function is normal. Plasma concentrations of magnesium should be measured daily. Treatment should be continued for 24 hours after delivery because of the risk of late fits.

In pre-eclamptic women without these features and in whom oral therapy is preferred, phenytoin is probably at least partly effective in reducing the occurrence of fits. A loading dose of 1.5 mg/kg body weight should be followed by regular daily dosing and plasma concentration determinations, bearing in mind that elimination of phenytoin is increased during the final stages of pregnancy (chapter 19) and that altered protein binding depresses the therapeutic range (p. 79).

Prevention of pre-eclampsia

The pathophysiology of pre-eclampsia is only partly understood, but seems to involve a loss of the resistance to vasoconstrictor influences that usually accompany pregnancy. One hypothesis is that this is due to an imbalance of vasoconstrictor and vasodilator prostanoids, and aspirin (75 mg daily) which inhibits thromboxane synthesis more than that of vasodilator prostaglandins such as prostacyclin, has been found to reduce the risk of pre-eclampsia in highly selected subsets of women at high risk of this disorder. The selection procedures in these studies involved tests such as pressor sensitivity to intravenous angiotensin II that could not be applied generally. Clinical trials to determine whether these encouraging findings can be extended to larger groups of women with simple risk factors have, however, been negative.

Pre-existing hypertension

The great majority of women with pre-existing hypertension have essential hypertension, although of course secondary hypertension is also encountered in pregnant women. Of secondary causes it is especially important to keep the possibility of pheochromocytoma in mind, as this can present during pregnancy in a clinically indistinguishable manner from pre-eclampsia, yet its successful management is very different from either pre-eclampsia or essential hypertension, and failure to make this diagnosis accounts for a disproportionate number of maternal deaths.

Women with essential hypertension are at increased risk of pre-eclampsia, but more than 85% of such women have uncomplicated pregnancies, so it is appropriate to provide general reassurance. If treatment is *initiated* during pregnancy it is appropriate to use methyldopa which has the longest record of use and follow up in children born to mothers following treatment. Information on use of first-line antihypertensive drugs during pregnancy is decidedly thin. One has to balance the risk of stopping such a drug against uncertainties about possible adverse effects on the fetus.

Angiotensin-converting enzyme inhibitors are absolutely contraindicated in later stages of pregnancy as they cause oligohydramnios and neonatal renal failure. For this reason we do not generally start women of reproductive potential with essential hypertension on these drugs. The use of diuretics during pregnancy is controversial: it is generally agreed that they should not be used to treat established pre-eclampsia or eclampsia (unless left ventricular failure has supervened), but some authorities recommend continuing them if they were being taken before conception. β-Blockers (especially atenolol and metoprolol) and the combined α- and β-blocker labetalol have been used successfully in pregnancy, although concerns about an effect of propranolol on fetal growth and of maternal hepatotoxicity of labetolol have been expressed. Trials of Ca^{2+} antagonists have been promising, but experience is limited, and we generally recommend substituting methyldopa in women taking these drugs who become pregnant.

ACCELERATED AND MALIGNANT HYPERTENSION

Malignant hypertension is diagnosed on the basis of high blood pressure accompanied by papilloedema and, usually, microscopic hematuria with red cell casts. Hypertension with grade III retinopathy (cotton wool spots and/or hemorrhages) is sometimes called accelerated hypertension. Both conditions are associated with a vasculitis characterized by fibrinoid necrosis in arterioles in brain and kidneys and progression to death within 1 year in 90% of cases if untreated. These are emergency situations, requiring immediate hospitalization. There are two principles for successful treatment:

1. To lower the blood pressure promptly, but
2. To avoid lowering the pressure too much.

The reason that excessive lowering of pressure is so dangerous in this situation is that cerebral autoregulation is severely impaired in this circumstance, so reducing the pressure to values that would be well tolerated in normotensive individuals causes an excessive reduction in blood flow in patients with malignant hypertension (Fig. 25.3). Inadequate cerebral blood flow causes infarction in watershed areas of the brain, and blindness or disconnection syndromes and other forms of stroke can follow a precipitate fall in blood pressure.

In most patients blood pressure should therefore be reduced over days rather than hours. The main indications for parenteral drugs are severe left ventricular failure or hypertensive encephalopathy. If these are absent the patient should be put to bed and oral treatment commenced with a β-blocker or slow release preparation of a calcium channel antagonist such as a slow-release preparation of nifedipine. It is important to realize that unpredictable and sometimes catastrophic (i.e. causing blindness or stroke) falls of blood pressure have been reported following intra-venous boluses of antihypertensive drugs and after buccal administration of nifedipine (e.g. following biting into a capsule of the regular formulation of this drug).

In mild left ventricular failure frusemide is used. More severe failure is an indication for sodium nitroprusside by constant rate infusion in an intensive care unit. If intensive care facilities are unavailable, an oral drug regime may be safer for the patient. Encephalopathy is present if convulsions or a fluctuating level of consciousness or chang-ing focal neurological signs occur. It is rare, and optimal management depends absolutely on intensive care unit facilities. Neurological features in hypertensive patients often result from cerebral infarction or hemorrhage due to thrombosis of a large vessel or rupture of a Charcot–Bouchard aneurysm rather than

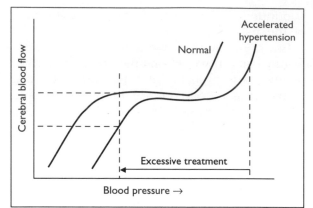

Fig. 25.3 Cerebral blood flow in accelerated hypertension. The autoregulation curve is shifted to the right. Cerebral blood flow is increased before treatment, but if blood pressure is reduced by treatment to a value that would be well tolerated in a normal subject this will cause a potentially catastrophic fall in cerebral blood fall in a patient with accelerated hypertension.

encephalopathy. These are contraindications to rapid blood pressure reduction which may exacerbate the neurological deficit. Sodium nitroprusside by constant rate infusion (0.5 μg/kg/min increasing to 8 μg/kg/min) is the best drug for treating hypertensive encephalopathy but it is mandatory to monitor the response frequently in an inten-sive care unit, and oral treatment should be started as soon as possible.

Once the immediate emergency is past, the possibility of secondary hypertension should be considered, particularly renal artery steno-sis which has been reported in around one-third of such patients in some modern series.

ACUTE AORTIC DISSECTION

Aortic dissection is extended by a wide pulse pressure and by a rapid rate of rise of arterial pressure (dP/dt). Vasodilators such as hydralazine (which increase pulse pressure and dP/dt) should therefore be avoided in the first instance. The ganglion-blocker trimetaphan decreases the rate and force of myocardial contraction as well as blood pressure and is appropriate. Alternatively a fast-acting parenteral β-receptor antagonist (e.g. esmolol) can be infused intravenously, supplemented by sodium nitroprusside once β-blockade has been achieved. Following stabilization the anatomy of the tear is defined and a surgical plan established. If operation is not indicated, medical therapy should include an oral β-blocker if possible.

DIABETES

Diabetes and hypertension often coexist. Hypertension is a risk factor for many of the complications of diabetes, and diabetics who are also hypertensive have a particularly high incidence of myocardial infarction, stroke and renal failure. The progression of renal impairment in diabetics can be slowed by treatment with antihypertensive drugs. It is therefore especially worth treating hypertension in diabetic patients.

Diuretics and β-adrenoceptor antagonists each have disadvantages in diabetic patients: thiazides worsen glucose tolerance in diabetics on oral agents or diet, and β-adrenoceptor antagonists may mask symptoms of hypoglycemia in patients who are treated with insulin. Each of these classes of agent have mild but potentially adverse effects on plasma lipid profiles that are theoretically especially undesirable in diabetic patients. Ca^{2+} antagonists and converting enzyme inhibitors are useful in diabetic patients, and there is evidence that converting enzyme inhibitors have a unique ability to reduce albumin excretion (a marker of diabetic glomerular injury) in such patients and hence perhaps to reduce the rate of progression of renal damage.

RENAL IMPAIRMENT

Although most patients with hypertension have normal or near-normal renal function, hypertension is a common cause and effect of renal failure. Although good control of blood pressure is not easy in many patients with renal failure, it should be sought vigorously as uncontrolled hypertension accelerates the deterioration of renal function and good control may delay the need for dialysis although, disappointingly, in some patients renal functional deterioration is inexorable despite apparently good control of blood pressure.

Thiazides are not effective in patients with renal failure and, in contrast to patients with normal renal function, a loop diuretic like frusemide is preferable in individuals with substantial degrees of renal dysfunction. Potassium-retaining diuretics such as amiloride or triamterene should be avoided in renal failure because of the danger of hyperkalemia (especially in patients receiving converting enzyme inhibitors).

Mild hypertension in patients with reduced renal function may respond to a β-adrenoceptor antagonist, calcium channel blocker, α_1-adrenoceptor antagonist or converting enzyme inhibitor. Renal function should be monitored closely when starting treatment with any of these drugs, because a reduction in mean arterial pressure may cause a further reduction in glomerular filtration. Converting enzyme inhibitors are a special case since these drugs predictably cause functional renal failure in patients with bilateral renal artery stenosis (or renal artery stenosis in an artery supplying a single functioning kidney) (see p. 293). This is due to the loss of efferent arteriolar tone on which glomerular filtration in these individuals depends. It is reversible if recognized promptly and the drug discontinued. More severe hypertension often requires the use of combinations of drugs, as in patients with normal renal function.

The blood pressure of patients on chronic dialysis can often be controlled by slow removal of water and salt during dialysis and by restriction of dietary salt and water between dialyses, supplemented with drug treatment if necessary.

Reference

Beevers DG, MacGregor GA. *Hypertension*. Volume 1. *The Causes and Consequences of Hypertension*. London: Martin Dunitz, 1987.

Ischemic Heart Disease

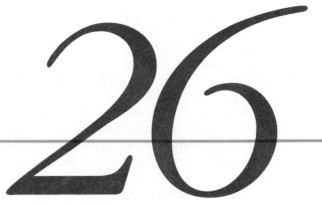

Pathophysiology **308**

Management of stable angina **309**

Management of unstable coronary disease **309**

Drugs used in ischemic heart disease **312**

PATHOPHYSIOLOGY

Rational use of drugs in patients with coronary artery disease depends on understanding the pathophysiology of the clinical syndromes to which this gives rise. Ischemic heart disease is nearly always caused by atheroma in one or more of the coronary arteries. Such disease is very common in western societies, and is often asymptomatic. When the obstruction caused by an uncomplicated atheromatous plaque exceeds a critical value, myocardial oxygen demand during exercise exceeds the ability of the stenosed vessel to supply oxygenated blood. Such patients complain of intermittent chest pain, brought on predictably by exertion and relieved within a few minutes on resting ('angina pectoris'). Such pain is probably caused by products of anaerobic metabolism in the working myocardium, formed as a result of the temporary imbalance between oxygen supply and demand.

Most patients with angina pectoris experience attacks of pain in a constant stable pattern, but in some patients attacks occur at rest, or occur with increasing frequency and severity on less and less exertion ('unstable angina'). Unstable angina may be a prelude to myocardial infarction, which can also occur unheralded. Both unstable angina and myocardial infarction occur as a result of fissuring of an atheromatous plaque in a coronary artery. Platelets adhere to the underlying subendothelium and white thrombus, consisting of platelet/fibrinogen/fibrin aggregates, extends into the lumen of the artery. Infarction results when such thrombus occludes the coronary vessel.

In addition to mechanical obstruction caused by atheroma, with or without adherent thrombus, spasm of smooth muscle in the vascular media can contribute to ischemia. The importance of such vascular spasm varies in different patients and at different times in the same patient, and its contribution is often hard to define clinically. The mechanism of such spasm also probably varies, and has been difficult to establish. Possible mediators include vasoconstrictors released from formed elements of blood (e.g. platelets or white cells) in relation to atheroma, or from nerve terminals. 5-Hydroxytryptamine (5HT, serotonin), thromboxane A_2, and various neuropeptides and endothelium-derived peptides (e.g. angiotensin II and endothelin), may each contribute alone or in combination in different circumstances. A relative *deficiency* of endothelium-derived *vasodilators*, including nitric oxide and prostacyclin, may be as important as release of vasoconstrictors.

Several of these mediators influence platelet function as well as vascular smooth muscle contraction: some vasoconstrictors, including 5HT and thromboxane A_2, are proaggregatory while several vasodilators including prostacyclin and nitric oxide are antiaggregatory. Consequently thrombosis as well as spasm is likely to be favored in situations characterized by an imbalance of these vasoactive mediators. There is currently intense interest in these issues, but the importance or otherwise of spasm in the majority of patients with acute coronary syndromes is unknown. Despite these uncertainties, modern treatment of patients with symptomatic ischemic heart disease, both angina and myocardial infarction, not only improves symptoms, but also prolongs life.

MANAGEMENT OF STABLE ANGINA

Modifiable risk factors

The object is to prevent progression (and, hopefully, cause regression) of coronary atheroma. Modifiable risk factors include smoking, hypertension, hypercholesterolemia, diabetes mellitus, obesity and lack of exercise. Their treatment is discussed in chapters 24, 25 and 34.

Pain relief

Angina is relieved by glyceryl trinitrate (GTN). However, in patients with chronic stable angina, pain usually resolves within a few minutes of stopping exercise even without treatment, so prophylaxis is usually more important than relief of an attack.

Prophylaxis

Glyceryl trinitrate is best used for 'acute' prophylaxis of angina. A dose is taken immediately before undertaking activity that usually brings on pain (e.g. climbing a hill) to prevent pain. Alternatively, long-acting nitrates (e.g. isosorbide mononitrate) may be taken regularly to reduce the frequency of attacks. β-Blockers or calcium channel blockers are also useful as regular prophylaxis.

Consideration of surgery/angioplasty

Cardiac catheterization can identify patients who would benefit from surgery or angioplasty. Patients with significant disease in the left main coronary artery survive longer if operated on, and so probably do patients with severe triple-vessel disease. Patients with strongly positive stress cardiograms have a relatively high incidence of such lesions, but unfortunately there is no foolproof method of making such anatomical diagnoses non-invasively, so the issue of which patients to subject to the small but real dangers of invasive study remains one of clinical judgment.

Patients for surgery usually undergo bypass grafting using their own saphenous vein, or, preferably, internal mammary artery, which is used to circumvent the diseased segment(s) of coronary artery. Angioplasty has yet to be shown to prolong life, but can be valuable as a less demanding alternative to surgery in patients with accessible lesions whose symptoms are not adequately controlled by medical therapy alone, despite concerns as to possible long-term adverse functional effects of de-endothelializing the arterial segment subjected to dilatation.

MANAGEMENT OF UNSTABLE CORONARY DISEASE

Unstable angina

Patients with unstable angina must stop smoking, and require urgent antiplatelet therapy, in the form of aspirin. This approximately halves the likelihood of myocardial infarction, and is the most effective known treatment for improving outcome in preinfarction syndromes. By contrast glyceryl trinitrate (GTN), while more effective than aspirin in relieving *pain* associated with unstable angina, is only marginally effective (as judged by meta-analysis of a number of individually inconclusive trials) in improving *outcome*. Glyceryl trinitrate is usually given as a constant rate intravenous infusion for this indication. Intravenous heparin is also used in unstable angina, and a β-adreno-ceptor antagonist prescribed if not contraindicated. Once the patient has stabilized, attention to modifiable risk factors and consideration of angiography and possible surgery are considered. Emergency angiography may be indicated in patients who do not stabilize, with a view to emergency surgery or angioplasty.

Myocardial infarction

Management entails:

I. OXYGEN

This is given in the highest concentration available (unless there is coincident pulmonary disease with carbon dioxide retention) delivered by nasal prongs or by face mask.

2. PAIN RELIEF

This usually requires an intravenous opiate (morphine or diamorphine) and concurrent treatment with an antiemetic (e.g. prochlorperazine or metaclopramide).

3. INFARCT LIMITATION

Aspirin and thrombolytic therapy reduce infarct size and improve survival, each to a similar extent; their beneficial effects are additive, and early fears as to the potential toxicity of the combination have proved unfounded so they are used together. Treatment with heparin to maintain patency of a vessel opened by aspirin plus thrombolysis is needed when recombinant tissue plasminogen activator is used for thrombolysis; it should not be used routinely after streptokinase since it was found not to confer overall benefit to such patients in the large ISIS III study. Heparin following streptokinase is used in patients judged to be at especially high risk of deep venous thrombosis. The use of β-blockers within the first few hours of infarction may limit myocardial damage or reduce mortality. The largest study (in patients who did *not* receive the now standard thrombolysis) showed that the 7-day mortality in treated patients was 3.7% compared with 4.3% in controls. The modest magnitude of this benefit probably does not warrant routine use of β-blockers for this indication (as opposed to their use in secondary prevention following recovery from acute infarction, which is discussed below).

4. TREATABLE COMPLICATIONS

These may occur early in the course of myocardial infarction and are best recognized and managed with the patient in a coronary care unit. Transfer from the admission room should therefore not be delayed by obtaining X-rays, since a portable film can be obtained on the unit if needed. Complications include cardiogenic shock (chapter 28) as well as acute tachy- or bradyarrhythmias (chapter 29) which may require treatment by cardioversion or pacing, or by drugs. Prophylactic treatment with antiarrhythmic drugs (i.e. before significant arrhythmia is documented) has not been found to improve survival, and is not recommended. In contrast, trials of magnesium supplementation (e.g. 40 mmol magnesium chloride intravenously over 4 hours followed by 40 mmol over the next 20 hours), have yielded promising but individually inconclusive results. A recent meta-analysis has supported the probable efficacy of magnesium in preventing arrhythmias and improving clinical outcome in patients with acute myocardial infarction. The large ISIS IV study failed to confirm a benefit of magnesium, the use of which is still actively debated. Magnesium treatment is safe in patients who are not in renal failure and without heart block, and in the absence of renal impairment or AV conduction delay the balance of evidence currently favors use of magnesium supplementation only if patients are treated within an hour or two of onset of symptoms. Timing in relation to thrombolysis (see below) may also prove to be critical. Plasma potassium concentration is difficult to interpret in the context of acute myocardial infarction: elevated plasma catecholamines cause redistribution of K+ into the intracellular compartment, so low plasma values neither correctly reflect total body potassium nor necessarily *per se* signify an increased risk of arrhythmia. Intravenous potassium replacement is not without hazard (it had the dubious honor of topping a list of fatal adverse reactions compiled by the Boston Collaborative Drug Surveillance program), and severe hypokalemia should be corrected cautiously, preferably by mouth.

5. PREVENTION OF FURTHER INFARCTION/SUDDEN DEATH

Drugs are used prophylactically following recovery from myocardial infarction to prevent sudden death or recurrence of myocardial infarction ('secondary prevention'). Pain prevention may be an added bonus if postinfarction angina is a problem in a particular patient. Aspirin and β-adrenoceptor antagonists each reduce the risk of recurrence or sudden death. It is unknown if their beneficial effects are additive, although this seems plausible, and in the absence of contraindications they are usually used together. Meta-analysis of the many clinical trials of aspirin has demonstrated an overwhelmingly significant effect of modest magnitude (approximately a 30% reduction in risk of reinfarction).

The effect of β-adrenoceptor antagonists has been studied in several large clinical trials that have shown benefit. These trials of β-adrenoceptor antagonists contained mainly patients who had recovered from *transmural* infarcts. Smaller trials have suggested that calcium channel antagonists may be more effective than β-adrenoceptor antagonists in patients who have recovered from *subendocardial* myocardial infarction, and some clinicians use one or other of these drugs in this circumstance. More definitive studies are awaited. The issue is important, especially as with increasing use of thrombolysis the proportion of patients with subendocardial as opposed to transmural infarction is likely to increase.

6. RISK FACTORS

Modifiable factors such as smoking, hypertension and hypercholesterolemia are sought and attended to where possible.

7. CONSIDERATION OF SURGERY/ANGIOPLASTY

Ideally all patients who are potentially operative candidates would have angiography at some stage, to identify those with lesions such as left main coronary artery disease that are known to fare best if managed surgically. In practice this is not economically or logistically feasible in many countries, and in the UK angiography is usually undertaken on the basis of a clinical judgment based on age, coexisting disease, presence or absence of postinfarction angina, and often on a stress test performed after recovery from the acute event.

8. PSYCHOLOGICAL AND SOCIAL FACTORS

After recovery from myocardial infarction, patients need explanation as to what has occurred, advice regarding activity in the short and long term, advice regarding work, driving and sexual activity, and help in regaining self-esteem. A supervised graded exercise program is often much appreciated by patients in this context. Neglect of these unglamorous aspects of management may cause prolonged and avoidable unhappiness.

DRUGS USED IN ISCHEMIC HEART DISEASE

ORGANIC NITRATES

Use and administration

Glyceryl trinitrate is used for relief of anginal pain, and in unstable angina. As explained above, it is generally best used as 'acute' prophylaxis, i.e. immediately before undertaking strenuous activity. It is usually given sublingually (0.3 or 0.5 mg tablets, or 0.4 mg spray), thereby assuring rapid absorption and avoiding presystemic metabolism (chapter 5), but in patients with unstable angina it may be given as an intravenous infusion (5–200 μg/min). The spray has a somewhat more rapid onset of action and longer shelf-life than tablets of GTN, but is more expensive. Glyceryl trinitrate is absorbed transdermally, and is available in a patch preparation for longer prophylaxis than the short-term benefit provided by a sublingual dose. Alternatively, a longer acting nitrate such as isosorbide mononitrate or isosorbide dinitrate (which is converted to the mononitrate in the body) may be used. Isosorbide mononitrate is less expensive than GTN patches and is taken by mouth.

Glyceryl trinitrate is volatile, so tablets have a limited life (around 6 weeks after the bottle is opened); they need to be stored in a cool place in a tightly capped dark container, without cotton wool or other tablets that may adsorb GTN. Adverse effects include headache, flushing and light headedness. Patients who experience headache may be warned that failure of their tablets to produce this symptom may signal that they are no longer active and that a new supply should be obtained. Adverse effects of GTN can be minimized by swallowing the tablet after the strenuous activity is completed, because of the low systemic bioavailability from the gut as opposed to the buccal mucosa.

Mechanism of action

Glyceryl trinitrate works by relaxing vascular smooth muscle. It is metabolized by smooth muscle cells with generation of nitric oxide (NO). This metabolic step apparently requires sulfydryl groups from a stereospecific intermediary. Exhaustion of this sulfydryl-containing intermediary occurs readily and causes loss of efficacy of GTN. This is clinically important with GTN patches and with longer acting organic nitrates (e.g. isosorbide dinitrate), and is called tolerance. Tolerance can be avoided by using these preparations intermittently, for example by omitting the evening dose in patients who do not experience angina at night. By contrast, sodium nitroprusside (an inorganic nitrovasodilator used to treat hypertensive encephalopathy (see chapter 25), and to reduce afterload following cardiopulmonary bypass operations) degrades *chemically* to yield NO (i.e. without any enzyme catalyzed step). Tolerance consequently does not occur, although prolonged use of sodium nitroprusside is undesirable for another reason (cyanide toxicity).

Nitric oxide mediates the action of nitrovasodilators (organic nitrates such as GTN, as well as inorganic nitrates such as sodium nitroprusside). It combines avidly with a heme group in guanylyl cyclase, activating this enzyme and thereby increasing the cytoplasmic concentration of the second messenger cGMP. Cyclic GMP causes sequestration of free calcium ions within sarcoplasmic reticulum, thereby relaxing smooth muscle. Glyceryl trinitrate can also inhibit platelet function via NO formed by vascular smooth muscle. This could be important in patients with inappropriate platelet activation (e.g. unstable angina), although it is not known to what extent it occurs *in vivo*.

Nitric oxide is synthesized from endogenous substrate (L-arginine) under physiological conditions by a constitutive enzyme in vascular endothelial cells, and is the 'endothelium-derived relaxing factor' described originally by Furchgott. This endogenous NO is responsible for the resting vasodilator tone present in human resistance arterioles under basal conditions. Nitro-vasodilator drugs provide NO in an endothelium *independent* manner, and hence are effective even if endothelial function is severely impaired, as in many patients with coronary artery disease. (Nitric oxide is also formed in other cells and by an enzyme in vascular tissue that is inducible by endotoxin: this is now believed to contribute to the progressive hypotension that characterizes septic shock.)

Hemodynamic effects

For reasons that are still uncertain, GTN is relatively selective for venous rather than arteriolar smooth muscle. Venodilatation reduces cardiac preload. Reduced venous return results in reduced ventricular filling and hence reduction in ventricular chamber diameter. Ventricular wall tension is directly proportional to chamber diameter (the Laplace relation), so wall tension is reduced by GTN which thereby reduces cardiac work and oxygen demand. In addition, coronary blood flow improves due to the decreased left ventricular end-diastolic pressure. This improves forward flow in the coronaries (which occurs during diastole), and any spasm of the diseased vessel is opposed by NO-mediated coronary artery relaxation. The mild reduction in arterial tone reduces after-load and thus also reduces myocardial oxygen demand. Nitrates also relax some non-vascular smooth muscles, and therefore sometimes relieve the pain of esophageal spasm and biliary or renal colic causing potential diagnostic confusion.

Adverse effects

As mentioned above GTN and the other organic nitrates are generally very safe drugs, although they can cause hypotension in patients with diminished cardiac reserve. Headache is a common problem and nitro-glycerine patches have not fared well when evaluated by 'quality of life' questionnaires. Another problem with continuous rather than intermittent therapy with organic nitrates is the occurrence of tolerance. This is minimized by removing the patch at night, except in patients with angina decubitus who may benefit more from nitrate administered last thing at night than during the day.

β-ADRENOCEPTOR ANTAGONISTS

Uses and administration

The main uses of β-blockers in patients with ischemic heart disease are in prophylaxis of angina, and in reducing the risk of sudden death or reinfarction following myocardial infarction ('secondary prevention'). In addition, β-blockers are used in treating hypertension (chapter 25), cardiac arrhythmias (chapter 29), in patients with essential tremor and to suppress symptoms of hyperthyroidism before more specific therapy has time to work (chapter 35).

Mechanism of action

β-Adrenoceptors are linked via stimulatory G-proteins to adenylyl cyclase, so endogenous β-agonists (noradrenaline or adrenaline) increase cytoplasmic cyclic adenosine monophosphate (cAMP). In cardiac tissue cAMP increases force of contraction and heart rate and is arrhythmogenic; in arteriolar vascular smooth muscle it causes vasodilatation in many vascular beds; in the juxta-glomerular cells in the kidney it causes renin release; in airways smooth muscle it causes relaxation. β-Blocking drugs work by competing with endogenous noradrenaline and adrenaline and thereby reduce their β-receptor-mediated effects. Consequently they slow the heart, are negatively inotropic and reduce arterial blood pressure, are antiarrhythmic, increase peripheral vascular resistance, reduce plasma renin activity and predispose to bronchoconstriction. Thyroxine increases cAMP in several kinds of cell, and β-blockers non-competitively antagonize several of the actions of thyroxine. They also have a number of minor metabolic effects including a small increase in plasma triglyceride concentration. Various drugs with some degree of selectivity for β_1-receptors (the type present in cardiac tissue) have been marketed, as have drugs with mixed actions (e.g. partial agonists, β-blockers with some α-blocking activity etc.). Partial agonists (e.g. oxprenolol, pindolol) cause less resting bradycardia because of their mild agonist efficacy, but do oppose further increases in rate caused by full agonists such as noradrenaline or adrenaline released during exercise or other sympathetic activation. These have not yet proved especially advantageous in practice.

Pharmacological effects

Sympathetic stimulation increases myocardial oxygen consumption. Increased sympathetic activity is associated with exercise, emotion and going out in the cold, all of which precipitate angina, and in most patients β-adrenoceptor blockade reduces the frequency of attacks. Drugs commonly used in this way include atenolol and metoprolol. Conversely, patients in whom coronary artery spasm is particularly important may paradoxically deteriorate if treated with β-blockers because of unopposed α-adrenoceptor-mediated coronary vasoconstriction, although this is uncommon. Studies in angina patients indicate that most β-blockers are similarly effective despite pharmacological differences.

Adverse effects and contraindications

Adverse effects are also similar among β-receptor antagonists. All such drugs can precipitate cardiac failure, irrespective of selectivity for β$_1$-receptors ('cardioselectivity'), partial agonist activity, concomitant α-adrenoceptor-blocking activity, β$_2$-receptor agonist activity etc. Obstructive airways disease is similarly worsened by all such drugs, and relatively contraindicates their use. Other contraindications to β-adrenoceptor antagonists include heart block (unless the patient is already paced) and Raynaud's disease. β-Adrenoceptor antagonists should be avoided if possible in patients with peripheral vascular disease (claudication is worsened by β-adrenoceptor antagonists which reduce the supply of oxygenated blood to muscle distal to a fixed atheromatous obstruction) and diabetes (symptoms of hypoglycemia may be masked in patients receiving insulin or sulfonylurea drugs, and insulin secretion further impaired in patients treated with diet alone).

Abrupt discontinuation of treatment with β-blockers sometimes provokes a rebound increase in frequency and severity of angina and instances of myocardial infarction have been documented in this setting. Such a clinically important 'withdrawal' syndrome, which may be caused by unmasking of receptor up-regulation that occurred during prolonged β-blockade, is unusual but real. It occurs most commonly in those patients who experienced the greatest relief when β-blockers were started and who continue strenuous activity during the first 1–2 days after stopping. Such patients should therefore be prescribed a tapering dose over 2–3 days and advised to avoid strenuous exertion for rather longer.

Dose-related unwanted effects are common: symptoms include fatigue (of particular concern to sportsmen) and, especially in women, cold hands and feet. Less commonly β-blockers cause vivid and horrible dreams, and, rarely, more florid psychiatric disturbances. Dreams occur most commonly with lipid-soluble non-polar drugs such as propranolol which readily penetrate the blood–brain barrier, but are, rarely, encountered when using more polar drugs such as atenolol.

The idiosyncratic occulomucocutaneous syndrome, characterized by involvement of cornea (sometimes leading to blindness), skin, mucous membranes and peritoneum (benign fibrous tumors concentrically encircling bowel), was caused by practolol. Practolol is a highly cardioselective drug and was the second β-blocker to be introduced into clinical use in the UK. There was considerable concern at the time that this syndrome might represent an adverse effect common to β-blockers as a class, but this has proved unfounded. The experience does, however, carry a more general lesson for prescribers: be conservative. The possible gain to patients from joining a new band wagon (however plausible the rationale based on animal pharmacology) must be tempered with awareness of the possibility of as yet undiscovered severe idiosyncratic reactions. There is still no known animal model or mechanism for the oculomucocutaneous syndrome caused by practolol, despite extensive further research by first rate pharmacologists backed by the resources of one of the world's leading chemical companies.

Pharmacokinetics

Propranolol was the first β-blocker to be introduced into clinical practice. It is a non-selective β-adrenoceptor antagonist (i.e. blocks both β_1- and β_2-receptors), and has substantial and highly variable presystemic metabolism, making dose titration particularly important. Atenolol and/or metoprolol have largely replaced propranolol. They were marketed initially on the basis of their 'cardioselectivity' (i.e. they are relatively selective for β_1-receptors). However, as explained above, this degree of selectivity is insufficient to have had much, if any, impact in clinical practice. Instead, their success has been due partly to the need for less frequent dosing, and partly because the clinically useful range of doses is much less wide than that of propranolol, making them rather easier to use. Atenolol is eliminated by the kidneys and is excreted largely unchanged in the urine, whereas metoprolol is inactivated by hepatic metabolism.

CALCIUM ANTAGONISTS

Uses

The main uses of calcium channel antagonists in patients with ischemic heart disease are for prophylaxis of angina, and possibly to provide secondary prevention following subendocardial myocardial infarction, as discussed above. In addition they are used to treat hypertension (chapter 25), supraventricular tachycardia (chapter 29), Raynaud's disease and (in the case of nimodipine) to prevent cerebral vasospasm following subarachnoid hemorrhage.

Mechanism of action

Calcium antagonists inhibit the passage of calcium ions through voltage-dependent L-type calcium channels in cell membranes in the heart and vascular smooth muscle as well as some other excitable tissues. These channels open more slowly than the voltage-dependent sodium channels responsible for the initial depolarization phase of the cardiac action potential, and are therefore sometimes called 'slow' channels. They contribute to the membrane current during the plateau phase of the cardiac action potential, and also to the slow initial depolarization that occurs during the initial phase of the action potential in tissue in the atrioventricular node. There are several chemically distinct classes of calcium antagonist: dihydropyridines (e.g. nifedipine, amlodipine, nicardipine), phenylalkylamines (e.g. verapamil) and benzothiazepines (e.g. diltiazem). All are absorbed from the gastrointestinal tract and metabolized in the liver, inactive metabolites being excreted in the urine.

Pharmacological effects

1. Relaxation of vascular smooth muscle causes arteriolar dilatation, reducing arterial blood pressure and cardiac afterload.
2. Reduced myocardial contractility (negative inotropic effect). This is partly offset by reduced afterload. All calcium channel antagonists have a negative inotropic effect; nicardipine is possibly least harmful in this regard, while verapamil is the most markedly negatively inotropic.
3. Relaxation of coronary vascular smooth muscle may be useful in patients with coronary vasospasm.
4. Effect on heart rate and cardiac conduction:

   (a) Dihydropyridines (e.g. nifedipine, amlodipine, nicardipine) have no direct effect on cardiac conduction and usually cause a mild increase in resting heart rate as a reflex response to peripheral vasodilatation.
   (b) Verapamil and diltiazem depress the cardiac conducting system. Reduction of sinus node automaticity usually produces a mild resting bradycardia. Prolongation of conduction through the atrioventricular node accounts for antiarrhythmic effects (verapamil is

sometimes used in treating supraventricular tachycardia). Lack of reflex tachycardia is useful in patients with unstable coronary artery disease (e.g. following subendocardial myocardial infarction), and diltiazem is often preferred over a dihydropyridine in this situation for this reason.

Adverse effects and contraindications

The main contraindication to calcium channel blocking drugs is cardiac failure, because of their negative inotropic effect. As noted above this is variably offset by their favorable effect on afterload. Trouble is most likely to occur when verapamil (or another calcium channel blocking drug) is used intravenously, especially in patients recently treated with β-antagonists. In contrast to β-blockers, calcium antagonists may be given safely to patients with asthma, chronic bronchitis, peripheral arterial disease or diabetes.

Verapamil and diltiazem must not be given to patients with heart block or bradycardia.

Common adverse effects are related to vasodilatation and include flushing and headache. These are most marked at peak plasma concentration, and are less troublesome in patients treated with amlodipine (which has a long half-life and consequently a relatively stable plasma concentration profile) than with nifedipine (which has a short plasma half-life, only partly offset by the use of slow-release formulations). Ankle swelling is another common effect of the dihydropyridine calcium channel blocking drugs. It appears to occur equally commonly with all members of this group. By contrast, ankle swelling is uncommon with verapamil. Verapamil frequently causes constipation, which may be severe, because of its effect on calcium channels in the gut. Occasionally patients experience increased frequency of micturition, partly because of a mild diuretic effect and perhaps also partly due to an effect on muscle in the bladder.

In addition to the pharmacodynamic interaction with β-blockers (and presumably also with other negative inotropes) mentioned above, verapamil has a clinically significant pharmacokinetic interaction with digoxin, increasing its plasma concentration and potentially causing toxicity. When chronic treatment with verapamil is started in a patient previously stabilized on digoxin it is therefore prudent to halve the digoxin dose when possible and to check plasma digoxin after around a week.

ASPIRIN

See also chapter 27.

Use in cardiovascular disease

The use of aspirin in cardiovascular disease depends on its effects on platelet function. Aspirin improves survival in patients with acute myocardial infarction and reduces the risk of myocardial infarction in patients with unstable angina and after recovery from myocardial infarction. It has not been adequately studied in patients with stable angina, but is probably beneficial in this group as well, since it reduces the risk of myocardial infarction in apparently healthy middle-aged men. (It is *not*, however, recommended generally as prophylaxis in asymptomatic men, because in this setting its benefits are probably outweighed by adverse effects.) Aspirin is also used in patients with transient cerebral ischemic attacks, in whom it reduces the risk of stroke. It reduces the risk of thromboembolism in patients with atrial fibrillation and following valve replacement.

Mechanism of action

Aspirin (acetylsalicylic acid) irreversibly inhibits fatty acid cyclo-oxygenase, a key enzyme in the biosynthesis of prostaglandins and thromboxanes. It achieves this by acetylation of a serine residue, thereby preventing access of substrate (arachidonic acid) to the active site by steric hindrance. Thromboxane (TX) A_2 is the main cyclo-oxygenase product of activated platelets, and is proaggregatory and a vasoconstrictor. Thromboxane A_2 can therefore work as a positive feedback, recruiting more platelets to sites of platelet activation. When platelets adhere to thrombogenic material in a ruptured atheromatous plaque they become activated and synthesize TXA_2, which causes further platelets to stick to one another ('aggregation') causing propagation of the thrombus and ultimately occlusion of the artery. Aspirin is believed to exert its antithrombotic effects by inhibiting platelet TXA_2 biosynthesis and thereby opposing thrombus extension. Although non-steroidal anti-inflammatory drugs such as ibuprofen and indomethacin also inhibit cyclo-oxygenase, they are much less effective than aspirin at inhibiting platelet TXA_2 biosynthesis, possibly because, unlike aspirin, they are reversible inhibitors of the enzyme. It should *not* therefore be assumed that patients receiving such drugs for another indication are thereby necessarily receiving adequate antiplatelet therapy. In this regard the uricosuric drug and cyclo-oxygenase inhibitor sulfinpyrazone appears to be a special case. There is some evidence of clinical efficacy of sulfinpyrazone following myocardial infarction (albeit much debated), and it causes only partial and reversible inhibition of cyclo-oxygenase (via a slowly formed sulfide metabolite). However, it has additional actions on platelets that distinguish it from other cyclo-oxygenase inhibitors, including inhibition of platelet-activating factor (PAF)-induced aggregation and normalization of shortened platelet survival in various clinical situations.

Pharmacological effects

The pharmacological effects of aspirin are explained by inhibition of fatty acid cyclo-oxygenase. These include anti-inflammatory, antipyretic and mild analgesic effects in addition to its effect on platelet function, which is evidenced by a mild prolongation of bleeding time. Many of the adverse effects of aspirin are also caused by inhibition of fatty acid cyclo-oxygenase (see below).

Pharmacokinetics and dose regimen

Aspirin is absorbed from the gastrointestinal tract, and rapidly deacetylated to yield salicylate, which has anti-inflammatory but little if any antiplatelet activity at ordinary doses. Salicylate is metabolized further (see Fig. 22.2, p. 234) and metabolites, together with some unchanged salicylate, are excreted in the urine. There has been considerable interest in the possibility that very low doses of aspirin (40 mg/day or less) may selectively inhibit platelet TXA_2 biosynthesis, without reducing prostacyclin (PGI_2) biosynthesis in blood vessels. This strategy has yet to be shown to result in increased antithrombotic efficacy, and it is possible that it will not produce uniformly satisfactory inhibition of platelet TXA_2 biosynthesis in all patients, especially older people with atheromatous disease.

A simpler approach is to use a substantial dose interval between larger doses of aspirin that reliably produce essentially complete inhibition of platelet TXA_2 biosynthesis in all subjects. Within limits, the longer the dose interval the greater the specificity for platelet TXA_2 biosynthesis, because platelets (which do not possess nuclei) can not resynthesize cyclo-oxygenase after inhibition by aspirin, whereas in human endothelium cyclo-oxygenase appears to be completely resynthesized within approximately 6 hours. Appreciable recovery of platelet TXA_2 biosynthesis occurs only after 48 hours, and then occurs over the time span with which new platelets enter the circulation from megakaryocytes (complete in 7–10 days). Consequently, if aspirin is given once every 24 or 48 hours platelet TX biosynthesis is essentially completely inhibited throughout the entire dose interval, whereas endothelial PGI_2 biosynthesis is inhibited on average only one-quarter or one-eighth of the dose interval. Aspirin was given in a dose of 150 mg every 24 hours in the ISIS II trial that demonstrated its efficacy in acute myocardial infarction, and in a dose of 320 mg every 48 hours in the American physicians' trial that showed that it approximately halved the risk of myocardial infarction in healthy male physicians. We generally employ one or other of these regimens (in the UK aspirin is available in 300 mg rather than 320 mg tablets: these doses are essentially the same). Aspirin was used in a dose of 75 mg daily in one positive study of unstable coronary disease. This is not selective for platelets but is worth considering using following an initial 'loading' dose of 300 mg in patients who are intolerant of the larger dose when given repeatedly.

Adverse effects and contraindications

Dose-related adverse effects consequent on the pharmacological effect of aspirin on cyclo-oxygenase ('type A') are common: approximately 25% of British physicians were intolerant of it in a trial that required regular prolonged use. Furthermore, although available over the counter for nearly a century some of its adverse effects are serious. The commonest severe adverse effect is upper gastrointestinal hemorrhage, and the commonest symptom is dyspepsia. These relate to inhibition of PGE_2 biosynthesis in the stomach. PGE_2 is the main cyclo-oxygenase product of the stomach, and has a number of effects that help protect this organ from ulceration, including mucus secretion, inhibition of acid secretion, vasodilatation of microvessels in the submucosa which carry away hydrogen ions that have diffused back through the mucosal barrier, and possibly a cytoprotective effect on the mucosal cells themselves. Inhibition of PGE_2 biosynthesis consequently predisposes to ulceration. Should such an ulcer occur, bleeding is exacerbated because of inhibition of platelet TXA_2 biosynthesis. Active ulcer disease contraindicates use of aspirin. A history of past ulcer disease also argues against aspirin use, although if the indication is strong enough the risk may be judged clinically acceptable. In such cases coincident treatment with an H_2 antagonist such as cimetidine and/or with a stable PGE analog (misoprostol) may be useful. Constipation is less well recognized as an unwanted effect of aspirin than are upper gastrointestinal symptoms, but is not uncommon. It may also relate to inhibition of PGE_2 biosynthesis, since PGE_2 increases gastrointestinal motility and causes a secretory diarrhea when administered therapeutically.

Some patients with asthma (especially those with a history of nasal polyps) are sensitive to aspirin. The mechanism is not fully established, although this adverse effect appears likely to be due to the pharmacology of the drug ('type A') rather than to an idiosyncrasy, since individuals who are aspirin sensitive are also sensitive to other structurally unrelated cyclo-oxygenase inhibitors (e.g. indomethacin, piroxicam). It is possible that it is caused by a disturbance in the usual balance in the lung between cyclo-oxygenase products and lipoxygenase products (which include the peptido-leukotrienes, which have potent bronchoconstrictor actions). In contrast, symptoms of salicylism (e.g. tinnitus, deafness) are unrelated to cyclo-oxygenase inhibition. These occur only in overdose (chapter 50), or when aspirin is used for high-dose anti-inflammatory indications and not with therapeutic regimens used to inhibit platelet function. Epidemiological evidence has linked aspirin use to Reye's syndrome in some but not all cases. This is a rare but devastatingly severe form of hepatic failure and encephalopathy in children usually aged less than 12 years old who have experienced a 'viral' prodrome. It is by no means clear that the association with aspirin is causal, but if it is it represents an unpredictable idiosyncratic ('type B') effect. Since paracetamol has not been associated with Reye's syndrome, and is a satisfactory alternative to aspirin for most indications that are relevant in children, aspirin is usually avoided in this age group.

FIBRINOLYTIC DRUGS

Several fibrinolytic drugs are used in acute myocardial infarction, including streptokinase (an enyme from streptococci that breaks down fibrin), anistreplase (APSAC: a prodrug that liberates streptokinase) and alteplase (human tissue plasminogen activator made in bacteria by recombinant DNA technology). In addition, urokinase (from human urine), while awaiting licensing for use in myocardial infarction, is sometimes used to dissolve blood clots in extracorporeal shunts or in the anterior chamber of the eye complicating hyphema. Streptokinase works indirectly, combining with plasminogen to form an activator complex that converts remaining free plasminogen to plasmin which dissolves fibrin clots. Alteplase is a direct acting plasminogen activator.

Use in myocardial infarction

Streptokinase has been available for many years, but its efficacy in reducing myocardial damage and mortality in myocardial infarction has only been appreciated in the last decade. This realization has revolutionized the management of acute myocardial infarction. The credit for this goes to GISSI, an Italian multicenter trial, and to ISIS II, a large multicenter trial coordinated from Oxford, that not only demonstrated the efficacy of streptokinase unequivocally but further showed that it is approximately equieffective as aspirin, and that its effect is additive with that of aspirin in this setting. The earlier streptokinase was used the greater the benefit, but some benefit was evident up to 24 hours after the onset of symptoms. Bleeding complications were much less than had been feared and, as expected, tended to occur mainly in patients who received invasive monitoring such as Swann–Ganz catheterization.

Streptokinase, used with aspirin, is thus effective and safe. It is also relatively inexpensive, and is the standard fibrinolytic for myocardial infarction. The other available fibrinolytics have distinctive features that hold some promise for the future, and in a few special situations in the present. It may, for instance, prove advantageous to initiate fibrinolytic therapy at home or in the ambulance before hospital admission, in order to gain the greatest benefit from early treatment. This is impracticable with streptokinase but may be feasible with anistreplase, because of its greater convenience of administration (see below). Studies of this approach are in progress, and the results will need to be examined critically before advocating a general move towards such home initiated treatment. It was argued that alteplase, which, unlike streptokinase, does not produce a generalized fibrinolytic state, but rather encourages the dissolution of a recently formed clot, would have a better therapeutic ratio than streptokinase. Disappointingly, this argument, although highly plausible in theory, did not appear to be correct in practice as evidenced by a direct comparison in a further large clinical trial called ISIS III, and this conclusion also accorded with the Italian GISSI studies. However, another large study (GUSTO) has recently demonstrated superiority of alteplase over streptokinase when it is given more rapidly than previous standard practice (over 30 min instead of over 3 hours) and immediately followed by heparin. Whether the cost of alteplase will be judged to justify the fairly small additional benefit of this approach remains to be seen. Alteplase or urokinase may also have a place in treating the increasing number of patients in whom streptokinase is contraindicated because of previous use. Hard evidence as to their usefulness in this situation would be valuable.

Administration

Fibrinolytic drugs are given intravenously. Streptokinase is given as an infusion of 1.5 megaunits over 60 min with regular monitoring of blood pressure, and reduction of rate if necessary. Anistreplase, 30 units, being a prodrug, is given over a shorter period (4–5 min). Alteplase has been given over 3 hours: adults over 67 kg are given a bolus dose of 10 mg followed by 50 mg over the next hour and 40 mg over the subsequent 2 hours (total dose 100 mg). Individuals of lower body weight are given a total of 1.5 mg/kg divided in the same proportions, i.e. 10% as a bolus, 50% infused over the next hour and 40% over the subsequent 2 hours. As mentioned above there appears to be a case for giving it over a 30 min rather than a 3 hour infusion period.

Adverse effects and contraindications

Bleeding may occur with any of the fibrinolytic drugs. Many of the contraindications to their use therefore relate to conditions that increase the risk of bleeding. These exclusions were originally applied more stringently than is now current practice, as increasing use has shown that early fears were exaggerated. Patients are not generally treated with fibrinolytic drugs if they have recently undergone surgery; are pregnant; have evidence of recent active gastrointestinal bleeding, symptoms of active peptic ulcer disease or evidence of severe liver disease (especially if complicated by the presence of varices); have recently suffered a stroke; have severe uncontrolled hypertension; have a significant bleeding diathesis; have diabetic or other proliferative retinopathy; have suffered recent substantial trauma including vigorous chest compression during resuscitation; or require invasive monitoring (e.g. for cardiogenic shock).

Immune reactions are important with streptokinase and its prodrug anistreplase. Streptokinase is a streptococcal protein, so individuals who have been exposed to it synthesize antibodies which can cause allergic reactions or loss of efficacy due to binding to and neutralization of the drug. Individuals who have received either of these drugs within perhaps the previous year, should not be retreated with them if they reinfarct. It is possible that such patients will benefit from alteplase. The situation regarding previous streptococcal infection is less certain. Such infections, usually in the form of sore throats, are quite common and often undiagnosed; despite this, ISIS III demonstrated similar efficacy of streptokinase and alteplase so it seems unlikely that such mild infections substantially reduce the efficacy of streptokinase. It is therefore our practice to exclude patients from treatment with streptokinase only if they have a history of bacteriologically proven severe streptococcal infection such as cellulitis or septicemia.

Hypotension may occur during infusion of streptokinase, partly as a result of activation of kinins and other vasodilator peptides. The important thing is tissue perfusion rather than the blood pressure *per se* and as long as the patient is warm and well perfused hypotension is not an absolute contraindication to the use of streptokinase, although it does indicate the need for especially careful monitoring, and sometimes for slowing or temporarily halting the infusion.

Drug interactions

Two useful interactions are important: as explained above aspirin has an additive effect with streptokinase. Secondly, heparin is needed after treatment with alteplase (but not streptokinase) to prevent early reocclusion of the thrombosed artery.

Anticoagulants and Antiplatelet Drugs

27

Introduction **322**

Pathophysiology of thrombosis **322**

Anticoagulants **324**

Antiplatelet drugs **331**

Anticoagulants in pregnancy and puerperium **334**

INTRODUCTION

The treatment and prevention of thrombosis involves three classes of drugs: anticoagulants, antiplatelet drugs and fibrinolytics. Aspirin (the main antiplatelet drug in clinical practice) and fibrinolytics are discussed in chapter 26. The clinical pharmacology of the anticoagulants and of antiplatelet drugs other than aspirin is described in this present chapter. Anticoagulants inhibit the coagulation cascade. Their main use is to treat and prevent venous thrombosis ('red thrombus') and its major complication pulmonary embolism, whereas antiplatelet and fibrinolytic drugs are used particularly in the treatment of platelet-rich coronary and other arterial thrombi ('white thrombus'). Nevertheless, there are many links between platelet activation and the coagulation cascade, so it is not surprising that anticoagulants can also have beneficial effects in the prevention of coronary artery disease or that antiplatelet drugs such as aspirin have some effect on venous thrombosis.

PATHOPHYSIOLOGY OF THROMBOSIS

Thrombosis is hemostasis occurring in the wrong place. Hemostasis is achieved by an exquisitely balanced series of interlocking control systems involving both positive feedbacks permitting very rapid responses to the threat of hemorrhage following sharp injury and negative feedbacks to prevent the clotting mechanism from running out of control and causing thrombus to propagate throughout the circulation following hemostasis at a site of injury. In addition there is an endogenous fibrinolytic system that dissolves thrombus that has done its job. Not surprisingly, these systems sometimes go wrong, leading to bleeding disorders such as hemophilia or thrombocytopenic purpura, or to thrombosis.

Thrombosis is caused by injury to the vessel wall, stasis of blood and activation of platelets and the coagulation cascade. Coagulation involves the sequential activation of a cascade of clotting factors which amplifies a small initial change in a single factor to produce splitting of large numbers of fibrinogen molecules to give a fibrin mesh. Each factor is present in blood as an inactive zymogen. Several of these factors (II, VII, IX and X) are glycoproteins which contain γ-carboxyglutamic acid residues that are the result of post-translational modification. This process requires vitamin K. After activation (indicated by the letter 'a' after the Roman numeral that designates the zymogen) several of the factors acquire proteolytic activity: thrombin and factors IXa, Xa, XIa and XIIa are all serine proteases.

There are two coagulation pathways (intrinsic and extrinsic) that converge on factor X (Fig. 27.1). There are several possible points of entry to the cascade. Blood vessels are lined with a continuous layer of endothelial cells that possess an array of mechanisms (e.g. the capacity to synthesize prostacyclin and nitric oxide and the presence of heparan and thrombomodulin – a receptor that binds thrombin and prevents its procoagulant effect while enabling it to activate anticoagulant protein C) whereby

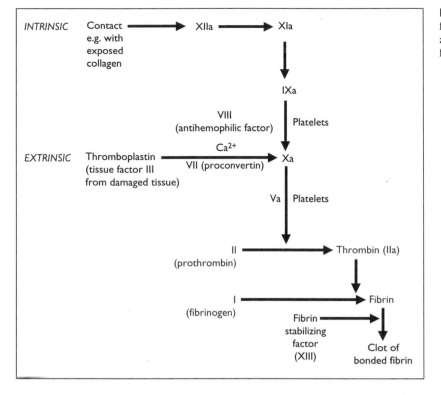

Fig. 27.1 Simplified clotting factor cascade. 'a' indicates activation of appropriate clotting factor.

blood is preserved in a fluid state. Damage to the endothelium exposes platelets to collagen and other subendothelial material to which they adhere and become activated. Activated platelets express glycoprotein receptors (IIb/IIIa) on their surface membranes that are dormant in quiescent platelets. Glycoprotein IIb/IIIa binds fibrinogen which links adjacent activated platelets in an aggregate. Activated platelets also synthesize thromboxane A_2 from arachidonic acid liberated from their membranes by phospholipase and secrete adenosine diphosphate and other preformed mediators that recruit further platelets and cause the aggregate to propagate. They also secrete clotting factors including factor Va, and negatively charged phospholipids (e.g. phosphatidyl serine) become exposed on their outer membranes and act as surface catalysts for factor Xa. Another way in which endothelial damage initiates coagulation is

by exposure of the blood to tissue factor in underlying fibroblasts. Tissue factor interacts with factor VII to initiate the extrinsic pathway.

Activated factor X catalyzes the conversion of prothrombin (factor II) to thrombin which is the most important enzyme of the cascade. It cleaves small peptides from the N-terminal region of fibrinogen dimers allowing them to polymerize to form strands of insoluble fibrin. It also acts on receptors on platelet surface membranes thereby causing platelet activation. Thrombus consists of platelets and other formed elements of the blood enmeshed within a fibrin network. Thrombus structure is not homogeneous, even in the red thrombus that forms in veins: typically there is a platelet-rich head attached to the vessel wall, and a tail of gelatinous material containing large numbers of red cells similar to the clot that forms when blood is allowed to coagulate in a glass tube *in vitro*.

Aɴᴛɪᴄᴏᴀɢᴜʟᴀɴᴛꜱ

HEPARIN

Heparin is a sulfated acidic mucopolysaccharide present in the granules of mast cells. It was discovered in liver (hence the name heparin) by McLean while doing a vacation project as a medical student at the Johns Hopkins Hospital. Currently it is prepared from lung or intestine of ox or pig, and is a mixture of polymers of varying molecular weights. Since the structure is variable dosage is given in terms of units of biological activity.

Use

Heparin is available either as the sodium or calcium salt. It is administered either as an intravenous infusion (to treat established disease), or by subcutaneous injection (as prophylaxis). Calcium heparin is less painful than sodium heparin when given subcutaneously. Intramuscular injection must not be used because it causes hematomas. Intermittent bolus intravenous injections cause a higher frequency of bleeding complications than does constant intravenous infusion and is no longer recommended for this reason. For prophylaxis 5000 units in 0.2 ml is injected via a fine (25 guage) needle into the fatty layer of the lower abdomen 8 or 12 hourly. An inch or so of skin is pinched up and pressure applied for 5 min after the injection to minimize bruising. Monitoring coagulation times is not routinely performed when heparin is used prophylactically in this way, but may be appropriate if long-term prophylaxis is contemplated using this method. Continuous intravenous infusion is initiated with a bolus of 5000 units for a 70 kg adult (proportionately less for a child on a weight basis) followed by 25 000 or 30 000 units in saline or 5% glucose infused over 24 hours. Therapy is monitored by measuring the kaolin cephalin clotting time (KCCT) or the activated partial thromboplastin time (APTT) 4–6 hours after starting treatment and then every 6 hours until two consecutive readings

Table 27.1 Dose adjustment guidelines for maintaining APPT or KCCT ratios at 1.5–2.5 (modified from *Drug and Therapeutics Bulletin*, Vol. 30 Number 20, 1994).

APPT or KCCT ratio	Change in heparin dose
>7.0	Stop for 1 hour and reduce by 10 000 U/24 h
5.1–7.0	Reduce by 10 000 U/24 h
4.1–5.0	Reduce by 5000 U/24 h
3.1–4.0	Reduce by 2000 U/24 h
2.6–3.0	Reduce by 1000 U/24 h
1.5–2.5	No change
1.2–1.4	Increase by 5000 U/24 h
<1.2	Increase by 10 000 U/24 h

APTT = activated partial thromboplastin time. KCCT = kaolin cephalin clotting time.

are within the target range, and thereafter at least daily. Dose adjustments are made to keep the APTT or the KCCT ratio (i.e. the ratio between the value for the patient to the value of a control) at 1.5–2.5. Table 27.1 gives guidelines to dose adjustment.

The main indications for heparin are:

1. To treat massive proximal deep venous thrombosis and/or pulmonary embolus by intravenous infusion of heparin. Treatment is for 7–10 days. For less massive and more distal disease oral anticoagulants are started at the same time and heparin infusion is discontinued once these have established their effect (usually about 5 days).

2. To prevent deep vein thrombosis and pulmonary embolus in individuals at increased risk of these problems such as those undergoing surgery (where the increased risk of bleeding must be balanced carefully against risk of thromboembolism) or while resting in bed during the early stages of treatment of severe heart failure. Low-dose subcutaneous heparin is highly effective in general surgical patients in whom the first dose is usually given 2 hours preoperatively. Certain major procedures constitute

especially high risk situations and adjusted dose intravenous heparin may be more effective in these situations. These include patients undergoing hip replacement, major amputations or open urological operations, and those with fractured neck of femur.

3. To prevent thrombosis in extracorporeal circulations (e.g. hemodialysis, hemoperfusion, membrane oxygenators, artificial organs) and in intravenous cannulae.

4. Following treatment of patients with acute myocardial infarction with anistreplase (recombinant human tissue plasminogen activator) heparin is used to maintain patency of the vessel, and may also reduce the risk of systemic embolization. However, the magnitude of any benefit of heparin in managing patients treated with streptokinase and aspirin (standard treatment in the UK) is very small, and is outweighed by the extra risk of bleeding in the judgment of many clinicians.

5. Disseminated intravascular coagulation. This is caused by a heterogeneous group of disorders, and treatment is aimed at the underlying cause (e.g. prostate cancer, sepsis, eclampsia). Heparin is sometimes used as an adjunct while such treatment has time to take effect, although it occasionally worsens the situation. Its use for this indication demands specialist input and meticulous laboratory control.

6. Heparin is sometimes used following peripheral or cerebral arterial embolus, but this use is incompletely validated.

Mechanism of action

The main action of heparin is on the coagulation cascade. It works by binding to antithrombin III, the naturally occurring inhibitor of thrombin and of the other serine proteases (factors IXa, Xa, XIa and XIIa) and enormously potentiating its inhibitory action. Consequently it is effective *in vitro* as well as *in vivo*, but is ineffective in (rare) patients with inherited or acquired deficiency of antithrombin III. A lower concentration of heparin is required to inhibit factor Xa and the other factors early in the cascade than is needed to antagonize the action of thrombin,

and this provides the rationale for the use of low-dose heparin in prophylaxis. (More specific directly acting thrombin antagonists are currently being developed, such as the leech anticoagulant hirudin prepared by recombinant gene technology in bacteria.) Heparin also has complex actions on platelets of uncertain importance: as an antithrombin drug it inhibits platelet activation by thrombin, but it also has the ability to potentiate platelet aggregation by increasing fibrinogen binding. It is possible that this contributes to the thrombocytopenia that is one of the adverse effects of heparin.

Adverse effects and contraindications

1. **Bleeding** is the chief side effect and was one of the commonest drug-induced adverse effects in hospital patients in the Boston Collaborative Drug Surveillance program. It may occur at any site and may be life threatening. Risk factors include old age, any other hemostatic defect (most commonly drug induced by aspirin or recent fibrinolytic therapy) and recent trauma. Contraindications to heparin generally relate to situations in which the risk of bleeding is judged to be unacceptable, as following a cerebral bleed, in the presence of bleeding or potential bleeding into an inaccessible space (thorax or abdomen) including recent liver or renal biopsy, lumbar puncture or epidural anesthesia, recent eye surgery and severe hemostatic disorders. Management of heparin associated bleeding is described below.

2. **Osteoporosis and vertebral collapse** is a rare complication described in young adult patients receiving heparin in doses of 10 000 units or more daily for longer than 10 weeks (usually longer than 3 months).

3. **Skin necrosis** at the site of subcutaneous injection after several days treatment.

4. **Alopecia** has been described.

5. **Thrombocytopenia** A modest decrease in platelet count within the first 2 days of treatment is common (approximately one-third of patients) but clinically unimportant. By contrast severe thrombocytopenia is rare. It occurs between 2 days and 2 weeks

of treatment and is associated with thrombotic as well as hemorrhagic complications. It is thought to be caused by antibodies directed against a platelet–heparin complex that causes platelet activation. Platelet counts should be obtained in patients treated for more than 5 days and treatment stopped if they develop thrombocytopenia. Low molecular weight heparin is an alternative if ongoing anticoagulation is needed but low molecular weight heparin has also caused thrombocytopenia.

6. **Hypersensitivity** reactions including chills, fever, urticaria, bronchospasm and anaphylactoid reactions occur rarely.

7. **Hypoaldosteronism** Heparin inhibits aldosterone biosynthesis. This is seldom clinically significant, but there have been case reports of fatal hyperkalemia and selective hypoaldosteronism with pathological changes in the zona glomerulosa of the adrenal cortex associated with heparin treatment.

There is no evidence that rebound hypercoagulability on discontinuing heparin (demonstrable *in vitro*) is clinically significant.

Management of severe heparin-associated bleeding

1. Compression of the bleeding site when this is accessible.
2. Protamine sulfate is given as a slow intravenous injection: rapid injection has caused anaphylactoid reactions. It is of no value if it is more than 3 hours since heparin was administered. An exact dose of protamine can be determined from a protamine titration *in vitro*. More commonly, a dose of 1 mg for every 100 units of heparin given over the preceding hour (maximum dose 50 mg, above which protamine itself has anticoagulant properties) can be used empirically.
3. If bleeding is very severe and continues despite protamine, fresh frozen plasma is given to provide uninhibited coagulation factors.

Pharmacokinetics

Heparin is not absorbed from the gastrointestinal tract, and is administered parenterally. Its half-life ($t_{1/2}$) varies from 0.5 to 2.5 hours and is dose dependent with a longer half-life at higher doses and wide interindividual variation. The short half-life probably reflects rapid uptake by the reticuloendothelial system, and there is no good evidence of hepatic metabolism. The mechanism underlying the dose-dependent clearance is unknown. The short half-life means that a stable plasma heparin concentration is best achieved by a constant infusion rather than intermittent bolus administration. Heparin does not cross the placental barrier or enter milk, and is the anticoagulant of choice in pregnancy because of the teratogenic effects of warfarin and other oral anticoagulants.

LOW MOLECULAR WEIGHT HEPARINS

Low molecular weight heparins preferentially inhibit factor Xa, and were developed in hopes of reducing the risk of major hemorrhage that accompanies the use of conventional unfractionated heparin. They do not prolong the APTT, and monitoring (which would require sophisticated factor Xa assays) is not needed in routine clinical practice. There is evidence that low molecular heparins such as enoxaparin and dalteparin are as at least as safe and effective as unfractionated heparin. They are effective in prophylaxis against deep venous thrombosis. Surprisingly, low molecular weight heparins have proved more effective than conventional heparin in preventing deep vein thrombosis (about one-third the incidence of venographically confirmed disease in a meta-analysis of six trials) and pulmonary embolism (about one-half the incidence) in patients undergoing orthopedic surgery, but with the same incidence of major bleeds. Once daily dosage makes them convenient, but they are more expensive than regular heparin.

HIRUDIN ANALOGS

Hirudin is the anticoagulant of the leech, and can now be synthesized in bulk by recombint DNA technology. It is a direct inhibitor of thrombin and is more specific than heparin. Unlike heparin it inhibits clot associated thrombin and is not dependent on antithrombin III. Early human studies showed that pharmacodynamic response is closely related to plasma concentration, and its pharmacokinetics are more predictable than those of heparin. Clinical trials are in progress to determine whether these promising properties will result in improved clinical performance compared with heparins.

WARFARIN AND OTHER ORAL ANTICOAGULANTS

Warfarin, a derivative of 4-hydroxycoumarin, is the most commonly used oral anticoagulant. Unless otherwise specified the following discussion refers specifically to warfarin rather than to other oral anticoagulants. Phenindione, an indane 1:3 dione derivative, is an alternative but is seldom used other than in rare cases of idiosyncratic sensitivity to warfarin.

Use

Warfarin is prescribed as a racemic mixture of R and S stereoisomers. The main indications for oral anticoagulation are:

1. Deep vein thrombosis and pulmonary embolism. There is evidence that recurrence may be prevented if oral anticoagulants are continued for at least 3 months after a single episode of deep vein thrombosis and for at least 6 months after a single episode of pulmonary embolism. Recurrent deep vein thrombosis probably requires life-long anticoagulation, and similarly recurrent pulmonary embolism with the attendant risk of secondary pulmonary hypertension may also be an indication for life-long treatment.
2. Atrial fibrillation. There is substantial evidence that the morbidity from embolism (especially stroke) is reduced by anticoagulation in patients with atrial fibrillation associated with many conditions including mitral stenosis, thyrotoxicosis, chronic sinoatrial disease, congestive cardiomyopathy and ischemic heart disease. Patients with atrial fibrillation without detectable underlying disease ('lone atrial fibrillation') are also at substantially increased risk of stroke compared to that of otherwise comparable individuals in sinus rhythm. There is also good evidence that moderate to severe mitral stenosis (with associated left atrial dilatation) in patients in sinus rhythm also carries a substantial risk of embolism that can be reduced by anticoagulants. Treatment of these groups of patients is usually life long, except for patients without valvular disease who convert from atrial fibrillation to stable sinus rhythm. Aspirin also reduces the risk of embolic stroke in patients with atrial fibrillation, and provides an alternative for patients with contraindications to warfarin.
3. Patients with prosthetic valve replacements require life-long anticoagulation but this does not invariably apply to tissue valves (xenografts). Recent evidence suggests that such patients at high risk of thrombosis (i.e. following artificial valve replacement, or tissue valves with atrial fibrillation or history of embolism) have markedly reduced mortality from vascular causes and reduced risk of embolization if aspirin (100 mg daily) is added to warfarin. The increased risk of bleeding from aspirin was modest in the setting of careful monitoring, and more than offset by the benefit.

Treatment of deep vein thrombosis and pulmonary embolus is usually started with heparin, because of its immediate effect. Warfarin is usually started on days 3–7 in patients with massive ileofemoral disease or pulmonary embolus, and on day 1 in patients with less extensive and more distal disease. Therapy is monitored by measuring the international normalized ratio (INR). This is the prothrombin time related to an international standard for thromboplastin reagents. The therapeutic range for most indications is 2–3, but in patients with recurrent disease or with prosthetic valves a greater effect is desirable and the recommended therapeutic range is 3–4.5. Before starting treatment a baseline value of INR is determined. This is not influenced by concurrent heparin treatment provided the APTT is <2.5. If APTT is >2.5 the laboratory can correct this by addition of protamine *in vitro* to neutralize the heparin before determination of the INR. Provided the baseline INR is normal the patient is started on two 10 mg doses of warfarin given at the same time of day (most conveniently in the evening) 24 hours apart. If the baseline INR is prolonged or the patient has risk factors for bleeding such as old age or debility, liver disease, heart failure, or recent major surgery treatment is started with a lower dose (e.g. 5 mg daily). The INR is measured daily; on the morning of day 3 about half of the patients will be within the therapeutic range and heparin can be discontinued. A useful guide for adjusting warfarin dose (from the *Drug and Therapeutics Bulletin*) is given in Table 27.2.

Once the maintenance dose is known and the patient stable, the INR is checked weekly for the first 6 weeks and then monthly or 2 monthly if control is good. The patient is warned to report immediately if there is evidence of bleeding, to avoid contact sports or other situations that put them at increased risk of trauma, to avoid alcohol (or at least to stick to a moderate and unvarying intake), to avoid over-the-counter drugs (other than paracetamol), and to check that any prescription drug is not expected to alter his or her anticoagulant requirement. Women of childbearing age should be warned of the risk of teratogenesis and given advice regarding contraception.

There is no convincing evidence that abrupt cessation of warfarin results in a rebound hypercoagulable state. It is therefore unnecessary to taper off the dose.

Mechanism of action

Oral anticoagulants prevent the synthesis in the liver of the vitamin K-dependent coagulation factors II, VII, IX and X. Preformed factors are present in blood, so unlike heparin the oral anticoagulants are not effective *in vitro* and are only active when given *in vivo*. Functional forms of factors II, VII, IX and X contain residues of γ-carboxyglutamic acid. This is formed by carboxylation of a

Table 27.2 Dose adjustment of warfarin with respect to INR.

Day	INR (9.00–11.00 am)	Dose (mg) (5.00–7.00 pm)
1	<1.4	10
2	<1.8	10
	1.8	1
	>1.8	0.5
3	<2	10
	2.0–2.1	5
	2.2–2.3	4.5
	2.4–2.5	4
	2.6–2.7	3.5
	2.8–2.9	3
	3.0–3.1	2.5
	3.2–3.3	2
	3.4	1.5
	3.5	1
	3.6–4.0	0.5
	>4.0	0
		Predicted maintenance dose:
4	<1.4	>8
	1.4	8
	1.5	7.5
	1.6–1.7	7
	1.8	6.5
	1.9	6
	2.0–2.1	5.5
	2.2–2.3	5
	2.4–2.6	4.5
	2.7–3.0	4
	3.1–3.5	3.5
	3.6–4.0	3
	4.1–4.5	Miss next dose then 2 mg
	>4.5	Miss two doses then 1 mg

INR = international normalized ratio.

glutamate residue in the peptide chain of the precursor. This process is accomplished by cycling of vitamin K between epoxide, quinone and hydroquinone forms. This cycle is interrupted by warfarin, which is structurally closely related to vitamin K, and inhibits vitamin K epoxide reductase.

Adverse effects

1. Hemorrhage is the chief adverse reaction. Intracranial bleeding is especially serious, although gastrointestinal bleeding can also be life threatening. The incidence depends on predisposing pathology in the patient (note contraindications below), and on the INR. If the INR is >4.5 but there is no

bleeding, warfarin is withheld and the INR followed daily, but if there is bleeding vitamin K is given. It is given intravenously over 3–5 min to avoid dysphoric reactions and hypotension, or orally (by which route it is rapidly absorbed in the absence of diarrhea or malabsorption from liver or other disease). Minor bleeding can be treated with as little as 1 mg vitamin K, which does not make the patient resistant to subsequent rewarfarinization. For life-threatening bleeding, vitamin K, 5 mg, is given intravenously together with a factor IX concentrate which also contains other vitamin K-dependent factors. (It should be noted that very highly purified factor IX concentrates are now becoming available which, while they have the advantage of causing less thrombotic complications in patients with hemophilia B for whom they are intended, are not effective in reversing warfarin toxicity.) Fresh frozen plasma is a less potent alternative.

2. Other adverse actions of warfarin:

(a) Teratogenesis, particularly osteodysplasia punctata, optic atrophy and microcephaly and intrauterine death.
(b) Alopecia.
(c) Rashes.
(d) Thrombosis is a rare but severe and well documented paradoxical effect of warfarin, and can result in extensive tissue necrosis usually in a fatty structure such as a breast or buttock. Peripheries (feet or penis) may become gangrenous in this way. Pathologically these lesions are associated with extensive thrombosis in venules. It is noteworthy that vitamin K is involved in the biosynthesis of anticoagulant proteins C and S as well as of the clotting factors, and deficiencies of these proteins are associated with thrombotic disease. It is tempting to try to explain this rare paradoxical effect of warfarin on the basis of an action on these factors, perhaps in individuals with an otherwise subclinical deficiency, although so far evidence is lacking.

3. Adverse effects of phenindiones:

(a) Interference with iodine uptake by the thyroid.
(b) Renal tubular damage.
(c) Hepatitis.
(d) Agranulocytosis.
(e) Dermatitis.
(f) Secretion into breast milk (unlike warfarin).
(g) Metabolites sometimes color urine pink or orange (distinguished from blood by adding a few drops of acetic acid which causes the color to fade).

Contraindications

Contraindications to oral anticoagulants include:

- Active bleeding from gastrointestinal, respiratory or genitourinary tracts, for example peptic ulceration, active ulcerative colitis.
- Blood dyscrasias with hemorrhagic diathesis (e.g. leukemia complicated by severe thrombocytopenia).
- Dissecting aneurysm of the aorta.
- Recent surgery of the central nervous system (CNS) or eye.
- Space-occupying CNS lesion.
- Pregnancy: first trimester (especially during organogenesis in weeks 6–9), and the final 4 weeks (because of intracranial bleeding in the infant at delivery, and *postpartum* hemorrhage in the mother).

Relative contraindications to oral anticoagulation include:

- History of potential bleeding lesion.
- High risk of head injury (poorly controlled epilepsy, history of recurrent falls).
- Severe uncontrolled hypertension.
- Diabetes with proliferative retinopathy.
- Alcoholism.
- Any stage of pregnancy.
- Hepatic or renal insufficiency.
- Lack of sufficient intelligence or cooperation on the part of the patient.
- Elderly or debilitated patients.

Pharmacokinetics of warfarin

Warfarin can be measured in plasma by high-performance liquid chromatography, but separation of the R and S enantiomers requires specialized methods. Following oral administration absorption is almost complete and maximum plasma concentrations are reached within 2–8 hours. Approximately 97% is bound to plasma albumin. Warfarin does gain access to the fetus, but does not appear in breast milk in clinically relevant amounts. The basal rate of warfarin metabolism is inherited and is under polygenic control. There is substantial variation between individuals in warfarin $t_{1/2}$, the active S enantiomer having a $t_{1/2}$ of 18–35 hours and the R enantiomer a $t_{1/2}$ of 20–60 hours. The R and S enantiomers are metabolized differently in the liver. The S enantiomer is metabolized to 7-hydroxywarfarin by a cytochrome P_{450}-dependent mixed function oxidase, while the less active R enantiomer is metabolized by soluble enzymes to RS warfarin alcohol. Hepatic metabolism is followed by conjugation and excretion into the gut in the bile. Deconjugation and reabsorption occur to complete the enterohepatic cycle.

Knowledge of the plasma concentration of warfarin is not useful in routine clinical practice because pharmacodynamic response (INR) can be measured accurately, but is valuable in the investigation of patients with unusual resistance to warfarin in whom it helps to distinguish poor compliance, abnormal pharmacokinetics and abnormal sensitivity. Since warfarin acts by inhibiting synthesis of active vitamin K-dependent clotting factors anticoagulation following dosing awaits the catabolism of preformed factors. Consequently the delay between dosing and effect can not be shortened by giving a loading dose. The $t_{1/2}$ of the factors involved are: II, 60 hours; VII, 6 hours; IX, 20 hours and X, 40 hours.

Drug interactions

Numerous clinically important drug interactions occur with oral anticoagulants which have a narrow therapeutic range and steep dose–response curves. They have the potential to cause life-threatening toxicity, but inadequate treatment can also result in death through progression of thromboembolic disease. Many reports of drug interactions with warfarin are poorly documented and are based on single case reports. It is, however, prudent to minimize the use of other drugs during oral anticoagulation, and when additional drugs are deemed essential to monitor the INR closely over the ensuing 2 weeks. Drugs that are often needed or useful in patients receiving warfarin that do *not* interact adversely include digoxin, frusemide and paracetamol.

Potentially important pharmacodynamic interactions with warfarin include those with antiplatelet drugs. Aspirin, the main such drug in clinical use, not only influences hemostasis by its effect on platelet function but also increases the likelihood of peptic ulceration, displaces warfarin from plasma albumin, and in high doses decreases prothrombin synthesis. Despite these potential problems recent clinical experience suggests that with close monitoring the increased risk of bleeding when low doses of aspirin (100 mg daily) are taken regularly with warfarin may be more than offset by clinical benefits to patients at high risk of thromboembolism following cardiac valve replacement. Broad-spectrum antibiotics potentiate warfarin action by suppressing the synthesis of vitamin K_1 by gut flora. Conversely some enteral feeding solutions contain vitamin K_1 and reduce the effect of warfarin.

There are several pharmacokinetic interactions with warfarin of clinical importance. It was thought that the major effect of phenylbutazone was exerted via competition for plasma albumin binding. Certainly competition between warfarin and phenylbutazone for binding to plasma albumin can be demonstrated *in vitro*. However, the mechanism underlying this interaction turns out to be more interesting, and is a well-documented instance of stereoselective metabolic inhibition (others include co-trimoxazole, metronidazole and erythromycin). Phenylbutazone increases the plasma clearance of R-warfarin approximately two-fold but decreases S-warfarin clearance. Confusingly, the clearance of racemic warfarin measured by methods that do not distinguish the enantiomers appears to be unchanged since the decrease in S-warfarin clearance masks the increased R-warfarin clearance. However, the relative amount of the more powerfully anticoagulant S-warfarin is increased so anticoagulant potency is enhanced. Restriction of the use of phenylbutazone (to patients with severe ankylosing spondylitis) has reduced the occurrence of this potentially fatal interaction, but some other non-steroidal anti-inflammatory drugs (NSAIDs) and dextropropoxyphene also inhibit warfarin metabolism, so care is needed in prescribing these drugs to patients treated with warfarin. The gastrotoxic and platelet inhibitory actions of the NSAIDs further increase the risk of serious hemorrhage. Cimetidine (but not ranitidine) and amiodarone also potently inhibit warfarin metabolism and potentiate its effect.

Cholestyramine impairs warfarin absorption and interrupts its enterohepatic recirculation. Drugs that induce hepatic microsomal enzymes including rifampicin, carbamazepine and phenobarbitone increase warfarin metabolism and increased doses are required to produce a therapeutic effect. Furthermore, if such increased doses are not reduced when such concurrent therapy is discontinued catastrophic over-anticoagulation and hemorrhage may ensue.

ANTIPLATELET DRUGS

ASPIRIN AND OTHER DRUGS ACTING ON THE THROMBOXANE PATHWAY

Aspirin is the most important antiplatelet drug in clinical use. It works by inhibiting the synthesis of thromboxane A_2, and its use in treatment and prevention of ischemic heart disease is described more fully in chapter 26. Numerous clinical trials, several of them large, have demonstrated its efficacy, with reductions in myocardial infarction and vascular death ranging from approximately 25% following myocardial infarction to approximately 50% in patients with unstable angina. Efficacy has not been clearly related to dose, doses of 320 mg on alternate days or 150 mg daily being effective. Aspirin also reduces the incidence of stroke in patients with transient ischemic attacks by approximately 10% and may reduce the incidence of pre-eclampsia in women at high risk, although the evidence for this is incomplete. Thromboxane A_2 is synthesized by activated platelets and acts on receptors on platelets (causing further platelet activation and propagation of the aggregate) and on vascular smooth · muscle (causing vasoconstriction). Figure 27.2 shows the pathway of its biosynthesis from arachidonic acid. Aspirin inhibits thromboxane synthesis: it acetylates a serine residue in the active site of cyclo-oxygenase, irreversibly blocking this enzyme. The most common side effect of aspirin is gastric intolerance, and the most common severe adverse reaction is upper gastrointestinal bleeding,

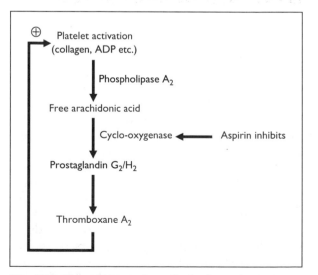

Fig. 27.2 Thromboxane A_2 and platelet activation. ADP = adenosine diphosphate.

effects that stem from inhibition of cyclo-oxygenase in the stomach.

Other drugs that act on the thromboxane pathway have considerable therapeutic potential, but have not yet been developed for clinical use. These include thromboxane receptor antagonists, which have the potential advantage over aspirin of greater selectivity. Thus they do not inhibit prostaglandin E_2 in the stomach (and so do not cause gastric toxicity of the kind caused by aspirin) and do not inhibit prostacyclin (and hence may have greater antithrombotic efficacy than aspirin). Thromboxane synthase inhibitors have the added potential benefit of increasing prostacyclin biosynthesis at the same time as inhibiting thromboxane biosynthesis. Drugs are available that simultaneously inhibit thromboxane A_2 synthesis and action (combined synthase inhibitors/receptor antagonists) which avoid one potential problem of pure thromboxane synthase inhibitors, namely that prostaglandin H_2, the precursor of thromboxane A_2 that accumulates when platelets are activated in the presence of thromboxane synthase inhibition, can also activate thromboxane receptors. Development of this potentially important class of drugs has been slow, perhaps because of the need to compete commercially with aspirin.

EPOPROSTENOL (PROSTACYCLIN)

Use

Epoprostenol is the approved drug name for synthetic prostacyclin, the principal endogenous prostaglandin of large and medium-sized blood vessels such as the aorta and coronary arteries. It is used *ex vivo* in the preparation of washed platelet concentrates. Epoprostenol relaxes pulmonary as well as systemic vasculature, and this underpins its use in patients with primary pulmonary hypertension. It has been administered chronically to such patients for periods of months or even years while awaiting heart–lung transplantation. Epoprostenol inhibits platelet activation during hemodialysis. It can be used with heparin, but is also effective as sole anticoagulant in this setting and is therefore particularly useful for haemodialysis in patients in whom heparin is contraindicated. It has also been used in other kinds of extracorporeal circuit (e.g. during cardiopulmonary bypass and during charcoal column hemoperfusion). Epoprostenol has been used with apparent benefit in acute retinal vessel thrombosis and in patients with critical limb ischemia and with platelet consumption due to multiple organ failure, especially those with meningococcal sepsis. Rigorous proof of efficacy is difficult to provide in such settings. It is dissolved immediately before use in a specially provided alkaline glycine buffer, and infused intravenously (or, in the case of hemodialysis, into the arterial limb supplying the dialyzer). The starting dose is 2 ng/kg body weight/min. This can be increased in stepwise increments of 2 ng/kg/min if necessary to 16 ng/kg/min, with frequent monitoring of blood pressure (usually with an automated indirect method) and heart rate during the period of dose titration. A modest reduction in diastolic pressure with an increase in systolic pressure (i.e. increased pulse pressure) and reflex tachycardia is the expected and desired hemodynamic effect; if bradycardia and hypotension occur the infusion should be temporarily discontinued and the patient's legs elevated if necessary.

Mechanism of action

Prostacyclin acts on specific receptors on the plasma membranes of platelets and vascular smooth muscle. These are coupled by G-proteins to adenylyl cyclase. Activation of this enzyme increases the biosynthesis of the second messenger cyclic adenosine monophosphate (cAMP), which causes inhibition of platelet aggregation to all agonists, and relaxes vascular smooth muscle.

Adverse effects

The vasodilator effect of prostacyclin causes flushing, headache, reduced diastolic blood pressure, increased pulse pressure and reflex tachycardia; unusually but of more concern, as mentioned above, vagally mediated bradycardia and hypotension occur. In addition it can cause nausea, abdominal discomfort, diarrhea and uterine cramps, but these effects are usually mild and much less pronounced than with the E-series prostaglandins. Crushing chest pain is, rarely, experienced by individuals with no evidence of ischemic heart disease; jaw pain is common during chronic administration. These effects usually resolve within minutes of stopping or reducing the infusion. Bleeding complications, which were anticipated, have in fact been rare, perhaps because whereas prostacyclin is very potent at inhibiting platelet aggregation, it is much less effective at inhibiting platelet adhesion. Consequently, the hemostatic function of platelets is little influenced by prostacyclin despite its antithrombotic action.

Pharmacokinetics

Prostacyclin is unstable under physiological conditions. It is therefore dissolved in base and infused intravenously. (Stable analogs such as carbacyclin and iloprost have been developed but not yet marketed in the UK.) The half-life of prostacyclin in the circulation is approximately 3 min, so steady state is achieved rapidly and dose increments can be made safely every 8–12 min. It hydrolyzes spontaneously to an inactive product (6-oxo-prostaglandin $F_{1\alpha}$) which is excreted in the urine both unchanged and as inactive enzyme derived oxidation products, of which the major metabolite is 2,3-dinor-6-oxo-prostaglandin $F_{1\alpha}$.

DIPYRIDAMOLE

Use

Dipyridamole was introduced as a vasodilator, but is now promoted, often in combination with aspirin, for its effects on platelet function. Clinical trials have not, however, supported any additional benefit over that of aspirin alone in the prevention of stroke or myocardial infarction. The combination with aspirin has been effective in reducing the incidence of graft occlusion following coronary artery bypass grafting, but has not been directly compared with aspirin alone. Addition of dipyridamole to warfarin in patients with prosthetic heart valves appeared

to reduce the risk of thrombembolism in one trial published in 1971, but the incidence of such events in the group treated with anticoagulation alone was unusually high, casting doubt on the reliability of this conclusion. Clinical use at the present time is therefore limited mainly to its intravenous use as a diagnostic agent in dipyridamole/thallium scanning of the heart. This is used in patients for whom a stress test is clinically indicated, but who are unable to cooperate with an exercise test (e.g. because of severe claudication or osteoarthrosis). In these individuals intravenous dipyridamole can act as a pharmacological stress and enable areas of reversible cardiac hypoperfusion to be identified.

Mechanism of action

Despite the lack of convincing evidence of clinical usefulness as an antithrombotic drug, there is no doubt that dipyridamole influences platelet function *in vitro* and *ex vivo*. The mechanism of these effects as well as of its vasodilator action is probably partly via inhibition of phosphodiesterase which leads to reduced breakdown of cyclic AMP, and partly to inhibition of adenosine uptake with consequent enhancement of the actions of this mediator on platelets and vascular smooth muscle.

Drug interactions

Dipyridamole increases the potency and duration of action of adenosine. This may be clinically important in patients receiving dipyridamole in whom adenosine is considered for treatment of arrhythmia (e.g. following bypass surgery).

TICLOPIDINE

Use

Ticlopidine is used in North America as prophylaxis against stroke or myocardial infarction in patients at high risk, in peripheral arterial disease, diabetic microangiopathy and to reduce platelet activation in extracorporeal circulations. It reduces the risk of recurrence in patients who have recovered from ischemic stroke, and even appears to be rather more effective than aspirin, 650 mg, twice daily for this indication, but at the expense of a substantial incidence of adverse events, some of them severe. Ticlopidine is also effective in reducing the risk of stroke and myocardial infarction in patients with intermittent claudication. In patients with unstable angina addition of ticlopidine to β-blockers, nitrates and calcium channel antagonists resulted in approximately a 50% reduction in myocardial infarction. This is similar to the effect of aspirin in unstable angina. Ticlopidine reduces the rate of progression of microaneurysms in patients with diabetes mellitus by about three-fold. The clinical importance of this is not known. Ticlopidine is given by mouth, 250 mg, twice daily. White blood cell counts are checked every 2 weeks for the first 12 weeks (see below).

Mechanism of action

Ticlopidine does not inhibit cyclo-oxygenase, and its mechanism is entirely different from that of aspirin. It is an inactive prodrug that is converted in the liver to unstable biologically active metabolite(s) that have not been characterized. Consequently it is inactive when added to platelet-rich plasma *in vitro*, but when platelet-rich plasma is prepared from a subject who has ingested the drug aggregation to a wide variety of agonists is inhibited. This wide spectrum of activity is explained by inhibition of fibrinogen binding to activated glycoprotein IIb/IIIa receptors. (It is this fibrinogen binding that causes platelets to stick together in response to aggregating agents of all kinds.) Ticlopidine also reduces fibrinogen concentrations by about 10% during chronic treatment, although the importance of this is unknown.

Adverse effects and contraindications

Neutropenia occurs in about 2.4% of patients, usually in the first 12 weeks, and is severe in 0.8%. Thrombocytopenia and pancytopenia have also been described but are less common than neutropenia. Cholestatic jaundice has occurred in the first few months, and is reversible on stopping the drug. Gastrointestinal symptoms are common (around 40%) and include nausea, anorexia, vomiting, epigastric pain and diarrhea. These usually occur early and may resolve despite continued treatment, or not recur on reinstituting treatment. Various rashes occur. Plasma lipid concentrations increase by about 10% during chronic treatment, the increases occurring in all fractions so that the low to high density lipoprotein (LDL/HDL) ratio is unchanged. Ticlopidine is contraindicated in patients with coagulation or platelet disorders, or diseases where local bleeding may occur such as hemorrhagic stroke or active peptic ulcer disease.

MONOCLONAL ANTIBODIES TO GLYCOPROTEIN IIb/IIIa

Use

Recent trials have shown such antibodies reduce restenosis following angioplasty, but can cause bleeding. Their clinical role remains to be established.

ANTICOAGULANTS IN PREGNANCY AND PUERPERIUM

There is an increased risk of thromboembolism in pregnancy and women at risk (e.g. those with prosthetic heart valves) must continue to be anticoagulated. However, warfarin crosses the placenta and when taken throughout pregnancy will result in complications in about one-third of cases: 16% of fetuses will be spontaneously aborted or still-born, 10% will have *postpartum* complications (usually due to bleeding) and 7% will suffer teratogenic effects.

Heparin does not cross the placenta, and may be self-administered subcutaneously. Its long-term use may cause osteoporosis or alopecia and there is an increased risk of retroplacental bleeding resulting in fetal death. One approach to the management of pregnancy in women on anticoagulants is to change to subcutaneous heparin from the time of the first missed period and remain on this until term, maintaining a high intake of elemental calcium and adequate, but not excessive, intake of vitamin D. Alternatively, once the critical period (6–9 weeks) has passed, the patient may be switched back to warfarin with very careful control to avoid overdosage with its attendant risk of bleeding. She is admitted to hospital at 36 weeks and changed back to heparin. Heparin may be reversed with protamine immediately before delivery, but heparin together with warfarin is restarted immediately *postpartum* and continued until the full effect of warfarin is re-established. If labor starts suddenly in a patient still receiving warfarin, she should be given fresh frozen plasma and the baby given vitamin K. Warfarin does not enter milk to an important extent, and mothers may nurse while anticoagulated in this way, in contrast to phenindione.

Heart Failure

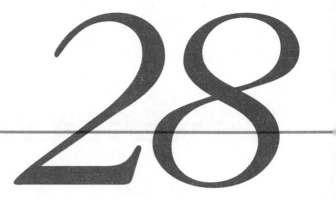

Introduction **338**

Pathophysiology **338**

Therapeutic objectives **339**

General measures **339**

Shock: general principles **340**

Drugs for cardiac failure **340**

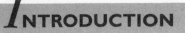

INTRODUCTION

Heart failure occurs when the heart fails to deliver adequate amounts of oxygenated blood to the tissues during exercise or, in severe cases, at rest. Such failure of pump function may be chronic, in which case symptoms of fatigue, ankle swelling, effort dyspnea and orthopnea predominate, or acute, with sudden onset of dyspnea at rest. Both acute and chronic heart failure severely reduce life expectancy.

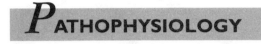

PATHOPHYSIOLOGY

Heart failure can be caused by diseases of the heart (myocardium: ischemic heart disease or idiopathic cardiomyopathy; conducting tissue: various arrhythmias; pericardium: constrictive pericarditis, pericardial effusion; or endocardium: valvular disease), by hypertension (systemic or pulmonary), by congenital defects (atrial or ventricular septal defects or patent ductus arteriosus) or by extracardiac disorders including fluid overload, anemia and thyrotoxicosis.

Heart failure causes several pathophysiological changes that are 'counter-regulatory', that is they make the situation worse not better. This puzzling situation is probably due to natural selection since our ancestors probably encountered low cardiac output during hemorrhage rather than because of heart failure. Mechanisms to conserve blood volume and maintain blood pressure would therefore have been of selective advantage. Reflex and endocrine changes that are protective in the setting of hemorrhage are, however, totally inappropriate in patients with low cardiac output due to pump failure rather than volume loss.

An important part of modern treatment of cardiac failure is therefore directed to reversing these counter-regulatory changes which include:

1. Activation of baroreflexes leading to increased sympathetic tone, tachycardia and vasoconstriction.

2. Activation of the renin–angiotensin–aldosterone system and renin release, with consequent increased production of angiotensin II (which increases peripheral resistance both by direct vasoconstriction and indirectly by synergy with the sympathetic nervous system) and aldosterone (which causes salt and water retention).

Important physiological factors determining cardiac performance include: preload, afterload, myocardial contractility and heart rate. Each of these may be adversely affected by the primary cause of heart failure, and be exacerbated by the counter-regulatory changes mentioned above.

PRELOAD

The filling pressure of the left ventricle determines the extent of stretch of myocardial fibers at the end of diastole. Up to a point, increased stretch results in increased force of contraction but, in the failing heart, beyond this point further increase in stretch results in reduced contraction (the Frank–Starling relation). Preload is increased directly if blood or physiological saline is transfused too rapidly. The major influences on preload are blood volume, which increases in heart failure due to salt and water retention, and increased capacitance vessel tone due to sympathetic nervous system activation. In heart failure, preload is usually excessive, and cardiac function is improved by drugs that reduce blood volume (diuretics) or reduce capacitance vessel tone (venodilators).

AFTERLOAD

This determines the tension that needs to be developed in the ventricular wall to eject the stroke volume. It is principally determined by the systemic vascular resistance: the lower this resistance, the less the impedance to ventricular emptying. Systemic vascular resistance is excessively high in patients with systemic hypertension, and in the majority of patients with heart failure, because of inappropriate activation of renin–angiotensin and sympathetic nervous systems as explained above. Drugs that reduce afterload (arteriodilators) therefore improve cardiac output in patients with heart failure.

MYOCARDIAL CONTRACTILITY

This describes the intrinsic contractility of the heart and is reduced following myocardial infarction or in idiopathic congestive cardiomyopathy. Positive inotropes (e.g. digoxin, phosphodiesterase inhibitors, β_1-adrenoceptor agonists) can improve cardiac performance temporarily by increasing contractility, but at the expense of increased work and oxygen consumption of viable cardiac muscle.

HEART RATE

Cardiac output is the product of heart rate and stroke volume, so increased heart rate increases cardiac output in the healthy heart. It does this at the expense of increased cardiac work and oxygen consumption. When there is coronary artery disease coronary blood flow may be reduced and ischemia worsened as rate increases. Furthermore, cardiac function deteriorates as rate increases beyond an optimum due to insufficient time for filling during diastole, and positive chronotropes are not useful clinically in the absence of specific bradyarrhythmia.

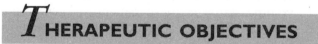

THERAPEUTIC OBJECTIVES

Therapy specific for the underlying disease may be available. Surgery (e.g. for valvular or congenital heart disease), pacing (for symptomatic bradyarrhythmias) or oxygen (for cor pulmonale) may be indicated in addition to drugs to improve hemodynamics by reducing cardiac load or increasing contractility. Selected patients with severe disease may benefit dramatically from cardiac transplantation. In addition to correction of specific defects where possible, the objectives of management are: (1) to improve symptoms, and (2) to prolong survival.

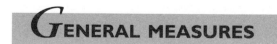

GENERAL MEASURES

These include:

1. Sitting the patient upright in acute heart failure.

2. Oxygen, to correct hypoxia if present.
3. Withdrawal of drugs that aggravate cardiac failure, i.e. negative inotropes (e.g. β-blockers, calcium channel blockers), direct

cardiac toxins (e.g. daunorubicin) or drugs that cause salt retention (e.g. non-steroidal anti-inflammatory drugs, stilbestrol, carbenoxolone).

4. Dietary salt and, less importantly, fluid restriction.

5. Anticoagulants: bed rest, vigorous diuresis and low cardiac output predispose to deep venous thrombosis and pulmonary embolism. Anticoagulation reduces this risk. Once patients are up and about anticoagulation may not be needed, provided they are in sinus rhythm. Aspirin should be considered in patients with ischemic heart disease to reduce the risk of reinfarction.

6. Bed rest: improves renal blood flow and is appropriate in acute, but seldom, if ever, in chronic heart failure.

SHOCK: GENERAL PRINCIPLES

Shock is life-threatening hypoperfusion of vital organs especially the brain and kidneys. The main types of shock are:

1. **Hypovolemic** Replacement of volume with blood, plasma, colloid (e.g. dextran or gelatin solutions) or crystalloid solutions (e.g. physiological saline) is the main therapeutic approach.

2. **Endotoxin** Appropriate antibiotics, in addition to fluids and pressors, are given as needed.

3. **Cardiogenic** This requires augmentation of myocardial contractility, although in many patients the pump is irreversibly damaged and no therapy is effective. A few patients with apparent cardiogenic shock have problems for which there is specific therapy which may be life saving. These are often readily diagnosed on Swann–Ganz catheterization, and include unrecognized hypovolemia, right ventricular infarction, cardiac tamponade, ventriculoseptal or papillary muscle rupture.

However, in the majority of patients with cardiogenic shock the problem is due to pump failure. Measurement of pulmonary capillary wedge pressure (a measure of left heart filling pressure) together with arterial blood pressure, cardiac output and urine output permit optimal use of pressor and vasodilator drugs as well as management of volume status in these patients. Management often entails a combination of dobutamine (a positive inotrope relatively free of chronotropic effects), low-dose dopamine (to improve renal blood flow) and an arterial vasodilator (e.g. sodium nitroprusside) to reduce cardiac load and improve tissue perfusion. These short-term measures permit recovery of function in some patients with reversible cardiac dysfunction (e.g. from so-called 'stunned' myocardium).

DRUGS FOR CARDIAC FAILURE

DIURETICS (SEE ALSO P. 439)

Use

A diuretic is usually the drug of first choice to control symptomatic edema and dyspnea in patients with heart failure. In mild cardiac failure, a thiazide (e.g. bendrofluazide, 5 mg, daily by mouth) is sometimes adequate, but more severe cases require a loop diuretic such as frusemide, started in a low dose (e.g. 20–40 mg by mouth and increased if necessary). Acute pulmonary edema requires treatment with intravenous frusemide (e.g. 40 mg, or if needed larger doses given slowly: not faster than 4 mg/min). Slow intravenous infusion of frusemide by syringe pump is useful in resistant severe cases. Combinations of a fixed dose of frusemide with a potassium-sparing diuretic such as amiloride ('co-amilofruse') are marketed aggressively, and enjoy considerable popularity. They are relatively expensive and are not without problems: they should not be prescribed uncritically and automatically in place of frusemide, but are useful in certain circumstances (see below).

Mechanism of action

Diuretics increase renal salt and water excretion. Thiazides do this by inhibiting Na^+ reabsorption in the early part of the distal convoluted tubule. Loop diuretics inhibit $Na^+/K^+/2Cl^-$ cotransport in the thick ascending limb of Henlé's loop. Both cause kaliuresis in addition to the desired natriuresis, because of increased delivery of Na^+ to the distal tubular and collecting duct segments where Na^+ is exchanged for K^+. Potassium-sparing diuretics (e.g. amiloride, triamterene) are relatively feeble diuretics but inhibit this distal Na^+/K^+ exchange. Increased elimination of salt and water reduces cardiac preload, and reduces edema. Frusemide also has an indirect vasodilator effect (probably via prostaglandin and vasodepressor neutral lipid mediators released from the kidneys), since diuresis begins some 10–20 min after an intravenous dose whereas dramatic symptomatic improvement in patients with pulmonary edema can occur more rapidly.

Adverse effects

Diuretics have several electrolyte/metabolic effects of uncertain clinical significance. They cause some degree of hypokalemia in many subjects, and sometimes also hypomagnesemia and hyponatremia. Increased elimination of sodium chloride (especially by loop diuretics) causes hypochloremic alkalosis, which can be important in patients with cor pulmonale from obstructive airways disease. Total body potassium may be little affected during chronic treatment, but many of the adverse interactions of diuretics with other drugs (see below) are probably mediated by hypokalemia and/or hypomagnesemia, although this issue remains controversial. Thiazide and loop diuretics reduce urate clearance, thereby increasing plasma urate concentration and precipitating gout in predisposed individuals. Thiazides impair glucose tolerance, and can cause hyperglycemia in non-insulin-dependent diabetics. Thiazide diuretics cause a small increase in plasma cholesterol concentration which is clinically unimportant in the great majority of patients.

Frusemide causes idiosyncratic reactions including rashes and rarely bone marrow depression, evidenced either by neutropenia or by thrombocytopenia in rare patients. These latter reactions require stopping the drug, and an alternative loop diuretic (e.g. bumetanide) may be useful in this circumstance. Thiazides can also cause rashes and/or thrombocytopenia. High doses of frusemide (particularly if given by rapid intravenous injection) are predictably ototoxic, causing deafness and tinnitus, because formation of endolymph in the inner ear involves a $Na^+/K^+/2Cl^-$ transporter.

Pharmacokinetics

Absorption of frusemide from the gastrointestinal tract is delayed in severe cardiac failure, due to edema of the intestinal mucosa (chapter 7), and frusemide is more effective when administered intravenously (ideally by syringe pump) than by the oral route in this circumstance. When the clinical situation improves the oral route can be used.

Frusemide is eliminated in the urine: it is secreted in the proximal tubule and becomes progressively more concentrated as water is reabsorbed in the proximal tubule, so that when it reaches its site of action in the ascending limb of the loop of Henle its concentration in the tubular fluid is much greater than plasma. Since the ion transporter that it inhibits is located on the luminal surface this explains the selectivity of frusemide for the $Na^+/K^+/2Cl^-$ exchanger in the kidney as opposed to other sites in the body such as the inner ear.

Drug interactions

Diuretic-induced hypokalemia increases the toxicity of several important cardiovascular drugs, notably digoxin. It increases the risk of *torsades de pointes* from antiarrhythmic drugs that prolong the cardiac action potential (quinidine, disopyramide, amiodarone, sotolol). Potassium supplements can counter this problem, but are unpleasant to take, and are present in totally inadequate amounts in 'combination' tablets. Concurrent use of a potassium sparing diuretic (e.g. amiloride or triamterene) with frusemide is sometimes justified in the treatment of heart failure, particularly if digoxin or one of the above antiarrhythmic drugs is also needed. However, amiloride and triamterene have important toxicities and can cause severe hyperkalemia, especially if given with converting enzyme inhibitors and/or to patients with renal impairment, which is a common accompaniment of heart failure. It is therefore important to monitor plasma concentrations of potassium during treatment with diuretics. In modern practice, converting enzyme inhibitors, which help conserve potassium, are used earlier than hitherto (see below) and digoxin is usually relegated to third-line treatment, so potassium-sparing diuretics are often unnecessary and it is unfortunate that expensive fixed dose combinations of frusemide or bumetanide with amiloride are prescribed so uncritically.

Non-steroidal anti-inflammatory drugs (NSAIDs) cause salt and water retention by inhibiting prostaglandin biosynthesis by the kidney (prostaglandin E_2 and prostacyclin are vasodilator and natriuretic). The NSAIDs therefore reduce the effectiveness of frusemide and other diuretics. Diuretics also interact with lithium by causing salt depletion, thereby increasing its proximal tubular reabsorption and plasma concentration and, hence, the likelihood of toxicity.

CONVERTING ENZYME INHIBITORS (SEE ALSO CHAPTER 25)

Angiotensin-converting enzyme (ACE) is inhibited by several synthetic peptides and peptide analogs derived originally from the toxin of a South American snake (*Bothrops jacaraca*).

Captopril (the first to be marketed) is shorter acting than enalapril, and in higher than therapeutic doses causes adverse effects related to its sulfydryl group (see p. 293). Many different ACE inhibitors are now marketed, and many more are in development. Much is made of differences between ACE inhibitors, but apart from duration of action few of these differences are of definite clinical importance in treatment of heart failure. (One study on quality of life in patients with hypertension has suggested that captopril is better than enalapril in such patients.)

Use

Angiotensin-converting enzyme inhibitors are a major advance in the treatment of cardiac failure. They reduce mortality as well as improving symptoms in patients with mild or severe heart failure, and are superior to other vasodilators that have been used to treat heart failure. When symptoms are mild diuretics can be temporarily discontinued a day or two before starting an ACE inhibitor, reducing the likelihood of first-dose hypotension. In these circumstances treatment with an ACE inhibitor can be started as an outpatient, as for hypertension (chapter 25). A small starting dose (which will have only a short effect) is used and the first dose taken last thing before retiring at night, with advice to sit on the side of the bed before standing if the patient needs to get up in the night. Starting doses of 2.5 mg are appropriate for enalapril, or of 6.25 mg for captopril. The dose is increased with careful monitoring of blood pressure and signs of heart failure to a maintenance dose that is individualized for each patient: usual doses are enalapril 10–20 mg daily or captopril 25 mg 2–3 times daily. Baseline evaluation with an objective measure of ventricular function (e.g. ejection fraction by echocardiography), is increasingly needed to detect evidence of subclinical heart failure as evidence of improved survival from treatment of such patients with ACE inhibitors increases.

Mechanism of action

Angiotensin-converting enzyme (also called kininase II) is located on the surface membrane of vascular endothelial cells as well as in other cells and in plasma. The lung (which possesses a huge surface area of endothelium) is particularly rich in ACE, but this enzyme is also present in many other organs, including the heart and systemic resistance vessels. Angiotensin-converting enzyme catalyzes the removal of two terminal amino acid residues from angiotensin I and from several other short peptides. This results in formation of angiotensin II (a potent vasoconstrictor) from its inactive precursor angiotensin I. Angiotensin II releases aldosterone from the zona glomerulosa of the adrenal cortex, as well as constricing vascular smooth muscle, and therefore causes salt and water retention and urinary loss of potassium. In addition to activating the vasoconstrictor/salt retaining angiotensin mechanism ACE also inactivates bradykinin, which is an endogenous vasodilator. Angiotensin-converting enzyme inhibitors therefore reduce angiotensin-mediated vasoconstriction and salt retention, mildly increase plasma potassium, and enhance bradykinin-mediated vasodilatation. They reduce cardiac preload and afterload, thereby improving the function of the failing heart.

Adverse effects

Hypotension can be a problem on starting treatment: patients with heart failure usually have high concentrations of circulating renin, and this is further increased by treatment with diuretics. Introduction of an ACE inhibitor can therefore cause dramatic 'first-dose' hypotension. This can be minimized as explained above. Patients in whom first-dose hypotension is marked may be those with the greatest activation of the renin–angiotensin system, and consequently those most likely to benefit from treatment with ACE inhibitors in the long term. Angiotensin-converting enzyme inhibitors are usually well tolerated during chronic treatment, although dry cough is common and occasionally unacceptable. This symptom may be caused by kinin accumulation stimulating cough afferents. The same explanation has been offered for the urticarial reactions and angioneurotic edema sometimes caused by ACE inhibitors. Functional renal failure is a predictable effect of ACE inhibitors in patients with hemodynamically significant bilateral renal artery stenoses or with renal artery stenosis in the vessel supplying a single functional kidney (p. 293). Angiotensin converting enzyme inhibitors are contraindicated in pregnancy from the second trimester until term because they cause renal failure in the fetus, oligohydramnios and also birth defects.

Angiotensin-converting enzyme inhibitors cause a modest increase in plasma potassium as a result of reduced aldosterone secretion. This may usefully counter the small reduction in potassium ion concentration caused by diuretics. Increased plasma potassium is, however, potentially hazardous in patients with renal impairment, and close monitoring of plasma potassium and creatinine is essential in this setting. This is particularly important when such patients are also prescribed potassium supplements and/or potassium-sparing diuretics including those marketed as fixed dose combinations (e.g. co-amilozide, coamilofruse) or NSAIDs which can reduce renin secretions.

When first introduced captopril caused a cluster of adverse effects including heavy proteinuria, rashes and neutropenia. These were identified as being related to its sulfydryl group. Similar effects occur with penicillamine, another drug that contains a sulfydryl group (p. 293). These dose-related effects seldom occur with the maximum doses of captopril that are now commonly regarded as useful (i.e. usually no more than 50 mg twice daily), and paradoxically converting enzyme inhibitors including captopril actually *reduce* albuminuria in patients with diabetic nephropathy (see chapter 34).

Pharmacokinetics

Currently available converting enzyme inhibitors are all active when administered orally, but are highly polar and are eliminated in the urine. Some (e.g. fosinopril) are also metabolized by the liver. Some (e.g. captopril) are active as the parent molecule, while some (e.g. enalapril) are inactive prodrugs (enalapril is converted to its active metabolite enalaprilat in the liver). This does not have important clinical consequences. No currently available ACE inhibitor penetrates the central nervous system particularly well, and none penetrates to inhibit the testicular enzyme. There is only a poor correlation between inhibition of plasma converting enzyme and hemodynamic effect, possibly because of the importance of ACE in resistance vessels rather than in the plasma in influencing vascular tone and hence cardiac load.

Drug interactions

The useful interaction with diuretics has already been alluded to: diuretic treatment increases plasma renin activity, and the consequent activation of angiotensin II and aldosterone limits the efficacy of diuretic treatment. Converting enzyme inhibitors interrupt this loop and so enhance the efficacy of diuretics. Adverse interactions with potassium-sparing diuretics and potassium supplements, leading to hyperkalemia especially in patients with renal impairment, have also been mentioned. Non-steroidal anti-inflammatory drugs are contraindicated in heart failure and may cause renal failure and severe hyperkalemia as well as fluid retention in heart failure patients receiving treatment with converting enzyme inhibitors.

OTHER VASODILATORS

Before the introduction of converting enzyme inhibitors several other vasodilators were found to be effective in heart failure. These include hydralazine and α-adrenoceptor antagonists (chapter 25) and organic nitrates (chapter 26). Converting enzyme inhibitors are more effective than these drugs, which are now reserved for patients with heart failure who cannot tolerate converting enzyme inhibitors.

CARDIAC GLYCOSIDES

William Withering published his description of the use of digitalis (an extract of the foxglove) as a cure for 'dropsy' (congestive cardiac failure) in 1785. 'Digitalis' is the name used for a group of cardiac glycosides that all possess an aglycone ring essential for activity. These share similar pharmacodynamic properties, differing in their pharmacokinetics. Among digitalis glycosides, digoxin is now used almost exclusively, although the faster acting ouabain is useful in urgent situations, and the longer half-life digitoxin can be useful when drugs have to be given under supervision (e.g. to a mildly demented patient by a visting nurse who can call only three times a week).

Use

The only undisputed indication for chronic digoxin in heart failure is control of ventricular rate in rapid atrial fibrillation. However, mild persistent hemodynamic benefit has been demonstrated in severely compromised patients in sinus rhythm who are inadequately controlled on diuretics, presumably as a consequence of its positive inotropic effect. It is therefore probably useful to control symptoms in such patients. Digoxin is usually given orally but if this is impossible, or if a rapid effect is required, it can be given intravenously. Since the half-life ($t_{1/2}$) is approximately 1–2 days, repeated administration of a once daily maintenance dose (usually 0.125–0.5 mg, depending on estimated renal function) results in a plateau level in about 5–10 days. The dose may need to be adjusted based on plasma concentration determinations once steady state has been reached. This is quite acceptable in many settings, but if clinical circumstances are more urgent a therapeutic plasma concentration can be attained more rapidly by administering a loading dose, e.g. a single dose of 0.5 mg followed by 0.25 mg 8 hourly for three doses followed by the estimated once daily maintenance dose. In still more urgent situations digitalization can be initiated by an intravenous loading dose of 0.5 mg.

Mechanism of action

Digoxin inhibits membrane Na⁺/K⁺ adenosine triphosphatase (ATPase) which actively extrudes Na^+ from myocardial as well as other cells. This causes accumulation of intracellular Na$^+$ which indirectly increases intracellular Ca^{2+} content via reduced Na$^+$/Ca^{2+} exchange and increased intracellular Ca^{2+} storage. The rise in availability of intracellular Ca^{2+} accounts for the positive inotropic effect of digoxin. Excessive poisoning of Na$^+$/K$^+$-ATPase causes numerous non-cardiac as well as cardiac (arrhythmogenic) toxic effects of digoxin. Ventricular slowing results from several mechanisms (chapter 29) particularly the effect of increased vagal activity on the AV node. Slowing of ventricular rate improves cardiac output in patients with atrial fibrillation by improving ventricular filling during diastole. Clinical progress is assessed by measuring heart rate (at the apex): successful control is usually gained at apical rates of 70–80/min.

Adverse effects and contraindications

Digoxin has a low therapeutic index. Studies of the prevalence of intoxication have yielded figures of 15–20% for hospital inpatients receiving the drug. As digoxin preparations have become more pure the incidence of gastrointestinal symptoms (nausea, vomiting and diarrhea) as the harbinger of toxicity has decreased, but today the initial indication of intoxication can be a fatal cardiac arrhythmia. Before using digoxin it is important to consider the possibility of Wolff–Parkinson–White (WPW) syndrome, in which digoxin is contraindicated. Digoxin can cause ventricular fibrillation in such patients.

Pharmacokinetics

Currently available preparations of digoxin disperse rapidly and uniformly, although this has not always been so in the past. Approximately 80% of administered digoxin is excreted unchanged in the urine in subjects with normal renal function. It is eliminated mainly by glomerular filtration, although a small amount is subject to both tubular secretion and reabsorption. A small amount of digoxin undergoes metabolism to inactive products or excretion via the bile and elimination in feces. The proportion eliminated by these non-renal clearance mechanisms increases in patients with renal impairment,

being 100% in anephric patients in whom $t_{1/2}$ is approximately 4.5 days.

It is sometimes useful to measure digoxin plasma concentration. Blood should be sampled more than 6 hours after an oral dose or immediately before the next dose is due (trough level). The usual therapeutic range is 1–2 ng/ml, although toxicity can occur at concentrations of less than 1.5 ng/ml in some individuals. Plasma concentration determination is useful in patients in sinus rhythm in whom there is no simple pharmacodynamic measure of response analogous to apical heart rate in patients with atrial fibrillation.

Drug interactions

Digoxin has a steep dose–response curve and narrow therapeutic range, and clinically important interactions are common (chapter 12 and p. 367). Pharmacokinetic interactions with digoxin include reduced absorption, which can result in loss of efficacy (e.g. antacid, bile acid binding resins, tetracyclines), and combined pharmacokinetic effects involving displacement from tissue binding sites and reduced renal elimination (e.g. digoxin toxicity due to concurrent treatment with quinidine, verapamil or amiodarone).

Pharmacodynamic interactions involving digoxin are also important: in particular, drugs causing hypokalemia (e.g. diuretics, β-agonists, carbenoxolone) predispose to digoxin toxicity by increasing its binding to (and effect on) Na$^+$/K$^+$-ATPase. Drugs causing hypomagnesemia (e.g. diuretics, alcohol excess) also predispose to digoxin toxicity.

SYMPATHOMIMETIC AMINES

Use

Sympathomimetic amines are sometimes used in acute severe heart failure with hypoperfusion (shock). Before sympathomimetic amines are employed to treat severe hypotension from any cause, hypovolemia must be corrected. This requires careful monitoring, particularly when the cause is severe heart failure due to myocardial infarction (cardiogenic shock), and when measurement of pulmonary artery wedge pressure as an indicator of left-sided filling pressure using a Swann–Ganz catheter is particularly helpful. Sympathomimetic amines are given by a central line. Reliable constant rate infusion pumps are essential to avoid inadvertent bolus administration with the risk of direct cardiac toxicity (arrhythmia and sudden death). Adrenaline is not used for heart failure, although it is important in treatment of cardiac arrest (chapter 29) and anaphylactic shock (chapter 47). Noradrenaline is a potent β- and, especially, α-agonist. When injected parenterally it can precipitate tachyarrhythmias because of its β-agonist action, but paradoxically it can also cause secondary reflex bradycardia, initiated by the carotid sinus baroreceptors and mediated by the vagus. Despite causing increased cardiac contractility and increased oxygen demand, it may actually decrease cardiac output, and is now seldom used in severe cardiac failure having been supplanted by newer drugs, notably dobutamine.

Dobutamine is related chemically to isoprenaline but is predominantly a β$_1$-receptor agonist. It exerts a more prominent inotropic than chronotropic action than does isoprenaline. It does not release endogenous catecholamines and is less likely to cause arrhythmias than pressor doses of dopamine. It is the pressor agent of choice in patients with shock caused by myocardial infarction or following cardiac surgery, and is usually given with invasive monitoring on the intensive care unit in doses of 5–40 µg/kg/min. Although it causes some peripheral vasodilatation it does not dilate the renal vasculature. Thus in cardiogenic shock, a combination of dobutamine (to increase cardiac output) with low-dose dopamine (for its renal effect, see below), or with low-dose sodium nitroprusside (to reduce cardiac afterload) is often appropriate.

Dopamine is the biochemical precursor of noradrenaline, but also has transmitter functions in its own right in the central nervous system and probably in the innervation of the renal vasculature. It releases endogenous catecholamines including noradrenaline when given in high pharmacological doses, and is markedly pro-arrhythmogenic, probably for this reason. However, at low doses it has a selective vasodilator effect on the renal vascular bed mediated via specific dopamine receptors, and is particularly useful for this reason. Low dose dopamine, 2–5 µg/kg/min, stimulates renal dopamine receptors producing increased renal perfusion and urine output. Dopamine at this dose is often given with intravenous frusemide to produce diuresis. Cardiac output is slightly increased and peripheral resistance is slightly decreased by dopamine, so mean blood pressure is little altered. Low doses of dopamine may be combined with dobutamine to obtain the benefit of a pressor together with reduced renal vascular resistance.

Mechanism of action

Cardiovascular responses to sympathomimetic amines are mediated by α- and β-adrenoceptors. β-Receptors are coupled to adenylyl cyclase, and many effects of β-receptor stimulation are mediated by cyclic AMP (chapter 3); the second messenger system involved in mediating the effects of α-receptor stimulation are less well understood. Pharmacological effects of α- and β-receptor stimulation include:

1. α-Receptor stimulation leads to vasoconstriction.
2. β$_1$-Receptors are located in the heart and stimulation leads to increased heart rate and contractility.
3. β$_2$-Receptor stimulation dilates peripheral and coronary arteries and arterioles.
4. Dopamine receptors selectively vasodilate renal vasculature.

Adverse effects

The main concerns with sympathomimetic drugs are arrhythmias and that increased oxygen demand may cause infarct extension. Extravasation can cause tissue necrosis and it is essential to establish good venous access.

Pharmacokinetics

Dobutamine has a short $t_{1/2}$ (2 min) and is mainly eliminated by hepatic metabolism to glucuronides and 3-O-methyldobutamine. Dopamine also has a short plasma $t_{1/2}$, and is taken up into sympathetic nerves by uptake 1. It may consequently displace endogenous catecholamines from the nerve terminals. It is taken up from the cytoplasm by synaptic vesicles and converted by dopamine β-hydroxylase in the vesicles into noradrenaline which is subsequently available for release in response to nerve impulses. Alternatively, it may not gain access to vesicles but be metabolized in the nerve terminals to yield vanillyl mandelic acid which is excreted in the urine.

Drug interactions

The valuable pharmacodynamic interactions between dobutamine and dopamine, and between dobutamine and vasodilators such as sodium nitroprusside have already been mentioned. Adrenoceptor and dopamine receptor antagonists (such as chlorpromazine or haloperidol) predictably reduce the potency of these drugs, and patients in cardiogenic shock who have received them may require increased doses of sympathomimetic amines to compete with such antagonists.

PHOSPHODIESTERASE INHIBITORS

Phosphodiesterase (PDE) inactivates cyclic AMP, so it might be anticipated that inhibitors of this enzyme would to some extent mimic the actions of β-agonists, increasing the force of contraction of the heart and relaxing vascular smooth muscle. Such actions might be therapeutically useful, especially since phosphodiesterase inhibitors are active when given orally, unlike the sympathomimetic amines discussed above. Xanthine alkaloids (e.g. theophylline) are phosphodiesterase inhibitors, and were used in the past to treat patients with heart failure, but they are toxic and not very effective. Furthermore, some of their pharmacological effects are due to competitive antagonism at adenosine (A_2) receptors and other biochemical actions distinct from their action on cyclic nucleotide phosphodiesterase.

Inhibitors with specificity for different isoenzymes of PDE have been developed, some of which have clinical potential. The most extensively studied isoenzyme is PDE III, and PDE III inhibitors (e.g. enoximone, amrinone, milrinone) are positively inotropic vasodilators, and also inhibit platelet aggregation. Short-term administration of amrinone to patients with heart failure increases cardiac output and lowers ventricular filling pressure. However, long-term administration has not been shown to be beneficial, and may indeed shorten survival. Adverse effects include hypotension (secondary to vasodilatation), cardiac arrhythmias (probably secondary to increased cAMP in cardiac cells), thrombocytopenia and, in the case of enoximone, hepatotoxicity. At present these drugs do not play a major role in the treatment of heart failure, although it is possible that more selective PDE III inhibitors presently under development will do so in future.

Cardiac Arrhythmias

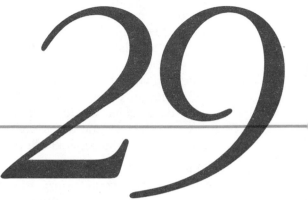

Pathophysiology **350**

Common arrhythmias **351**

General principles of management **352**

Classification of antiarrhythmic drugs **353**

Cardiopulmonary resuscitation: basic life support **354**

Cardiac arrest: advanced life support **354**

Treatment of other specific arrhythmias **355**

Selected antiarrhythmic drugs **358**

PATHOPHYSIOLOGY

The chambers of the heart contract in a coordinated manner, pumping blood efficiently around the body. Coordination is achieved by a specialized conducting system. Excitation involves triggering a propagated action potential, which is coupled to contraction by changes in cytoplasmic Ca^{2+} concentration. Cardiac cells share some of the properties of other excitable tissues such as nerve and striated muscle, including:

1. An inside negative 'resting' potential caused by the concentration gradient of K^+ across a relatively K^+ permeable plasma membrane; and
2. A propagated action potential during which the potential inside the cells becomes positive with respect to the outside due to a rapid but transient increase in Na^+ permeability in the presence of high external Na^+ concentration and low cytoplasmic Na^+ concentration.

Cardiac tissues also have distinctive features of their own, including:

1. A prolonged depolarization phase of the action potential during which Ca^{2+} enters through voltage-dependent Ca^{2+} channels; and
2. The capacity of some cardiac tissues to develop spontaneous pacemaker activity.

Some cardiac tissues have the capacity to develop pacemaker activity: the most rapid pacemaker, usually the sinoatrial (SA) node, captures the system and determines the heart rate. Action potentials propagate from the SA node to atrial myocytes and also through specialized pathways in the atria to the atrioventricular (AV) node, then via the bundle of His and Purkinje fibers to the ventricular myocytes. Repolarization follows depolarization, leaving the cells refractory for a brief interval, after which the cycle is repeated. This cycle of orderly propagated depolarization originating in the SA node followed by repolarization is called sinus rhythm. Sinus rhythm is influenced by nervous activity (e.g. it is slowed by the vagus nerve which releases acetylcholine that acts on muscarinic receptors to increase the K^+ permeability of the cardiac membrane, and accelerated by sympathetic nerves which release noradrenaline that acts on cardiac β-receptors) and by endocrine mechanisms (e.g. circulating catecholamines and thyroxine). These control mechanisms permit the heart rate to adapt appropriately in accord with varying physiological demands, such as exercise.

The cycle of propagated orderly depolarization followed by repolarization is generally extremely reliable, occurring some 2.5–3 $\times 10^9$ times in a human lifetime. This reliability depends on a 'fall-back' mechanism, whereby if impulse generation in the SA node fails, another pacemaker lower down the conducting system takes over, and if *that* pacemaker fails, it is in turn supplanted by another and so on. The cost of this safety net is the innate tendency of cells throughout the heart to initiate independent 'ectopic' (i.e. outside the SA node) pacemakers. Occasional ectopic beats are not sinister. Rarely, however, because of the innate automaticity of cardiac tissue, ectopic beats initiate repetitive activity resulting in an *arrhythmia*. Under pathological circumstances (e.g. in the presence of an abnormal anatomical pathway, or following myocardial infarction, or if there is an abnormal balance of inorganic ions or of chemical mediators) this arrhythmia can temporarily or permanently interrupt sinus rhythm.

COMMON ARRHYTHMIAS

Supraventricular

ARISING FROM THE SINUS NODE
Sinus tachycardia
In sinus tachycardia the rate is 100–150/min with normal P waves and PR interval. Treatment is directed to the underlying cause: for example, pain, anxiety, left ventricular failure, asthma, thyrotoxicosis, iatrogenic.

Sinus bradycardia
The rate is less than 60/min with normal complexes in sinus bradycardia. It is a common finding in athletes, young healthy individuals and patients taking β-blockers. It also occurs in patients with raised intracranial pressure or SA node disease ('sick-sinus syndrome'). It requires treatment only if it causes or threatens hemodynamic compromise.

ATRIAL ARRHYTHMIAS
Atrial fibrillation
The atrial rate in atrial fibrillation is >350/min with variable AV conduction resulting in an irregular pulse. If the AV node conducts rapidly, ventricular response is also rapid. Ventricular filling is consequently inadequate and cardiac output falls. The most important methods of treating atrial fibrillation are either to convert it to sinus rhythm, or to slow conduction through the AV node, slowing ventricular rate and improving cardiac output even though the rhythm remains abnormal.

Atrial flutter
Atrial flutter has a rate of 250–350/min with fixed ventricular conduction, for example atrial rate 300/min with 3:1 block gives a ventricular rate of 100/min.

NODAL AND OTHER SUPRAVENTRICULAR ARRHYTHMIAS
Atrioventricular block
- **First degree** prolongation of the PR interval.
- **Second degree** is of two types, Mobitz type I in which the PR interval lengthens progressively until a P wave fails to be conducted to the ventricles (Wenckebach phenomenon) and Mobitz type II in which there is a constant PR interval with variable failure to conduct to the ventricles.
- **Third degree** complete AV dissociation with emergence of an idioventricular rhythm (usually <50/min). Severe cerebral underperfusion with syncope sometimes followed by convulsions (Stokes–Adams attacks) results. The importance of first and second degree block is that they may presage complete heart block. Sinoatrial block can also cause symptomatic bradycardia in patients with 'sick-sinus syndrome'.

Supraventricular tachycardias
Supraventricular tachycardia (SVT) is caused by re-entry circuits and leads to rapid, narrow complex tachycardias at rates of approximately 150/min. Not uncommonly in older patients the rapid rate leads to failure of conduction in one or other bundle and 'aberrant' conduction with broad complexes because of the rate-dependent bundle branch block. This can be difficult to distinguish from ventricular tachycardia, treatment of which is different in important respects. In cases of broad complex tachycardia where the diagnosis is uncertain bolus injections of *adenosine* (see below) can be diagnostically helpful.

Distinct types of SVT include intranodal and extranodal.

Intranodal supraventricular tachycardia

Fiber tracts in the AV node are arranged longitudinally and if differences in refractoriness develop between adjacent fibers then an atrial impulse may be conducted antegradely through one set of fibers and retrogradely through another leading to a re-entry ('circus') tachycardia.

Extranodal supraventricular tachycardia

An anatomically separate accessory pathway is present through which conduction is faster and the refractory period shorter than in the AV node. The cardiogram usually shows a shortened PR interval (because the abnormal pathway conducts more rapidly from atria to ventricle than does the AV node) sometimes with a widened QRS complex with a slurred upstroke or delta wave, due to arrival of the impulse in part of the ventricle where it must pass through unspecialized slowly conducting ventricular myocytes instead of through specialized Purkinje fibers (Wolff–Parkinson–White or WPW syndrome). Alternatively there may be a short PR interval but a normal QRS complex (Lown–Ganong–Levine syndrome) if the abnormal pathway connects with the physiological conducting system distal to the AV node.

VENTRICULAR ARRHYTHMIAS

1. **Ventricular ectopic beats** are abnormal QRS complexes originating irregularly from ectopic foci within the ventricles.
2. **Ventricular tachycardia** the cardiogram shows rapid, wide QRS complexes (>0.14 s); the patient is usually, but not always, hypotensive and poorly perfused. This rhythm may presage ventricular fibrillation.
3. **Ventricular fibrillation** the cardiogram is chaotic; circulatory arrest occurs immediately.

GENERAL PRINCIPLES OF MANAGEMENT

1. Antiarrhythmic drugs are among the most dangerous at the clinician's disposal. Always think carefully before prescribing one.
2. If the patient is acutely very ill on account of a cardiac arrhythmia, the most appropriate treatment is almost never a drug: in bradyarrhythmia consider pacing; in tachyarrhythmia consider DC cardioversion. Consider the possibility of hyperkalemia or other electrolyte disorder, especially in renal disease, and treat accordingly.
3. Treat the patient not the cardiogram: remember that unattractive looking electrocardiographic (ECG) abnormalities may not necessarily be bad prognostic signs in themselves, and that several antiarrhythmic drugs can themselves cause arrhythmias and shorten life. When arrhythmias are prognostically bad, this often reflects severe underlying cardiac disease which is not improved by an antiarrhythmic drug but may be improved by, for example, a converting enzyme inhibitor (for heart failure) or by aspirin or oxygen (for ischemic heart disease) or by operation (valvular heart disease).
4. In an acutely ill patient consider the possible immediate cause of the rhythm disturbance. This may be within the heart, for example myocardial infarction, ventricular aneurysm, valvular or congenital heart disease, or elswhere in the body, for example pulmonary embolism, infection or pain (e.g. from a distended bladder in a stuporose patient).
5. Look for reversible processes that contribute to the maintenance of the rhythm disturbance (e.g. hypoxia, acidosis, pain, electrolyte disturbance including Mg^{2+} as well as K^+ and Ca^{2+}, thyrotoxicosis, excessive alcohol or caffeine intake or proarrhythmic drugs), and correct them.
6. Avoid 'cocktails' of drugs.

CLASSIFICATION OF ANTIARRHYTHMIC DRUGS

The classification of antiarrhythmic drugs is not very satisfactory. The Singh–Vaughan Williams classification (I–IV) based on *in vitro* effects on the cardiac action potential is widely used, but unfortunately does not predict reliably which rhythm disturbances will respond to which drug. Consequently selection of what antiarrhythmic drug to use in a particular patient remains largely empirical. Furthermore, this classification does not include some of the most clinically useful antiarrhythmic drugs, such as digoxin, atropine or adenosine.

Class I

Class I drugs block fast Na^+ channels, thereby slowing the upstroke of the cardiac action potential and are sometimes referred to as 'membrane stabilizing'. These are subdivided into classes Ia and Ib. Class Ia are quinidine-like drugs which additionally slow repolarization hence slightly prolonging the action potential; disopyramide is an example that is used clinically. Class Ib drugs, in addition to blocking Na^+ channels, also speed repolarization. Lignocaine is a clinically important example, but has to be given intravenously. Attempts to discover an 'orally active lignocaine' have yielded several drugs with superficially similar electrophysiological effects such as tocainide and mexilitene, but despite being 'class Ib' agents these behave clinically quite unlike lignocaine. Phenytoin has antiarrhythmic properties on the heart as well as on the brain, and is also a class Ib drug. It is however seldom used for its cardiac properties, although it has been used in patients with digoxin-induced arrhythmias. Class Ic drugs (e.g. flecainide, encainide, propafenone) inhibit conduction in the His–Purkinje system, thereby prolonging the QRS interval, in addition to blocking Na^+ channels. There is concern that these drugs predispose to polymorphic ventricular tachycardia which can degenerate into ventricular fibrillation, and indeed clinical trials indicate that they shorten life in some patients.

Class II

Class II drugs are β-adrenoceptor antagonists which reduce the rate of rise of the pacemaker potential.

Class III

These drugs prolong the plateau phase of the cardiac action potential, thereby increasing the absolute refractory period (i.e. the time that must elapse after an action potential before the tissue is again capable of generating an action potential). Such drugs reduce the likelihood of an ectopic pacemaker capturing the system or of a re-entrant pathway becoming perpetuated, and indeed amiodarone and sotalol, the most important drugs of this class, are extremely effective against both ventricular and supraventricular arrhythmias.

Class IV

Class IV drugs are Ca^{2+} antagonists which block voltage-dependent L-type Ca^{2+} channels. Verapamil, a phenylalkylamine, is particularly effective at blocking such channels in AV conducting tissues, and is used acutely to terminate SVT (although this has decreased with the increased availability of adenosine) or chronically in prophylaxis. In conjunction with digoxin it controls

ventricular rate in patients with rapid atrial fibrillation inadequately responsive to digoxin alone.

CARDIOPULMONARY RESUSCITATION: BASIC LIFE SUPPORT

When a person is found collapsed, make a quick check to make sure no live power lines are in the immediate vicinity. Call 'are you all right?'. If there is no response, call for help. Do not move the patient if neck trauma is suspected. Otherwise roll them on their back (on a firm surface if possible) and loosen clothing round the throat. Assess **A**irway, **B**reathing, **C**irculation (ABC).

Tilt the head and lift the chin, and sweep an index finger through the mouth to clear any obstruction (e.g. dentures). Tight fitting dentures need not be removed, and may help maintain the mouth sealed during assisted ventillation.

If the patient is not breathing spontaneously, start mouth to mouth (or, if available, mouth to mask) ventilation. Inflate the lungs with two expirations (1–1.5 s), and check that the chest falls between respirations. One

hundred per cent oxygen should be used if available.

Check for a pulse by feeling carefully for the carotid or femoral artery before diagnosing cardiac arrest. If the arrest has been witnessed, administer a single thump to the precordium. Start cardiac compression two finger breadths above the xiphisternum at a rate of 60–80/min and an excursion of 1.5–2 in. For a single operator allow two breaths per 15 chest compressions, if there are two operators give one breath every five compressions. Drugs can cause fixed dilated pupils so do not give up on this account if drug overdose is a possibility. Hypothermia is protective of tissue function so do not give up too readily if the patient is severely hypothermic (e.g. after being pulled out of a freezing lake): mobilize facilities for active warming.

CARDIAC ARREST: ADVANCED LIFE SUPPORT

Basic cardiopulmonary resuscitation is continued throughout as described above; it should not be interrupted for more than 10 s (except for administration of DC shock when personnel apart from the operator must stand well back). 'Advanced' life support refers to the treatment of cardiac arrhythmias in the setting of cardiopulmonary arrest. The electrocardiogram is likely to show asystole, severe bradycardia or ventricular fibrillation; occasionally narrow complexes are present but there is no detectable cardiac output

('electromechanical dissociation'). These are considered in this section, the doses suggested being for an average sized adult; during the course of an arrest other rhythm disturbances are frequently encountered in addition (e.g. sinus bradycardia) and these are considered in the next section on other specific arrhythmias. If intravenous access cannot be established giving double doses of adrenaline, atropine or lignocaine as appropriate via an endotracheal tube can be life saving.

Asystole

Make sure ECG leads are attached properly, and that the rhythm is not ventricular fibrillation, which is sometimes mistaken for asystole if the fibrillation waves are of low amplitude. If there is doubt DC countershock (200 J). Once the diagnosis is *definite* administer adrenaline, 1 mg, intravenously, followed by atropine, 2 mg, intravenously. If P waves (or other electrical activity) are present consider pacing.

Ventricular fibrillation

The following sequence is used until a rhythm (hopefully sinus) is achieved that sustains a cardiac output: DC countershock (200 J) is delivered as soon as a defibrillator is available and repeated (200 J, then 360 J) if necessary, followed by adrenaline, 1 mg, intravenously and further defibrillation (360 J) repeated as necessary. Consider varying the paddle positions and consider other antiarrhythmic drugs, notably amiodarone, 300 mg, intravenously or bretylium, 500–1000 mg.

During prolonged resuscitation attempts adrenaline, 1 mg, intravenously is recommended every 5 min. Calcium salts should not be given into the same line as sodium bicarbonate (which is used only in severe acidosis) as this combination results in precipitation in the line.

Electromechanical dissociation

When the pulse is absent but the ECG shows QRS complexes this is known as electromechanical dissociation. This may be the result of severe global damage to the left ventricle in which case the outlook is bleak. If caused by some potentially reversible pathology such as hypovolemia, pneumothorax, pericardial tamponade or pulmonary embolus, volume replacement or other specific measures may be dramatically effective. Adrenaline, 1 mg, intravenously followed by calcium chloride, 10 ml of 10% solution, should be considered.

*T*REATMENT OF OTHER SPECIFIC ARRHYTHMIAS

Tachyarrhythmias

SUPRAVENTRICULAR TACHYCARDIA

Atrial fibrillation/flutter

Acute
DC cardioversion is the treatment of choice when the patient is in shock.

Digoxin (orally or intravenously) is useful if the patient is not in shock. It slows ventricular rate by increasing AV block, and about half of such patients revert to sinus rhythm. Intravenous verapamil (given slowly) is an effective alternative but is a negative inotrope and can precipitate acute heart failure.

DC shock can cause dangerous arrhythmias in patients who are overdigitalized. To avoid this, the plasma concentration of digoxin should be measured and if possible >24 hours should elapse after the last dose of digoxin, unless cardioversion is required as an emergency. Low-energy countershock can be used in this situation, followed by higher energy shocks if necessary.

Long-term treatment
Patients who have not been in atrial fibrillation for too long and in whom the left atrium

is not irreversibly distended may revert 'spontaneously' to sinus rhythm. If this does not occur, such patients benefit from elective DC cardioversion, following which many remain in sinus rhythm. The main hazard is embolization of cerebral or peripheral arteries from thrombus that may have accumulated in the left atrial appendage. Patients should therefore be anticoagulated before elective cardioversion (usually for 4–6 weeks) to prevent new and friable thrombus from accumulating and permit any existing thrombus to organize, thereby reducing the risk of embolization. An alternative currently undergoing controlled clinical trial is to perform early cardioversion following acute anticoagulation, provided transesophageal echocardiography shows no evidence of thrombus in the left atrial appendage, anticoagulation being continued for 1 month if the patient remains in sinus rhythm. Anticoagulation should be continued long term if fibrillation persists or intermittent episodes of arrhythmia recur.

In patients in whom cardioversion is inappropriate (e.g. patients with a chronically enlarged left atrium caused by mitral stenosis in whom sinus rhythm is unlikely to persist even if it can be achieved), digoxin (given by mouth) is the drug of choice. Digoxin is not always adequate to control ventricular rate and verapamil or a β-blocker (particularly sotalol, because of its additional class III action) may be added. Amiodarone is very effective in atrial fibrillation, but is only used when other drugs have failed because of its toxicity (see below).

Paroxysmal supraventricular tachycardias

Vagal stimulation (e.g. by carotid sinus massage, facial immersion in cold water, Valsalva maneuver or pressure on the eyeballs) may be effective in terminating the arrhythmia abruptly. If vagal maneuvers are ineffective, the next choice is adenosine, given as a rapid intravenous bolus (in increasing doses if necessary). Although negatively inotropic it is cleared rapidly and this effect is brief. Verapamil (10 mg intravenously over 5–10 min) is also a negative

inotrope, and is cleared much less rapidly than adenosine. It is still sometimes used to terminate SVT in the absence of hemodynamic compromise, although it must be avoided if the patient has been treated with a β-adrenoceptor antagonist as this combination causes circulatory collapse. β-Adrenoceptor antagonists are themselves effective in terminating SVT, but are contraindicated in the presence of hemodynamic compromise or following treatment with verapamil and are now seldom used.

Patients with underlying heart disease may be hemodynamically compromised by SVT. The best treatment in such cases is usually DC cardioversion, as most drugs used to terminate SVT are negatively inotropic and can be disastrous in this setting. Cardiac glycosides are an important exception, and intravenous ouabain (the most rapidly acting glycoside) or digoxin can be considered in circumstances where DC shock is relatively contraindicated (e.g. postoperatively in cardiac patients who have undergone sternotomy). The decision is often not easy, because of (1) the extra risk of DC shock if this has to be undertaken in a patient after administration of a glycoside mentioned above, and (2) the possibility of previously undiagnosed WPW syndrome. Supraventricular tachycardia in WPW may be worsened by cardiac glycosides and verapamil because they may dangerously accelerate anterograde conduction and thus increase ventricular rate. Delta waves are not present on the ECG in patients with WPW during attacks when conduction through the pathological pathway is retrogradal, so the syndrome can be very difficult to recognize. The rapidity of the ventricular response may warn the clinician of this possibility, and thus that digoxin is contraindicated. Amiodarone is effective in SVT as well as in VT, and can be given slowly intravenously; it is less negatively inotropic than verapamil or β-adrenoceptor antagonists, but is not without hazard. If used, blood pressure should be monitored carefully.

Recurrence of SVT may not occur. Overindulgence in caffeine or alcohol should be avoided, and smoking prohibited. If attacks do recur frequently and do not respond to simple vagal maneuvers, prophylactic treatment with an oral β-adrenoceptor antagonist or verapamil may be effective.

Ventricular arrhythmias

Ventricular ectopic beats

Electrolyte disturbance, smoking, alcohol abuse and excessive caffeine consumption should be sought and corrected if present. The only justification for treating patients with antiarrhythmic drugs in an attempt to reduce the frequency of ventricular ectopic beats (VE) in a chronic setting is if the ectopic beats cause intolerable palpitations, or if they precipitate attacks of more serious tachyarrhythmia such as ventricular tachycardia or fibrillation, which is seldom the case. If palpitations are so unpleasant as to warrant treatment despite the suspicion that this may shorten rather than prolong life, an oral agent class I such as disopyramide or quinidine may be considered. Sotalol with its combination of class II and III actions is a more attractive alternative, although long-term trials with hard clinical endpoints such as survival are still awaited.

In an acute setting (most commonly the immediate aftermath of myocardial infarction), treatment to suppress ventricular ectopic beats may be warranted if these are running together to form brief recurrent episodes of ventricular tachycardia, or if frequent ectopic beats are present following cardioversion from ventricular fibrillation. Lignocaine is used in such situations, being given as an intravenous bolus followed by an infusion to attempt to reduce the risk of sustained ventricular tachycardia or ventricular fibrillation.

Ventricular tachycardia

If the differential diagnosis from a supraventricular broad complex tachycardia (above) is not in doubt, treatment is usually by DC cardioversion. As an alternative, a bolus of 50–100 mg lignocaine followed by an infusion (1–4 mg/min) with constant monitoring in an intensive care unit may be considered if the rate is less than 170/min and the blood pressure well maintained. If the tachycardia is refractory or poorly tolerated, DC cardioversion followed by lignocaine infusion is indicated. Intravenous amiodarone is used for patients refractory to lignocaine.

Ventricular fibrillation

See above under 'Advanced life support'.

Bradyarrhythmias

ASYSTOLE

See above under 'Cardiac arrest'.

SINUS BRADYCARDIA

1. Raising the foot of the bed may be successful in increasing cardiac output and cerebral perfusion.
2. Atropine (see below).
3. Discontinue digoxin, β-blockers, verapamil or other drugs that exacerbate bradycardia.
4. Pacemaker insertion is indicated if bradycardia is unresponsive to atropine and is causing significant hypotension.

SICK SINUS SYNDROME (TACHYCARDIA–BRADYCARDIA SYNDROME)

Treatment is difficult. If the patient is symptomatic from bradycardia, atropine may be used. Digoxin or other drugs may be used for the tachycardias. However, drugs useful for one rhythm state often aggravate the other and a pacemaker is often used to control bradycardia so that the tachycardias can be treated with appropriate drugs.

ATRIOVENTRICULAR CONDUCTION BLOCK

- **First-degree** heart block by itself does not require treatment, but if associated with sinus bradycardia it may be treated with atropine.
- **Second-degree** Mobitz type I block (Wenckebach block) is relatively benign and often transient. If complete block occurs the escape pacemaker is situated

relatively high up in the bundle so that the rate is 50–60/min with narrow QRS complexes. Atropine (0.6–1.2 mg intravenously) is usually effective. Mobitz type II block is more serious and may progress unpredictably to complete block with a slow escape ventricular rate. The only reliable treatment is a pacemaker.

- **Third-degree** heart block (complete AV dissociation) can cause cardiac failure. Treatment is by electrical pacing; if delay in arranging this is absolutely unavoidable isoprenaline may be used as a temporizing measure. Congenital complete heart block, diagnosed incidentally, does not usually require treatment.

SELECTED ANTIARRHYTHMIC DRUGS

LIGNOCAINE AND OTHER CLASS I DRUGS

Use

Lignocaine is the drug of first choice for the treatment of ventricular tachycardia and fibrillation. The therapeutic plasma concentration range is 1.5–4.0 mg/l. This is achieved rapidly by giving a bolus of 50–100 mg intravenously over 1 min followed by an infusion of 4 mg/min for 1 hour reducing to 2 mg/min for 2 hours and to 1 mg/min thereafter for a period not usually exceeding 36–48 hours. Lower doses are required in patients with shock or severe hepatic dysfunction in whom the initial infusion should not exceed 1 mg/min. The difference between therapeutic and toxic plasma concentrations is small.

If the patient shows no signs of lignocaine toxicity and break-through ventricular tachycardia or fibrillation occur, then a further 100 mg bolus may be given over 2 min and the infusion rate increased to 4 mg/min as appropriate to suppress the arrhythmia.

Mechanism of action

Lignocaine is a class Ib agent that blocks Na^+ channels, reducing the rate of rise of the cardiac action potential and increasing the effective refractory period.

Adverse effects

1. **Central nervous system** drowsiness, twitching, paresthesia, nausea and vomiting, focal followed by generalized seizures.
2. **Cardiovascular system** bradycardia, cardiac depression (negative inotropic effect), asystole.

Pharmacokinetics

Oral bioavailability is poor (30%) and lignocaine is given intravenously. It is metabolized in the liver, its clearance being limited by hepatic blood flow. Heart failure reduces lignocaine clearance predisposing to toxicity unless the dose is reduced. Monoethylglycylxylidide (MEGX) and glycylxylidide (GX) are active metabolites with less antiarrhythmic action than lignocaine but with central nervous system toxicity. Mean lignocaine half-life is approximately 2 hours in healthy subjects with an apparent volume of distribution of approximately 1.5 l/kg.

Drug interactions

Negative inotropes reduce the clearance of lignocaine by reducing hepatic blood flow, and consequently predispose to lignocaine accumulation and toxicity.

Other class I drugs

Other class I drugs have been widely used in the past, but are now used much less frequently. Physicians will however continue to encounter patients treated chronically with one or other of these agents and so a brief account of quinidine, disopyramide and flecainide is provided here.

Quinidine

Quinidine is used to reduce the frequency of ventricular ectopic beats that are causing intolerable palpitations and for prevention of recurrent ventricular arrhythmias. Its use has been largely curtailed because of its unpleasant and potentially dangerous adverse effects. Quinidine is usually given orally as a sustained-release preparation (500 mg twice daily). The intravenous route is dangerous and is avoided (except to treat comatose patients for chloroquine-resistant falciparum malaria, Chapter 44).

Quinidine is the D-isomer of quinine (and is itself a potent antimalarial drug). It has class Ia activity, reducing the rate of rise of the cardiac action potential by inhibiting Na^+ channels, and interfering with repolarization thereby modestly prolonging action potential duration. These effects cause prolongation of the effective refractory period, which probably accounts for its antiarrhythmic action.

Concurrent administration of quinidine with digoxin leads to a two- to three-fold increase in plasma digoxin levels. The mechanism is complex: quinidine displaces digoxin from tissue binding sites, so transiently increasing its plasma concentration even if the first dose of quinidine is administered after discontinuing digoxin some hours previously. In addition, quinidine reduces the renal clearance of digoxin so the maintenance dose of digoxin must be reduced to avoid its plasma concentration climbing to a new steady-state level. This interaction was probably responsible for many of the severe dysrhythmias once attributed solely to quinidine. Quinidine potentiates warfarin.

Adverse effects effects of quinidine are common:

1. Cardiovascular effects are important and can be fatal, including atrioventricular and ventricular block, ventricular arrhythmias and depressed myocardial contractility. Quinidine syncope is due to ventricular tachycardia and can occur with plasma concentrations within or below the therapeutic range. The major effect of quinidine on the ECG is prolongation of the QRS and QT intervals. (It should be discontinued if QRS duration exceeds 0.14 s or widens by >50%.)
2. Cinchonism is the complex of symptoms caused by excessive doses of quinidine or quinine (which is extracted from cinchona bark, hence the term 'cinchonism'). These comprise tinnitus, headache, nausea, visual disturbances including altered color perception, diplopia and night blindness. Vertigo and deafness occur with large doses.
3. Gastrointestinal disturbances (nausea, diarrhea and vomiting) are the most common problems in clinical use.
4. Thrombocytopenia is due to hypersensitivity reaction involving antibodies against a plasma protein–quinidine complex. Bone marrow suppression also occurs as a direct effect on the marrow.

Quinidine is contraindicated in heart block, hyperkalemia, digitalis intoxication, heart failure and hypotensive states.

Disopyramide

Disopyramide is used for similar indications as quinidine. Intravenous use is seldom indicated except during electrodiagnostic studies. It is a class Ia drug but also has pronounced antimuscarinic activity which is probably more relevant to its adverse effects than to its efficacy.

Adverse effects of disopyramide include atropine-like (antimuscarinic) effects which occur at therapeutic doses, consisting of dry mouth, blurred vision, raised intraocular pressure, urinary hesitancy and constipation. Disopyramide is therefore contraindicated in men with prostatic symptoms and in patients with glaucoma. It is a pronounced negative inotrope and a history of heart failure is a contraindication to its use. QT prolongation and various intracardiac blocks occur, and bundle branch block or hemiblock is consequently also a contraindication.

Disopyramide potentiates the action of coumarin anticoagulants. Unlike quinidine, it does not interact with digoxin. Hypokalemia (e.g. from diuretics) antagonizes disopyramide.

Flecainide

Flecainide is given by mouth or intravenously, with continuous electrocardiographic monitoring, for the rapid control of arrhythmias. Flecainide suppresses premature ventricular beats, but it is not justified to use it solely for this indication in view of evidence that it increases mortality during chronic treatment of patients with ventricular ectopics or runs of asymptomatic non-sustained ventricular tachycardia. Flecainide does, however, continue to have a place in treating SVT, atrial flutter and atrial fibrillation in patients with WPW syndrome. It is a class Ic drug.

Adverse effects of flecainide may be fatal and include heart failure, conduction system block or ventricular proarrhythmic effects. The drug is generally well tolerated, but symptomatic effects related to its local anesthetic properties occur, including light headedness, ataxia, blurred vision, nausea, vomiting, headache and anxiety. It is contraindicated in patients with heart failure or with disease of the conducting system.

β-ADRENOCEPTOR ANTAGONISTS

Use (see chapter 25 for use in hypertension)

The antiarrhythmic properties of β-adrenoceptor antagonists are useful in several clinical situations:

1. Inappropriate sinus tachycardia (e.g. in association with panic attacks).
2. Paroxysmal supraventricular tachycardias that are precipitated by emotion or exercise.
3. Rapid atrial fibrillation that is inadequately controlled by digoxin.
4. Tachyarrhythmias of thyrotoxicosis.
5. Tachyarrhythmias of pheochromocytoma, after adequate α-receptor blockade.
6. Patients who have survived myocardial infarction, irrespective of any ECG evidence of arrhythmia. β-Adrenoceptor antagonists are effective in prolonging life

in such individuals. (Evidence is strongest following Q wave infarction.)

Atenolol, 2.5 mg, over 2.5 min, repeated at 5 min intervals as needed to a maximum total dose of 10 mg is available for intravenous use after myocardial infarction. Esmolol is a cardioselective β-adrenoceptor antagonist for intravenous use with a short duration of action (half-life, $t_{1/2}$, approximately 10 min). β-Adrenoceptor antagonists are given more commonly by mouth when used for the above indications. Oral doses of atenolol greater than 100 mg or of metoprolol greater than 200 mg are seldom needed.

Varieties of β-adrenoceptor blockers

β-Adrenoceptor antagonists may have several properties in addition to their primary effect of competitive antagonism of agonists at β-adrenoceptors. Adrenoceptors are classified α or β, with further subdivisions into α_1/α_2 and β_1/β_2 based on the effects of different agonists and antagonists (see chapter 25). Some β-adrenoceptor antagonists have additional actions on α-receptors. Cardioselective β-blockers (e.g. atenolol, metoprolol) inhibit β_1-receptors. Some β-blockers (e.g. oxprenolol, pindolol) are partial agonists and some have membrane stabilizing or vasodilator activity. Several such drugs are racemates, and their different properties may be contributed in differing degrees by the different isomers, raising the possibility of more selective products in future. The importance of these pharmacological differences has not yet proved great in clinical practice, however.

Mechanism of action

Excessive concentrations of cyclic adenosine monophosphate (cAMP) in cardiac myocytes are arrhythmogenic. β-Agonists cause arrhythmias by increasing cyclic AMP by activating adenylyl cyclase. β-Adrenoceptor antagonists inhibit this. Ancillary properties of β-adrenoceptor antagonists (e.g. cardioselectivity, partial agonist action, membrane stabilizing action) are not generally important in determining their antiarrhythmic activity. Optical isomers with similar membrane stabilizing but markedly different β-antagonist potencies have antiarrhythmic activities that closely parallel their β-blocking potencies.

Adverse effects

In addition to causing serious problems in patients in whom β-blockers are contraindicated (below), β-blocking drugs cause a variety of symptoms in healthy individuals. Fatigue, cold extremities, sexual dysfunction and loss of motivation and *joie de vivre* are common. Less commonly β-adrenoceptor antagonists cause hallucinations or vivid and sometimes horrible dreams. β-Adrenoceptor antagonists may mask symptoms of hypoglycemia in insulin-dependent diabetics.

Contraindications

β-Blocking drugs, whether non-selective or cardioselective, can cause catastrophic airways obstruction in patients with pre-existing obstructive airways disease whether asthma, emphysema or chronic bronchitis, and are contraindicated in these conditions. Their negative inotropic action renders them dangerous in patients with heart failure. They also predictably worsen symptoms of claudication in patients with symptomatic atheromatous peripheral vascular disease. Patients with peripheral vasospasm should also not be prescribed β-blockers, as these will worsen symptoms of Raynaud's phenomenon.

Pharmacokinetics

β-Blockers are well absorbed when administered orally. Atenolol is highly polar and is eliminated by renal excretion, whereas metoprolol is less polar and is largely inactivated by hepatic metabolism.

Drug interactions

- β-Blockers inhibit drug metabolism indirectly by decreasing hepatic blood flow secondary to decreased cardiac output. This causes accumulation of drugs such as lignocaine that have so high a hepatic extraction ratio that their clearance reflects hepatic blood flow.

- Pharmacodynamic interactions: increased negative inotropic effects occur with verapamil (given intravenously this can be fatal), lignocaine, disopyramide or other negative inotropes. Exaggerated and prolonged hypoglycemia occurs with insulin and oral hypoglycemic drugs.

AMIODARONE

Use

Amiodarone is highly effective but its use is limited by the severity of its adverse effects. Amiodarone is effective in a wide variety of arrhythmias including:

1. **Supraventricular**: resistant atrial fibrillation or flutter, re-entrant tachycardias (e.g. WPW syndrome).
2. **Ventricular**: recurrent ventricular tachycardia or fibrillation.

Amiodarone administration does not preclude the use of DC cardioversion and may be used to maintain sinus rhythm if cardioversion is successful. Amiodarone is given intravenously via a central line to avoid thrombophlebitis. Initially 5 mg/kg in 250 ml of 5% glucose is infused over 20 min to 2 hours (to avoid hypotension) and may be repeated as needed up to 15 mg/kg/24 hours. In cardiac arrest with refractory or recurrent ventricular fibrillation amiodarone is given as a slow injection of 150–300 mg over 1–2 min. Oral treatment is started when response is established. For patients who have not received intravenous treatment, 200 mg three times a day for 7 days followed by 200 mg twice daily for a week and 200 mg once daily for a week (or until the desired effect is achieved) helps to establish adequate tissue levels reasonably quickly. The lowest effective dose, usually 100–200 mg daily, is used for maintenance.

Mechanism of action

Amiodarone is a class III agent, prolonging the duration of the action potential but with no effect on its rate of rise, prolonging repolarization by reducing the permeability of the cell membrane to outward potassium current. It also reduces the slope of diastolic depolarization (i.e. the pacemaker potential) and at the sinus node this action reduces the resting heart rate. Amiodarone delays atrial and AV nodal conduction but has no effect on ventricular conduction.

Adverse effects and contraindications

Adverse effects are many and varied and are common when plasma amiodarone concentration exceeds 2.5 mg/l.

1. **Cardiac effects** The ECG may show U waves or deformed T waves but these are not in themselves an indication to discontinue treatment. Amiodarone can cause ventricular tachycardia of the variety known as *torsades de pointes*. Care is needed in patients with heart failure and amiodarone is contraindicated in the presence of sinus bradycardia or AV block.
2. **Eye** Amiodarone causes corneal microdeposits eventually in almost all patients. Electron microscopy shows deposits (possibly of drug or metabolite) in tissue macrophages. These deposits form linear opacities radiating in a fan-like manner throughout the corneal epithelium from a point below the centre of the cornea (described as 'une image de la moustache du chat'). Patients may report colored haloes without change in visual acuity. The deposits are seen only on slit lamp examination and gradually regress if the drug is stopped.
3. **Skin** Photosensitivity rashes occur in 10–30% of patients. They are a phototoxic response to wavelengths in both the long ultraviolet (UVA) and visible parts of the spectrum so ordinary sunscreens (which only protect against UV below 320 nm) are ineffective. Topical compounds which reflect both UVA and visible light are needed (for example zinc oxide) and patients should be advised to forego exposure to direct sunlight and to wear a broad-brimmed hat in sunny weather. Patients sometimes develop blue-gray pigmentation of exposed areas. This is a separate phenomenon from phototoxicity.

4. **Thyroid** Amiodarone contains 37% iodine by weight and may precipitate hyperthyroidism in susceptible subjects, or conversely cause hypothyroidism. Amiodarone alters thyroid function tests and specific methods must be used. Usually there is a rise in thyroxine (T4) and reverse 3,5,3'-tri-iodothyronine (rT3) with a normal or low T3 and a flat thyroid-stimulating hormone (TSH) response to thyroid-relaxing hormone (TRH). Thyroid function (T3, T4 and TSH) should be assessed before starting treatment and thereafter annually, or more often if the clinical picture suggests thyroid dysfunction.
5. **Pulmonary fibrosis** (evidenced by dyspnea with interstitial infiltrates on chest X-ray) may develop with prolonged use. This usually but not always improves on stopping the drug. Improvement may be accelerated by prednisolone.
6. **Hepatitis** Transient elevation of hepatic enzymes may occur, and occasionally severe hepatitis develops.
7. **Peripheral neuropathy** occurs in the first month of treatment, and reverses on stopping amiodarone. Proximal muscle weakness, ataxia, tremor, nightmares, insomnia and headache are also reported.
8. **Gastrointestinal intolerance** and **cardiac failure** are unusual, but can be severe.

Pharmacokinetics

Amiodarone is variably absorbed (20–80%) when administered orally. However, both amiodarone and its main metabolite, desethyl amiodarone (the plasma concentration of which exceeds that of the parent drug), are highly lipid soluble. This is reflected in a very large volume of distribution (approximately 5000 litres). Amiodarone is highly plasma protein bound (>90%) and accumulates in all tissues, particularly heart. It is only slowly eliminated via the liver with a $t_{1/2}$ of 28–45 days. Consequently antiarrhythmic activity may continue for several months after amiodarone is stopped. The therapeutic range is 0.5–1.5 mg/l.

Drug interactions

Amiodarone potentiates warfarin by inhibiting its metabolism. It can precipitate digoxin toxicity (digoxin dose should be reduced by 50% when amiodarone is added), and cause severe bradycardia if used with β-adrenoceptor antagonists or verapamil.

SOTALOL

Use

Sotalol is safer than amiodarone, except in patients in whom β-adrenoceptor antagonists are contraindicated, and may be comparable to it in efficacy. The usual dose is 120–240 mg as a single dose by mouth daily. In urgent situations it can be given by slow intravenous injection: 20–60 mg over 3 min or longer with ECG monitoring, repeated if necessary after 10 min.

Mechanism of action

Sotalol is unique among β-adrenoceptor antagonists in possessing substantial class III activity. It is a racemate, the D-isomer possesses exclusively class III activity.

Adverse effects and contraindications

Sotalol appears to be considerably safer than amiodarone, but since it does prolong the cardiac action potential (detected on the ECG as a prolonged QT interval), it can cause ventricular tachycardia of the *torsade de pointes* variety like amiodarone. The β-blocking activity of sotolol contraindicates its use in patients with obstructive airways disease, heart failure, peripheral vascular disease or heart block.

Pharmacokinetics

Sotalol may be given by mouth once daily. It is extremely polar and is excreted unchanged in the urine. The dose should be reduced in patients with renal impairment (glomerular filtration rate <20 ml/min).

Drug interactions

Diuretics predispose to *torsades de pointes* by causing electrolyte disturbance (hypokalemia/ hypomagnesemia). Similarly other drugs that prolong the QT interval should be avoided. These include class Ia antiarrhythmic drugs (quinidine, disopyramide), which slow cardiac repolarization as well as depolarization, as well as several important psychotropic drugs including tricyclic antidepressants and phenothiazines. Histamine H_1 antagonists (terfenadine, astemizole) should be avoided for the same reason.

VERAPAMIL

Use

Verapamil is used as an antiarrhythmic:

1. To terminate SVT in patients who are not hemodynamically compromised. In this setting it is given intravenously over 5 min.
2. Prophylactically to reduce the risk of recurrent SVT by mouth (40–120 mg three times daily or a slow-release preparation once daily, with dose titration).
3. To reduce ventricular rate in patients with atrial fibrillation who are not adequately controlled by digoxin on its own.

Intravenous verapamil is given during continuous monitoring; 10 mg may be given over 5 min, followed if necessary by a further 5 mg after 5 min. The oral dose is 40–120 mg three times daily, or more conveniently 240 mg of a sustained release preparation once daily. This is about 10 times the intravenous dose, the difference being because of extensive presystemic metabolism when verapamil is given by mouth.

Intravenous verapamil must not be given to patients receiving β-blockers as this combination can cause severe AV block and asystole.

Oral verapamil is used as an alternative to a β-adrenoceptor antagonist for patients in whom digoxin alone has failed to control ventricular rate in atrial fibrillation. This requires care, because verapamil reduces digoxin excretion and the dose of digoxin should therefore be halved when these drugs are combined. For this same reason verapamil is contraindicated in patients with digoxin toxicity, especially as these drugs also have a potentially fatal additive effect on the AV node.

Mechanism of action

Verapamil blocks L-type voltage-dependent Ca^{2+} channels in cardiac tissues. It is a class IV drug and has greater effects on cardiac conducting tissue than other Ca^{2+} antagonists. In common with other calcium antagonists verapamil also relaxes smooth muscle of peripheral arterioles and veins and of coronary arteries. It is a negative inotrope since Ca^{2+} is crucial for cardiac contraction. As an antiarrhythmic drug its major effect is to slow intracardiac conduction, particularly through the AV node. This reduces ventricular response in atrial fibrillation and flutter and abolishes most re-entry nodal tachycardias. Mild resting bradycardia is common, together with prolongation of the PR interval.

Adverse effects and contraindications

1. **Cardiovascular** Verapamil is contraindicated in cardiac failure because of the negative inotropic effect. Verapamil is also contraindicated in sick sinus syndrome or intracardiac conduction block. It can cause hypotension, AV block or other bradyarrhythmias (calcium gluconate, atropine and/or isoprenaline may be useful in emergency situations precipitated by verapamil toxicity). It is contraindicated in WPW syndrome complicated by supraventricular tachycardia, atrial flutter or atrial fibrillation, as it can increase the rate of conduction through the accessory pathway. Verapamil is ineffective in ventricular arrhythmias, and its negative inotropic effect makes its inadvertent use in such arrhythmias extremely hazardous.
2. **Gastrointestinal tract** As many as one-third of patients treated with verapamil experience constipation, although this can usually be prevented or managed successfully with advice about increased dietary intake of fiber, and laxatives if necessary.
3. **Other adverse effects** Headache, dizziness and facial flushing are related to vasodilatation (cf. similar or worse symptoms caused by other Ca^{2+} channel blockers). Drug rashes, pain in the gums and a metallic taste in the mouth are uncommon.

Pharmacokinetics

Verapamil is a racemic mixture of (–) and (+) verapamil. The (–) isomer is much more potent than the (+). Although verapamil is well absorbed after oral administration its bioavailability is only 10–20% due to presystemic elimination which is stereoselective, the (–) isomer being preferentially metabolized. This explains the observation that even when equivalent total verapamil concentrations are achieved, the effect on the PR interval is greater for the same total plasma concentration after intravenous than after oral dosing: this is due to higher concentrations of the more active (–) isomer after an intravenous dose. Verapamil is highly protein bound in plasma. It is metabolized by the liver, one of the metabolites (norverapamil) being active. Mean $t_{1/2}$ is 3–7 hours in healthy individuals, but is significantly prolonged in patients with liver disease. Sustained release preparations permit the use of once daily dosing.

Drug interactions

The important pharmacodynamic interaction of verapamil with β-adrenoceptor antagonists which occurs especially when one or other member of the pair is administered intravenously contraindicates their combined use by this route. The pharmacokinetic interaction whereby verapamil increases digoxin concentrations and toxicity and the pharmacodynamic interaction of verapamil with digoxin are described above.

ADENOSINE

Use

Adenosine is used to terminate SVT. In addition to use in regular narrow complex tachycardia, it is particularly useful diagnostically in patients with regular broad complex tachycardia which is suspected of being SVT with aberrant conduction. If adenosine terminates the tachycardia this implies that the AV node is indeed involved. If, however, this diagnosis is wrong (as it not infrequently is) and the patient actually has VT, little or no harm results, in contrast to the use of verapamil in VT. Adenosine is administered into a peripheral vein as a bolus followed by a saline flush; the starting dose is 0.05 mg/kg increasing in increments of 0.05 mg/kg at intervals of 1 min or more until the SVT terminates or a total dose of approximately 20 mg has been given.

Mechanism of action

Adenosine acts on specific adenosine receptors. A_1-Receptors block AV nodal conduction. Adenosine also constricts bronchial smooth muscle by an A_1 effect, especially in asthmatics. It relaxes vascular smooth muscle, stimulates nociceptive afferent neurons in the heart and inhibits platelet aggregation via A_2-receptors.

Adverse effects and contraindications

Chest pain, flushing, shortness of breath, dizziness and nausea are common but short lived. Chest pain can be alarming if the patient is not warned of its benign nature before administering the drug. Adenosine is contraindicated in patients with asthma or heart block (unless already paced), and should be used with care in patients with WPW syndrome in whom ventricular rate during atrial fibrillation may be accelerated as a result of blocking the normal AV nodal pathway and hence favoring conduction through the abnormal pathway. This theoretically increases the risk of ventricular fibrillation; however, a recent report suggests that this risk is small and should not discourage the use of adenosine in patients with broad complex tachycardias of uncertain origin.

Pharmacokinetics

Adenosine is rapidly cleared from the circulation by uptake into red blood cells and by enzymes on the luminal surface of endothelial cells. It is deaminated to inosine. The circulatory effects of a bolus dose of a therapeutic dose of adenosine last 20–30 s, although effects on the airways in asthmatics persist longer.

Drug interactions

Dipyridamole blocks cellular adenosine uptake, and potentiates its action. Theophylline blocks adenosine receptors, and inhibits its action.

DIGOXIN

See also chapter 28.

Use

The main use of digoxin as an antiarrhythmic drug is to control the ventricular rate (and hence improve cardiac output) in patients with atrial fibrillation. It can also be used to terminate SVT and in patients with atrial flutter. Digoxin is usually given orally but if this is impossible, or if a rapid effect is needed, it can be given intravenously (0.5 mg given over 30 min). Since the $t_{1/2}$ is approximately 1–2 days in patients with normal renal function, repeated administration of a maintenance dose results in a plateau concentration in about 3–6 days. This is acceptable in many settings, but if clinical circumstances are more urgent a therapeutic plasma concentration can be attained more rapidly by administering a loading dose; for example, 0.5 mg followed by 0.25 mg 8 hourly for three doses followed by a maintenance dose of 0.0625–0.5 mg daily depending on response sometimes supplemented by plasma concentration measurement.

Mechanism of action

1. Digoxin inhibits membrane Na^+/K^+-adenosine triphosphatase (ATPase) which is responsible for the active extrusion of Na^+ from myocardial as well as other cells. This results in accumulation of intracellular Na^+ which indirectly increases intracellular Ca^{2+} content via Na^+/Ca^{2+} exchange and intracellular Ca^{2+} storage. The rise in availability of intracellular Ca^{2+} accounts for the positive inotropic effect of digoxin. Excessive

poisoning of Na^+/K^+-ATPase causes numerous non-cardiac as well as cardiac (arrhythmogenic) toxic effects of digoxin.

2. Slowing of ventricular rate results from several mechanisms, particularly increased vagal activity:

   (a) Delayed conduction through the atrioventricular node and bundle of His. This is particularly important in atrial fibrillation where the atria discharge at very high rates (350/min) and the ventricles follow irregularly with some degree of block. Delaying AV conduction increases the degree of block and slows ventricular response.

   (b) Increased cardiac output due to the positive inotropic effect of digoxin reduces reflex sympathetic tone.

   (c) Small doses of digitalis sensitize the sinoatrial node to vagal impulses.

Adverse effects and contraindications

1. **Cardiovascular** Second degree heart block or sinus bradycardia may presage complete heart block, and digoxin should usually be withheld in these circumstances. Almost any arrhythmia can be precipitated by digoxin toxicity (e.g. coupled beats, nodal tachycardias, ventricular or supraventicular ectopics). Supraventricular tachycardia caused by WPW syndrome can be worsened by digoxin, which slows conduction in the AV node without affecting that in the pathological accessory bundle and therefore favors very rapid transmission from atria to ventricles via this route. Patients with WPW who develop rapid atrial rates (e.g. atrial fibrillation) are thus at increased risk of consequent ventricular fibrillation if treated with digoxin. Digitalized patients (especially those with digoxin toxicity) are at risk of developing serious ventricular arrhythmias following attempted DC cardioversion. If possible, digoxin should be withheld for 24 hours before cardioversion, and the smallest effective shock employed. In an emergency, however, digoxin is no bar to attempting electrical cardioversion.

2. **Gastrointestinal symptoms** Especially nausea, vomiting and diarrhea.

3. Distortion of **color vision**, especially yellow vision ('xanthopsia').

Some of these effects are potentially serious, so treatment of digitalis toxicity is important. Discontinuation of digoxin may be all that is needed, particularly if signs of toxicity are confined to the gastrointestinal tract or some non-dangerous arrhythmia such as ectopic beats. If there are serious cardiac manifestations active treatment may be needed. Hypokalemia should be corrected either by giving oral potassium chloride, or in more serious toxicity potassium chloride diluted in 5% dextrose or physiological saline can be given intravenously at a rate up to 0.5 mmol/min with constant electrocardiographic monitoring.

Intravenous magnesium (as sulfate or chloride salt) terminates several digoxin-induced arrhythmias, and is safe provided the patient has normal renal function. Other antiarrhythmic drugs, in particular phenytoin or lignocaine, are sometimes used in the hope of controlling digoxin-induced arrhythmias.

Wherever the patient is adequately perfused and passing urine we prefer close monitoring on a coronary care unit without active intervention other than correction of electrolyte disturbances and administration of magnesium while excessive digoxin is eliminated. DC countershock is used only as a last resort if ventricular fibrillation or tachycardia unresponsive to other measures occurs. Pacing is required for complete heart block with hypoperfusion. Severe cases of digoxin poisoning have been successfully treated with the Fab fragments of digoxin-specific antibodies. This can be life saving in the rare cases in which it is indicated: usually in massive deliberate overdose with suicidal intent. The Fab fragments bind digoxin, preventing it from binding to Na^+/K^+ ATPase and hence preventing its toxic effects, and the complexes are excreted by the kidneys.

Pharmacokinetics

Gastrointestinal absorption of digoxin is greatly influenced by the pharmaceutical characteristics of tablet preparations, and in the past differences between preparations have led to marked variations in bioavailability resulting in digoxin toxicity (chapter 4). Modern manufacturing processes ensure that the currently available preparations disperse rapidly and uniformly.

Digoxin is widely distributed throughout the body, entering the central nervous system but not fat. The apparent volume of distribution varies from about 4 to 12 l/kg and is reduced in renal failure, myxedema and the elderly.

Eighty per cent of administered digoxin is excreted unchanged in the urine in subjects with normal renal function. It is eliminated mainly by glomerular filtration, although a fraction is subject to both tubular secretion and reabsorption. A small amount of digoxin undergoes metabolism to inactive products or excretion via the bile and elimination in feces. The proportion eliminated by these non-renal means increases in patients with renal impairment, being 100% in anephric patients in whom $t_{1/2}$ is approximately 4.5 days.

Plasma digoxin concentration determination is useful in patients with arrhythmias when toxicity is suspected or in checking compliance. Blood should be sampled more than 7 hours after an oral dose (4 hours after an intravenous dose). The usual therapeutic range is 1–2 ng/ml, although toxicity can occur at concentrations <1.5 ng/ml in some individuals. In most patients with atrial fibrillation apical heart rate provides the most useful clinical pharmacodynamic measure of response.

Drug interactions

- Reduced absorption can result in loss of efficacy (e.g. antacid, bile acid binding resins, tetracycline).
- Drugs causing hypokalemia (e.g. diuretics, β-agonists, carbenoxolone) predispose to toxicity by increasing digoxin binding to Na^+/K^+ ATPase.
- Quinidine, verapamil and amiodarone predispose to toxicity by complex pharmacokinetic effects (displacement from tissue binding sites and reduced renal secretion into urine).

ATROPINE

Use

Atropine is administered intravenously (0.3–0.6 mg doses, repeated if necessary up to a maximum of 2.4 mg) to patients with hemodynamic compromise due to inappropriate sinus bradycardia. (It is also used for several other non-cardiological indications, including anesthetic premedication, topical application to the eye to produce mydriasis, and for patients who have been poisoned with organophosphorous anticholinesterase drugs (chapter 50).

Mechanism of action

Acetylcholine released as the neurotransmitter from the vagus nerve acts on muscarinic receptors in atrial and cardiac conducting tissues. This increases K^+ permeability of the plasma membranes of these cells, thereby shortening the cardiac action potential and slowing the rate of rise of pacemaker potentials and cardiac rate. Atropine is a highly selective antagonist of acetylcholine at muscarinic receptors. It thereby counters these actions of acetylcholine, accelerating heart rate in patients with sinus bradycardia by inhibiting excessive vagal tone.

Adverse effects and contraindications

Parasympathetic blockade by atropine produces widespread effects: reduced salivation, lachrymation and sweating, decreased secretions in the gut and respiratory tract, tachycardia, urinary retention, constipation, pupillary dilatation and ciliary paralysis. It is contraindicated in patients with narrow angle glaucoma. Many of the acetylcholine receptors in the brain are antagonized by atropine (atropine-like drugs are used to prevent motion sickness and to treat some of the manifestations of Parkinsonism). Atropine can cause central nervous system effects including hallucinations. (It is the active alkaloid in deadly and enchanters' nightshade.)

Pharmacokinetics

Although atropine is completely absorbed after oral administration it is used intravenously to treat sinus bradycardia when this is causing hemodynamic compromise following myocardial infarction.

ADRENALINE

Use

Although not usually classed as an 'antiarrhythmic' drug (it is of course powerfully proarrhythmogenic in healthy individuals), adrenaline is used in the emergency treatment of patients with cardiac arrest due to asystole or ventricular fibrillation. For these indications it is administered intravenously (or sometimes directly into the heart or down an endotracheal tube) (see above in the section on cardiac arrest). Adrenaline is the most important drug for treatment of anaphylactic shock (chapter 47, p. 644). Adrenaline is also sometimes used in combination with local anesthetics to reduce their rate of removal from their injection site (chapter 21).

Mechanism of action

Adrenaline is a potent and non-selective agonist at both α- and β-receptors. It causes an increased rate of depolarization of cardiac pacemaker potentials, in addition to increasing the force of contraction of the heart and intense peripheral vasoconstriction (thereby causing a very marked pressor response). The mechanisms underlying its beneficial effects in cardiac arrest are poorly understood.

Adverse effects

Adrenaline is powerfully proarrhythmogenic and increases the work of the heart (and hence its oxygen requirement). Its peripheral vasoconstrictor effect can reduce tissue perfusion. For these reasons it is used systemically only in emergency situations.

Pharmacokinetics

Adrenaline is rapidly eliminated from the circulation by a high affinity/low capacity uptake process into sympathetic nerve terminals ('uptake 1'), and a lower affinity larger capacity process into a variety of tissues called uptake 2. It is subsequently metabo-lized, and is excreted in the urine as inactive metabolites including vanillyl mandelic acid.

Drug interactions

Tricyclic antidepressants block uptake 1, and so may potentiate the action of adrenaline. Adrenoceptor antagonists, both α and β, block its actions at these receptors.

ISOPRENALINE

Use

Isoprenaline is used to speed the heart in those few patients who are hemodynamically compromised because of complete heart block in whom pacing is impractical. It is a temporizing measure while pacing facilities are mobilized. Although it can speed the idioventricular rhythm in such patients thereby improving cardiac output the disadvantage is increased oxygen demand and hence possible extension of myocardial infarction and increased risk of serious ventricular tachyarrhythmia. Isoprenaline therefore tends to be used as a last resort. It is given by intravenous infusion (starting dose 1 μg/min, increasing if necessary by 1 μg/min increments up to a maximum of 5 μg/min). Isoprenaline is also sometimes used after myocardial infarction or cardiac arrest when complicated by other severe bradyarrhythmias unresponsive to atropine. It may also be useful in managing patients poisoned with β-adrenoceptor antagonists, with verapamil or with disopyramide.

Mechanism of action

Isoprenaline is a potent non-selective β-receptor agonist. β_1-Receptors in ventricular tissue are coupled via stimulatory G-proteins to adenylyl cyclase. Isoprenaline therefore increases cytoplasmic cyclic AMP which increases the rate of depolarization of the pacemaker potential and hence the rate of firing of the ventricular pacemaker. It also inevitably increases the risk of tachyarrhythmia and increases the force of contraction and hence oxygen demand of the heart.

It relaxes airways smooth muscle and vascular smooth muscle. Unlike adrenaline it therefore usually *lowers* blood pressure by reducing peripheral vascular resistance, especially in blood vessels supplying striated muscle.

Adverse effects

As explained above isoprenaline predisposes to tachyarrhythmias and may cause infarct extension. Its use is therefore limited.

Pharmacokinetics

Isoprenaline is rapidly taken up by uptake 2, terminating its action and is subsequently metabolized by catechol-O-methyl transferase and monoamine oxidase. It is absorbed from the intestine, and indeed oral preparations are still available. This route is, however, seldom if ever justified since isoprenaline is reserved for short-term emergency use.

CALCIUM CHLORIDE

Use

Calcium chloride is uniquely valuable in treating the broad complex ('sine wave') ventricular tachycardia that is a preterminal event in patients with severe hyperkalemia (often secondary to renal failure, see chapter 33). Its use may 'buy time' during which other measures to lower the plasma potassium concentration (glucose with insulin, ion binding resins, dialysis) can take effect or be mobilized. Calcium chloride is given as a slow intravenous injection of 5–10 ml (not more than 2 ml/min of 10% solution of the dihydrate, which is what is provided in prefilled syringes in most cardiac arrest boxes: 10 ml contains 6.8 mmol calcium). Calcium chloride is used in patients with cardiac arrest due to electromechanical dissociation. Calcium chloride is also used in patients with hypocalcemia, but these usually present with tetany rather than with cardiac arrhythmia. It is also suggested that calcium chloride may be useful in treating patients overdosed with Ca^{2+} antagonists such as verapamil or diltiazem.

Mechanism of action

Ca^{2+} is a divalent cation. Divalent cations are involved in maintaining the stability of the membrane potential in excitable tissues, including the heart. The outer aspects of cell membranes contain fixed negative charges that influence the electric field in the membrane, and hence the state of activation of voltage-dependent ion channels (Na^+ and Ca^{2+}) in the membrane. Divalent cations bind to the outer membrane, neutralizing the negative charges and in effect hyperpolarizing the membrane. Conversely, if the extracellular concentration of Ca^{2+} falls, Ca^{2+} dissociates from the membrane rendering it more unstable: in consequence a single stimulus to a nerve axon can give rise to a train of action potentials (tetany), and presumably similar instability underlies the cardiac arrhythmias that can accompany hypocalcemia and hypomagnesemia.

Adverse effects and contraindications

Calcium phosphate can precipitate in the kidneys of patients with hyperphosphatemia, worsening renal function. This consideration is, however, irrelevant when faced with a hyperkalemic patient with broad complex tachycardia.

Drug interactions

Calcium carbonate precipitates if calcium chloride solution is mixed with sodium bicarbonate. These agents should not be given simultaneously through the same line, nor consecutively without an intervening saline flush. Calcium increases digoxin toxicity, and calcium chloride must not be administered if digoxin toxicity is suspected.

MAGNESIUM

Use

Intravenous magnesium chloride (or sulfate) is of benefit in several situations. It is sometimes effective in treating arrhythmias caused by digoxin, and in drug-induced *torsades de pointes*. It is also valuable in eclampsia. The precise place of magnesium therapy, especially in the context of acute myocardial infarction, is still being worked out, and the best dose is uncertain: one recommendation is for 50 mmol magnesium added to 5% dextrose and infused over 12 hours in patients following acute myocardial infarction. In urgent situations 8 mmol may be given intravenously by slow injection. Magnesium chloride may be particularly useful in settings where magnesium deficiency is common. These include: prior chronic diuretic treatment, hypocalcemia, hypokalemia, alcoholism, diarrhea, vomiting, drainage from a fistula, pancreatitis, hyperaldosteronism or prolonged infusion of intravenous fluid without magnesium supplementation. There is no simple test currently available to detect total body magnesium deficiency, since Mg^{2+} is predominantly an intracellular cation; serial plasma magnesium determinations may, however, be useful in preventing excessive dosing with accumulation and toxicity.

Mechanism of action

Mg^{2+} is a divalent cation, and some at least of its beneficial effects are probably due to the consequent neutralization of fixed negative charges on the outer aspect of the cardiac cell membranes. In addition Mg^{2+} is a vasodilator, and can release prostacyclin from damaged vascular tissue *in vitro*. Unlike Ca^{2+}, Mg^{2+} does *not* trigger transmitter release or excitation contraction coupling, and indeed it blocks excitatory actions of glutamate on central NMDA (N-methyl D-aspartate) receptors by preventing Ca^{2+} entry.

Adverse effects and contraindications

Excessively high extracellular concentrations of Mg^{2+} can cause neuromuscular blockade. Magnesium chloride should be used with great caution in patients with renal impairment or hypotension. It should also be used with caution in patients receiving drugs with neuromuscular blocking activity, including aminoglycoside antibiotics. Mg^{2+} can cause AV block.

Pharmacokinetics

Magnesium salts are not well absorbed from the gastrointestinal tract, accounting for their efficacy as osmotic laxatives when given by mouth. Mg^{2+} is eliminated in the urine, and therapy with magnesium salts should be avoided or the dose reduced (and frequency of determination of plasma Mg^{2+} concentration increased) in patients with glomerular filtration rates <20 ml/min.

Drug interactions

Magnesium salts form precipitates if mixed with sodium bicarbonate, and as with calcium chloride magnesium salts should not be administered at the same time as sodium bicarbonate or through the same line without an intervening saline flush. Hypermagnesemia increases neuromuscular blockade caused by drugs with nicotinic receptor antagonist properties (e.g. pancuronium, aminoglycosides).

BRETYLIUM

Use

Bretylium is used to treat recurrent ventricular fibrillation or ventricular tachycardia after DC cardioversion and lignocaine have failed. We generally prefer amiodarone in this situation, although there are no controlled data. In a controlled comparison with lignocaine in 147 patients with out of hospital cardiac arrest bretylium and lignocaine were similarly effective. Bretylium tosylate is given as a rapid intravenous bolus (5 mg/kg) in cardiac arrest, and this dose can be repeated once if necessary.

Mechanism of action

Bretylium is taken up rapidly by the uptake 1 mechanism in adrenergic nerve terminals. It causes release of endogenous noradrenaline, followed by blockade of further release ('adrenergic neuron blockade'), probably because the high concentration in the nerve terminal acts as a local anesthetic, preventing propagation of action potentials in the sympathetic nerve axons into the terminals. This latter property underlies its hypotensive effect (it used to be given by mouth to treat hypertension, but often caused unacceptable postural hypotension). It is also said to have a class III action on Purkinje fibers and to a lesser extent on ventricular myocytes. The precise mechanism of its action in terminating ventricular fibrillation or tachycardia is unknown: type II action (i.e. antiadrenergic) has been invoked but seems unlikely as it can have a rapid effect on ventricular fibrillation whereas its adrenergic neuron blocking action is delayed, and because its behavior is so different qualitatively from other class II agents. Release of endogenous noradrenaline perhaps combined with class III effect is probably responsible for the therapeutic effect of bretylium.

Adverse effects

Nausea and vomiting are common after rapid intravenous injection, and hypotension is inevitable.

Pharmacokinetics

Bretylium is secreted rapidly into the tubular lumen and excreted entirely by the kidneys. The half-life is normally 7–9 hours, and this is much prolonged in renal failure.

Drug interactions

Prior treatment with drugs that block uptake 1 (e.g. tricyclic antidepressants) is likely to render bretylium ineffective. Conversely an uptake 1 blocker (protriptyline, 5 mg 6 hourly) has been used to treat the hypotension that follows its successful use. Noradrenaline infusion has also been used in this situation.

The
Respiratory
System

V

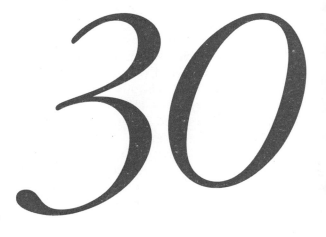Asthma and Other Respiratory Disorders

30

Pathophysiology of asthma **376**

Principles of management of asthma, bronchitis and emphysema **377**

Drugs used to treat asthma **380**

Future directions in drug therapy of asthma **387**

Respiratory failure **387**

Cough **388**

Respiratory surfactant **389**

α_1-Antitrypsin **390**

Respiratory stimulants **390**

Drug-induced pulmonary disease **391**

PATHOPHYSIOLOGY OF ASTHMA

Asthma is characterized by variable airways obstruction. This manifests as wheeze, cough and/or breathlessness, due to a combination of constriction of bronchial smooth muscle, edema of the mucosa lining small bronchi and plugging of the bronchial lumen with viscous mucus-containing inflammatory cells. Although the process is initially reversible secondary changes in the lungs and bronchi lead ultimately to irreversible airways obstruction. Two forms of asthma are recognized: non-allergic and allergic. Patients with non-allergic (late onset) asthma do not appear to be sensitive to any well-defined antigen although infection (usually viral) often precipitates an attack. In allergic asthma, which is usually of early onset, extrinsic allergens produce a type I allergic reaction in atopic subjects (chapter 47). Type I reactions are associated with the presence of reaginic antibodies (IgE) on the surface of mast cells. When a specific antigen comes into contact with such sensitized cells, chemical mediators of the asthmatic reaction are released. Even in allergic asthma the airways are hyper-responsive to a variety of stimuli, and specific immunotherapy has consequently been disappointing.

Biochemical mediators that are believed to be important in asthma include histamine, 5-hydroxytryptamine (5HT, serotonin), prostaglandin D_2, platelet-activating factor, kinins and leukotrienes (LT). These mediators

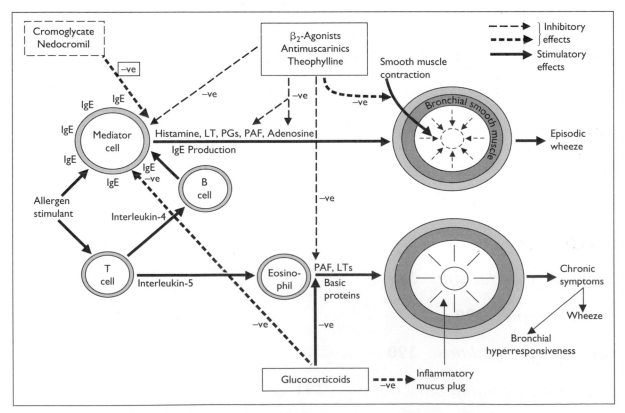

Fig. 30.1 Pathophysiology of asthma and sites of drug action. PAF = platelet-activating factor. LTs = leukotrienes. PGs = prostaglandins.

interact with one another, and the precise role of each is consequently hard to establish. Leukotriene B_4 is a powerful chemoattractant and may be involved in the inflammatory response. Leukotriene C_4, LTD_4 and LTE_4 (sulfidopeptide LT) collectively comprise the factor historically known as 'slow-reacting substance of anaphylaxis' or SRS-A, which is a powerful bronchoconstrictor. The most powerful bronchoconstrictor leukotriene is LTD_4 (Fig. 30.1). Cholinergic stimuli also cause bronchoconstriction.

PRINCIPLES OF MANAGEMENT OF ASTHMA, BRONCHITIS AND EMPHYSEMA

Management of acute severe asthma

See Table 30.1.

1. The patient should be admitted to hospital, and observed both clinically and with objective measures of airflow obstruction, for example peak expiratory flow rate (PEFR) and blood gases.
2. Maximum percentage oxygen (40–60%) should be given. Bronchodilators improve respiratory function, but this may be preceded by a transient fall in arterial oxygen tension. This fall occurs both with β_2-agonists and aminophylline and may predispose to cardiac arrhythmia. It is believed to be due to changes in ventilation/perfusion matching. Arterial hypoxemia is prevented by oxygen which should therefore be given with these drugs.
3. An intravenous infusion is initiated to prevent or correct dehydration. Five per cent glucose is infused and serum potassium monitored since hypokalemia is caused by corticosteroid and β_2-agonist administration.
4. A β_2-agonist is given via a nebulizer, for example 5.0 mg salbutamol 2–4 hourly depending on severity and response. Higher doses increase the incidence of adverse effects. Intravenous salbutamol, 250 µg over 5–10 min, followed by 10–20 µg/min) is seldom more effective, but may be necessary in patients who cannot tolerate a nebulizer or whose inspiratory effort is very poor due to the severity of airflow obstruction.
5. Intravenous hydrocortisone, 200 mg, 6 hourly or 40 mg once daily of prednisolone should be given. Glucocorticosteroids take 4–6 hours to act.
6. An antibiotic such as amoxycillin or trimethoprim or co-amoxiclav is given if there is reasonable suspicion of bacterial infection.
7. Nebulized anticholinergics (e.g. ipratropium bromide) are given with β_2-agonists to improve resistant bronchoconstriction.

Table 30.1 Management of acute severe asthma.

1. Admit patient to hospital
2. Continuous high percentage oxygen – 40% or more
3. Nebulized β_2-agonist, e.g. salbutamol, 5 mg, 2–4 hourly
4. Intravenous or oral corticosteroids – intravenous hydrocortisone, 5 mg/kg, 6 hourly or oral prednisolone, 0.6 mg/kg (40 mg) daily
5. Nebulized anticholinergics, e.g. ipratropium bromide, 500 µg, 8 hourly
6. Antibiotics, e.g. amoxycillin if sputum is purulent
7. In a refractory case not responding to the above give either intravenous β_2-agonist – salbutamol, 250 µg, over 5 min then 5–20 µg/min, or aminophylline, loading dose 5 mg/kg no more than 350 mg over 20–30 min followed by 0.5 mg/kg/hour maintenance infusion. If the patient is on oral theophylline omit the loading dose
8. If the patient is still no better or worsening consider IPPV
9. Never give any asthmatic a sedative, unless already receiving IPPV

IPPV = intermittent positive pressure ventilation.

8. The role of intravenous theophylline (aminophylline) is controversial. It can be effective, but acutely it is difficult to achieve optimal therapeutic plasma concentrations, and the therapeutic index is low. Aminophylline may perhaps best be reserved for patients who fail to respond to the above initial regime. The method of loading and maintenance is described below and in Table 30.1.

9. If the patient fails to respond and develops a rising pulse rate, increasing respiratory rate and fall in PaO_2 to <6.5 kPa or rise in $PaCO_2$ to >6 kPa, assisted ventilation will probably be needed.

10. **Except when assisted ventilation is used, no sedation should be given**: even small doses can cause fatal respiratory depression in this situation.

Chronic asthma

1. Bronchodilators are used to treat chronic wheeziness and to abort acute episodes. Metered dose inhalers of β_2-agonists are convenient, and with correct usage little drug enters the circulation. The patient should be warned to contact the physician promptly if the clinical state deteriorates and the frequency of inhalations is rising. Aerosols are particularly useful in treating an acute episode of breathlessness, and recent studies suggest that 'on demand' medication (i.e. taken only when symptomatic) may be more beneficial in the long term rather than regular β_2-agonist therapy. Oral preparations of β_2-agonists or theophylline have a role in pediatric practice, because young children cannot coordinate inhalation with depression of an inhaler device.

2. Patients, particularly children, with asthma provoked by allergy, exercise or physical agents (e.g. cold air, sulfur dioxide) sufficient to need bronchodilator drugs may be given a trial of sodium cromoglycate for at least 1 month. History and lung function tests before and after exercise are used to determine whether the drug effect is of sufficient magnitude to continue. Some patients with intrinsic asthma respond to this drug.

3. Steroids are used in chronic asthma when:

   (a) Bronchodilators (one dose of short-acting inhaled β_2-agonist daily on a regular basis) fail to allow normal activity and sleep.
   (b) Repeated attacks interfere with work or school.
   (c) The growth of a child is impaired.

   Systemic side effects are minimized by using the inhaler route. The inhaled steroid should be tried for 2–3 weeks in doses of beclomethasone up to 500 µg, twice daily; or budesonide, 400 µg, twice daily. Severely affected patients (forced expiratory volume in 1 s (FEV1) <1.5 l for adults) do not usually respond but frequently improve on oral prednisolone. During a chest infection 30–40 mg prednisolone may be required daily until a response is attained. The drug is then reduced rapidly or tapered more slowly. Some patients need continuous steroid therapy with increased dosage during exacerbations. If a patient eventually improves to such an extent that withdrawal of steroids can be tried, this should be done gradually (2.5 mg prednisolone/week). After complete withdrawal steroids are again required if another attack does not respond readily to bronchodilators. Alternate morning administration of glucocorticoids causes less adrenal and growth suppression than daily administration (chapter 37).

4. Asthma associated with bacterial chest infection is treated with a broad-spectrum penicillin (amoxycillin), trimethoprim, or ciprofloxacin or one of the macrolides.

5. Hypnotics and sedatives should not be used and are **absolutely contraindicated** in the presence of respiratory failure and acute severe asthma attacks.

6. Home peak flow monoitoring. Patients can perform peak flow monitoring first thing in the morning and last thing at night, as soon as asthmatic symptoms develop or

worsen. With a knowledge of their best peak flow this allows adjustment of inhaled medication, or appropriate urgent medical assessment if peak flow falls to below 50% of normal or diurnal variation exceeds 20%.

Late-onset asthma

This is often difficult to treat and long-term steroid treatment may be the only way to control the disease. Nevertheless, bronchodilators, inhaled corticosteroids and sodium cromoglycate should be tried, particularly if sputum eosinophilia is present.

Acute bronchitis

Acute bronchitis commonly presents to general practitioners. There is little evidence that antibiotics confer benefit in otherwise fit patients presenting with cough and purulent sputum, and the most important step is to stop smoking. In the absence of fever or evidence of pneumonia it seems best to avoid antibiotics for this self-limiting condition.

Chronic bronchitis and emphysema

Chronic simple bronchitis is associated with chronic or recurrent increase in the volume of mucoid bronchial secretions sufficient to cause expectoration. At this stage there need be no disability and measures such as giving up smoking (this may be aided by the use of nicotine, chapter 49) and avoidance of air pollution improve prognosis. Simple hypersecretion may be complicated by infection or

the development of airways obstruction. Bacterial infection is usually due to commensal organisms including *Hemophilus influenzae*, although pneumococci, staphylococci or occasionally branhamella or coliforms may also be responsible. The commonly encountered acute bronchitic exacerbation is due to bacterial infection in only about one-third of cases; in the rest other factors such as increased air pollution, environmental temperature changes, or viruses, are presumably responsible. *Mycoplasma pneumoniae* infections may be responsible for some cases and these usually respond to erythromycin or tetracyclines. In practice bacterial infection is assumed to be present when sputum becomes purulent and treatment with antibiotics initiated promptly. Appropriate antibiotic therapy is based on adequate sputum penetration and the suspected organisms. The decision is seldom assisted by sputum culture or Gram stain, in contrast with pneumonias.

1. Ampicillin penetrates purulent more readily than mucoid sputum. Nevertheless, 1 g 6 hourly is required to achieve bactericidal levels against *H. influenzae*.
2. Amoxycillin produces sputum concentrations twice those from the same dose of ampicillin.
3. Most tetracyclines must be given in doses of 500 mg 6 hourly to achieve adequate sputum penetration. Doxycycline given as 200 mg initially followed by 100 mg daily penetrates well into sputum; it is also suitable for the older patient with renal insufficiency in whom other tetracyclines are contraindicated.
4. Co-amoxiclav (amoxycillin, 250 mg, and potassium clavulanate,125 mg), one tablet 8 hourly for 5–7 days, is often used because of its efficacy against β-lactamase-producing organisms.
5. Trimethoprim is as effective as co-trimoxazole for this indication and less toxic. The dose is 200 mg twice daily.
6. Cefuroxime penetrates sputum poorly but has some role in the management of bronchitis because of its activity against *H. influenzae*.

In the absence of respiratory disability, antibiotics alone may be sufficient treatment. Increased respiratory difficulty may be caused by sputum retention. Physiotherapy is traditional and possibly effective in this situation.

Prevention of acute exacerbations is difficult. Stopping smoking and avoidance of climatic extremes are beneficial. Patients should be given a supply of antibiotic to take as soon as their sputum becomes purulent. Despite recovery from an acute attack, patients are at greatly increased risk of death or serious illness from intercurrent respiratory infections and administration of influenza and pneumococcal vaccines to such patients is important.

Airways obstruction is invariably present in chronic bronchitis but is of variable severity. Bronchodilators, either β-adrenoreceptor agonists or aminophylline, are often used but frequently fail since much of the obstruction is irreversible. In some patients, however, there is a reversible element and a trial of these drugs is usually justified to assess whether benefit will be obtained. Similarly a therapeutic trial of corticosteroids (40 mg prednisolone daily for 2 weeks followed by a rapid reduction in dose if no benefit is obtained) may be used in more severe cases of airways obstruction unresponsive to conventional bronchodilators.

Intermittent use of oxygen at low concentration by patients at home is ineffective, dangerous and expensive. Long-term oxygen therapy (LTOT), 15 hours or more daily, in severely disabled bronchitics with pulmonary hypertension decreases mortality and morbidity. The mortality of such patients is related to pulmonary hypertension which is increased by chronic hypoxia. Relief of hypoxia on a long-term basis by increasing the concentration of inspired oxygen reverses the vasoconstriction in the pulmonary arteries and decreases pulmonary hypertension. Long-term oxygen therapy cannot be safely offered to patients who continue to smoke because of the hazards of fire and explosion.

DRUGS USED TO TREAT ASTHMA

β₂-Agonists

Use

β₂-Agonists (e.g. salbutamol, terbutaline) are used to treat the symptoms of asthma both in an acute attack and as maintenance therapy. These drugs are given via inhalation, wherever possible. The benefits of this are that the drugs are delivered directly into the bronchi, the desired site of action, with little systemic absorption and consequently fewer systemic side effects. Commonly used inhaler devices include various metered dose inhaler (MDI) devices (delivering 8–12% of the administered dose to the bronchi). Plastic 'spacer' devices (known as the 'Nebuhaler' or 'Volumatic'), which are easier for the elderly and the young to use, deliver between 15 and 20% of the administered dose to the bronchi. Salbutamol is used widely.

1. Inhalation methods:

   (a) Metered dose inhaler – aerosol (100 μg/puff), usual dose one to two puffs up to six times daily.
   (b) Aerosol administered via a nebulizer – 2.5–5 mg salbutamol in sterile saline are given over 5–15 min between 2 and 6 hourly.
   (c) As a dry powder ('Rotahaler' or 'Diskhaler'). Whereas some 15% of adults on aerosol inhalations may use these devices inefficiently despite careful instruction almost all patients can use a dry-powder inhaler correctly, in doses up to 800 μg 4 hourly.

2. Oral – 8–16 mg daily as tablets or sustained release preparations.
3. Subcutaneous – 500 µg 8 hourly.

The increase in FEV1 after inhalation of 200 µg salbutamol begins within 15 min, peaks at 1 hour and persists for 4–6 hours. Following intravenous injection of 100–300 µg over 5 min airways resistance usually falls to a minimum in 5–10 min although in severely affected patients response may be delayed by 30 min. Intravenous β_2-agonists are also used in obstetric practice to inhibit premature labor, for up to 48 hours. Salbutamol is given initially at 10 µg/min increasing to a maximum of 45 µg/min; an alternative is ritodrin given as 50 µg/min increasing to 150–350 µg/min.

Pharmacological effects and mechanism of action

Agonists occupying β-adrenoceptors increase cyclic adenosine monophosphate (cAMP) by stimulating adenylyl cyclase via a membrane-bound G-protein. Cyclic AMP phosphorylates a cascade of enzymes (Fig. 30.2). This causes a wide variety of effects in different tissues:

1. Relaxation of bronchial smooth muscle.
2. Inhibition of release of mast cell and other inflammatory mediators.
3. Relaxation of uterine smooth muscle.
4. Increase in heart rate, force of myocardial contraction, speed of impulse conduction and enhanced production of ectopic foci in the myocardium and automaticity in pacemaker tissue.
5. Muscle tremor.
6. Vasodilatation in skeletal and myocardial muscle.
7. Metabolic effects, for example increased glucose release by hepatocytes, increased release of insulin and increased cellular uptake of K^+.
8. Increased mucociliary clearance.

Adverse effects

1. **Neuromuscular and central nervous system** muscle tremor (30%), headache and insomnia.
2. **Cardiovascular system** tachycardia, flushing, palpitations and cardiac arrhythmias. Caution is essential when any β_2-adrenoreceptor agonist is used intravenously as the risk of cardiac arrhythmias is increased. There is a risk of precipitating or exacerbating angina in patients with ischemic heart disease.
3. **Metabolic**:

   (a) Hypokalemia.
   (b) Raised free fatty acid concentrations.
   (c) Increased insulin secretion but increased glycogenolysis which overall increases blood sugar.

4. Tolerance to β_2-agonists occurs *in vitro* but the importance of this in asthmatic patients is unknown.

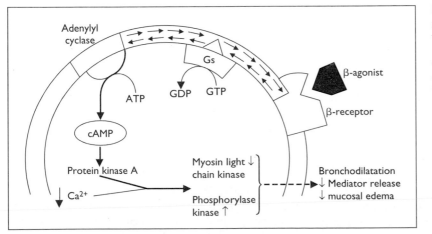

Fig. 30.2 Membrane and intracellular events triggered when β-agonists stimulate β-receptors. Gs = stimulating G-protein. GDP = guanidine diphosphate. GTP = guanidine triphosphate. cAMP = 3',5'-cyclic adenosine monophosphate.

Pharmacokinetics

Salbutamol is not metabolized by catechol-O-methyl transferase or monoamine oxidase and is effective when given by mouth in sufficient dose. When absorbed from the gut it undergoes pronounced presystemic metabolism in intestinal mucosa (sulfation) and hepatic conjugation to form an inactive metabolite that is excreted in urine. Most (80%) of the dose administererd by aerosol is swallowed but the fraction which is inhaled (10–20%) largely remains as free salbutamol in the bronchi and even following absorption into plasma. Plasma half-life ($t_{1/2}$) is 2–4 hours but a decrease in airways obstruction persists when no drug can be detected in plasma, due to local deposition in the airways.

TERBUTALINE

Terbutaline is an alternative β_2 selective agonist to salbutamol, with a longer plasma $t_{1/2}$ of 3–4 hours. It may be given orally, by injection or by inhalation via a 'Turbohaler' inhalation device which delivers 20–30% of the dose to the lungs.

SALMETEROL

Salmeterol xinafoate is an analog of salbutamol, with approximately 4000 times greater potency at the β_2-receptor. It is very long acting, with a pharmacodynamic $t_{1/2}$ of at least 12 hours. It is believed that this is because the lipophilic side chain of salmeterol binds closely adjacent to the β_2-receptor, such that the agonist can interact with the receptor so that it functions essentially as an irreversible agonist. This allows twice daily administration. The onset of bronchodilatation is slow taking 17 min to produce a 15% increase in FEV1 and 3–4 hours to peak effect. Salmeterol should not therefore be used to treat acute attacks of bronchospasm. It is used as prophylactic therapy, especially overnight with additional 'top ups' with shorter acting β_2-agonists, but it is expensive and it has been suggested that it may actually worsen the progression of the underlying inflammatory disease, so its place in treatment remains controversial. Plasma $t_{1/2}$ is several days after oral dosing.

Muscarinic receptor antagonists

Use

Inhaled muscarinic receptor antagonists are effective bronchodilators. Anticholinergic drugs are most effective in older patients. Atropine has a bronchodilator action in bronchitics and asthmatics, with some benefit in patients with exercise-induced asthma. (Osler recommended stramonium – which contains atropine – cigarettes for asthmatics!). Atropine is precluded by its systemic side effects and modern drugs of this type are quaternary ammonium analogs of atropine that are minimally absorbed.

IPRATROPIUM BROMIDE

Use

Ipratropium is given as 1–2 puffs (20 or 40 µg) three or four times daily from a metered dose inhaler. It can be given via a nebulizer (stock solution 0.25 mg/ml; 2 ml (500 µg) diluted with 2 ml saline, nebulized and inhaled). The degree and rate of onset of bronchodilatation is somewhat less than that of salbutamol or terbutaline, but the duration of response is longer. Ipratropium has a place in maintenance therapy and in acute severe attacks of asthma. Some benefit for patients with exercise-induced asthma has also been demonstrated, but its slower onset of action makes it most useful in maintenance therapy, especially in chronic bronchitis. It is useful for patients with heart disease or thyrotoxicosis in whom β-agonists are unsuitable. It is compatible with β_2-agonists and such combinations are additive.

Mechanism of action

There is increased parasympathetic activity in patients with reversible airways obstruction resulting in bronchoconstriction through effects of acetylcholine on M1, M2 and M3 muscarinic cholinoreceptors in the bronchi. The final common pathway is via a membrane-bound G-protein which leads to a fall in cAMP and increased intracellular calcium with consequent bronchoconstriction.

Adverse effects

1. Bitter taste (this may compromise compliance).
2. Acute urinary retention may be precipitated by high doses in patients with prostatic hypertrophy.
3. Acute glaucoma has been precipitated when nebulized doses are given via a facemask.
4. Paradoxical bronchoconstriction has occasionally been reported, due to sensitivity to benzalkonium chloride which is the preservative in the nebulizer solution.

Pharmacokinetics

When administered by aerosol plasma concentrations of ipratropium are some 1000 times lower than when the same degree of bronchodilatation is produced by systemic administration. Ipratropium appears in the blood approximately 2 min after inhalation and the plasma concentrations continue to rise for 1–3 hours thereafter, because of the small amount of swallowed drug absorbed from the gut. Plasma $t_{1/2}$ is 3–4 hours. Ipratropium is excreted in both feces and urine as metabolites and unchanged compound.

OXITROPIUM

Oxitropium bromide is similar to ipratropium, but with a longer duration of action (biological half-life 12 hours) allowing twice daily dosing (200 µg via a metered dose inhaler).

Methylxanthines

THEOPHYLLINE AND ITS DERIVATIVES

These are the only phosphodiesterase inhibitors currently in common therapeutic use for asthma. Aminophylline is a mixture of 80% theophylline and 20% ethylene diamine which increases theophylline solubility but is the likely culprit for occasional allergic reactions.

Use

Aminophylline is used intravenously in patients with severe asthma or severe chronic obstructive airways disease (COAD) and is used orally in less severe cases or to reduce symptoms, especially at night. Oral theophylline preparations are widely available, mainly in the form of sustained release preparations allowing twice daily dosing (at night and in the morning).

1. Intravenous aminophylline (Table 30.1) usually produces rapid relief of asthmatic symptoms:

   (a) A loading dose of 350mg initially given over 20–30 min for moderately severe asthma (for large or small adults this dose should be adjusted to approximately 5.0 mg/kg) is used.
   (b) A continuous infusion of 0.5 mg/kg/hour follows. A solution of 250 mg aminophylline can be diluted in 500 ml saline and given by infusion preferably using a pump. Infusion rates must be reviewed and adjusted frequently according to plasma theophylline concentrations (chapter 8), and if rapid theophylline determinations are unavailable this substantially reduces the safety of the drug. In patients with impaired liver function or heart failure the dose should be halved. It should also be reduced in the elderly. It is essential to enquire about oral theophylline administration prior to intravenous injection. If the patient is receiving oral theophylline the plasma concentration should be measured and the dose modified accordingly.

2. Oral theophylline is obtainable in many different forms and there is great variation in the bioavailability of different preparations. Sustained release preparations of aminophylline are available which provide

effective therapeutic levels for up to 12 hours following a single dose. Because of their slow release rate they have a reduced incidence of gastrointestinal side effects. Oral theophylline is useful in patients whose airways obstruction increases in the early hours of the morning (morning 'dippers').

Mechanism of action and pharmacological effects

It is still not clear exactly how theophylline produces its beneficial bronchodilating effects at the therapeutic concentrations achieved in humans. Pharmacologcical actions include:

- Theophylline is a powerful relaxant of smooth muscle and inhibits mediator release from mast cells. It raises intracellular cAMP concentrations by non-specifically inhibiting all isoenzymes of phosphodiesterase. However, the degree of inhibition of phosphodiesterase at therapeutic concentrations is relatively small.
- Antagonism of adenosine (a potent bronchoconstrictor) at A_2-receptors by theophylline may be a further mechanism of bronchodilatation.
- Anti-inflammatory activity on T lymphocytes by reducing release of platelet-activating factor (PAF), reduced calcium entry via receptor-operated channels, and inhibition of calcium release from stores by inositol trisphosphate.
- Theophylline increases the tone and contractility of the diaphragm and respiratory muscles.
- Central stimulation of respiration.

Adverse effects

Adverse effects of theophylline are generally related to its plasma concentration.

1. **Gastrointestinal tract**: Nausea and vomiting are common and related both to stimulation of the medullary emetic centre and a local gastric effect, and can occur with plasma concentrations of 10–15 µg/ml.

2. **Cardiovascular system**: Some adverse effects resemble those of catecholamines since both drugs raise intracellular cAMP concentrations. These include tachycardia, cardiac arrhythmias (atrial and ventricular), and occur at plasma concentrations of 20–40 mg/l.

3. **Central nervous system:** Insomnia, anxiety, agitation hyperventilation, headache and ultimately fits (>40 mg/l).

4. Dilatation of vascular **smooth muscle:** Flushing and hypotension.

Pharmacokinetics

Theophylline is well absorbed from the small intestine (oral administration) or rectum (suppositories), but intravenous administration is most effective for acute severe asthma. The volume of distribution is about 0.3–0.8 l/kg and at therapeutic concentrations 60% is bound to plasma proteins. The therapeutic range is 5–20 µg/ml, but it is preferable not to exceed 10 mg/l in children. Theophylline is largely metabolized (85–90%) in the liver. Fixed dose regimes may lead to high blood levels and toxicity in the presence of liver disease.

Drug interactions

Although synergism between β_2-adrenergic agonists and theophylline has been demonstrated *in vitro* this does not occur in patients where the effect of these combinations is at best additive. This may none the less be useful in patients who experience unacceptable side effects from high doses of either drug alone but who may achieve comparable bronchodilatation without side effects from low doses of the combined agents. Many drugs inhibit or enhance theophylline metabolism (Table 30.2). Perhaps most noteworthy is the inhibition of theophylline metabolism by erythromycin and ciprofloxacin, since these are commonly used to treat respiratory infections. Thus concomitant prescription of these agents with theophylline can increase plasma theophylline concentration and cause toxicity.

Table 30.2 Factors influencing theophylline clearance (see also p. 71).

Factors decreasing theophylline clearance and suggested dose (assuming normal dose is 100%)	*Factors increasing theophylline clearance and suggested dose (assuming normal dose is 100%)*
Congestive cardiac failure (40%)	Smoking (150%)
Hepatic disease, cirrhosis (40%)	Marijauna (150%)
Old age (80%)	Barbecued meat (130%)
Neonates (60%)	Hyperthyroidism (150%)
Pneumonia (70%)	Drugs
Drugs	Carbamazepine (150%)
Cimetidine (50%)	Phenytoin (150%)
Erythromycin (75%)	Rifampicin (150%)
Chloramphenicol (75%)	Ethanol (120%)
Propranolol (70%)	High protein, low carbohydrate diet (150%)
Ciprofloxacin (50%)	
Interferon (75%)	

Corticosteroids

Glucocorticoids are used in asthma for their potent anti-inflammatory effect. They are effective both in prophylaxis and in treatment of the acute severe attack.

SYSTEMIC GLUCOCORTICOIDS

See chapter 37.

Hydrocortisone is given intravenously in emergency situations. Following an initial loading dose of 200 mg hydrocortisone hemisuccinate, further doses are usually given by intermittent intravenous injections. The plasma $t_{1/2}$ is approximately 120 min. Although high cortisol levels are rapidly attained, subjective improvement is not experienced for several hours and objective improvement (rise in FEV1 and forced vital capacity (FVC)) does not begin until 6 hours and is usually maximal at about 13 hours after the start of treatment. This delay is due to the pharmacodynamics of glucocorticoids, which work via new protein synthesis (chapter 37) which takes several hours. Oral corticosteroids are usually started within 12–24 hours. Prednisolone, 40–60 mg per day, or methyl prednisolone are given once daily in the mornings most commonly for a short course of 10–14 days.

INHALED CORTICOSTEROIDS

Use

These drugs are often used alone as prophylaxis or in conjunction with oral corticosteroids, when they allow reduction of the oral maintenance dose of prednisolone by up to 10 mg per day. Beclomethasone, 400 µg, is equivalent to 5 mg prednisolone. With newer more efficient inhaler devices delivery to the lung may reach 30% of total dose. Beclomethasone is given at a dose of 500 µg twice daily from an inhaler and budesonide is given at a dose of 200 µg twice daily. The budesonide metered aerosol canister can be used with a collapsible spacer or with a 750 ml plastic cone. Beclomethasone (and salbutamol) may also be administered via a plastic cone spacer device – the 'Volumatic'. Such devices deliver 15–20% of the dose to the lungs.

- Beclomethasone dipropionate dose: 50–2000 µg/day.
- Budesonide dose: 100–2000 µg/day.
- Fluticasone propionate (Diskhaler) – potency approximately twice that of beclomethasone: dose 100–2000 µg/daily.

These are fluorinated steroids which are inhaled via a metered dose inhaler. Halogenation increases polarity, so reducing absorption through membranes (these steroids were originally developed for topical use on the skin). They are extremely powerful anti-inflammatory agents and mainly exert a local action although some systemic absorption occurs. About 10–20% enters the lungs, the rest being swallowed to be rapidly converted to inactive metabolites by the liver. Fluticasone (<1%) and budesonide have the lowest systemic oral bioavailability of the three drugs above; following inhalation they are almost 100% metabolized. All these agents are administered twice daily to help compliance and minimize side effects. A nebulized formulation of budesonide (250 µg/ml, 2 ml units) has been produced and is currently under investigation as an alternative to oral steroid therapy and appears to be of benefit in growing children.

Adverse effects of inhaled steroids

1. At the lowest recommended daily dose of 400 µg there is no prolonged suppression of the hypothalamic–pituitary–adrenal (HPA) axis, although after cessation of treatment the blood cortisol concentration is suppressed for 48 hours. Higher doses (800–1600 µg) produce more prolonged depression of adrenal function. Doses >2000 µg/day beclomethasone cause significant adrenal suppression. Even at the higher doses of fluticasone (1000–2000 µg/day) significant HPA axis suppression is unproven.
2. Candidiasis of the pharynx (13% of patients) or larynx (5%). Reducing administration frequency and using mouthwashes can alleviate this problem. Occasionally nystatin or amphotericin lozenges are required. The incidence of candidiasis is reduced by administering the inhaled steroid via a spacer device.
3. Hoarse voice due to a laryngeal myopathy at high doses. This is dose dependent and reversible and its occurrence is minimized by the use of a spacer device.
4. Bruising and skin atrophy at high dose.
5. Reversible inhibition of long bone growth in children at doses of 400–800 µg/day.

Cromoglycate and nedocromil

Use

Sodium cromoglycate is administered by inhalation of a powder liberated from a 20 mg capsule and dispersed by devices containing an inspiration-driven propeller or by spinning of the punctured capsule in a plastic chamber. Cromoglycate produces no benefit during an asthmatic attack but taken regularly (e.g. 20–40 mg 6 hourly) will diminish the frequency of attacks of allergic asthma. Exercise-provoked attacks may also be prevented. Bronchospasm due to chest infection is not affected. A good response to cromoglycate may allow a rapid reduction in the dose of corticosteroid. At present there is no absolute method of predicting which patients will benefit and in view of its excellent tolerance a therapeutic trial is often warranted. Cromoglycate is also used as nose drops and spray for perennial and allergic rhinitis and as eye drops in allergic conjunctivitis. Nedocromil sodium is an alternative to cromoglycate.

Mechanism of action

These drugs do not prevent antigen–antibody combination, but if given before exposure to an antigen they can prevent type I and III allergic reactions. They inhibit mediator release from sensitized mast cells *in vitro* and used to be called 'mast cell stabilizers' for this reason. This action does not, however, account for their efficacy in allergic disorders, since congeners that are more potent in this regard are without therapeutic efficacy. These drugs reduce firing of sensory C fibers in response to kinins, but the mechanism underlying their therapeutic efficacy is uncertain.

Adverse effects

1. Cromoglycate is virtually non-toxic. The powder produces bronchospasm and hoarseness in approximately 1:10 000 people. The former can be treated with an inhalation of salbutamol and the latter usually responds to a drink of water.

2. Nedocromil sodium has a bitter taste (14%), and nausea and/or headaches occur following either of these drugs in up to 5% of patients.

Pharmacokinetics

Sodium cromoglycate is not appreciably absorbed from the gut and is given as an inhaled powder. The powder is mainly swallowed but some 10% reaches the alveoli where it acts and a small amount is absorbed. It is not metabolized, unchanged drug appearing mainly in feces (because it has been swallowed) together with a small amount in urine. Nedocromil sodium is also poorly absorbed from the gut and is given as an inhaled aerosol, its duration of action allows administration to be two to four times daily.

Antihistamines
H$_1$-blockers

See chapter 47.

TERFENADINE

Antihistaminies are not widely used in the treatment of asthma, but may have an adjunctive role in a few asthmatics with hay fever. Terfenadine is a relatively non-sedating H$_1$ antagonist with a long plasma half-life of 16–23 hours. There is a potential for dangerous interactions with drugs that inhibit its metabolism (e.g. erythromycin) or prolong the QT interval (e.g. amiodarone).

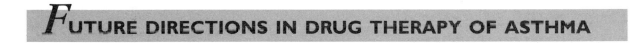

FUTURE DIRECTIONS IN DRUG THERAPY OF ASTHMA

Other anti-inflammatory drugs such as methotrexate, 7.5–15 mg, weekly or cyclosporin A reduce glucocorticosteroid requirement in chronic asthmatics, but because of their long-term toxicities (chapters 23 and 47) they are not used routinely. Promising drugs at present undergoing development for asthma therapy include specific phosphodiesterase III and IV inhibitors, potassium channel activators, and lipoxygenase inhibitors. The efficacy of various antagonists of specific mediators (e.g. PAF antagonists, leukotriene antagonists) has so far been disappointing.

RESPIRATORY FAILURE

Respiratory failure is the result of impaired gas exchange. It is defined as a PaO_2 below 8 kPa (60 mmHg) with or without a $PaCO_2$ above 6.3 kPa (47 mmHg). Two kinds are recognized:

1. Type I respiratory failure is characterized by a combination of a low PaO_2 and a normal or lowered $PaCO_2$. This is characteristic of ventilation/perfusion inequality (as in pneumonia, left ventricular failure, pulmonary fibrosis and shock lung).
2. Type II respiratory failure is characterized by a combination of low PaO_2 and raised $PaCO_2$ (ventilatory failure). This occurs with chronic airways obstruction (as in obstructive bronchitis), reduced activity of the respiratory center (e.g. from drug overdose or in association with morbid obesity and somnolence – Pickwickian

syndrome) and peripheral neuromuscular disorders (e.g. Guillain–Barré syndrome or myasthenia gravis), leading to a pure failure of ventilation.

Treatment of type I respiratory failure

The treatment of ventilation/perfusion inequality is that of the underlying lesion and in such cases there is no danger of precipitating carbon dioxide retention so that oxygen at high flow rate can be given (by nasal cannulae or mask). Shock lung is treated by controlled ventilation, oxygenation and positive end expiratory pressure (PEEP).

Treatment of type II respiratory failure

Sedatives must never be used. Benzodiazepines can produce fatal respiratory depression in patients with ventilatory failure.

SUPPORTIVE MEASURES

Physiotherapy

Physiotherapy is used to encourage coughing to remove tracheobronchial secretions and encourage deep breathing to preserve patency of airways.

Oxygen

Oxygen improves tissue oxygenation but high concentrations may depress respiration by removing the hypoxic respiratory drive. A small increase in the concentration of inspired oxygen to 24% using a Venturi-type mask is tried. If $PaCO_2$ does not increase or increases by <0.66 kPa and the level of consciousness is unimpaired, the inspired oxygen concentration is increased to 28%, and after further assessment to 35%. If oxygen produces respiratory depression, assisted ventilation may be needed urgently.

SPECIFIC MEASURES

Respiratory failure can be precipitated in chronic bronchitis by infection, fluid retention and bronchoconstriction. Antibacterial drugs are used if the sputum has become purulent. A loop diuretic is indicated if there is pulmonary edema (chapter 33). Bronchospasm may respond to 5 mg salbutamol given 6 hourly in a nebulizer via a tight fitting mask. If this fails to reduce bronchospasm, hydrocortisone, 800–1200 mg/day, is infused intravenously. If, despite the above treatment, PaO_2 continues to fall and $PaCO_2$ to rise and consciousness becomes impaired, endotracheal intubation and suction with controlled respiration should be considered.

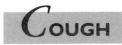

COUGH

Cough suppressants

Cough is a normal physiological reflex that frees the respiratory tract of accumulated secretions and removes particulate matter. The reflex is usually initiated by irritation of the mucous membrane of the respiratory tract and is coordinated by a center in the medulla. Ideally treatment should not impair elimination of bronchopulmonary secretions. A number of antitussive drugs are available but critical evaluation of their efficacy is difficult. Cough can be produced in volunteers by inhalation of irritants such as sulfur dioxide or citric acid or capsaicin and the effect of a potential cough suppressant on such induced cough measured. Patients with chronic cough usually have little idea of the effects of drugs on their cough or of its spontaneous variation in intensity from day to day. Using objective recording methods it has been possible to show dose-dependent efficacy for some cough suppressants. Coughing should not normally be suppressed except in a few circumstances such as intractable cough in carcinoma of the bronchus, and when an unproductive cough interferes with sleep, or exhausts the patient. In many patients cough can be relieved by a bland demulcent syrup (e.g. simple linctus BPC) containing no active drug. Codeine depresses the medullary cough center, is effective and frequently used.

Expectorants

Difficulty in clearing the chest of viscous sputum is associated with chronic cough in many patients. Various expectorants and mucolytic agents are available although there is little evidence of efficacy.

1. Drugs which increase production of watery bronchial secretions by reflex stimulation of stomach and duodenum. These include squill and ammonium chloride or bicarbonate. Mixtures containing a demulcent and an antihistamine, a decongestant such as pseudoephedrine and sometimes a cough suppressant such as codeine phosphate are often prescribed. This cocktail is less harmful than anticipated probably because the dose of most of its components is too low to exert much effect.

2. Drugs which reduce the viscosity of sputum by altering the nature of its organic components are also available. They are sometimes called mucolytics, and the traditional agents are unhelpful because they reduce the efficacy of mucociliary clearance (which depends on beating cilia being mechanically coupled to viscous mucus). The increased viscosity of infected sputum is due to nucleic acids rather than mucopolysaccharides and is not affected by drugs such as bromhexine or acetyl cysteine, which are therefore ineffective. Nebulized recombinant DNAase enzyme therapy to break down viscous DNA polymers is being assessed in patients with cystic fibrosis and chronically infected sputum, with encouraging results.

RESPIRATORY SURFACTANT

COLFOSCERIL PALMITATE

This consists of phospholipid, dipalmitoylphosphatidylcholine with hexadecanol and tyloxapol.

Use

Colfosceril palmitate is used in newborn infants (4–24 hours after birth) who are 700 g or more undergoing mechanical ventilation for respiratory distress syndrome (RDS) to reduce the severity of RDS and its complications (pneumothorax, bronchopulmonary dysplasia and death). It supplements the natural surfactants in the lung which are deficient in premature babies. Infants who are treated must be continuously monitored for heart rate and arterial blood oxygenation. The synthetic surfactant is given as 67.5 mg/kg via the endotracheal tube; if still intubated the dose may be repeated after 12 hours. All the administered surfactant is rapidly dispersed and undergoes the same recycling as natural surfactant, without evidence of inhibiting synthesis of natural phospholipids.

Adverse effects

1. Obstruction of the endotracheal tube.

2. Increased incidence of pulmonary hemorrhage.

3. Acute hyperoxemia due to rapid improvement if not monitored.

α_1-ANTITRYPSIN

α_1-Antitrypsin is a serine protease produced by the liver. It inhibits neutrophil elastase in lungs. In patients deficient in α_1-antitrypsin neutrophil elastase destroys the alveolar wall leading to early onset emphysema which is rapidly progressive. Such patients usually die of respiratory failure. Diagnosis is by measuring α_1-antitrypsin in blood. Replacement therapy with α_1-antitrypsin can be considered. At present in the USA, replacement therapy with heat treated (human immunodeficiency and hepatitis virus negative) pooled plasma from donors is given intravenously weekly or four times the weekly dose given monthly. The half-life of α_1-antitrypsin is 5.2 days and the only adverse effect is postinfusion fever. Plasma concentrations rise into the normal range and longitudinal clinical studies are in progress to establish efficacy. Aerosolized administration on a weekly basis is also being studied and the use of recombinant α_1-antitrypsin is being investigated.

RESPIRATORY STIMULANTS

Respiratory stimulants (analeptic drugs) stimulate the central nervous system. Small doses produce respiratory and cardiovascular stimulation, but larger amounts are convulsant. Analeptic drugs are of possible short-term value in acute exacerbations of chronic lung disease.

DOXAPRAM

This is a non-specific central nervous system stimulant. The ratio of convulsant to respiratory stimulant dose is 70:1 but large doses of doxapram produce general central nervous stimulation and tachycardia, palpitations, sweating and tremor. Doxapram is contraindicated in epilepsy, hypertension, cerebral edema and hyperthyroidism and should not be used with monoamine oxidase inhibitors or sympathomimetic drugs. Doxapram is given intravenously 0.5–1.5 mg/kg over 30 s followed by an infusion of 2–4 mg/min. The half-life is 2.5–4.0 hours.

ALMITRINE

Almitrine bimesylate (not licensed in the UK) is given as 10 mg orally in patients with chronic respiratory failure and cor pulmonale, increasing ventilation via stimulation of peripheral chemoreceptors. It also affects the pulmonary vasculature and may improve alveolar ventilation/perfusion matching in some patients. Almitrine may retard the progression of cor pulmonale and perhaps has an adjunctive role to chronic oxygen therapy. Its major side effect is reversible painful neuropathy.

Respiratory stimulants in ventilatory failure

The standard treatment of ventilatory failure with controlled administration of oxygen in low concentrations is usually successful. Doxapram is considered in the short term for treating patients with acute exacerbations of chronic bronchitis with accompanying type II respiratory failure, i.e. hypercapnia and hypoxia, when ventilation is unavailable or not deemed suitable. Doxapram is also effective (over short periods) in reversing the fall in PaO_2 which may result from oxygen administration in such patients.

DRUG-INDUCED PULMONARY DISEASE

The lungs may be adversely affected by drugs in several important ways. Physical irritation by the powder of disodium cromoglycate can precipitate bronchospasm in asthmatics. Allergy to drugs of the immediate variety (type I) is particularly common in atopic individuals. Specific reaginic antibodies (IgE) to drugs can produce disturbances ranging from mild wheezing to laryngeal edema or anaphylactic shock. Delayed bronchospasm may be due to drug interactions involving IgG antibodies (type III). Any drug may be responsible for allergic reactions, but several antibiotics are powerful allergens.

β-Blockers can produce prolonged and dangerous, often fatal, bronchospasm in asthma and hay fever sufferers. Aspirin and other non-steroidal anti-inflammatory drugs (chapter 23) cause bronchoconstriction in sensitive individuals with asthma, nasal polyps and urticaria (up to 3% of asthmatics). Parasympathomimetic drugs and acetylcholinesterase inhibitors such as physostigmine can increase bronchial secretions and raise airways resistance. Angiotensin-converting enzyme (ACE) inhibitors (chapters 25 and 28) commonly (9–30% of patients) cause a chronic dry cough which is dose dependent and unresponsive to simple remedies. It is probably caused by inhibition of pulmonary ACE which is also responsible for the breakdown of bradykinin and tachykinin in the tissues.

Pulmonary eosinophilia presents as dyspnea, cough and fever. The chest X ray shows widespread patchy changing shadows and there is usually eosinophilia in the peripheral blood. The pathogenesis of the condition is not fully understood but several drugs have been implicated in this reaction, including aspirin, nitrofurantoin, imipramine, isoniazid, penicillins and streptomycin. Polyarteritis nodosa is sometimes associated with hepatitis B acquired by abuse of amphetamines ('skin popping'). Sulfonamides have also been implicated in such reactions.

The lungs can be involved by pleuritic reactions, pneumonia-like illness and impaired respiratory function due to small, stiff lungs in drug-induced systemic lupus erythematosus. Examples of drugs that cause this include hydralazine and procainamide.

Several drugs can produce pulmonary fibrosis. Drugs implicated include amiodarone, bleomycin, busulphan, cyclophosphamide, gold salts, methotrexate and nitrofurantoin.

The Alimentary System

VI

Alimentary System and Liver

31

(*with Dipti Amin*)

Peptic ulceration **396**

Esophageal disorders **404**

Antiemetics **405**

Inflammatory bowel disease **409**

Constipation **411**

Diarrhea **415**

Irritable bowel syndrome **416**

Pancreatic disease **416**

Liver disease **418**

Gallstones **422**

Drugs modifying appetite **423**

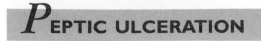

*P*EPTIC ULCERATION

Pathophysiology

Peptic ulcer disease is a chronic disorder characterized by frequent recurrences over a period of many years. It affects approximately 10% of the population of western countries.

The incidence of duodenal ulcer is four to five times higher than that of gastric ulcer. Up to 1 million of the UK population suffer from peptic ulceration in a 12-month period.

Figure 31.1 illustrates the mechanisms regulating gastric acid secretion. Peptic ulceration occurs in a number of clinical settings

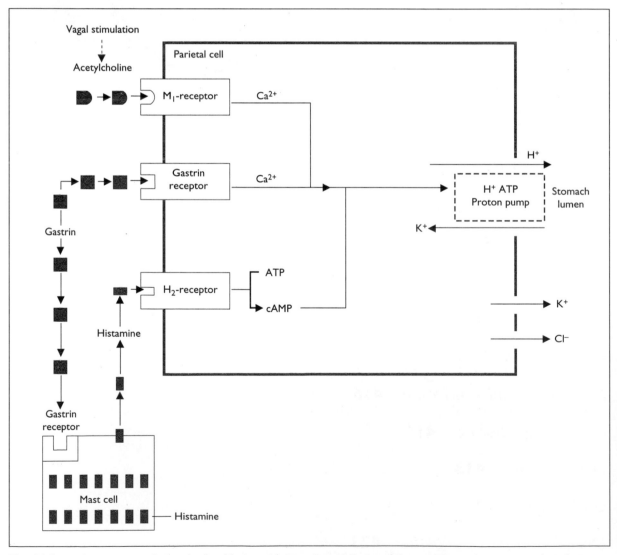

Fig. 31.1 Mechanisms regulating hydrochloric acid secretion. Ca^{2+} = calcium. ATP = adenosine triphosphate. cAMP = cyclic adenosine monophosphate. K^+ = potassium. Cl^- = chloride.

and it is unlikely that a single drug will be universally effective. The etiology of ulceration is not understood well but there are four major factors of known importance:

1. Acid–pepsin secretion.
2. Mucosal resistance to attack by acid and pepsin.
3. Non-steroidal anti-inflammatory drugs (NSAIDs).
4. The presence of *Helicobacter pylori*.

ACID–PEPSIN SECRETION

Gastric parietal (oxyntic) cells secrete isotonic hydrochloric acid (pH<1). Acid secretion is stimulated by gastrin, acetylcholine, and histamine. Gastrin is secreted by endocrine cells in the gastric antrum and duodenum. Zollinger–Ellison syndrome is an uncommon disorder caused by a gastrin-secreting adenoma associated with very severe peptic ulcer disease.

MUCOSAL RESISTANCE

Some endogenous mediators suppress acid secretion and protect the gastric mucosa. Prostaglandin E_2 (the principal prostaglandin synthesized in the stomach) is an important gastroprotective mediator. It inhibits secretion of acid, promotes secretion of protective mucus and causes vasodilatation of submucosal blood vessels. The gastric and duodenal mucosa is protected against acid–pepsin digestion by a mucus layer into which bicarbonate is secreted. Agents such as salicylate, ethanol and bile impair the protective function of this layer. Acid diffuses from the lumen into the stomach wall at sites of damage where the protective layer of mucus is defective. The presence of strong acid in the submucosa causes further damage, and persistence of hydrogen ions in the interstitium initiates or perpetuates peptic ulceration. Hydrogen ions are cleared from the submucosa by diffusion into blood vessels and are then buffered in circulating blood. Local vasodilatation in the stomach wall is thus an important part of the protective mechanism against acid–pepsin damage.

NON-STEROIDAL ANTI-INFLAMMATIORY DRUGS

Aspirin and other NSAIDs inhibit the biosynthesis of prostaglandin E_2 as well as causing direct irritation and damage to the gastric mucosa.

HELICOBACTER PYLORI

Helicobacter pylori is a bacterium that is strongly linked to the development and recurrence of duodenal ulcer. This organism is usually found in the gastric antrum but may also colonize other areas of the stomach and patches of gastric metaplasia in the duodenum. It is a common cause of antral gastritis and its eradication may alleviate symptoms in dyspeptic patients. However it is very common even in asymptomatic subjects and the relationship between *Helicobacter* infection of the stomach and symptoms remains controversial. Antral gastritis is, however, closely associated with duodenal ulcer, and *Helicobacter* is present in the stomach of 95% of patients with duodenal ulcer. Furthermore, clearance of *H. pylori* in ulcer patients is accompanied by a reduced rate of relapse and its reappearance is associated with recurrent ulceration.

Principles of management

Therapeutic objectives are:

1. Symptomatic relief.
2. Promotion of ulcer healing.
3. Prevention of recurrence once healing has occurred.
4. Prevention of complications.

GENERAL MANAGEMENT

1. Bed rest accelerates healing in gastric ulcers but is no longer appropriate following the advent of effective drugs.
2. Stopping smoking increases the healing rate of gastric ulcers and is more effective

in preventing the recurrence of duodenal ulcers than H_2-receptor antagonists.

3. Diet is of symptomatic importance only. Patients usually discover for themselves which foods upset them. A healthy diet should be recommended as for other individuals (chapter 24).

4. Avoidance of 'ulcerogenic' drugs. These include caffeine (as strong coffee or tea), alcohol, aspirin and other NSAIDs (paracetamol is a safe minor analgesic in these cases) and corticosteroids.

5. Drug therapy. Several drugs (see below) are effective. These are used in various ways.

Duodenal ulcer

Antacids are used to relieve symptoms. The existence of ulceration is confirmed by endoscopy and 1 month's treatment with an H_2 antagonist given. If symptoms resolve, treatment is stopped. If symptoms persist, treatment is continued for another month and endoscopy repeated to confirm the persistence of an ulcer. If the ulcer has failed to heal a change to sucralfate or omeprazole may be useful. An alternative approach is to look for gastric infection with *H. pylori* and, if present, to treat with bismuth and antibiotics. If there is a recurrence of identical symptoms, a repeat course of treatment is given. A few patients require continuous maintenance therapy.

Gastric ulcer

Before treatment with an H_2 antagonist all gastric ulcers require endoscopy and biopsy to exclude malignancy. Treatment is as for duodenal ulcers, but healing should be confirmed by repeat endoscopy. Large ulcers take longer to heal.

Non-steroidal anti-inflammatory drug-associated ulcer

Ulcers associated with NSAIDs usually heal rapidly if the NSAID is withdrawn and an H_2 antagonist given. If it is necessary to continue giving a NSAID in the presence of peptic ulceration, high dose H_2-receptor antagonists or misoprostol should be prescribed concurrently. Whilst many drugs have given the clinical impression that they may produce gastric irritation, ulceration or bleeding, with the exception of aspirin and other NSAIDs, the evidence is currently inadequate.

Drugs reducing acidity

ANTACIDS

Use and adverse effects

Antacids react with gastric acid to form a neutral salt and produce prompt pain relief in the majority of patients. Large doses increase healing of duodenal ulcers at a similar rate to H_2 antagonists, but are less convenient. Antacids are less effective at healing gastric ulcers. Alkalis leave the stomach too quickly to be very effective and the doses commonly taken to suppress symptoms usually produce only a transient reduction in gastric acidity lasting less than an hour, although pain relief lasts longer. Several preparations are available, the choice generally depending on patient preference based on effects on bowel habit. Sodium bicarbonate is rapid in action but produces carbon dioxide by reacting with acid, and so causes belching and distension. Excessive doses produce systemic alkalosis, and sodium intake should be considered in patients with hypertension or heart failure. Calcium carbonate is also rapidly acting and produces carbon dioxide. Absorption of excess calcium resulting in hypercalemia (milk-alkali syndrome) and gastric hypersecretion occur only at very high doses. Magnesium salts (oxide, trisilicate, hydroxide) have a relatively slow action due to their insolubility and may produce diarrhea, whereas aluminum salts (hydroxide, phosphaté, glycinate) are constipating. Aluminum ions are neurotoxic at high concentrations but only minimal absorption occurs from antacid formulations and accumulation is a potential problem only in renal failure, in which they are, however, useful as phosphate binders (chapter 33).

Large doses of aluminum or magnesium antacids taken at fixed intervals (30 ml, 1 and

3 hours after meals and at bedtime) reduce gastric acidity to a degree comparable to cimetidine, with comparable effect on duodenal ulcer healing and pain relief. These doses are larger than the usual (10 ml as required) dosage used for symptomatic relief and cause adverse effects due to alteration of bowel habit. The full regime requires an intensely obsessional patient and a suitcase in which to carry the drugs home.

Drug interactions

Magnesium and aluminum salts can bind other drugs in the stomach, reducing the rate and extent of absorption of antibacterials such as erythromycin, ciprofloxacin, isoniazid, norfloxacin, ofloxacin, pivampicillin, rifampicin, and most tetracyclines, and other drugs such as phenytoin, itraconazole, ketoconazole, chloroquine, hydroxychloroquine, phenothiazines, iron, and penicillamine. They increase the excretion of aspirin (in alkaline urine).

H$_2$-RECEPTOR ANTAGONISTS

Use

H$_2$-receptors stimulate gastric acid secretion and are also present in human heart, blood vessels and uterus (and probably brain). Competitive H$_2$-receptor antagonists in clinical use include cimetidine and ranitidine. The uses of these are similar and are considered together in this section. Because each is so widely prescribed, separate sections on their individual adverse effects, pharmacokinetics and interactions are given below, followed by a brief consideration of the choice between them.

1. In cases of duodenal ulcer H$_2$ antagonists achieve endoscopically verified healing of up to 85% of ulcers after 8 weeks' treatment compared to 30% healing in placebo-treated patients. At least 4 weeks' treatment is required to achieve healing although pain may be relieved within a few days. The usual course of treatment is cimetidine, 400 mg, twice daily after meals (this slows absorption but does not reduce bioavailability) or 800 mg as a single dose at night, or ranitidine, 150 mg, twice daily or a single 300 mg bedtime dose. Larger doses supplemented with other drugs may be used in resistant cases. Acid rebound after cessation of therapy does not occur when the drug is discontinued, although relapse may occur, often quite rapidly. Maintenance treatment with 400 mg cimetidine or 150 mg ranitidine at night reduces the relapse rate from 80–90% per year to about 25% but the required duration of such maintenance is still not clearly defined. If this maintenance dose is discontinued there is a risk of relapse. The question of whether an indefinitely prolonged course of therapy will be necessary is unresolved though the long-term safety of H$_2$-blockade has now been well established. Usually if a patient has less than two relapses per year then each occurrence is treated on an individual basis with approximately 8 weeks' treatment with an H$_2$-blocker. Four or more relapses per year probably warrant continuous low-dose maintenance therapy.

2. In cases of gastric ulcer rates of healing of around 75–80% have been reported together with rapid pain relief, although the associated chronic gastritis is unaffected. Relapse may occur after stopping therapy. It is essential to exclude carcinoma endoscopically since H$_2$-blockers can improve symptoms caused by malignant ulcers.

3. Esophagitis may be treated with H$_2$ antagonists but omeprazole is more effective.

4. In cases of acute upper gastrointestinal hemorrhage and stress ulceration the use of H$_2$-blockers is rational although their efficacy has not been clearly proven.

5. Replacement of pancreatic enzymes in steatorrhea due to pancreatic insufficiency is often unsatisfactory due to destruction of the enzymes by acid and pepsin in the stomach. H$_2$-blockers improve the effectiveness of these enzymes in such cases.

6. In anesthesia, H$_2$-receptor blockers can be given before emergency surgery to prevent aspiration of acid gastric contents particularly in obstetric practice (Mendelson's syndrome).

CIMETIDINE

Adverse effects

Cimetidine has few adverse effects. Diarrhea, rashes, dizziness, fatigue, constipation and muscular pain (usually mild and transient) have all been reported. Mental confusion can occur in the elderly. Cimetidine transiently increases serum prolactin, but the significance of this is unknown. Decreased libido and impotence have occasionally been reported during cimetidine treatment. Chronic cimetidine administration can cause gynecomastia which is reversible and appears with a frequency of 0.1–0.2%. Rapid intravenous injection of cimetidine has rarely been associated with bradycardia, tachycardia, asystole or hypotension. There have been rare reports of interstitial nephritis, urticaria and angioedema.

Pharmacokinetics

Cimetidine is well absorbed (70–80%) orally and is subject to a small hepatic first-pass effect. Intramuscular and intravenous injections produce equivalent blood levels. The plasma $t_{1/2}$ is 2 hours. Cimetidine is only 15–20% protein bound and is removed by hemodialysis. It crosses the placenta and the blood–brain barrier, particularly in seriously ill and elderly patients. Elimination is mainly renal as the unchanged compound but some is excreted as metabolites, mainly the sulfoxide. Renal tubular secretion (by the non-specific base transport carrier, chapter 8) occurs so renal clearance exceeds glomerular filtration rate. Cimetidine blocks the tubular secretion of creatinine and this explains the transient rise in serum creatinine that occurs during the first few weeks of cimetidine treatment. There is a minor excretory pathway into the gut which may become important in renal failure.

Drug interactions

- Absorption of ketoconazole (which requires a low pH) and itraconazole is reduced by cimetidine.
- Metabolism of several drugs is reduced by cimetidine due to inhibition of cytochrome P_{450}, resulting in raised plasma drug concentrations. Interactions of potential clinical importance include warfarin, theophylline, phenytoin, carbamazepine, pethidine and other opioid analgesics, tricyclic antidepressants, lignocaine (cimetidine-induced reduction of hepatic blood flow is also a factor in this interaction), terfenadine, amiodarone, flecainide, quinidine and fluorouracil.
- Cimetidine inhibits the renal excretion of metformin and procainamide resulting in increased plasma concentrations.

RANITIDINE

Adverse effects

Ranitidine has a similar profile of minor side effects to cimetidine. There have been some very rare reports of breast swelling and tenderness in men; however, unlike cimetidine, ranitidine does not bind to androgen receptors, and impotence and gynecomastia in patients on high doses of cimetidine have resolved when they were switched to ranitidine. Cardiovascular effects have been even more infrequently reported than with cimetidine. Small amounts of ranitidine penetrate the central nervous system (CNS) and (like but less commonly than cimetidine) it can rarely cause mental confusion, mainly in the elderly and in patients with hepatic or renal impairment.

Pharmacokinetics

Ranitidine is well absorbed after oral administration but its bioavailability is only 50% suggesting appreciable first-pass metabolism. Absorption is not affected by food. Like cimetidine, the half-life is about 2 hours and some 70% is excreted unchanged by the kidneys by tubular secretion and filtration.

In elderly patients the half-life is prolonged by about 50%, probably because of reduced renal excretion. Clearance is only slightly reduced in patients with liver disease and alteration in the dose is unnecessary. In severe renal failure (creatinine clearance <20 ml/min), therapeutic levels can be achieved with half the usual dose of ranitidine (75 mg twice daily).

Drug interactions

Ranitidine has lower affinity for cytochrome P_{450} than cimetidine and does not inhibit the metabolism of warfarin, phenytoin and theophylline to a clinically significant degree.

Choice of H_2 antagonist

All the H_2-receptor antagonists currently available in the UK are effective in peptic ulceration and are well tolerated. Cimetidine and ranitidine are most commonly prescribed, and have been available for the longest time. Cimetidine is the least expensive but in young men requiring prolonged treatment ranitidine may be preferable due to a lower reported incidence of impotence and gynecomastia. Ranitidine is also preferable in the elderly where cimetidine occasionally causes confusion and also when the patient is on drugs whose metabolism is inhibited by cimetidine (e.g. warfarin, phenytoin or theophylline).

PROTON PUMP INHIBITOR: OMEPRAZOLE

Use

1. Duodenal ulcer: At a dose of 20 mg once daily omeprazole heals over 90% of duodenal ulcers after 4 weeks.
2. Gastric ulcer: An 8 week course of omeprazole, 20 mg, once daily heals 85–90% of gastric ulcers.
3. Esophagitis: Omeprazole, 20 mg, once daily heals erosive esophagitis in approximately 80% of patients after 4 weeks and is licensed for long-term use in peptic esophagitis.
4. Zollinger–Ellison syndrome: Omeprazole is the drug of choice for suppressing acid secretion in this rare disorder. Such patients may need treatment for long periods at high doses (up to 120 mg daily).
5. Other indications: Omeprazole may also have a place in the prevention of stress ulceration in acutely ill and burns patients as well as in the prevention of aspiration syndromes where emergency anesthesia is necessary. There is as yet no clear evidence that omeprazole reduces morbidity or mortality from upper gastrointestinal bleeding but further work on this is awaited.

Omeprazole degrades in the presence of moisture, and capsules are supplied in special containers with a desiccant in the lid, and once the container has been opened the contents should be used within 3 months. To prevent degradation by gastric acid, granules in each capsule are enteric coated.

Mechanism of action

Omeprazole is an irreversible inhibitor of the H^+/K^+ adenosine triphosphatase (ATPase) locus of the gastric parietal cell – the 'proton pump' which secretes acid into the gastric lumen.

Adverse effects

Minor side effects include diarrhea and headache (although both may be severe), nausea, constipation and flatulence. Other less common side effects include muscle and joint pains, skin reactions some of which are serious, blurred vision, peripheral edema, gynecomastia, loss of taste and blood disorders. Severely ill patients may develop reversible mental confusion, depression and hallucinations.

Pharmacokinetics

Bioavailability is very variable and depends on the formulation. The time to maximum plasma concentration ranges from 20 min for a solution to over 2 hours for enteric-coated granules. Plasma half-life is between 0.5 and 1.5 hours with a mean of 1 hour. Volume of distribution is $0.3 - 0.4$ l/kg. Omeprazole is 95% plasma protein bound. Although there is a clear dose-related inhibition of gastric acid secretion with omeprazole, peak concentrations of the drug in plasma do not correlate with antisecretory activity.

Omeprazole undergoes rapid and almost complete metabolism and unchanged drug is not excreted in the urine although nearly 20% of unchanged drug may be recovered in the feces. Clearance is not influenced by renal disease or by hemodialysis.

Drug interactions

Omeprazole inhibits drug metabolism and thereby enhances the effects of warfarin, phenytoin and diazepam.

Antisecretory drugs and gastric cancer

It has been suggested that the chronic use of drugs that suppress gastric acid secretion may produce gastric cancer. The hypothesis is that reduced gastric acidity could allow bacterial colonization of the stomach by nitrate-reducing bacteria. These could produce nitrite from dietary nitrates and could form N-nitroso compounds with food amines. Some N-nitroso compounds are mutagenic and resemble animal carcinogens. All of these steps could theoretically follow any antiulcer treatment and it is certainly the case that carcinoma of the gastric remnant has followed some ulcer operations and occurs in 0.5–20% of patients in several studies. Similarly, there is an increased risk of gastric carcinoma with Addisonian pernicious anemia with associated achlorhydria. Vagotomy, however, is not associated with this problem and similarly no causal link has been established between chronic administration of H_2-blocking drugs and gastric cancer in humans or animals; as yet there is also no definite evidence linking omeprazole to gastric cancer in humans or animals. A potential problem of the use of antisecretory drugs is their effectiveness in producing transient symptomatic relief in gastric cancer hence causing delay in diagnosis.

PROSTAGLANDIN ANALOGS: MISOPROSTOL

Use

Misoprostol is a synthetic analog of prostaglandin E_1 which inhibits gastric acid secretion, causes vasodilatation in the submucosa and stimulates production of protective mucus. It is used:

1. For prophylaxis of gastric and duodenal ulceration in patients on NSAID therapy.
2. In the treatment of NSAID-induced gastric damage.
3. To heal non-NSAID-induced gastric and duodenal ulcers, albeit less effectively than H_2 antagonists and omeprazole.

Adverse effects

Diarrhea, abdominal pain, nausea and vomiting, abnormal vaginal bleeding, rashes and dizziness may occur. The most frequent adverse effects are gastrointestinal ones which are usually dose dependent.

Contraindications

Pregnancy is an absolute contraindication to the use of misoprostol as it causes abortion.

Pharmacokinetics

Misoprostol is rapidly and nearly completely absorbed and extensively metabolized to inactive products that are excreted in urine.

MUSCARINIC RECEPTOR ANTAGONISTS

Use

Acetylcholine acts on muscarinic receptors in gastrointestinal smooth muscle and stomach to cause contractions and acid secretion. Antimuscarinic drugs are used in non-ulcer dyspepsia, irritable bowel syndrome and diverticular disease. Antimuscarinic drugs decrease gastric motility and possibly spasm produced by irritation from ulceration (hence they have been termed antispasmodics). Dose is limited by antimuscarinic side effects and only pirenzepine, a selective M_1 receptor antagonist, has significant antisecretory effects at a tolerated dose.

Adverse effects and contraindications

Adverse effects are predictable from their actions on muscarinic receptors:

1. Dryness of the mouth (decreased salivation).
2. Blurring of vision and photophobia (paralysis of accommodation and dilatation of the pupil); precipitation of glaucoma.
3. Constipation.

4. Urinary retention and difficulty with micturition.
5. Tachycardia.
6. Impotence.

Contraindications include glaucoma, prostatic enlargement, coronary artery disease and pyloric stenosis. Pirenzepine produces fewer such effects than other antimuscarinic drugs because of its higher selectivity for M_1 receptors but some patients notice mild difficulty with accommodation and dry mouth. Anticholinergic drugs alter the rate of absorption of other drugs if given concurrently (chapter 12).

Drugs enhancing mucosal resistance

BISMUTH CHELATE

Colloidal tripotassium dicitratobismuthate precipitates at acid pH to form a layer over the mucosal surface and ulcer base where it combines with the proteins of the ulcer exudate. This coat is protective against acid and pepsin digestion. It also stimulates mucus production and may chelate with pepsin thus speeding ulcer healing. Several studies show it to be as active as cimetidine in the healing of duodenal and gastric ulcers after 4–8 weeks of treatment.

It has a direct toxic effect on *H. pylori* and the greatest current interest in bismuth chelate is as part of triple therapy for the treatment of duodenal ulcer thought to be caused by this organism. In attempting to eradicate *H. pylori* it is important to use combination therapy as there is widespread resistance to antibiotics. The combination that is most commonly used is colloidal bismuth with either tetracycline or amoxycillin and metronidazole for 2 weeks. This is sufficient to eradicate bacteria in 90% of patients. Side effects are common and compliance is difficult. Adverse effects of such triple therapy include malaise, nausea, diarrhea, sore throat, fungal infection and pseudomembranous colitis.

Bismuth chelate elixir is given as 5 ml diluted with 15 ml of water 30 min before meals and 2 hours after the last meal of the day. This liquid has an ammoniacal, metallic taste and odor which is unacceptable to some patients, and chewable tablets can be used instead. Antacids or milk should not be taken concurrently.

Adverse effects

Adverse effects are mainly trivial, consisting of blackening of the tongue, teeth and stools (causing potential confusion with melena) and nausea. The latter may limit dosing. Bismuth is potentially neurotoxic. Urine bismuth levels rise with increasing oral dosage indicating some intestinal absorption. Although with usual doses the blood concentration remains well below the toxic threshold, bismuth should not be used in renal failure or for maintenance treatment. (See also effects of triple therapy of bismuth with antibiotics above.)

SUCRALFATE

Use

Sucralfate is used in the management of benign gastric and duodenal ulceration and chronic gastritis. Its action is entirely local with minimal if any systemic absorption. It is a basic aluminum salt of sucrose octasulfate which, in the presence of acid, becomes a sticky adherent paste that retains antacid efficacy. This material coats the floor of ulcer craters exerting its acid neutralizing properties locally, unlike conventional antacid gels which form a diffusely distributed antacid dispersion. In addition it binds to pepsin and bile salts and prevents their contact with the ulcer base. Sucralfate compares favorably with cimetidine for healing both gastric and duodenal ulcers and is equally effective in symptom relief. The dose is 1 g (1 tablet) four times daily for 4–6 weeks. Antacids may be given concurrently.

Adverse effects

It is well tolerated but, because it contains aluminum, constipation can occur and in severe renal failure accumulation is a potential hazard.

CARBENOXOLONE

Use

Carbenoxolone is a liqorice derivative used to treat benign gastric ulceration. Its mode of action is complex and it increases mucosal resistance without affecting acid secretion or motility. It is now seldom used because there are more effective and better tolerated alternatives.

Adverse effects

Side effects are frequent and hazardous. Those particularly at risk are the elderly and patients with cardiac, renal and hepatic disease.

1. Sodium retention is common due to an aldosterone-like action. Headache, edema, dyspnea, cardiac failure, hypertension and epilepsy have all been reported. Mild fluid retention can be corrected with a thiazide diuretic but spironolactone cannot be used since, although effective, it interferes with the ulcer-healing effects.
2. Hypokalemia occurs in 30–40% of patients. This can be so severe as to present with muscle weakness, myositis, myasthenia, myoglobinuria and peripheral neuropathy and a diagnosis of hyperaldosteronism or Guillain–Barré syndrome may be considered. The drug must be stopped and potassium supplements may be needed temporarily.

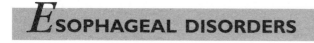

ESOPHAGEAL DISORDERS

Reflux esophagitis

Reflux esophagitis is a common problem: it causes heartburn and acid regurgitation and predisposes to stricture formation.

Non-drug measures

Non-drug measures which may be useful include:

1. Sleeping with the bed head raised. Most damage to the esophagus occurs at night when swallowing is much reduced and acid can remain in contact with the mucosa for long periods.
2. Avoid:
   (a) Large meals.
   (b) Alcohol and/or food before bed.
   (c) Smoking, which lowers the lower esophageal sphincter (LES) pressure and coffee.
   (d) Aspirin and NSAIDs.
   (e) Constricting clothing around the abdomen

3. Weight reduction.
4. Bending from knees not the spine.

Drug therapy

Drugs that may be useful include:

1. Metoclopramide or cisapride (see below), which raise LES pressure.
2. A mixture of alginate with antacids is symptomatically useful. The alginate forms a viscous layer floating on the gastric contents.
3. A mixture of silicon with an antacid (e.g. dimethicone, aluminum hydroxide and sorbitol). These mixtures are supposed to lower surface tension and thus allow formation of large and easily expelled gas bubbles from the stomach without encouraging reflux. It is not clear why this helps in reflux: possibly the silicon coats the lower esophagus and 'protects' it from acid/bile. It is of uncertain value.

4. Symptomatic relief may be obtained with antacids, but there is a risk of chronic aspiration of poorly soluble particles of magnesium or aluminum salts if these are taken at night.
5. H$_2$ antagonists.
6. Proton pump inhibitors. Omeprazole is the most effective agent currently available for reflux esophagitis and is the drug of choice for erosive reflux esophagitis.

CISAPRIDE

Use

Cisapride is a motility stimulant that releases acetylcholine in the gut wall; unlike metoclopramide it does not have central dopamine antagonist properties. It is costly. It is used in:

1. Gastroesophageal reflux: Cisapride (10 mg three times a day for up to 12 weeks) is more effective than placebo and about as effective as H$_2$ antagonists in reducing the symptoms and healing reflux esophagitis.
2. Dyspepsia: Patients who have dyspeptic symptoms without an identifiable lesion on endoscopy. Cisapride (10 mg three times daily for between 2 and 4 weeks) causes relief of symptoms in more than 80% of such patients, compared with only about 35% of those on placebo.
3. Delayed gastric emptying: This may be due to chronic administration of other drugs such as alcohol, opiates, anticholinergics, or in association with systemic diseases causing disorders of motility such as the autonomic neuropathy of diabetes mellitus. A trial of cisapride, 10 mg, three times daily for 6 weeks or longer may prove effective.

Adverse effects

These are predominantly those of increased gut motility such as abdominal cramps, borborygmi, diarrhea and loose stools. Other minor effects include headache and dizziness and there have been rare reports of headache and extrapyramidal effects.

Pharmacokinetics

There is rapid and extensive absorption (94–96%) following oral administration of cisapride with a peak concentration at 1–2 hours. Plasma half-life is 7–10 hours and it has a volume of distribution of 2.4 l/kg. It is 98% protein bound, predominantly to albumin. The predominant site of metabolism is the liver. Half-life is prolonged in elderly patients and in those with renal failure and cirrhosis, and it is important to reduce the dose in these patients.

Drug interactions

These are mainly as a consequence of increased rate of gastric emptying, which can increase the rate of absorption of other drugs. This is seldom a problem in practice.

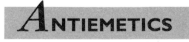

ANTIEMETICS

Complex processes underlie nausea and vomiting. Nausea is associated with autonomic effects (sweating, bradycardia, pallor and profuse salivary secretion). Vomiting is preceded by rhythmic muscular contractions of the 'respiratory' muscles of the abdomen (retching) and is a somatic rather than an autonomic function. Central coordination of these processes occurs in a group of cells in the dorsolateral reticular formation in the floor of the fourth ventricle of the medulla oblongata in close proximity to the cardiovascular and respiratory centers with which it has synaptic connections. This vomiting center (Fig. 31.2) is not directly responsive to chemical emetic stimuli but is activated by one or more inputs. The major efferent pathways from the vomiting center

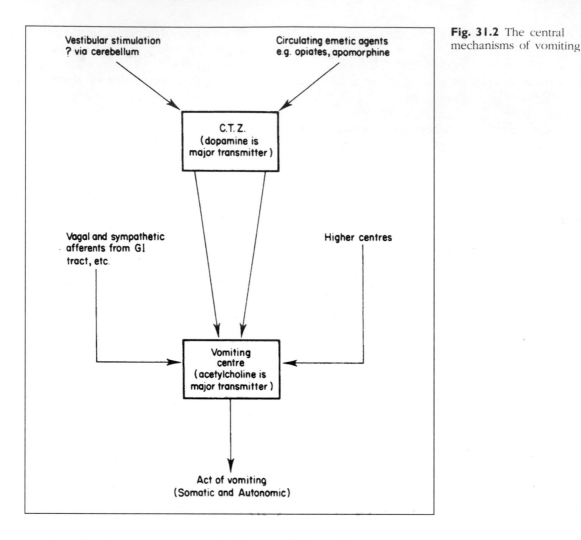

Fig. 31.2 The central mechanisms of vomiting

are the phrenic nerve, visceral efferent of the vagus to the stomach and esophagus and the spinal nerves to the abdominal musculature.

An important receptor area for emetic stimuli, the chemoreceptor trigger zone (CTZ), is a group of neurones in the area postrema of the fourth ventricle which is sensitive to emetic stimuli such as radiation, bacterial toxins and uremia. Dopamine excites CTZ neurones which in turn activate the vomiting center and cause emesis. Emetic stimuli originating in the pharynx, esophagus and gut are transmitted directly to the vomiting center via the vagus and glossopharyngeal nerves. Those from the vestibular organs (in travel sickness and Ménière's disease) act indirectly via the CTZ. A histamine pathway is apparently involved in labyrinthine vomiting. Naloxone, an opioid antagonist, can block the antiemetic

effect of nabilone on the vomiting produced by apomorphine and nitrogen mustard in cats. This and other evidence suggests that opioid receptors may be involved in centrally induced emesis involving higher centers. Drugs may act at more than one site to provoke emesis, for example nitrogen mustard (CTZ, cortex,

Table 31.1 Classification of antiemetics.

Anticholinergics, e.g. hyoscine
Antihistamines (H_1-blockers), e.g. promethazine
Dopamine antagonists, e.g. metoclopramide
5-Hydroxytryptamine receptor ($5HT_3$) antagonists, e.g. ondansetron
Cannabinoids, e.g. nabilone
Miscellaneous: Corticosteroids
               Benzodiazepines
               Trimethobenzamide

gut), digitalis (CTZ and gut). Antiemetic drugs are classified pharmacologically in Table 31.1.

Antiemetics should only be used when the cause of nausea or vomiting is known lest the symptomatic relief produced should delay diagnosis of a remediable and serious cause. Nausea and sickness during the first trimester of pregnancy will respond to most antiemetics but should rarely be treated with drugs because of possible dangers (unquantifiable) of teratogenesis.

Muscarinic receptor antagonists

These act partly by their antimuscarinic action on the gut as described above, but also have some central action. Hyoscine, 0.3 mg, is effective in preventing motion sickness. It is useful in single doses for short journeys but the anticholinergic side effects (dry mouth, blurred vision, drowsiness) are too troublesome for chronic use.

Antihistamines (H_1-blockers)

These are most effective in preventing motion sickness and treating vertigo and vomiting from labyrinthine disorders. They have additional anticholinergic actions and this contributes to their antiemetic effect. They include cyclizine, promethezine, betahistine and cinnarizine. The main limitations of these drugs are their modest efficacy and common dose-related adverse effects in addition to antimuscarinic effects.

1. Cyclizine given either orally or by injection is effective in opiate-induced vomiting and has been given widely in pregnancy without any untoward effects on the fetus. The main side effects are drowsiness and a dry mouth.
2. Promethazine is also an effective antiemetic. It is more sedative than cyclizine.
3. Betahistine is used in vertigo, tinnitus and hearing loss associated with Ménières disease, the dose being 8–16 mg three times daily after meals.
4. Cinnarizine is an antihistamine and calcium antagonist. It has an action on the labyrinth and is effective in motion sickness and in vertigo. The dose is 30 mg three times daily orally.

Dopamine antagonists

METOCLOPRAMIDE

Use

Metoclopramide is effective for:

1. Postoperative vomiting.
2. Radiation sickness.
3. Drug-induced nausea.
4. Migraine (chapter 18).
5. Diagnostic radiology of the small intestine is facilitated by metoclopramide, which reduces the time required for barium to reach the cecum and reduces the number of films required.
6. Duodenal intubation and endoscopy are facilitated.
7. Emergency anesthesia (including in pregnancy) to clear gastric contents.
8. Symptoms of reflux esophagitis may be improved since it prevents nausea, regurgitation and reflux.

The usual effective dose is 10 mg orally three to four times daily; intramuscularly or intravenously it is given 10 mg one to three times daily depending on the severity of the condition. It should be avoided for 3–4 days following gastrointestinal surgery.

Adverse effects

Adverse effects are usually mild but can be severe. Extrapyramidal effects (about 1% of patients) consist of dystonic effects including akathisia, oculogyric crises, trismus, torticollis and opisthotonos, but Parkinsonian features are absent. These effects are commoner in females and the young. They are treated by stopping metoclopramide and giving benztropine or diazepam acutely if necessary. Overdosage in infants, in whom the maximum dose is 0.5 mg/kg, has produced convulsions, hypertonia and irritability. Milder effects include dizziness, drowsiness, lassitude and bowel disturbances.

Mechanism of action

Metoclopramide increases the amount of acetylcholine released at postganglionic terminals.

Metoclopramide is a central dopamine antagonist and raises the threshold of the CTZ. It also decreases the sensitivity of the visceral nerves carrying impulses from the gut to the emetic centre. It is relatively ineffective in motion sickness and other forms of centrally mediated vomiting.

High doses of metoclopramide block $5HT_3$ receptors.

Pharmacokinetics

Metoclopramide is well absorbed orally and is also given by intravenous or intramuscular injection. It undergoes metabolism by dealkylation and amide hydrolysis, about 75% being excreted as metabolites in the urine. Mean plasma $t_{1/2}$ is 4 hours.

Drug interactions

Metoclopramide potentiates the extrapyramidal effects of phenothiazines and butyrophenones. Its effects on intestinal motility result in numerous alterations in drug absorption which include increased rates of absorption of several drugs including aspirin, tetracycline and paracetamol.

DOMPERIDONE

Domperidone is a dopamine receptor antagonist similar to metoclopramide. It does not penetrate the blood–brain barrier and seldom causes sedation or extrapyramidal effects. The CTZ, however, lies functionally outside the barrier and thus domperidone is an effective antiemetic which can logically be given with centrally acting dopamine agonists or levodopa to counter their emetogenic effect (e.g. apomorphine for severe Parkinsonism, chapter 16). The dose is 10–20 mg orally or by injection 4–8 hourly.

PHENOTHIAZINES

Use

Phenothiazines (chapter 16) act on the CTZ, and larger doses depress the vomiting center as well. The following have established uses as antiemetics:

1. Chlorpromazine, 10–25 mg, orally or 25 mg by i.m injection; 100 mg by suppository causes sedation (unlicensed).
2. Prochlorperazine, 5–25 mg, orally; 12.5 mg by intramuscular injection; 25 mg by suppository.
3. Perphenazine, 2–5 mg.

These are effective against opioid- and radiation-induced vomiting and sometimes are helpful in vestibular disturbances. They are least effective in motion sickness. All carry a risk of extrapyramidal disturbances, dyskinesia and restlessness. Perphenazine is probably the most soporific of this group.

BUTYROPHENONES

See chapter 16.

Droperidol is used as an antiemetic. It is given by intramuscular or intravenous injection in a dose of 2.5–10 mg. Its use is largely restricted to opioid-induced vomiting. Extrapyramidal effects and oculogyric crises are a particular risk.

5-Hydroxytryptamine ($5HT_3$)-receptor antagonists

Use

Ondansetron is a highly selective 5-hydroxytryptamine ($5HT_3$)-receptor antagonist, licensed in 1990 for use in the treatment of nausea and vomiting occurring due to cancer chemotherapy and radiotherapy and subsequently for use in the treatment of postoperative nausea and vomiting. It is predominantly used in patients who have not achieved adequate control with other antiemetics or who have experienced side effects with other drugs such as dystonic reactions with metoclopramide, and for very emetogenic chemotherapy regimes which include cisplatin.

Mechanism of action

The site of action of $5HT_3$-receptor antagonists is uncertain. This may be peripheral at abdominal visceral afferent neurones, or central within the area postrema of the brain or a combination of both.

Adverse effects

Serious side effects are very rare. The most common complaint is one of constipation due to slowing of intestinal transit. A less frequent complaint is of headache as well as flushing or a sensation of warmth, sedation, abdominal discomfort and diarrhea. Transient elevation of liver transaminases has been reported.

Pharmacokinetics

Ondansetron is rapidly absorbed after oral administration with a peak plasma concentration at 1–1.5 hours. It is approximately 70–75% bound to plasma proteins with a plasma half-life of approximately 3 hours. It is extensively metabolized in liver with very little excreted unchanged in the urine. Ondansetron is available as both an oral and an intravenous preparation.

Granisetron is similar to ondansetron. Both drugs are expensive, compared to other antiemetics.

Cannabinoids

Cannabis and its major constituent, Δ^9-tetra-hydrocannabinol (THC) have antiemetic properties and have been used to prevent vomiting caused by cytotoxic therapy. In an attempt to reduce side effects and increase efficacy, a number of analogs, including nabilone, have been synthesized. The site of action of nabilone is not known but an action on cortical centers affecting vomiting via descending pathways seems probable. There is some evidence that opioid pathways are involved in these actions. There appears to be very little to choose between the members of the group both in terms of efficacy and side effects. They are only moderately effective.

Adverse effects

Adverse effects include sedation, confusion, incoordination, dry mouth and hypotension. These are more prominent in older patients.

Miscellaneous agents

Large doses of corticosteroids exert some antiemetic action when used with cytotoxic drugs. Their mode of action is not known. Benzodiazepines given before treatment with cytotoxics reduce vomiting. Whether this a specific antiemetic action or is due to reduced anxiety is unknown.

INFLAMMATORY BOWEL DISEASE

Mediators of the inflammatory response in ulcerative colitis and Crohn's disease include kinins and prostaglandins. The latter stimulate adenylyl cyclase which induces active ion secretion and thus diarrhea. Synthesis of prostaglandin E_2, thromboxane A_2 and prostacyclin by the gut increases during disease activity but not during remission. Sulfasalazine and its active metabolite 5-aminosalicylic acid influence the synthesis and metabolism of these eicosonoids, and influence the course of disease activity.

Apart from correction of dehydration, nutritional and electrolyte imbalance (which in an acute exacerbation is potentially life-saving) and other non-specific treatment, corticosteroids, aminosalicylates and immunosuppressive drugs are valuable.

Corticosteroids

Steroids modify every part of the inflammatory response and corticosteroids (chapter 35) remain the standard by which other drugs are judged. Prednisolone and hydrocortisone given orally or intravenously are of proven value in the treatment of acute colitis or exacerbation of Crohn's disease. Topical therapy in the form of a rectal drip or enema of hydrocortisone or prednisolone is very effective in milder attacks of ulcerative colitis. Corticosteroid enemas are less effective in Crohn's colitis. Systemic absorption may occur.

Steroids are not useful in maintaining remission in ulcerative colitis. They may have some efficacy in this respect in Crohn's disease but their hazards are such that failure to maintain remission below 15 mg prednisolone per day necessitates adoption of alternative steroid sparing therapy.

Prednisolone is preferred to hydrocortisone as it has less mineralocorticoid effect at equipotent anti-inflammatory doses. The dose, route of administration (oral or rectal) and duration of treatment will vary according to the extent of the disease during relapse and the response to therapy. The usual initial oral dose is 40 mg once daily and the initial rectal dose is 20 mg once or twice daily.

Recently steroids which are poorly absorbed from the gastrointestinal tract or have a very high first-pass effect (e.g. budesonide) have been studied in the hope that they would produce similar therapeutic efficacy but fewer systemic side effects. As yet such drugs have mainly been used in local preparations but they may also prove effective as oral preparations.

Aminosalicylates

5-Aminosalicylic acid (5ASA) acts at many points in the inflammatory process and has a local effect on the colonic mucosa. However, as it is very readily absorbed from the small intestine, it has to be attached to another compound or coated in resin to ensure that it is released in the large bowel. Though these drugs are only effective in controlling mild to moderate ulcerative colitis when given orally they are very effective in reducing the incidence of relapse per year from about 70 to 20%. The aminosalicylates are not effective in small bowel Crohn's disease. For rectosigmoid disease, suppository or enema preparations are as effective as systemic steroids.

Currently available drugs of this group include sulfasalazine, mesalazine and olsalazine. Sulfasalazine remains the standard agent but mesalazine and olsalazine avoid the unwanted effects of the sulfonamide carrier molecule of sulfasalazine whilst delivering 5ASA to the colon. Both of these newer agents are useful in patients intolerant to sulfasalazine and in men who wish to be fertile.

SULFASALAZINE

See also chapter 23.

Use

Sulfasalazine is a prodrug which is broken down to the active moiety (5-aminosalicylate) and sulfapyridine. It is used for maintenance treatment of ulcerative colitis, where it reduces the number of relapses. This effect persists for as long as the drug is taken. Rapid acetylators of sulfapyridine achieve therapeutic levels (20 $\mu g/ml$) when given 3–4 g sulfasalazine orally daily, but slow acetylators are likely to experience side effects on this dose because their serum level often reaches 50 $\mu g/ml$. They usually require only 2.5–3 g per day. It is best tolerated by all patients if it is begun in a small dose of 0.5 g twice daily. Sulfasalazine does not help any but the mildest acute attacks for which steroids are the treatment of choice. Sulfasalazine is available as a suppository for use when disease is confined to the rectum or as an adjunct to oral treatment in total colitis. Enteric-coated tablets are also available. Although partially effective in treatment of acute Crohn's disease, it does not maintain remission. It is not effective in patients with disease confined to the small bowel. The use of aminosalicylates in rheumatological disease is discussed in chapter 23.

Adverse effects

Nausea, vomiting, epigastric discomfort, headache and rashes may occur but sulfa-salazine is generally well tolerated. All of the adverse effects associated with sulfonamides can occur with sulfasalazine: they are more pronounced in slow acetylators. Toxic effects on the red cells are common (70%) and in some cases lead to hemolysis, anisocytosis and methemoglobinemia. Sulfasalazine should be avoided in glucose-6-phosphate dehydrogenase (G6PD) deficiency. Temporary oligo-spermia with decreased sperm motility and infertility occurs in up to 70% of males treated for over 3 years. Uncommon effects include pancreatitis, hepatitis, thrombocytopenia, agranulocytosis, Stevens–Johnson syndrome, neurotoxicity, photosensitization, a systemic lupus erythematosus (SLE) like syndrome, and renal effects including proteinuria, hematuria and nephrotic syndrome.

Pharmacokinetics

Sulfasalazine is poorly absorbed from the ileum; bacterial flora in the colon reduce the azo link to liberate the active aminosalicylate moiety. This acts locally in the bowel. Patients with an ileostomy lack the appropriate gut flora and do not split sulfasalazine so that it has little place in their management. Sulfapyridine has little therapeutic effect in the context of inflammatory bowel disease, although it is responsible for some of the adverse effects.

MESALAZINE

This is 5-aminosalicylic acid coated with a resin which dissolves at the pH found in the terminal ileum and colon. It has few side effects, namely nausea, diarrhea, abdominal pain and headache although there have been rare reports of reversible pancreatitis, hepatitis and interstitial nephritis.

OLSALAZINE

This is a prodrug consisting of a dimer of two 5-aminosalicylic acid (5ASA) molecules linked by an azo bond. Less than 1% is absorbed unchanged from the small bowel. The azo bond is split by colonic bacteria and about 20% of the 5ASA is absorbed, acetylated and then excreted in the urine. Diarrhea, rash, nausea and abdominal pain cause 20% of patients to stop the drug.

Immunosuppressive drugs

Other than corticosteroids, the immuno-suppressive drug used most commonly for inflammatory bowel disease is azathioprine (chapter 47) which is metabolized to 6-mercaptopurine. It is most valuable in patients who have frequent relapses and for those whose chronic active disease flares up when steroids are reduced.

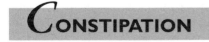

CONSTIPATION

Bowel function and constipation

Under normal circumstances the rectum is empty and fecal material is stored in the descending and pelvic colon. Under the appropriate stimulation, which may include food or drink, certain surroundings and specific times of the day, the colon contracts and feces enter the rectum. Sensors in the rectal wall are activated by the rise in pressure and also probably by tactile stimulus and this results in the call to stool. If this is answered the rectum and distal portion of the colon are emptied by complex coordinated activity consisting of:

1. Colonic contraction.
2. Relaxation of the anal sphincter.
3. Voluntary elevation of the intra-abdominal pressure.

There is considerable variation among healthy people in the frequency of bowel evacuation and anything between three times weekly to 3 times daily may be considered the normal range, but a significant *change* in bowel habit is an important symptom that demands investigation. The term 'constipation' when used by patients describes what they consider to be abnormal bowel function, and it is important to determine whether indeed their bowels are behaving abnormally.

Two main mechanisms lead to constipation: (1) decreased colonic activity and (2) decreased sensitivity of the rectal sensors.

DECREASED COLONIC ACTIVITY

This causes the bowel contents to pass slowly through the colon and become dehydrated and hard and of small volume. Under these circumstances emptying of the colon into the rectum is infrequent and rectal stimulation is minimal. This may be due to a variety of factors:

1. Old age, immobility.
2. Low bulk diet, dehydration.
3. Metabolic disorders – hypercalcemia, myxedema.
4. Depression, confusional states.
5. Various local conditions of the colon large bowel including carcinoma.
6. Drugs (see Table 31.2).

Table 31.2 Drugs that cause constipation.

| Aluminum hydroxide |
| Amiodarone |
| Anticholinergics |
| Disopyramide |
| Diuretics |
| Iron preparations |
| Opioids |
| Tricyclic antidepressants |
| Verapamil |

DECREASED SENSITIVITY OF THE RECTAL SENSORS

This usually occurs when the call to stool is neglected. After a while the stimulus dies away and the rectum becomes chronically full of fecal material. The condition is called dyschezia. It may occur in an acute form in patients who are too ill to appreciate or to respond to the 'call to stool' or when bowel evacuation is painful, or in a chronic form in which for domestic or other reasons the patient has not the time, inclination or opportunity to open the bowels at the appropriate time. This is especially a problem with some children and elderly persons.

Management of constipation

When constipation occurs it is important first to exclude both local and systemic disease which may be responsible for the symptoms.

In general patients with constipation present in two ways:

1. Long-standing constipation in otherwise healthy people. This may be due to decreased colon motility or to dyschezia or a combination of both. It is usually sufficient to reassure the patient and to instruct them in the importance of re-establishing a regular bowel habit. This should be combined with an increased fluid intake and increased bulk in the diet. Bran is cheap and often satisfactory. As an alternative, non-absorbed bulk substances such as methylcellulose are helpful. The other laxatives described below should only be tried if these more 'natural' treatments fail.
2. Loaded colon or fecal impaction. Sometimes it is necessary to evacuate the bowel before it is possible to start re-education. This is particularly so in the elderly or those who are ill. In these cases a laxative such as senna combined with glycerol suppositories is appropriate.

Laxatives

Laxatives are still widely, although often inappropriately, used by the public and in hospital. There is now a greater knowledge of intestinal pathophysiology and of outstanding importance is the finding that the fiber content of the diet has a marked regulatory action on gut transit time and motility and on defecation performance.

As a general rule laxatives should be avoided. They are employed:

1. If straining at stool will cause damage, for example postoperatively, in patients with hemorrhoids or after myocardial infarction.
2. In hepatocellular failure to reduce formation and/or absorption of neurotoxins produced in the bowel.
3. Occasionally in drug-induced constipation.

BULK LAXATIVES

Plant fiber

Plant fiber is the portion of the walls of plant cells that resists digestion in the intestine. The main effect of increasing the amount of fiber in the diet is to increase the bulk of the stools and to decrease the bowel transit time; this is probably due to the ability of fiber to take up water and swell. It also binds organic molecules including bile salts. Fiber does not increase the effective caloric content of the diet since it is not digested or absorbed.

The main uses of plain fiber (e.g. bran) are:

1. Constipation, particularly if combined with a spastic colon. By increasing the bulk of the intestinal contents, fibers slowly distend the wall of the colon and this causes an increase in useful propulsive contraction. The main result is a return of the large bowel function towards normal. Similar results are obtained in diverticular disease in which there is colon overactivity associated with a high intraluminal pressure.
2. Proposed effects of fiber in preventing large bowel carcinoma, piles, appendicitis,

coronary artery disease and varicose veins are still speculative.

The starting 'dose' of bran is a dessert spoonful daily and this can be increased at weekly intervals until a satisfactory result is obtained. It may be mixed with food as it is difficult to swallow if taken neat.

Adverse effects and contraindications

Bran usually causes some flatulence which is dose related. Phytates in bran could theoretically bind calcium and zinc ions. Bran should be avoided in gluten enteropathy and is contraindicated in bowel obstruction.

Other bulk laxatives

Methylcellulose takes up water in the bowel and swells thus stimulating peristalsis. If bran is not satisfactory, it is a reasonable substitute.

Osmotic agents

These have been thought for many years to act by retaining fluid in the bowel by virtue of the osmotic activity of their unabsorbed ions. The increased bulk in the lumen would then stimulate peristalsis. However, 5 g magnesium sulfate would be isotonic in only 130 ml and acts within 1–2 hours, well before it could have reached the colon, so mechanisms other than osmotic effects must account for its laxative properties. It has been postulated that, because magnesium ions can also contract the gallbladder, relax the sphincter of Oddi and increase gastric, intestinal and pancreatic enzyme secretion, they may act indirectly via cholecystokinin. Magnesium ions themselves may also have direct pharmacological effects on intestinal function. Sodium sulfate or magnesium sulfate (Epsom salts) are commonly used. It should be remembered that a certain amount of magnesium may be absorbed and accumulation can occur in renal failure. There is little, if any, rational medical use for these saline purges apart from in hepatocellular failure and following activated charcoal in the treatment of overdose (chapter 50).

LACTULOSE

Use

Lactulose is a disaccharide. It passes through the small intestine unchanged but is broken down in the colon by carbohydrate fermenting bacteria to unabsorbed organic anions (largely acetic and lactic acids) which retain fluid in the gut lumen and also make the colonic contents more acid. This produces a laxative effect after 2–3 days. It is effective and well tolerated. It is of particular value in the treatment of hepatic encephalopathy as it discourages the proliferation of ammonia-producing organisms and the absorption of ammonia. The usual dose is 30 ml by mouth after breakfast. In liver failure, larger doses are required, usually between 30 and 50 ml three times daily.

Lubricants and stool softeners

These were believed to act by softening or lubricating the feces but they act at least in part similarly to stimulant purgatives by inhibition of intestinal electrolyte transport.

DIOCTYL SODIUM SULFOSUCCINATE

This is a surface-active agent that acts on hard fecal masses and allows more water to penetrate the mass and thus soften it. Its use should be confined to patients with fecal impaction and it should not be given over long periods.

LIQUID PARAFFIN

Although still available this is obsolete and should not be used. Disadvantages of habitual use include malabsorption of fat-soluble vitamins, inhalation pneumonitis, and leakage

through the anus. Mineral oil cannot be cleared from the tissues and can cause chronic granulomas.

Chemical stimulants

Many of this class (e.g. castor oil, phenolphthalein) are now obsolete because of toxicity, but senna, co-danthramer and bisacodyl are still useful if bulk laxatives are ineffective.

SENNA

Use

Senna in the form of pods or leaves has been used as a laxative for many years. The important constituents are glycosides, which are hydrolyzed by colonic bacteria to the active principles sennoside A and sennoside B. Their main effect is to enhance the response of the colon to normal stimuli so it is important to combine them with a high bulk diet to ensure an adequate physiological stimulus. Senna acts directly on the intramucosal plexus of the gut wall and possibly also on electrolyte transport systems. Sennosides are absorbed in the small intestine and secreted into the colon, so senna takes about 8 hours to produce an effect. It is taken before retiring to bed.

Adverse effects

Colic (spasm) and diarrhea occur if the dose is too large. If given to nursing mothers it enters the milk and can cause diarrhea in the baby. Senna causes a yellow or red discoloration of the urine. Melanosis coli (a benign condition due to deposition of anthroquinone pigment derived from the drug) may also occur.

CO-DANTHRAMER

Co-danthramer has similar properties to senna.

BISACODYL

Bisacodyl (10 mg by mouth as an enteric-coated preparation) is given at night and the effect seen in about 10 hours. Suppositories produce bowel evacuation in about half an hour. The drug is deacetylated in the gut and then absorbed undergoing transformation to the glucuronide in the liver. This is excreted in the bile and converted back to the deacetylated drug which acts on the colon. It thus has an enterohepatic cycle.

GLYCEROL

Glycerol suppositories act as a rectal stimulant due to the local irritant action of glycerol and are useful if a rapid effect is required.

PHOSPHATE

Phosphate enemas are similarly useful.

Laxative abuse

Persistent use of laxatives, particularly in increasing doses, causes ill health.

After prolonged use of stimulant laxatives, the colon becomes dilated and atonic with diminished activity. The cause is not clear but is perhaps due to damage to the intrinsic nerve plexus of the colon. The disorder of bowel motility may improve after withdrawing the laxative and using a high-residue diet.

Some people, mainly women, take purgatives secretly. This probably bears some relationship to disorders such as anorexia nervosa, concerned with weight loss and is also associated with self-induced vomiting and with diuretic abuse. The clinical and biochemical features can closely mimic Bartter's syndrome, and this possibility should always be investigated in patients in whom the diagnosis of this rare disorder is entertained, especially adults in whom true Bartter's syndrome almost never arises *de novo*. Features include:

1. Sodium depletion: hypotension, cramps, secondary hyperaldosteronism.
2. Potassium depletion: weakness, polyuria and nocturia and renal damage.

In addition there may be features suggestive of enteropathy and osteomalacia.

Diagnosis and treatment are difficult; melanosis coli may provide a diagnostic clue. Urinary electrolyte determinations may help, but can be confounded if the patient is also surreptitiously taking diuretics.

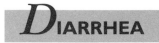

*D*IARRHEA

The most important aspect of the treatment of acute diarrhea is the maintenance of fluid and electrolyte balance, particularly in children and in the elderly. In non-pathogenic diarrhea or viral gastroenteritis, antibiotics and antidiarrheal drugs are best avoided. Initial therapy should be with oral rehydration preparations (such as 'Dioralyte'® or 'Electrolade'®) which contain electrolytes and glucose. Antibiotic treatment is indicated for patients with systemic illness and evidence of bacterial infection.

Adjunctive symptomatic treatment is sometimes indicated. Two main types of drug may be employed, ones that either decrease intestinal transit time or increase bulk and viscosity of gut contents.

Drugs decreasing intestinal transit time

OPIOIDS

See chapter 22.

Codeine is widely used for this purpose in doses of 15–60 mg. Morphine is also given, usually as a kaolin and morphine mixture BPC, which contains 700 µg of anhydrous morphine in every 10 ml dose. Diphenoxylate is related to pethidine and also has structural similarities to anticholinergic drugs. Diphenoxylate may cause drug dependence and euphoria. It is usually prescribed as

'Lomotil' (diphenoxylate 2.5 mg; atropine sulfate 0.025 mg). Overdose with this in children causes features of both opioid and atropine intoxication and may be fatal.

LOPERAMIDE

Loperamide is an effective, well-tolerated antidiarrheal agent. It antagonizes peristalsis, possibly by antagonizing acetylcholine release in the intramural nerve plexus of the gut, although non-cholinergic effects may also be involved. It is poorly absorbed and probably acts directly on the bowel. The dose is 4 mg initially followed by 2 mg after each loose stool up to a total dose of 16 mg/day. Adverse effects are unusual but include dry mouth, dizziness, skin rashes and gastric disturbances. Excessive use (especially in children) is to be deplored.

Drugs increasing bulk and viscosity of gut contents

These are usually satisfactory for milder cases of diarrhea. Preparations include kaolin compound powder BPC, which includes kaolin (a natural form of aluminum silicate), sodium bicarbonate and magnesium carbonate (dose 2–10 g 4 hourly).

Travelers' diarrhea

This is a syndrome of acute watery diarrhea lasting 1–3 days and associated with vomiting, abdominal cramps and other non-specific symptoms, resulting from infection by one of a number of enteropathogens, the most common being enterotoxigenic *Escherichia coli*. It probably reflects colonization of the bowel by 'unfamiliar' organisms. Because of the variable nature of the pathogen there is no specific treatment. Doxycycline prevents most episodes of traveler's diarrhea. There is a danger that widespread use might encourage bacterial antibiotic resistance. Antibacterials can also create problems for the traveler due to their side effects. Early treatment of diarrhea with co-trimoxazole or trimethoprim alone will control 90% of cases and this, with oral replacement of salts and water, is the presently preferred approach.

*I*RRITABLE BOWEL SYNDROME

This motility disorder of the gut affects approximately 10% of the population. Although the symptoms are mostly colonic, patients with the syndrome have abnormal motility throughout the gut and this may be precipitated by dietary items such as alcohol or wheat flour. The important management principles are firstly to exclude a serious cause for the symptoms and to determine whether exclusion of certain foods or alcohol would be worthwhile. An increase in dietary fiber over the course of several weeks may also reduce symptoms. Drug treatment is symptomatic and often disappointing.

1. Anticholinergic drugs such as hyoscine have been used for many years although evidence of efficacy is lacking. The oral use of better absorbed anticholinergics such as atropine is limited by side effects. Pirenzapine is effective in some patients.
2. Mebeverine (135 mg before meals three times daily) directly relaxes intestinal smooth muscle without anticholinergic effects. Efficacy is marginal.
3. Peppermint oil relaxes intestinal smooth muscle and is given in an enteric-coated capsule which releases its contents in the

distal small bowel. It is given before meals three times daily.
4. Antidiarrheal drugs such as loperamide reduce associated diarrhea.
5. Psychotropic drugs such as antipsychotics and antidepressants with anticholinergic properties have also been effective in some patients. In general, however, they should be avoided for such a chronic and benign condition because of their serious adverse effects (chapters 15 and 16).

PANCREATIC DISEASE

Acute pancreatitis has a high mortality. Replacement of fluid and electrolytes can be life-saving. Pain may be severe and is treated with an opioid (e.g. pethidine). Surgery should usually be reserved for complications (e.g. drainage of a related pseudocyst). Underlying disease (e.g. alcoholism, gallstones, hypertriglyceridemia or drugs, Table 31.3) should be sought and treated.

More specific modes of medical management have been disappointing. Drugs recently or currently under investigation include:

1. Aprotinin, a polypeptide (58 amino acids) extracted from bovine lungs which is a proteolytic enzyme inhibitor. A multicenter trial carried out by the Medical Research Council (MRC) has failed to show that it affects mortality. It is uncertain whether the complication rate is altered. Aprotinin is expensive. It is well tolerated, although being a polypeptide it occasionally produces hypersensitivity and rarely anaphylaxis. (It has an unrelated use in preventing bleeding in repeat cardiac surgery.)
2. Glucagon reduces the volume and enzyme concentration of pancreatic juice. The MRC multicenter trial failed to demonstrate benefit in pancreatitis.

3. Anticholinergic drugs are useless in pancreatitis since the excess pancreatic enzyme release is not vagally mediated.
4. Corticosteroids have sometimes been advocated as part of treatment for 'shock'. There is no scientific basis for this and they could be harmful.
5. Octreotide (a somatostatin analog) is undergoing clinical trials.
6. Bradykinin B_2-receptor antagonists have shown activity in animal models.

Pancreatic insufficiency

Exocrine pancreatic insufficiency is an important cause of steatorrhea. The pancreas has a large functional reserve and malabsorption does not usually occur until enzyme output is reduced to 10% or less of normal. This type of malabsorption is usually treated by replacement therapy using pancreatic extracts usually of porcine origin. Unfortunately, although useful, these preparations rarely abolish steatorrhea. A number of preparations are available but the enzyme activity varies between preparations: one with a high lipase activity is most likely to reduce steatorrhea. Unfortunately less than 10% of the lipase activity and 25% of the tryptic activity is recoverable from the duodenum regardless of the dose schedule. This limited effectiveness of oral enzymes is partly due to acid—peptic inactivation in the stomach and duodenum. H_2 antagonists decrease both acidity and volume of secretion and retard inactivation of exogenous pancreatic enzymes and are given as an adjunct to these preparations.

Table 31.3 Drugs associated with pancreatitis (this is uncommon).

Asparaginase	Estrogens
Azathioprine	Pentamidine
Corticosteroids	Sodium valproate
Dideoxyinosine (DDI)	Sulfonamides and sulfasalazine
Thiazides	Tetracycline

*L*IVER DISEASE

Principles underlying drug treatment of hepatic encephalopathy and liver failure

In severe liver disease neuropsychiatric changes occur and can progress to coma. The mechanism which produces these changes is not established but it is known that in hepatic coma and precoma the blood ammonia concentration rises. In many patients the progress of encephalopathy parallels the rise in blood ammonia. Orally administered nitrogenous compounds (e.g. protein, amino acids, ammonium chloride) yield ammonia in the gut, raise blood ammonia concentrations, and provoke encephalopathy. The liver is the only organ that extracts ammonia from the blood and converts it to urea. Bacterial degradation products of nitrogenous material within the gut enter the systemic circulation because of a failure of first-pass hepatic extraction (due to hepatocellular damage) or due to bypass of the hepatocytes by collateral circulation or intrahepatic shunting. About 4 g of ammonia per day is normally produced by bacteria from protein in the gut. Another source is urea which undergoes enterohepatic circulation and yields about 3.5 g/day of ammonia (Fig. 31.3).

Ammonia diffuses into the blood across the large bowel wall where it is trapped by becoming ionized due to the lower pH of blood compared with colonic contents. Ammonia is not the only toxin involved since perhaps 20% of patients with encephalopathy have normal blood ammonia levels and methionine can provoke encephalopathy without causing a significant rise in blood ammonia. Furthermore, ammonia toxicity affects the cortex but not the brain stem which is also involved in encephalopathy.

Other toxins of potential relevance:

1. Intestinal bacterial decarboxylation produces hydroxyphenyl amines such as octopamine (from tyramine) which could replace normal transmitters at nerve endings in the central and peripheral nervous systems, thus acting as 'false transmitters' and changing the balance of inhibition and excitation at central synapses.
2. Changes in fatty acid metabolism increase plasma free fatty acids, some of which

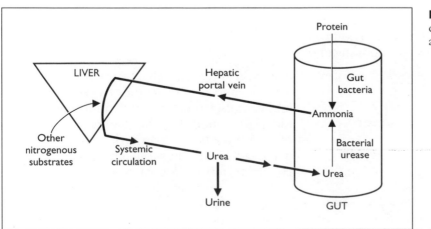

Fig. 31.3 Enterohepatic circulation of urea and ammonia.

have anesthetic properties. In addition, these determine the availability of tryptophan to the brain and hence have an effect on 5-hydroxytryptamine.

Glutathione synthesis is impaired in severe liver disease. Cellular damage due to free radical excess can produce multi-organ dysfunction. Intravenous administration of acetylcysteine is used prophylactically to enhance glutathione synthesis and thereby reduce oxidant (free radical) stresses by scavenging these reactive entities.

Treatment of hepatic encephalopathy includes the following measures:

1. Dietary protein restriction to as little as 20 g/day whilst ensuring an adequate intake of essential amino acids.
2. Emptying the lower bowel by enemas and purgatives to reduce the bacterial sources of ammonia.
3. Oral or rectal administration of non-absorbable antibiotics such as neomycin to reduce the bacterial population of the large bowel. Neomycin, 1–2 g, four times daily is often used: it should be remembered that a 2 g dose produces appreciable absorption and that if the patient also has renal impairment neomycin may accumulate and produce toxicity.
4. Oral lactulose, 50–100 g/day, improves encephalopathy. This disaccharide is not a normal dietary constituent and humans do not possess a lactulase enzyme, so that lactulose is neither digested nor absorbed but reaches the colon unchanged where the bacterial flora splits it to lactate, acetate and other acid products. These trap ammonia and other toxins within the lumen by reducing its pH and in addition act as a cathartic and reduce ammonia absorption by reducing colonic transit time.
5. Bleeding may occur due to interference with clotting factor synthesis or thrombocytopenia. Vitamin K is given and fresh frozen plasma or platelets used as required. Ranitidine is often used to prevent gastric erosions and bleeding.
6. Sedatives should be avoided since patients with liver disease are extremely sensitive to such drugs. If sedation is essential (e.g. because of agitation due to alcohol withdrawal) small doses of oxazepam are preferred to benzodiazepines with longer lived metabolites. The hazards of narcotic analgesics to the patient with acute or chronic liver disease cannot be stressed too strongly.
7. Prophylactic broad-spectrum intravenous antibiotics, especially if there is evidence of infection (e.g. spontaneous peritonitis).
8. Intravenous acetylcysteine.

Drug therapy of portal hypertension and esophageal varices

Esophageal varices form a collateral circulation in response to raised pressure in the portal system and are of clinical importance because of their tendency to bleed. Two-thirds of patients with varices die as a result, and of these one-third die of the first bleed, one-third re-bleed within 6 weeks and only one-third survive 1 year. Sclerotherapy and surgical shunt procedures are the mainstay of treatment and drug therapy must be judged against these gloomy survival figures. In addition to resuscitation, volume replacement and when necessary balloon tamponade using a Sengstaken-Blakemore tube the emergency treatment of bleeding varices may include vasoconstrictor drugs. These reduce portal blood flow through splanchnic arterial constriction:

1. Octreotide (chapter 38): this is a long-acting somatostatin that is now widely used in bleeding varices. Side effects include nausea, vomiting, abdominal pain and diarrhea.
2. Vasopressin (chapter 38): this posterior pituitary hormone and its derivative, terlipressin may also be used. Generalized vasoconstriction may precipitate coronary ischaemia (reduced by co-administration

of nitrates) in addition to abdominal pain, pallor and nausea.

Prevention of bleeding may be achieved by propranolol given orally. Propranolol lowers portal pressure by decreasing cardiac output, reducing splanchnic blood flow (via β_2-receptor blockade in mesenteric arterioles) and decreasing hepatic artery flow (again via β_2-blockade). This treatment is not effective in all patients and does not reduce portal pressure in decompensated cirrhotics. Nitrates are an alternative for patients in whom β-blockers are contraindicated.

Management of chronic viral hepatitis

The carrier rate for hepatitis B in the UK is 0.1–1% (it is particularly prevalent in socially deprived areas of inner cities) and seroprevalence for hepatitis C is 0.1–0.7%. Chronic viral hepatitis is diagnosed when there is evidence of continuing hepatic damage and infection for at least 6 months after initial viral infection. In hepatitis C the liver function may remain normal for months to years whilst the patient's blood remains infectious (confirmed by hepatitis C virus RNA detection). The course of the liver damage often fluctuates. While up to 90% of patients with acute hepatitis B clear the virus spontaneously, up to 60% of those with hepatitis C virus do not. About 20% of those with chronic active hepatitis progress insidiously to cirrhosis, and about 2–3% go on to develop hepatocellular carcinoma.

Hepatitis B virus is a DNA virus that is not directly cytopathic and hepatic damage occurs as a result of the host immune response. Hepatocytes infected with hepatitis B virus produce a variety of viral proteins, of which the 'e' antigen (HBeAg) is clinically the most important. HBeAg is a marker for continued viral replication and therefore for infectivity. Hepatitis C virus is a single-stranded RNA virus.

Several controlled trials have shown that α-interferon is beneficial in chronic hepatitis B virus infection. It is also being used in trials for chronic hepatitis C virus infection.

INTERFERONS

Use (see also pp. 562 and 611)

Interferons are a heterogeneous group of proteins that are produced by the body in response to viral infection. α-Interferon, of which at least 14 subtypes exist, is released by lymphocytes. β-Interferon originates primarily from fibroblasts and γ-interferon is produced by activated T cells. α-Interferon treatment is offered to patients with chronic hepatitis B virus who are HBeAg positive. There is some evidence that the sooner interferon therapy is started, the greater the probability of response. Treatment regimes are currently still being evaluated but therapy is usually continued 4–6 months. The therapeutic response is judged by the loss of hepatitis B 'e' antigen and this occurs in about 40% of those treated with α-interferon compared with 10% of untreated patients. Even those patients who do not achieve seroconversion do show an improvement in liver function. Comparing responders with non-responders suggests certain features that produce a low likelihood of seroconversion and these are:

1. No history of acute hepatitis.
2. Prolonged infection.
3. High serum hepatitis B virus DNA concentrations.
4. Near normal transaminase values.
5. Minimal inflammation on the pretreatment liver biopsy.
6. Human immunodeficiency virus (HIV) infection.

α-Interferon is also effective in hepatitis C virus infections, as judged by normalization of serum transaminase levels which occurs in approximately 50% of those treated compared with 10% in the control groups. The improvement in transaminase levels usually occurs within 4 weeks of starting therapy and is accompanied by an improvement in liver histology.

With both chronic hepatitis B and hepatitis C virus infections, there may be a reactivation when treatment is stopped.

Table 31.4 Dose-dependent hepatotoxicity.

Drug	Mechanism	Comment/predisposing factors
Paracetamol	Hepatitis	See chapter 50
Salicylates	Focal hepatocellular necrosis Reyes syndrome	Autoimmune disease (especially SLE) In children – viral infection
Tetracycline	Central and mid-zonal necrosis with fat droplets	–
Azathioprine	Cholestasis + hepatitis	Underlying liver disease
Methotrexate	Hepatic fibrosis	–
Fusidic acid	Cholestasis, conjugated hyperbilirubinemia	Rare
Rifampicin	Cholestasis, mixed conjugated and unconjugated hyperbilirubinemia	Transient
Synthetic estrogens	Cholestasis, may precipitate gallstone disease	Underlying liver disease, rare now low-dose estrogens are generally given
HMGCoA reductase inhibitors	Unknown	Usually mild and asymptomatic

SLE = systemic lupus erythematosus.

Adverse effects

The side effect profile of α-interferon is divided into early and late effects. Initial side effects which occur soon after the first injection are an influenza-like syndrome with fever, chills, myalgia, malaise and immense fatigue; tolerance to this tends to develop with continued therapy. The later side effects usually occur after days or weeks of treatment and include malaise, myalgia, tiredness, irritability, anxiety and depression, poor appetite and weight loss, alopecia, thrombocytopenia and leukopenia. Effects on the bone marrow are reversible and reducing the dose is often sufficient to allow recovery.

Drug-induced liver disease

After oral administration the entire absorbed dose of drug is exposed to the liver during the first pass through the body. The drug itself or its metabolites may affect liver function. Metabolic pathways may become saturated at high concentrations and drug or metabolites may accumulate leading to toxicity. The drugs shown in Table 31.4 predictably cause hepatotoxicity at excessive doses. Although traditionally hepatotoxicity is divided into dose-dependent and dose-independent hepatotoxicity, the relationship is not always clear cut; for example, even with predictable hepatotoxins there is considerable interindividual variation to susceptibility to hepatic damage. This can sometimes be attributed to genetic polymorphism or to environmental stimuli affecting hepatic microsomal enzymes or to previous liver disease. Although dose-independent hepatotoxicity is used to classify those reactions that are 'idiosyncratic' and usually unpredictable (Table 31.5), the severity of the resulting liver disease may be related to dose or to duration of therapy. Particular drugs tend to produce distinctive patterns of liver injury but this is not invariable.

Table 31.5 Dose-independent hepatotoxicity.

Drug	Mechanism	Comment/predisposing factors
Chlorpromazine	Cholestatic hepatitis	Estimated incidence 0.5%, associated with fever, abdominal pain, pruritus; subclinical hepatic dysfunction is more common
Chlorpropramide Tolbutamide	Cholestatic jaundice	–
Isoniazid	Hepatitis	Mild and self-limiting in 20%, severe hepatitis in <0.1%. Possibly more common in rapid acetylators
Pyrazinamide	Hepatitis	Similar to isoniazid but more clearly related to dose
Methyldopa	Hepatitis	5% have subclinical, raised transaminases, clinical hepatitis rare
Phenytoin	Hypersensitivity reaction	Resembles infectious mononucleosis. Pharmacogenetic predisposition, cross-reaction with carbamazepine
Isoniazid Methyldopa Nitrofurantoin Dantrolene	Chronic active hepatitis	Associated with prolonged treatment, usually regresses when drug discontinued
Halothane	Hepatitis/hepatic necrosis	See chapter 21, p. 214.

Investigation and management of hepatic drug reactions

Depending on the clinical presentation the most important differential diagnoses are hepatic dysfunction due to viral infection (which may be asymptomatic), malignant disease, alcohol and left ventricular failure. The etiology of a minor elevation of transaminases is often undetermined. If the patient is being treated for a disease associated with hepatic dysfunction, particularly with multiple drugs, identification of the responsible agent is particularly difficult. Minor elevations in transaminases are often picked up on routine biochemical profiles. If considered drug related, and further treatment is indicated, it is reasonable to continue the drug with regular monitoring of liver enzymes if a better alternative therapy is not available. If the transaminases reach twice the upper limit of the normal range it is prudent to stop the drug if the clinical situation permits (see also chapter 7).

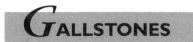

GALLSTONES

Gallstone dissolution

Chenodeoxycholic acid or ursodeoxycholic acid may be considered in patients who cannot be treated by laproscopic chole-cystectomy or endoscopic biliary techniques and who have mild symptoms, unimpaired gallbladder function, and small or medium-sized radiolucent stones. Radiological monitoring is required. Side effects include diarrhea, pruritus and minor hepatic abnormalities. Recurrence is common.

DRUGS MODIFYING APPETITE

Anorectic drugs (see also p. 267)

The commonest form of malnutrition in western society is obesity. Obesity is a killing disease and is preventable since the obese are fat because they eat too much for their needs. Cure is ostensibly simple: they must eat less. In practice, however, treatment is much more difficult. Naturally a calorie controlled diet and sensible amounts of exercise are the essentials of treatment. Unfortunately the results of treating patients at weight-reduction clinics are disappointing: many patients default at an early stage, there is a high relapse rate and only a few achieve permanent weight loss. There has accordingly been a great deal of interest in the possibility of altering appetite pharmacologically so as to help the patient reduce his/her calorie intake. Unfortunately the causes of obesity are not understood. There is conflicting evidence concerning the relative role of overeating, lack of exercise and individual variation in the utilization of food energy. One hypothesis is that lean people do not become obese when they overeat because their tissues preferentially liberate heat (in particular from brown fat). Despite this uncertainty, there is no doubt that starvation leads to weight loss. Therefore, research into drugs for obesity has concentrated on finding substances that inhibit appetite.

Social conditioning plays only a minor role in signalling normal satiety, but learned behavior probably is important in determining the frequency of eating and whether food is taken between major meals. Stretch receptors in the stomach are stimulated by distention, but the main factors that terminate eating are humoral. Bombesin and somatostatin are two candidates for humoral satiety factors released by the stomach. The most important satiety factor released from the gastrointestinal tract beyond the stomach is cholecystokinin (CCK). A small peptide fragment of this (CCK-8) has been synthesized, and has been found to cause humans to reduce their food intake, possibly by acting on the appetite/satiety center in the hypothalamus, but this is not in clinical use.

Amphetamine was shown to be anorectic in humans in 1938 and since that time a number of congeners have been employed for this purpose. The site of action of these compounds appears to be in the hypothalamus, where they increase noradrenaline and dopamine levels by causing transmitter release and blocking reuptake. Some members of this group are diethylpropion, phentermine, fenfluramine and mazindol. The central effects of diethylpropion and phentermine are those of excitation, anxiety and tremor. There is a high incidence of dependence and abuse with amphetamine and it must never be used for obesity. Dependence has also been described for diethylpropion and it would be unwise to assume that it cannot occur with the others. Cardiovascular effects are frequently observed with these drugs, a dose-related increase in heart rate and blood pressure being the most common.

Fenfluramine probably increases 5HT rather than noradrenaline levels in the brain and it may have a peripheral effect by enhancing lipolysis and increasing glucose uptake in fat cells. Although related to amphetamine this drug is not metabolized to amphetamine but is present in the blood and excreted in the urine, partly as unchanged fenfluramine. Although qualitatively its cardiovascular effects are similar to amphetamine they are less marked. Both stimulation and more commonly depression of the central nervous system including drowsiness and dysphoria have been described. Habituation and dependence are rare, but withdrawal may cause depression for several days. Nightmares may occur and it interferes with sleep electroencephalogram (EEG) patterns. It has been described as a drug of dependence but not of abuse. Unlike amphetamine it causes diarrhea. Acute confusional states may arise if given with a monoamine oxidase inhibitor, and it may potentiate the action of antihypertensive, antidiabetic, sedative and other anorectic drugs.

Mazindol appears to increase central dopamine levels but its effects closely resemble those of amphetamine. Its biochemical novelty does not appear to confer any superiority over other agents.

The long-term efficacy of all these agents has never been established and none can be recommended.

Fluoxetine has shown useful activity in patients with bulimia.

BULK AGENTS

Substances such as methylcellulose and guar gum acting as bulking agents in the diet are ineffective. A high-fiber diet may help weight loss, provided total caloric intake is reduced, and is desirable for other reasons as well.

MISCELLANEOUS

Diuretics cause a transient loss of weight through fluid loss. Their use for such an effect is to be deplored. Myxedema is associated with weight gain. Thyroxine has been used to increase the basic metabolic rate and reduce weight in euthyroid obese patients. This is dangerous and irrational.

Appetite stimulation

This is often difficult since patients with a poor appetite may have a debilitating systemic illness or an underlying psychiatric disorder. Drugs that inhibit serotonin (5HT) receptors, for example cyproheptadine, pizotifen, increase appetite and cause weight gain. Weight gain occurs during treatment with some other drugs: chlorpromazine (but not other phenothiazines or butyrophenones), amitriptyline, lithium, corticosteroids and ACTH, and the oral contraceptive pill. Corticosteroids may help appetite in terminally ill patients, but in general these affects are not therapeutically useful, but rather the reverse.

Vitamins and Other Nutrients

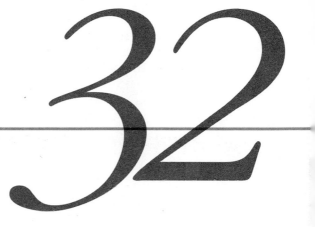

32

Introduction   **426**

Physiology of vitamins   **426**

Vitamin A (retinoic acid) and its derivatives   **426**

Vitamin B₁ (thiamin)   **428**

Vitamin B₂ (riboflavin)   **429**

Niacin (nicotinic acid) and nicotinamide   **430**

Vitamin B₆ (pyridoxine)   **430**

Vitamin C (ascorbic acid)   **431**

Vitamin E (tocopherol)   **432**

Vitamins D and K   **432**

Essential fatty acids   **433**

Trace elements   **433**

INTRODUCTION

Vitamins were first defined more than a century ago by a group of clinical syndromes relating to deficiency states (e.g. scurvy, beriberi). They are nutrients that are essential for health but are required in much smaller quantities than the aliments (carbohydrates, fats and proteins). Vitamins are essential components of cofactors that are needed for intermediary metabolism of the aliments and for numerous other biochemical and cellular control processes.

PHYSIOLOGY OF VITAMINS

Humans are incapable of synthesizing adequate amounts of vitamins. Vitamin deficiency usually results from:

1. Inadequate dietary intake.
2. Increased demand, for example during pregnancy, or growth.
3. Decreased absorption, for example in malabsorption syndrome.

Vitamin deficiency states are often multiple, and several multivitamin preparations are available for oral or parenteral use. Vitamin deficiencies are rarely diagnosed in the UK, but their true incidence is unknown and may be underrecognized in view of their association with poverty, particularly in elderly people and ethnic minorities.

In recent years the concept has emerged that dietary supplements with various vitamins might decrease the incidence of a variety of diseases, including cancer and atheroma. Several clinical trials address this hypothesis, but to date evidence is inconclusive. Not all vitamins are harmless when taken in excess (particularly vitamins A and D) and in general vitamins should therefore only be prescribed for specific indications of prevention or treatment of vitamin deficiency.

Vitamins fall into two groups:

1. Water soluble: the B complex and C.
2. Fat soluble: A, D, E and K. Essential fatty acids are also fat-soluble nutrients which were not classed as vitamins due to historical accident. The absorption of fat-soluble nutrients is impaired in steatorrhea since they are sequestered in the bowel lumen in solution in the fatty stool.

Vitamins B_{12} and folate are discussed in chapter 46, vitamin D in chapter 36 and vitamin K in chapter 27.

VITAMIN A (RETINOIC ACID) AND ITS DERIVATIVES

Physiology

This vitamin exists in several forms that are interconverted: retinol (vitamin A_1) is a primary alcohol and is present in the tissues of animals and seawater fishes; 3-dehydroretinol (vitamin A_2) is present in freshwater fishes; retinoic acid shares some but not all the actions of retinol; retinol ethers and esters also show retinol-type activity. The plant pigment carotene is provitamin A and is readily converted into the vitamin in the body. Vitamin A has several physiological functions: it is essential for the integrity of epithelial cells; it stabilizes membranes; it is an essential component of the visual pigment rhodopsin; and is required for skeletal and soft tissue growth. It acts as a cofactor in mucopolysaccharide synthesis, sulfate activation, hydroxysteroid dehydrogenation, cholesterol synthesis and microsomal drug-metabolizing enzyme function. There is some evidence that vitamin A inhibits tumor formation and encourages the regression of epithelial tumors by enhancing the immune system. Vitamin A deficiency retards growth and development, causes night blindness, keratomalacia, dry eyes and keratinization and drying of the skin. Dietary sources of vitamin A include eggs, fish liver oil, liver, milk and vegetables.

Use

Vitamin A is used to prevent and treat deficiency states. Dietary supplementation with halibut liver oil capsules BP (containing vitamin A 4000–5250 IU and vitamin D 450 IU) are used to prevent vitamin A deficiency. The normal adult daily requirement is about 2500–3000 IU, but for nursing mothers this is estimated to be about 4000 IU. Carotene, as a precursor of vitamin A, can replace the vitamin in the diet; 0.6 μg is equivalent to 1 IU vitamin A.

Large doses of vitamin A are given in clinical deficiency, for example 5000 IU/kg daily (thus 25 000–200 000 IU may be given daily). Although a single large intramuscular injection of retinol palmitate (30 000 μg retinol) has been used in severe malnutrition, this should be followed by oral therapy. In vulnerable and malnourished communities intramuscular doses of 60 000–120 000 μg retinol should be given to children 6 monthly. Continuous dietary or injected supplementation of vitamin A may be necessary in steatorrhea, for example in patients with cystic fibrosis.

Retinoic acid (vitamin A) is irritating when applied to the skin and is used in the treatment of acne to promote peeling. There is evidence that vitamin A accelerates the healing of wounds in normally nourished patients. Large amounts of vitamin A have been given orally to patients with ichthyosis and other skin disorders (chapter 48).

Adverse effects

Long-term ingestion of more than double the recommended daily intake of vitamin A can lead to toxicity. Vitamin E protects against hypervitaminosis A. The effects seen in chronic hypervitaminosis A include:

1. Anorexia, irritability, vomiting, headache.
2. Itching and dry skin.
3. Raised intracranial pressure (benign intracranial hypertension).
4. Tender hyperostoses in the skull and long bones.
5. Hepatotoxicity.
6. Congenital abnormalities.

Acute poisoning (as after eating polar bear liver or injection of more than 500 000 μg) causes:

1. Headache, vomiting and papilloedema.
2. Desquamation.

Excess vitamin A during pregnancy causes birth defects (closely related compounds are involved in controlling morphogenesis in the fetus). Pregnant women should therefore not take vitamin A supplements and should perhaps also avoid liver in their diet.

Pharmacokinetics

Retinol is well absorbed from the normal intestine by a saturable active transport process. Vitamin A absorption is impaired in patients with steatorrhea and under these circumstances water-miscible preparations of vitamin A can be administered. Carotene is converted to vitamin A by first-pass metabolism in the intestine. Esterified retinol reaches peak plasma levels 4 hours after ingestion. About 100 μg/g is stored in the parenchymal and Kupffer cells of the liver. Vitamin E enhances vitamin A storage. Retinol released from the liver is bound to globulin (retinol-binding protein) in the plasma. Retinol is partly conjugated to a glucuronide and undergoes enterohepatic circulation. The normal plasma concentration of vitamin A is 30–70 µg/100 ml. When a vitamin A deficient diet is taken, plasma concentrations are maintained for several months until hepatic stores have been depleted. Clinical evidence of vitamin A deficiency appears when the plasma concentration falls below 20 µg/100 ml. Low plasma concentrations of vitamin A may be present in pregnancy, liver disease and kwashiorkor without a corresponding reduction in liver stores.

Derivatives of vitamin A (retinoids)

Etretinate (chapter 48) is a derivative of retinoic acid. It produces desquamation (as does natural vitamin A) but at doses that do not raise intracranial pressure or cause organ damage. Etretinate is remarkably effective in severe psoriasis (including pustular psoriasis) and in congenital ichthysiform dermatoses. Isotretinoin (chapter 48) is 13-*cis*-retinoic acid. It has a strikingly beneficial effect in severe refractory acne in doses that do not affect psoriasis and ichthyosis.

Retinoids and cancer

Retinoids have powerful effects on cell differentiation and proliferation and can inhibit or retard malignant transformation of cells *in vitro*. In animals they can prevent the action of carcinogens and there is limited epidemiological evidence that retinoid status is a determinant of the risk of developing cancer. Clinical trials on retinoid therapy as primary prevention of cancer are nearing completion. Retinoids, either alone or in combination with established anticancer drugs (e.g. anthracyclines) are also being investigated as therapy for cancer.

VITAMIN B₁ (THIAMIN)

Physiology

All plant and animal cells require thiamin (in the form of thiamin pyrophosphate) for carbohydrate metabolism. Its most important role is as a coenzyme for decarboxylases. Thiamin deficiency leads to the various manifestations of beri-beri including peripheral neuropathy and cardiac failure. Increased carbohydrate utilization requires increased intake because thiamin is consumed during carbohydrate metabolism. It is therefore useful to express thiamin needs in relation to the calorie intake. Diets associated with beri-beri contain less than 0.3 mg thiamin/1000 kcal. If the diet provides more than this the excess is excreted in the urine. Thus the recommended daily intake of 0.4 mg/1000 kcal provides a considerable safety margin. The body possesses little ability to store thiamin and if the vitamin is withdrawn completely from the diet beri-beri develops in a few weeks.

Acute thiamin deficiency is precipitated by a carbohydrate load in patients who have been on a marginally deficient diet. This is especially important in alcoholics, and thiamin replacement should always precede intravenous dextrose in alcoholic patients with a depressed conscious level. Failure to do this may result in worsening encephalopathy and permanent sequelae (e.g. Korsakoff's psychosis). Thiamin is found in many plant and animal foods, for example yeast and pork. The outer coating of grains is rich in thiamin which is lost in the preparation of refined foods such as white flour or polished rice.

Use

The parenteral route of administration is used in confused patients, up to 30 mg is injected intramuscularly or intravenously 8 hourly. Once the deficiency state has been corrected the oral route is preferred, unless gastrointestinal disease interferes with ingestion or absorption of the vitamin. Thiamin hydrochloride tablets range from 3 to 300 mg but a generous oral dose is 5 mg daily. Thiamin is used in the treatment of beri-beri and other states due to thiamin deficiency. These include alcoholic neuritis, Wernicke's encephalopathy and the neuritis of pregnancy. Prophylactic use of thiamin is particularly indicated in chronic diarrheal states and following intestinal resections.

Adverse effects

Severe allergic reactions following parenteral administration of thiamin preparations have been reported, but are uncommon.

Pharmacokinetics

Absorption of thiamin is rapid and complete following intramuscular injection. Absorption from the intestine is limited to a maximum of 8–15 mg in 1 day. Thiamin is absorbed through the mucosa of the upper part of the small intestine by both active and passive mechanisms. Surplus intake is excreted in the urine as unchanged vitamin.

VITAMIN B₂ (RIBOFLAVIN)

Physiology

Riboflavin is converted in the body into two essential coenzymes: flavine mononucleotide and flavine adenine dinucleotide. These are coenzymes for respiratory electron transport proteins and a variety of enzymes that are flavoproteins (e.g. nitric oxide synthase). Riboflavin is present in significant amounts in yeast, green vegetables, liver, eggs and milk. The minimum daily requirement to prevent the signs of riboflavin deficiency is about 0.3 mg/1000 kcal. Riboflavin deficiency is common in developing countries and occurs sporadically amongst the poor and in alcoholics in the UK. It rarely occurs in isolation from deficiencies of other B vitamins. Angular stomatitis and a sore tongue are early findings and are followed by seborrheic dermatitis, itching and burning of the eyes with photophobia and corneal vascularization. Late findings include neuropathy and mild anemia.

Use

The only therapeutic application for riboflavin is in the prevention or treatment of deficiency. Riboflavin deficiency usually occurs with other dietary deficiencies but specific therapy consists of giving 5–10 mg riboflavin orally daily.

Pharmacokinetics

Riboflavin is well absorbed via the small intestine. Absorption is impaired in patients with liver disease. Excellent absorption occurs from intramuscular injections. Very little is stored in the tissues and when amounts in excess of daily requirements are taken the surplus appears unchanged in the urine. On an average UK diet only about 10% is excreted in the urine. Riboflavin in the feces is probably due to bacterial synthesis in the large intestine (from which riboflavin is not absorbed).

Niacin (nicotinic acid) and nicotinamide

Physiology

Niacin is a B vitamin. Its vital metabolic role is as a component of nicotinamide adenine dinucleotide (NAD) and of nicotinamide adenine dinucleotide phosphate (NADP). It is thus essential in numerous hydrogen-transport steps within the cell including drug metabolism. Deficiency causes pellagra, clinical manifestations of which are dementia, dermatitis and diarrhea. Niacin can be generated in the body in small amounts from tryptophan, 60 mg of the amino acid yielding 1 mg niacin. Consequently the pellagra-preventing properties of a diet are expressed as 'niacin equivalents' made up of niacin itself plus tryptophan. Patients with carcinoid syndrome are liable to develop pellagra because the large bulk of metastatic carcinoid tumors utilize substantial amounts of tryptophan in the synthesis of 5-hydroxytryptamine (5HT). Pellagra may develop on diets containing less than 5.0 mg niacin equivalents/1000 kcal. When 5.5 mg niacin equivalents/1000 kcal are taken, large amounts of nicotinamide are excreted in the urine. The recommended dietary intake includes an added safety margin to account for individual variation and is 6.6 niacin equivalents/1000 kcal. Niacin is found in yeast, rice, liver and other meats.

Use

1. Niacin is used to treat and prevent pellagra. In the acute disease the oral dose is 50 mg up to 10 times daily. If oral treatment is not possible, intravenous injections of 25 mg are given two or three times daily. The commonest causes of pellagra in the UK are alcoholism and gastrointestinal disease, multiple vitamin deficiency states often coexist and require treatment simultaneously. The response in acute pellagra is rapid and swelling and soreness of the tongue, mental state disturbance and diarrhea improve within 24 hours, skin lesions responding more slowly.
2. Niacin is sometimes used in pharmacological doses to treat hyperlipidemia (chapter 24).

Adverse effects

In replacement therapy for pellagra adverse effects are uncommon. High dose (as used for hyperlipidemia) causes:

1. Flushing, generalized vasodilatation with syncope; this is caused by prostaglandin D_2, and can be prevented by premedication with aspirin.
2. Nausea, vomiting and itching.
3. Impaired glucose tolerance.
4. Aggravation of hyperuricemia.

Pharmacokinetics

Both niacin and nicotinamide are well absorbed via the intestine and distributed widely to all tissues. When the usual dietary amounts are administered, a high proportion is excreted as N-methyl nicotinamide, and other metabolites. When increased doses are administered, a higher proportion is excreted unchanged in the urine.

Vitamin B₆ (pyridoxine)

Physiology

Pyridoxine is one of the three forms of naturally occurring vitamin B_6. The other two forms are pyridoxal and pyridoxamine. All three forms are converted in the body into pyridoxal phosphate, which is an essential cofactor in several metabolic reactions including decarboxylation, transamination, and other steps in amino acid metabolism. Deficiency causes glossitis, seborrhea, fits, peripheral neuropathy and sideroblastic anemia. Isoniazid prevents the activation of pyridoxal to pyridoxal phosphate by inhibiting the enzyme pyridoxal kinase and slow acetylators of isoniazid are at an increased risk of developing peripheral neuropathy for this reason (chapter 13). The minimal daily requirement is 1.25 mg/day/100 g of dietary protein. Pyridoxine is present in wheat-germ, yeast, bran, rice and liver.

Use

Pyridoxine hydrochloride, 10–50 mg, may be given to patients receiving long-term therapy with isoniazid to prevent peripheral neuropathy and in other deficiency states. In sideroblastic anemias pyridoxine is given as 400 mg day. It is also used with limited efficacy in the premenstrual tension syndrome (50–100 mg daily) and to treat certain uncommon inborn errors of metabolism, for example homocystinuria and primary hyperoxaluria.

Adverse effects

Megadoses of pyridoxine, 2 g daily for more than 2 months, cause ataxia and sensory neuropathy.

VITAMIN C (ASCORBIC ACID)

Physiology

Vitamin C is essential to humans, monkeys and guinea pigs, who unlike other mammals cannot synthesize it from glucose. Dietary lack of vitamin C causes scurvy which is characterized by bleeding gums and perifollicular purpura. Ascorbic acid is involved in several metabolic processes, including collagen biosynthesis, steroid metabolism, mitochondrial electron transport chain function, activation of folic acid and in the cytochrome P_{450} system of drug metabolism and is a potent antioxidant. Ascorbic acid is present in large quantities in citrus fruits, tomatoes and green vegetables.

Nutritional status of vitamin C can be assessed by measuring the intracellular leukocyte concentration, but this is not routinely available. Daily intakes of 40–100 mg vitamin C give whole blood concentrations of 34–68 μmol/l when the tissues are saturated. When the daily intake is less than 40 mg tissue saturation falls. A daily intake of 10–15 mg results in approximately 50% of tissue saturation.

Use

1. Ascorbic acid is used in the prophylaxis and treatment of scurvy. (Perhaps the first recorded clinical trial involved the distribution of limes to some, but not all, British naval vessels and observation of the incidence of scurvy. The admiralty were impressed and British sailors were subsequently provided with limes – whence the term 'limeys'.) Normal dietary requirements are less than 70 mg daily, but this may double in the presence of infection. Daily ingestion of 120 mg meets the highest requirements in non-scorbutic individuals. In fully developed scurvy, the dose is 1 g daily.
2. Ascorbic acid increases the absorption of orally administered iron.
3. The reducing properties of ascorbate may be used in the treatment of methemoglobinemia; methylene blue, however, is more effective in emergencies.
4. Large amounts of ascorbic acid (0.5–2 g daily) are ingested by some individuals who hope thereby to reduce their susceptibility to the common cold and similar

respiratory illnesses. Clinical trials have indicated a small degree of protection. Nevertheless, prolonged intake of such doses of ascorbic acid are not recommended and may predispose to oxalate renal calculi. Similar hopes are nurtured regarding the prophylactic effect of ascorbic acid against cancer, but hard evidence is lacking.

5. In normally nourished patients ascorbic acid does not accelerate wound healing. In scorbutic patients wound healing is delayed and this is restored to normal by administration of ascorbic acid.

Adverse effects

Ascorbic acid is generally non-toxic. However, administration of 4 g daily raises the excretion of oxalate by 12 mg and a daily intake of 9 g results in a 68 mg increase in oxalate excretion. Such large doses of vitamin C have resulted in calcium oxalate urolithiasis.

Pharmacokinetics

Ascorbic acid is well absorbed following oral administration. In the presence of vomiting or malabsorption the sodium salt can be given by intramuscular or intravenous injection. Ascorbic acid is mainly metabolized by oxidation to oxalic acid. Normally about 40% of urinary oxalate is derived from ascorbic acid. When the body stores of ascorbic acid are saturated some ingested ascorbic acid is excreted in the urine unchanged. Excretion is by both glomerular filtration and tubular secretion. Plasma clearance of ascorbic acid is greatly reduced in scorbutic patients.

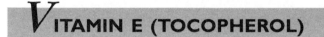

VITAMIN E (TOCOPHEROL)

This is present in nuts, wheat-germ and many foods. Deficiency in animals causes abortion and degeneration of the germinal epithelium of the testes. No defined deficiency syndrome exists in humans, but it can lead to anemia, particularly in premature and malnouruished infants. In an experiment in which volunteers took a diet containing only one-third of the normal vitamin E content over 8 years there were no effects apart from a minor reduction in erythrocyte survival time, although the blood concentrations of vitamin E fell by 80%. Feeding large amounts of polyunsaturated fatty acids increases vitamin E requirements. Vitamin E protects erythrocytes against hemolysis and is an antioxidant. It detoxifies free radicals. Free radicals cause membrane and epithelial injury and have been implicated in the pathophysiology of numerous diseases including cancer and atheroma, and epidemiological evidence suggests that reduced intake is associated with increased atherogenesis (chapter 24). Clinical trials of prevention in cancer and ischemic heart disease are ongoing. Despite the paucity of knowledge of its functions, vitamin E is widely consumed as part of the multiple vitamin therapies taken by some enthusiasts. Fortunately large doses of the vitamin are apparently harmless.

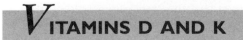

VITAMINS D AND K

These are described in chapter 36 and 27, respectively.

Essential Fatty Acids

Several naturally occurring unsaturated fatty acids are essential dietary components. Linoleic and linolenic acids occur in vegetable oils and nuts, arachidonic acid in meat and longer chain fatty acids (eicosapentanoic acid and docosahexanoic acid) in cold water oily fish. Humans can synthesize arachidonic acid (C20:4) from shorter chain (C18:2) essential fatty acids by chain elongation and desaturation. Arachidonic acid is present in the lipid component of cell membranes throughout the body. It is esterified on the 2 position of glycerol in membrane phospholipids and is liberated by phospholipases when cells are injured or otherwise stimulated. Such free arachidonic acid is the precursor of the 2-series of prostaglandins and thromboxanes and of the 4-series leukotrienes, and so is important in many mediator functions including inflammatory and hemostatic processes. Deficiency states have been described in patients receiving long-term parenteral nutrition, and are prevented by the use of lipid emulsions.

Trace Elements

Fourteen nutritionally essential trace elements are recognized: fluorine, silicon, vanadium, chromium, manganese, iron, cobalt, nickel, copper, zinc, selenium, tin and iodine. These are required in the human body at <0.01% body weight. Most are highly reactive chemically and one or more of these elements is present at the active site of over 50% of the enzymes in humans and help catalyze or inhibit chemical reactions. They are present in small but adequate amounts in a normal diet, but evidence is accumulating that in addition to iron, cobalt (chapter 46) and iodine (chapter 35), zinc, copper and selenium deficiencies can contribute to disease.

ZINC

Zinc deficiency occurs in several situations, including a congenital defect of zinc absorption which presents as acrodermatitis enteropathica; a maternal defect in the transport of zinc into breast milk that causes growth retardation in the infant; patients receiving highly refined therapeutic diets either enterally or intravenously; and patients with malabsorption. In each case characteristic skin lesions appear, associated with hair thinning, chronic diarrhea and mental apathy. Chronic infections occur due to impaired T cell function. Zinc is not stored in the body. Low plasma zinc concentrations occur in zinc deficiency, infection or trauma. The concentration of a plasma metallothionein protein (a sulfur-rich zinc binding protein) is low in zinc deficiency and high in infection. The daily replacement dose is 135 mg of elemental zinc (the recommended daily dietary allowance is 12–15 mg). The response to zinc supplementation is rapid. Adverse effects of oral zinc include dyspepsia and abdominal pain.

COPPER

Copper stores are built up by the fetus, and premature infants are copper deficient. Other causes of copper deficiency are malnutrition, and refined therapeutic diets are low in copper. Copper is bound to ceruloplasmin in the plasma (an acute phase protein synthesized by the liver), thus plasma copper does not reflect copper status as 90% is bound to ceruloplasmin. Copper deficiency presents with osteoporosis, costochondral cartilage cupping, hypochromic anemia and leukopenia. Copper deficency may be suspected if there is a reduction in red cell superoxide dismutase, which is linked to both copper and zinc but is only responsive to copper status. The daily safe copper dietary intake is 1.5–3 mg in adults, doses of copper sulfate of up to 0.1 mg/kg have been safely given orally.

SELENIUM

Selenium deficiency occurs in malabsorption and was endemic in parts of China. Clinically selenium deficiency causes acute or chronic heart failure with multiple foci of myocardial necrosis. Selenium is at the active site of glutathione peroxidase, which catalyzes the removal of hydrogen peroxide and organic peroxides from fatty acids during free radical damage. Selenium has a broad role in helping protect against oxidant stresses. Selenium deficiency may only present when several protective mechanisms are compromised. Selenium toxicity is diagnosed by measuring plasma selenium concentration or by assay of red cell or platelet glutathione peroxidase activity. The diagnosis of selenium deficiency must be confirmed because replacement therapy is toxic and the margin between an adequate and toxic selenium intake is narrow. The safe daily dietary intake of selenium is 45–75 µg.

Fluids and Electrolytes

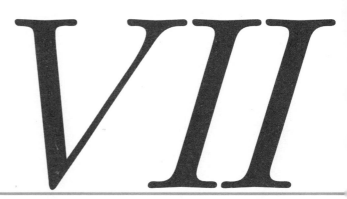

Drugs and the Renal and Genitourinary Systems: Fluid and Electrolyte Disorders

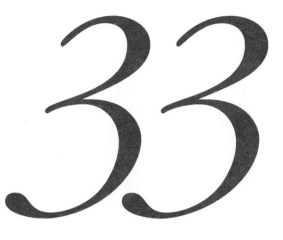

Volume overload (salt and water excess) **438**

Diuretics **439**

Overhydration **446**

Volume depletion **447**

Potassium **449**

Drugs that alter urine pH **451**

Drugs affecting the bladder and genitourinary system **452**

VOLUME OVERLOAD (SALT AND WATER EXCESS)

Volume overload is usually caused by an excess of sodium chloride with accompanying water. Effective treatment is directed at the underlying cause (e.g. heart failure or renal failure) in addition to measures directed toward improving volume status *per se*. These include reducing salt intake and increasing its elimination by the use of diuretics. Limiting water intake is seldom useful in patients with volume overload, although modest limitation is of value in patients with ascites due to advanced liver disease.

Diuretics increase urine production and Na$^+$ excretion. They are among the most widely prescribed drugs and are of central importance in managing hypertension (see chapter 25) as well as the many diseases associated with edema and volume overload that include heart failure (see chapter 28), cirrhosis, renal failure and nephrotic syndrome. In all these disorders, it is important to assess the distribution of salt and water excess in different body compartments: a patient with gross peripheral edema and ascites due to cirrhosis may none the less have a relatively contracted blood volume. Glomerular filtrate derives from plasma so diuretic treatment primarily reduces plasma volume. Tissue fluid takes time to re-equilibrate after an acute change in blood volume caused by a diuretic. Consequently attempts at vigorous diuresis using potent loop diuretics are inappropriate in some edematous states, and may lead to cardiovascular collapse and prerenal renal failure. The principles of using diuretics in the management of hypertension and heart failure are described in other chapters, but before considering individual classes of diuretic drugs in more detail it is appropriate to describe briefly the management of nephrotic syndrome and of cirrhosis of the liver. In both of these conditions there is hypoalbuminemia, which affects the kinetics of several drugs through its effects on protein binding and, paradoxically, an apparently inadequate intravascular volume in the face of fluid overload in the body as a whole. This results in an increased risk of nephrotoxicity from several common drugs, in particular non-steroidal anti-inflammatory drugs and converting enzyme inhibitors. Consequently particular caution is needed in prescribing and monitoring the effects of therapy for intercurrent problems in such patients.

Nephrotic syndrome

The primary problem in nephrotic syndrome is loss of the barrier function of glomerular membranes with leakage of plasma albumin into the urine. The oncotic pressure exerted by plasma falls because of the resulting hypoalbuminemia and water passes from the circulation into the tissue spaces, producing edema. The fall in effective blood volume stimulates the renin–angiotensin–aldosterone system causing sodium retention. Depending on the nature of the glomerular pathology it may be possible to reduce albumin loss with corticosteroid or other immunosuppressive drugs. However, in nephrotic syndrome caused by many kinds of glomerular pathology treatment is only symptomatic. Diuretics are only of limited value. Diet is important. Individuals vary in their ability to compensate for increased urinary protein loss by increased hepatic synthesis of albumin, and a high protein intake should be established in patients with an adequate glomerular filtration rate while minimizing salt intake.

Cirrhosis of the liver

Fluid retention in cirrhosis of the liver usually takes the form of ascites, the localization of the fluid being due to portal hypertension leading to exudation of fluid from the portal system, although dependent edema also occurs. Other important factors are the low concentration of albumin in the plasma (caused by failure of synthesis by the diseased liver) and hyperaldosteronism (due to activation of volume receptors and reduced hepatic aldosterone catabolism). Cirrhosis is an irreversible pathological state, and no current medical therapy is effective in improving the damaged hepatic architecture. Transplantation may be appropriate in cases where the underlying pathology (most commonly alcoholism) is judged to have been cured or (as in some rare inherited metabolic disorders) will not recur in the donor liver. Nevertheless, symptomatic treatment is all that is available for most patients.

Diet is especially important. Protein is restricted because of the risk of precipitating hepatic encephalopathy. What protein is consumed should be of high quality to provide an adequate supply of essential amino acids. High energy is desirable to minimize catabolism of body protein, and is provided by supplementary carbohydrate. Salt restriction and some degree of water restriction are essential. Frequent accurate weighing is the best way of monitoring progress as regards volume status. Diuretics should be used with especial care in this situation, as excessively rapid diuresis may precipitate renal failure as explained above. A loss of approximately 0.5 kg daily is ideal.

Because of aldosterone excess thiazides or loop diuretics cause especially marked potassium depletion and alkalosis in these patients, in whom these disturbances are more important than in patients with other diseases (such as hypertension) because they may precipitate hepatic encephalopathy by altering amino acid metabolism and increasing renal ammonia production. Amiloride or spironolactone can be used in this setting (see below), but if these are not adequate, more powerful diuretics may be given with potassium supplements while monitoring plasma potassium levels. Salt-free albumin (25–50 g/day intravenously given slowly) increases the response to diuretics in cirrhotic patients by causing extracellular fluid to redistribute from tissue spaces to plasma, but it is rapidly metabolized so its effects are short lived and it is expensive.

*D*IURETICS

Diuretics cause natriuresis, and are therefore used to treat patients with volume overload. As well as uses related to their natriuretic effect, there are several therapeutic niches occupied by individual agents because of particular actions within the kidney (e.g. the use of frusemide in treating hypercalcemia, or of thiazide diuretics to treat nephrogenic diabetes insipidus) or elsewhere in the body (e.g. the use of acetazolamide to treat glaucoma, or of mannitol to treat cerebral edema).

Thiazides

Use

Thiazide diuretics in common clinical use include bendrofluazide, hydrochlorothiazide and metolazone, which has a long duration of action and is used in the treatment of resistant edema in combination with a loop diuretic (see below). Except for some differences in duration of action and potency per unit weight (rather than in maximum effect achievable at the top of the dose–response curve) there is little to choose between them with the excellent exception of metolazone. Thiazides are usually taken orally in the morning and produce a mild to moderate diuresis throughout the day: diuresis starts after about 2 hours and lasts for 8–20 hours depending on the drug. They are used in:

1. Hypertension: This is currently the main indication for thiazide diuretics, and their clinical use for this indication is more extensively discussed in chapter 25.
2. Cardiac failure: Thiazides are seldom potent enough to treat heart failure, although they are sometimes useful when this is very mild.
3. Resistant edema: Thiazides, despite being mild when used alone, may be extremely effective in treating resistant edema when combined with a loop diuretic. Metolazone is particularly effective in this regard.
4. Reduction of urinary calcium excretion: This effect of thiazides is exploited to reduce urinary stone formation in patients with idiopathic hypercalciuria. Regular treatment with a thiazide together with maintaining a high urine output (>2.5 l/day) approximately halves the rate of recurrence in patients with recurrent stones and idiopathic hypercalciuria.
5. Diabetes insipidus: Paradoxically thiazides reduce urinary volume in diabetes insipidus by preventing the formation of hypotonic fluid in the distal tubule; they are therefore sometimes used to treat nephrogenic diabetes insipidus.

Thiazides are also sometimes prescribed for premenstrual edema: This may worsen cyclical edema and lead to diuretic abuse and should be avoided.

Mechanism of action

Originally discovered by modification of the sulfonamide structure of inhibitors of carbonic anhydrase, thiazides have a weak inhibitory effect on this enzyme in the proximal tubule. However, their main effect is to decrease sodium chloride reabsorption in the early part of the distal convoluted tubule, thus increasing excretion of sodium, chloride and water. Only about 8% of filtered sodium is reabsorbed by this mechanism, limiting the potency of thiazide diuretics. Thiazides also relax vascular smooth muscle by indirect mechanisms that are not understood. This may contribute to their therapeutic effect in hypertension. They cause increased sodium to reach the distal potassium–sodium exchange site, so increasing potassium excretion, and mild degrees of hypokalemia are common. Thiazides decrease urinary calcium excretion, but this does not lead to hypercalcemia except when hyperparathyroidism coexists, a possibility that must be considered before initiating treatment with a thiazide to reduce hypercalciuria in patients with a history of renal stones. Thiazides increase urinary magnesium excretion, an effect of uncertain clinical significance.

Pharmacokinetics

Thiazides are given orally. The duration of action of individual agents depends on their water solubility and protein binding. They are highly tissue and plasma protein bound and gain access to their renal site of action via the proximal tubular non-selective organic acid secretory mechanism. Thiazides are variably metabolized: for example bendrofluazide is 30% excreted unchanged in the urine and 70% metabolized, whilst hydrochlorothiazide is 95% excreted unchanged.

Adverse effects and contraindications

1. Thiazide diuretics impair glucose tolerance contraindicating their use in patients with non-insulin-dependent diabetes mellitus. After 6 years of continuous thiazide therapy up to 10% of hypertensive patients develop a frankly diabetic glucose tolerance curve. Risk increases with age and obesity. The effect is dose related and usually reversible; where glucose intolerance that occurs during treatment with a thiazide persists after treatment is discontinued this is probably due to the independent onset of non-insulin-dependent diabetes.

2. Thiazide diuretics cause hyperuricemia contraindicating their use in patients with a history of gout. Competition with uric acid at the non-specific acid secretion site in the proximal tubule results in uric acid retention which, combined with a decreased extracellular fluid volume, causes a rise in plasma uric acid concentration. Uricosuric agents act more distally in the nephron to block reabsorption of uric acid. They remain effective during thiazide treatment, as does allopurinol.

3. Hyponatremia, which may be severe, especially in elderly persons.

4. Hypokalemia and hypomagnesemia occur commonly during treatment with thiazide diuretics, but are usually of uncertain clinical significance. In practice they warrant attention in situations where there is increased risk of arrhythmia as during concurrent treatment with digoxin.

5. Allergy (including non-thrombocytopenic purpura and photosensitivity) and blood dyscrasias (including thrombocytopenia) occur rarely during treatment with thiazide diuretics.

6. Thiazide diuretics can cause impotence. This is common, dose related and reversible (provided it is indeed drug related).

Drug interactions

Thiazide diuretics are usefully combined with various other drugs in treating patients with moderate or severe hypertension, including β-adrenoceptor antagonists, converting enzyme inhibitors and α_1-adrenoceptor antagonists. Thiazides reduce the excretion of lithium, so a reduced dose of lithium carbonate is needed to avoid life-threatening lithium toxicity if these drugs are coadministered.

Loop diuretics

Use

The main clinical use of loop diuretics is in the treatment of heart failure, and this is described more fully in chapter 28. Several loop diuretics are marketed including frusemide and bumetanide. In the absence of idiosyncratic or other adverse effects frusemide is the standard agent. Frusemide is given intravenously in initial doses of 20–80 mg to patients with pulmonary edema caused by acute left ventricular failure, in whom it may produce dramatic symptomatic relief within a few minutes. It is also taken orally to treat patients with chronic congestive heart failure, in doses usually between 20 and 120 mg daily. Diuresis begins about 30 min after oral dosage and lasts for about 6 hours.

In refractory edema frusemide is sometimes administered by continuous infusion (4–16 mg/hour). An alternative in refractory edema is to combine frusemide (or bumetanide) with diuretics that act at different sites in the nephron including potassium-sparing distally acting drugs (e.g. amiloride), thiazides (e.g. metolazone), or (rarely) carbonic anhydrase inhibitors (e.g. acetazolamide).

Frusemide is useful in patients with chronic renal failure who are suffering from fluid overload and/or hypertension. Unlike thiazides which are ineffective in patients with a glomerular filtration rate (GFR) less than 25 ml/min, frusemide can produce some diuresis despite a low GFR when large doses (e.g. 0.25–2.0 g daily) are used. In patients with incipient acute renal failure, frusemide in doses of 250–500 mg intravenously sometimes produces diuresis and may prevent the development of established failure, although this is hard to prove.

Loop diuretics increase urinary calcium excretion (in contrast to thiazides which reduce it) and the hypercalciuric effect of frusemide is exploited in the treatment of hypercalcemia when it is given following volume replacement with physiological saline.

Mechanism of action

Loop diuretics are the most potent diuretics currently available. They have steep dose–response curves, and much higher maximum effects than thiazide or other diuretics, being capable of increasing fractional sodium excretion (i.e. the fraction of sodium filtered at the glomerulus appearing in the urine) to as much as 35%. They act from within the tubular fluid to inhibit a transport mechanism in the thick ascending limb of the loop of Henlé which transports Na^+ and K^+ together with $2Cl^-$ ions from the lumen ('Na^+ K^+ $2Cl^-$ cotransport').

Pharmacokinetics

Frusemide is rapidly and extensively absorbed from the gut. It is 95% bound to plasma protein and elimination is mainly via the kidneys, both filtration and proximal tubular secretion being involved. It is not reabsorbed substantially from the luminal fluid. Approximately two-thirds of water reabsorption occurs isosmotically in the proximal convoluted tubule, so frusemide and other loop diuretics are substantially concentrated before reaching their site of action in the thick ascending limb, accounting for their selectivity for the renal Na^+ K^+ $2Cl^-$ cotransport mechanism as opposed to Na^+ K^+ $2Cl^-$ cotransport at other sites such as the inner ear. The luminal site of action of these drugs also contributes to the resistance to their effect in patients with nephrotic syndrome, in whom heavy proteinuria results in substantial protein binding within the lumen. After intravenous injection 77% of a dose of frusemide is excreted in the urine within 4 hours, most of the remainder being metabolized or excreted in feces. The plasma $t_{1/2}$ is 1.5–3.5 hours. In renal failure $t_{1/2}$ is prolonged to 10 hours or more but toxicity is unusual. In these circumstances non-renal clearance increases and may account for up to 98% of total elimination.

Adverse effects

1. Loop diuretics in high dose cause massive diuresis, urine flow rate increasing up to 35% of GFR, that is approximately 2.5 litres per hour! This causes a profound decrease in blood and extracellular fluid volume. Normal blood volume in an adult is approximately 5 litres. Acute hypovolemia can precipitate prerenal renal failure, especially in elderly or debilitated patients. Those receiving other potentially nephrotoxic drugs such as gentamicin, non-steroidal anti-

inflammatory drugs or angiotensin-converting enzyme (ACE) inhibitors are especially at risk. Loop diuretics may also precipitate acute urinary retention in men with pre-existing prostate disease.

2. Loop diuretics cause hyperuricemia and can precipitate gout.

3. Inhibition of K^+ reabsorption in the loop of Henlé as well as increased delivery of Na^+ to the distal nephron (where it can be exchanged for K^+) results in increased urinary potassium loss, and some degree of hypokalemia is common, although as with thiazide-induced hypokalemia this is often clinically unimportant in the absence of additional risk factors for arrhythmia such as digoxin treatment. Digoxin is now less commonly used in treatment of heart failure than hitherto, whereas the early use of converting enzyme inhibitors (which increase plasma potassium concentration) is widely accepted, so the uncritical and excessive use of combination preparations such as Frumil™ and Burinex-A™ is to be deplored.

4. Magnesium clearance is also increased and loop diuretics can cause hypomagnesemia. Alcoholism and a diet low in magnesium are exacerbating factors. Magnesium and potassium metabolism are linked and correction of potassium deficiency is impeded by coexistent magnesium deficiency. The most important clinical features of magnesium deficiency are increased cardiac excitability with ventricular arrhythmias and refractory atrial fibrillation. Digitalis toxicity is increased. Other symptoms are depression and muscle weakness.

5. Carbohydrate intolerance may occur, but is less of a problem than with thiazide diuretics.

6. Ototoxicity with hearing loss is associated with excessive peak plasma concentrations caused by too rapid intravenous injection. It may be caused by inhibition of Na^+ K^+ $2Cl^-$ cotransport which is involved in the formation of endolymph, and is usually reversible. This is probably not the full story, however, since irreversible hearing loss has been caused by ethacrynic acid (another loop diuretic, now seldom used).

Loop diuretics potentiate the ototoxic effects of aminoglycoside antibiotics.

7. The increased water and chloride excretion caused by loop diuretics results in so-called contraction alkalosis, i.e. the extracellular fluid contracts with an increase in plasma bicarbonate concentration. This is seldom of clinical importance, although it can be a problem in patients with heart failure caused by chronic lung disease ('cor pulmonale') in whom plasma bicarbonate is high in compensation for respiratory acidosis.

8. Idiosyncratic blood dyscrasias occur rarely.

Drug interactions

Loop diuretics increase the nephrotoxicity of cephaloridine; more recently introduced cephalosporins are less nephrotoxic than cephaloridine, and less likely to interact in this way with loop diuretics. Renal prostaglandins including PGE_2 and PGI_2 are natriuretic, and non-steroidal anti-inflammatory drugs such as indomethacin inhibit prostaglandin biosynthesis and oppose the diuretic effect of loop diuretics as well as inhibiting their secretion into the tubule by competition for the transport mechanism. As with the thiazides, lithium reabsorption is reduced by loop diuretics necessitating plasma level monitoring and often dose reduction of lithium carbonate as indicated by plasma lithium concentration.

Potassium-sparing diuretics

Natriuresis caused by diuretics is usually accompanied by increased excretion of potassium, as described above. However, some diuretics inhibit distal Na^+/K^+ exchange, thereby causing potassium retention at the same time as mild natriuresis. These are not potent diuretics, but have been aggressively marketed in combination with thiazide or loop diuretics which have long outlived their patent lives when prescribed as single agents.

The commercial implications of this have been substantial, but clinical benefits are less certain. This is not to say that these drugs lack a valuable niche in therapeutics when used appropriately. They fall into two categories: competitive antagonists of aldosterone (of which only one, spironolactone, is available), and Na^+/K^+ exchange antagonists that do not compete with aldosterone, of which there are two, amiloride and triamterene.

SPIRONOLACTONE

Aldosterone promotes sodium retention and potassium loss by increasing the amount of sodium exchanged for potassium in the distal tubule. Spironolactone is structurally related to aldosterone and competes with it at receptors in the distal tubule. It increases sodium and water excretion and conserves potassium in patients with elevated circulating aldosterone concentrations. Hyperaldosteronism plays a key part in Conn's syndrome (primary hyperaldosteronism) and in ascites and fluid overload caused by cirrhosis (secondary hyperaldosteronism). The use of spironolactone is currently limited to these situations. This is partly because it is poorly tolerated, causing gynecomastia and breast tenderness in men and menstrual irregularity in women, probably because it is structurally related to estrogens. It also causes tumors in rodents. Even in Conn's syndrome and in ascites secondary to cirrhosis, the other class of potassium-sparing diuretic may be as effective and better tolerated.

AMILORIDE

Amiloride is a non-competitive antagonist of aldosterone in the distal nephron. Its effect on sodium transport at this site is responsible for its therapeutic effect, although at higher concentrations than are encountered therapeutically it also has other actions on sodium transport, including inhibition of Na^+/H^+ and Na^+/Ca^{2+} exchange. It is most commonly used in combination with frusemide (co-amilofruse), in which setting it should be restricted to patients with heart failure who develop clinically significant hypokalemia when treated with a loop diuretic as sole agent, or with a thiazide (co-amilozide) for hypertension. Such combinations often cause hyponatremia. Only 20% is absorbed after oral administration. It is not given intravenously since it can cause severe hypotension by this route, possibly via histamine liberation. It is not metabolized and is excreted unchanged by the kidneys. Plasma $t_{1/2}$ is 6 hours, but its action following a 10–20 mg dose lasts approximately 24 hours.

Adverse effects and drug interactions

The main danger with amiloride is potassium retention leading to dangerous hyperkalemia. Plasma potassium and creatinine should be monitored carefully as the indications for which diuretics are used including heart failure and hypertension are important causes of progressive renal impairment, especially in the elderly, and severe hyperkalemia can occur in patients treated with potassium-sparing drugs in whom renal impairment supervenes. Diabetics are especially prone to hyperkalemia because of hyporeninemic hypoaldosteronism. Patients taking potassium supplements or ACE inhibitors (which increase plasma potassium by inhibiting angiotensin II-stimulated aldosterone secretion) or NSAID (which block PGI_2-induced renin release) are especially at risk. Hyponatremia may occur particularly if amiloride is combined with a thiazide, again especially in the elderly.

TRIAMTERENE

This is a substituted pteridine with only weak natriuretic properties, the maximum fractional excretion of sodium that it causes being less than 2% of the filtered load. Like amiloride it acts on Na^+/K^+ exchange in the distal tubule, but not by aldosterone antagonism. It can be used like amiloride in conjunction with thiazides or loop diuretics to potentiate their diuretic effect and to prevent hypokalemic alkalosis. In combination with a thiazide (co-triamterzide) it has been intensively studied in elderly patients in the European working party on hypertension in the elderly study,

which demonstrated a beneficial effect of treatment in reducing the occurrence of myocardial infarction. Absorption after oral administration is rapid (the drug is not used parenterally). It is rapidly metabolized, 90% circulating as metabolites, and both drug and metabolites appear in urine and bile. Plasma $t_{1/2}$ is 1.5–2 hours. Diuresis starts within 2 hours of administration and is complete within 8–10 hours. Considerations regarding adverse effects are similar to those for amiloride.

Carbonic anhydrase inhibitors

Use and mechanism of action

The only carbonic anhydrase inhibitor used as such in clinical practice is acetazolamide. Acetazolamide is a sulfonamide and is a noncompetitive enzyme inhibitor. Carbonic anhydrase plays an important part in bicarbonate reabsorption from the proximal tubule. Consequently acetazolamide inhibits reabsorption of sodium bicarbonate resulting in an alkaline diuresis with loss of sodium and bicarbonate in the urine. Urinary alkalinization with acetazolamide has been used in the treatment of children with cysteine stones due to cysteinuria since cysteine is more soluble at alkaline than at acid pH. In the past it was suggested that urinary alkalinization with acetazolamide could also be used to increase salicylate elimination in cases of aspirin overdose; however, although salicylate elimination is indeed increased in an alkaline urine (chapter 50), the effects of acetazolamide on acid–base status (see below) are such as to increase salicylate toxicity by favoring its entry across the blood–brain barrier. Bicarbonate administration and not acetazolamide is therefore recommended for treating appropriately selected cases of salicylate overdose.

As a consequence of increased urinary elimination of bicarbonate during acetazolamide treatment, plasma bicarbonate concentration falls without accumulation of any unmeasured anions, giving a normal anion gap metabolic acidosis, the hallmark of a renal tubular acidosis. The reduction in plasma bicarbonate leads to a reduced filtered load of bicarbonate, so less bicarbonate is available for reabsorption from proximal tubular fluid. The diuretic effect of acetazolamide is therefore self limiting. However, the metabolic effect of acetazolamide is capitalized on in the prevention of mountain sickness, since it permits rapid acclimatization to altitude (which entails renal compensation for respiratory alkalosis caused by hyperventilation) by facilitating bicarbonate excretion. It may also be useful in patients with cor pulmonale in whom edema is accompanied by respiratory acidosis compensated by renal bicarbonate retention.

More importantly than its diuretic effect, acetazolamide inhibits carbonic anhydrase in the eye and thereby decreases the rate of secretion of the aqueous humor in the anterior chamber and lowers intraocular pressure. Treatment of glaucoma is currently the major use of acetazolamide; in acute closed angle glaucoma 250 mg is given intravenously, followed by 250 mg four times daily; in open angle glaucoma 125 mg three times daily is used. In the lower dose range acetazolamide can be given for long periods and fortunately the change in acid–base status does not interfere with its action on aqueous humor formation. A topical preparation for use in the eye is in development.

Carbonic anhydrase is also present in the brain and acetazolamide has anticonvulsant properties. It reduces formation of cerebrospinal fluid by carbonic anhydrase inhibition in the choroid plexus, and is therefore occasionally used in the management of so-called 'benign' intracranial hypertension.

Pharmacokinetics

Acetazolamide is well absorbed from the intestine. It is renally excreted and has a plasma half-life of about 3 hours; however, its effect on the kidney lasts about 6 hours, and sustained release tablets allow twice daily dosing.

Adverse effects

Adverse effects are common when acetazolamide is used in large doses, and relate to its metabolic effects and to the fact that it is a sulfonamide. Large doses cause paresthesia, fatigue and dyspepsia. Prolonged use predisposes to renal stone formation due to reduced urinary citrate (citrate increases the solubility of calcium in urine). Hypersensitivity reactions and blood dyscrasias occur.

Osmotic diuretics

USE AND MECHANISM OF ACTION

Osmotic diuretics undergo glomerular filtration but are poorly reabsorbed from the renal tubular fluid. Their main diuretic action is exerted on the proximal tubule. This section of the tubule is freely permeable to water and under normal circumstances sodium is actively reabsorbed accompanied by an isosmotic quantity of water. The presence of a substantial quantity of a poorly absorbable solute opposes this, since as water is reabsorbed the concentration and hence the osmotic activity of the solute increases. Osmotic diuretics also interfere with the establishment of the medullary osmotic gradient which is necessary for the formation of a concentrated urine. Mannitol (an alcohol) is an example of such an osmotic diuretic. It is poorly absorbed from the intestine and is given intravenously as a 10 or 20% solution and a single infusion contains 25–50 g. It is not metabolized but is filtered by renal glomeruli and is not reabsorbed from the tubules.

Unlike other diuretics, osmotic diuretics increase plasma volume (by increasing the entry of water to the circulation as a result of increasing intravascular osmolarity) so they are unsuitable for the treatment of most causes of edema, especially cardiac failure. It is possible that if used early in the course of incipient acute renal failure osmotic diuretics may stave off the occurrence of acute tubular necrosis by increasing tubular fluid flow and reducing accretion of material that would otherwise plug the tubules. Indeed it has been suggested that the rarity of acute tubular necrosis in diabetic ketoacidosis is a consequence of the osmotic diuresis caused by heavy glycosuria. If mannitol is used in patients with incipient acute renal failure intensive monitoring is needed to avoid precipitating pulmonary edema secondary to the osmotic load if renal function in fact deteriorates. In practice, low dose infusion of dopamine (chapter 28) which causes diuresis by selectively dilating renal vasculature is now commonly used in this situation. Osmotic diuretics are consequently used principally for reasons unconnected with their ability to cause diuresis. Because they do not enter cells or some anatomical areas such as the eye and brain, they cause water to leave cells down the osmotic gradient. This 'dehydrating' action is used in two circumstances:

1. Reduction of intraocular pressure preoperatively in closed angle glaucoma. Urea, 1.5 g/kg, intravenously or glycerol, 1.5 g/kg orally are used for this purpose as alternatives to mannitol.
2. Emergency reduction of intracranial pressure in conditions such as brain tumor.

OVERHYDRATION

Overhydration without excess salt is much less common than salt and water overload, but occurs when antidiuretic hormone (ADH) is secreted inappropriately, for instance by a neoplasm or following head injury or neurosurgery, giving rise to the syndrome of inappropriate secretion of ADH: 'SIADH'. This secretion of ADH is sometimes caused by drugs, notably the anticonvulsant carbamazepine which stimulates ADH release from the posterior pituitary, and sulfonylureas which potentiate its action on renal collecting ducts. Antidiuretic hormone secretion results in a concentrated urine, while continued drinking (as a result of dietary habit) leads to progressive dilution of plasma which becomes hypo-osmolar and hyponatremic. Plasma volume is only slightly increased, so volume receptors are not activated and urinary sodium loss continues. Some causes of SIADH resolve spontaneously (e.g. some cases of head injury), whereas others may improve after specific treatment of the underlying cause (e.g. following chemotherapy for small cell carcinoma of bronchus). Hyponatremia that has arisen gradually can be corrected gradually by restricting fluid intake, a measure that does not cause thirst (because of the hypoosmolality), but which may not be well tolerated because of habit. Rapid correction of hyponatremia to levels greater than 125 mmol/l is potentially harmful and has been associated with severe central nervous system toxicity including central pontine myelinolysis, with resultant devasting loss of brainstem function, sometimes with cortical function preserved (so-called 'locked-in syndrome').

Demeclocycline inhibits collecting duct adenylyl cyclase (thereby producing a nephrogenic diabetes insipidus) and has been used to treat SIADH. In common with other tetracyclines it increases plasma urea and can produce deterioration of renal function and increased loss of sodium in the urine. Electrolytes and renal function should therefore be monitored during treatment.

VOLUME DEPLETION

Principles of fluid replacement

Volume depletion is seldom treated with drugs. Even in situations such as Addisonian crisis where ultimately the definitive treatment is replacement with glucocorticoid and mineralocorticoid hormones, emergency treatment pivots on replacement of what is depleted, i.e. salt and water in the form of adequate volumes of isotonic (physiologically 'normal', i.e. 140 mM) sodium chloride solution (chapter 37). The same is true in treating diabetic ketoacidosis where the critical life-saving intervention is the rapid infusion of large volumes of isotonic saline at the same time as giving low doses of insulin by intravenous infusion (p. 463). In patients with hypovolemia due to acute and rapid blood loss the appropriate fluid with which to replace is blood. Whole blood is now not always available because blood transfusion centers frequently separate plasma as a source of clotting factors. Consequently a combination of 'packed' red cells with isotonic saline may be appropriate. In some situations, particularly when hypoalbuminemia and edema coexist with acute blood volume depletion, infusion of solutions of high molecular weight colloid (e.g. dextran or gelatin) may be preferable to low molecular weight readily diffusible crystalloid (e.g. isotonic saline). Anaphylactoid reactions are an unusual but severe adverse effect of such treatment. As mentioned above human serum albumin from which salt has been extracted is a seemingly logical but expensive alternative to artificial colloid solutions when there is hypoalbuminemia. Its beneficial effect is short lived.

Diabetes insipidus and vasopressin

'Pure' water deprivation, i.e. true dehydration, is much less common than loss of salt and water, i.e. desalination. If we fail to drink adequate water to make up insensible losses, which may be increased as in a desert climate, plasma osmolality rapidly increases. This causes thirst which leads to drinking and restoration of plasma osmolality, and to secretion of antidiuretic hormone (ADH, arginine vasopressin) by the posterior pituitary, which leads to the formation of a small volume of concentrated urine. Vasopressin acts at the cellular level by combining with specific receptors coupled to G-proteins. The most physiologically important actions of vasopressin, including its antidiuretic and vasodilator effects and its ability to release factor VIII and von Willebrand factor, are mediated by V_2 receptors which are coupled to adenylyl cyclase. V_1 receptors activate the phosphatidyl inositol signalling system in vascular smooth muscle, mobilizing cytoplasmic calcium and causing intense vasoconstriction. V_{1a} receptors are also present in liver, kidney and brain causing glycogenolysis, stimulating prostaglandin synthesis and inhibiting renin release, and influencing central functions such as memory, cerebrospinal fluid formation and the central control of blood pressure. V_{1b} receptors in anterior pituitary stimulate release of corticotropin.

Vasopressin renders collecting ducts permeable to water. Consequently water leaves the collecting ducts passively down its osmotic gradient from tubular fluid (which is hypotonic at the beginning of the distal tubule) into the highly concentrated papillary interstitium. This process results in the formation of a small volume of highly concentrated urine under the influence of vasopressin.

These homeostatic mechanisms fail when a patient is denied oral fluid, usually because of surgery ('nil by mouth'). Fluid must then be administered parenterally if dehydration with increased plasma sodium ion concentration is to be prevented. Pure water must not be given intravenously because this would cause hemolysis. Instead, an isotonic (5%) solution of glucose is used in this circumstance since the glucose is rapidly metabolized to carbon dioxide leaving water unaccompanied by solute. Surgical patients also lose salt, but, unless they have been vomiting or losing electrolyte-rich fluid from the gastrointestinal tract via a drain or fistula, at a lower rate than the loss of water. Consequently, postoperative surgical patients are often given two or three volumes of 5% glucose for every volume of isotonic saline, modified if necessary depending on the results of serial serum electrolyte determinations.

Diabetes insipidus is an uncommon disorder in which either the secretion of ADH is deficient ('central' diabetes insipidus), as following neurosurgery or head injury, or in some infiltrating diseases, for example sarcoid, that involve the posterior pituitary or the nuclei or tracts that innervate it, or the sensitivity of the collecting ducts to ADH is deficient ('nephrogenic' diabetes insipidus). Nephrogenic diabetes insipidus can be caused by a mutation in the gene for the vasopressin V_2 receptor. Dehydration is not invariably a problem in diabetes insipidus, because increasing plasma osmolality is still able to stimulate thirst. Consequently polydipsia occurs and prevents dehydration and increased plasma sodium ion concentration. Patients with diabetes insipidus are, however, at greatly increased risk of dehydration if they become unconscious for any reason such as anesthesia for an intercurrent surgical problem. Polydipsia and polyuria in central diabetes insipidus can be prevented by treatment with vasopressin. However, ADH is not well absorbed across mucous membranes so treatment necessitates the inconvenience of repeated injections. Currently, the usual treatment is therefore with a stable analog desamino-D-arginine vasopressin (DDAVP, desmopressin). This is sufficiently well absorbed through nasal mucosa that it is administered intranasally (adult dose 10–40 µg per day, given as one or two doses). Furthermore, it is selective for V_2 receptors, which are responsible for the effects of vasopressin on collecting ducts, and lacks the pressor effect of arginine vasopressin which is mediated by V_1 receptors on vascular smooth muscle cells in resistance arterioles. In addition to its use in diabetes insipidus, desmopressin is also used for nocturnal enuresis (20–40 µg intranasally at bed time in children over the age of 7), although caution is needed when the drug is used for this indication in adults with co-existing cardiovascular disease. (Children over 5 years old with regular enuresis may be helped by training using an enuresis alarm.) Desmopressin is also used intravenously in patients with von Willebrand's disease before undergoing elective surgery, because it increases circulating von Willebrand factor, and also increases factor VIII concentrations in patients with mild/moderate hemophilia.

Nephrogenic diabetes insipidus is sometimes drug induced, lithium being a common cause. If so, use of an alternative treatment may be possible. Severe nephrogenic diabetes insipidus is a rare X-linked disease caused by a mutation in the V_2 receptor gene. In such cases exogenous vasopressin or DDAVP is ineffective. Paradoxically, thiazide diuretics can reduce polyuria in nephrogenic diabetes insipidus, and are combined with mild salt restriction.

POTASSIUM

Hypokalemia

Hypokalemia commonly accompanies loss of fluid from the gastrointestinal tract (e.g. following profuse vomiting or diarrhea), or loss of potassium ions into urine due to diuretic therapy. Hypokalemia in untreated patients with hypertension is suggestive of mineralocorticoid excess (e.g. Conn's syndrome, liqorice abuse). Barter's syndrome is a rare cause of severe hypokalemia in normotensive children who are not vomiting. Severe hypokalemia causes symptoms of fatigue and nocturia (because of loss of renal concentrating ability), and can cause arrhythmias. Mild degrees of hypokalemia (often associated with diuretic use) are generally well tolerated and of little clinical importance. Patients at risk of developing more serious hypokalemia include:

1. Those receiving large doses of diuretics, especially combinations of loop diuretics and thiazides.
2. Patients receiving other drugs that cause increased potassium loss (e.g. systemic steroids or chronic laxative treatment).
3. Those with a low potassium intake, notably poor and/or elderly people.
4. Patients with diseases associated with high circulating aldosterone concentrations, particularly those with cirrhosis (in whom hypokalemia may precipitate hepatic encephalopathy), as well as those with nephrotic syndrome and severe cardiac failure. Relatively mild potassium depletion exacerbates the toxicity of digoxin, incurring the risk of serious arrhythmias.

Against this background a practical approach is:

1. Potassium replacement is not usually required in hypertensive patients on small doses of diuretics and taking a full mixed diet. Plasma potassium should be estimated after approximately 2–3 months of treatment as a markedly low concentration (<3.0 mmol/l) justifies replacement treatment. If replacement with items of food high in potassium (notably fruit and vegetables) is ineffective, replacement with an effervescent potassium supplement may be appropriate. These are not particularly palatable, but contain larger amounts of potassium (e.g. 14 mmol per tablet) than do conventional slow release potassium preparations (approximately 7 mmol per tablet, formulated in a wax matrix). Slow-release preparations are usually inadequate (see below) unless impractically large numbers of tablets are prescribed, and carry the risk of causing gastrointestinal injury if held up within the gastrointestinal tract (e.g. in the esophagus in an enlarged left atrium pressing backward on the esophagus in patients with mitral stenosis). Effervescent potassium preparations taste less awful if they are dissolved in fruit juice.
2. Plasma potassium should be monitored regularly (and replacements given if needed) in patients with congestive cardiac failure and/or nephrotic syndrome. In particular, patients treated with digoxin should receive potassium replacement therapy if there is clinically significant hypokalemia.
3. Patients with cirrhosis are especially likely to require potassium replacement.
4. Patients on diuretics who develop cardiac arrhythmias and/or who have recently had a myocardial infarct should have relatively aggressive potassium replacement, together with consideration of magnesium supplementation.
5. Patients with other risk factors should be monitored and given replacements as required.

POTASSIUM REPLACEMENT

There are two ways of increasing plasma potassium: by potassium supplements or by use of potassium-sparing diuretics.

Potassium supplements

To be effective 30–50 mmol potassium daily is required. Combined diuretic and potassium tablets are inadequate as they contain only 7–8 mmol. Potassium salts may be given orally either as an effervescent or slow-release preparation. Diet can be supplemented by foods with a high potassium content such as fruit and vegetables. Intravenous potassium is usually given in the form of potassium chloride and is used either to maintain body potassium in patients receiving intravenous feeding or to restore potassium levels in severely depleted patients (e.g. those with diabetic ketoacidosis). The main danger of intravenous potassium is hyperkalemia, which can cause any type of arrhythmia, including cardiac arrest. Potassium chloride caused 12 adverse effects per 100 exposures in the Boston Collaborative Drug Surveillance Program, and had the dubious distinction of the highest frequency of fatal adverse reactions of any drug. Potassium chloride solution is infused at a maximum rate of 10 mmol/hour unless there is severe depletion when 20 mmol/hour can be given with plasma level and electrocardiograph (ECG) monitoring. The dose should not usually exceed 120 mmol/24 hours unless there is severe depletion. Especial care is required if there is impaired renal function. Potassium chloride for intravenous replacement should be diluted with saline or glucose in the bag before infusion. Potassium chloride should not be combined with blood, mannitol, amino acids or lipids.

Potassium-sparing diuretics

An alternative to potassium supplementation is to combine a thiazide or loop diuretic with a potassium-retaining diuretic (p. 443). Potassium-retaining diuretics are better tolerated than potassium supplements but are not without risk (especially of hyperkalemia if renal impairment supervenes and/or other potassium-retaining drugs such as angiotensin-converting enzyme (ACE) inhibitors are prescribed) and add to the cost of treatment.

Hyperkalemia

Hyperkalemia in untreated patients suggests the possibility of renal failure or of mineralocorticoid deficiency (e.g. Addison's disease, hyporeninemic hypoaldosteronism). Most commonly, however, it is caused by drugs. Hyperkalemia can develop either with potassium supplements or potassium-sparing diuretics (still more so in patients treated with both!). Hyperkalemia is particularly liable to occur in patients with impaired renal function, in the elderly (in whom renal functional impairment may be unrecognized because the plasma creatinine may be within the normal range) and in patients receiving ACE inhibitors (in whom plasma aldosterone is suppressed). Regular estimations of plasma potassium are advised in these situations.

TREATMENT

The effects of an abnormal intracellular/extracellular K^+ ratio may be counteracted by the following:

1. Calcium injection is life saving in patients with arrhythmias caused by hyperkalemia (see p. 369). Ten per cent calcium gluconate, 10–30 ml, is given over 5 min with ECG monitoring. Calcium ions decrease membrane excitability. The beneficial effects are transient, however, so emergency measures to reduce hyperkalemia must be instituted without delay.
2. Glucose and insulin are given to shift extracellular potassium into cells. Over 30 min 200–500 ml of 10% glucose is given accompanied by 10 units of soluble insulin. Over the course of an hour the plasma potassium may fall by 1–2 mmol/l.
3. Sodium bicarbonate 100–150 mmol, given intravenously also shifts potassium into cells.

4. The above measures may buy a brief period of time that can be used to mobilize emergency dialysis.

5. Ion exchange resin made of sodium polystyrene sulfonate exchanges sodium for potassium ions in the gut lumen. It is given as a retention enema (30 g) or by mouth (15 g, three or four times daily). It removes potassium from the body rather than altering its distribution. This effect usually begins about an hour after administration. In a few patients the sodium ion exchanged for potassium may lead to sodium overload and heart failure. For such cases a calcium resin is available. Ion exchange resins are useful for preventing hyperkalemia in patients with chronic renal failure. The main adverse effect when resins are given chronically in this way is constipation, which can be avoided if they are suspended in a solution of sorbitol.

DRUGS THAT ALTER URINE pH

Acidifying drugs

AMMONIUM CHLORIDE

Ammonium chloride is given orally and after absorption the ammonium ion is converted to urea by the liver with the release of hydrogen and chloride ions. This produces a metabolic acidosis to which the kidney responds by excreting acid urine. There is also increased excretion of chloride ions together with a balancing cation (largely sodium) and water which results in a transient diuresis.

Use

Ammonium chloride is used in the investigation of renal tubular acidosis, to determine the ability of the kidney to form an acid urine. It is given in doses of 8–12 g. It is a gastric irritant and is given as enteric-coated tablets. The elimination of some basic drugs such as morphine and amphetamine is enhanced by acidification of the urine, but this has not lead to routine use of urinary acidification in the treatment of overdose with these drugs.

Adverse effects

Ammonium chloride should not be given in hepatic failure as it may precipitate encephalopathy. It will exacerbate the acidosis of renal failure. It is a gastric irritant and causes nausea, vomiting and abdominal pain. Acidifying drugs should not be used if the urine is alkaline because of infection by a urea-splitting organism such as *Proteus* (which liberates free ammonia in the urine).

VITAMIN C (ASCORBIC ACID)

Vitamin C is excreted in the urine, which it acidifies if given in sufficiently large dose (>2 g). It is safer than ammonium chloride.

Alkalinizing drugs

Sodium bicarbonate causes urinary alkalinization, but if given by mouth it reacts with hydrochloric acid in the stomach to produce carbon dioxide, so it is poorly tolerated and poorly effective. Instead, citric acid/potassium citrate mixture can be used since citrate is absorbed from the gut and metabolized via the tricarboxylic acid cycle with generation of bicarbonate. The usual dose is 3–6 g every 4–6 hours until the urine pH is >7. Potassium must be avoided in renal failure as retention of potassium ions may cause hyperkalemia.

Use

Alkalinization of the urine is used to give symptomatic relief for the dysuria of cystitis, and to prevent the formation of uric acid stones, especially in patients about to undergo cancer chemotherapy. The use of forced alkaline diuresis to increase urinary excretion of salicylate following overdose is discussed in chapter 50.

DRUGS AFFECTING THE BLADDER AND GENITOURINARY SYSTEM

Drugs for urological pain

The acute pain of ureteric colic may be relieved by morphine or pethidine. Recently it has been shown that diclofenac (a non-steroidal anti-inflammatory drug) compares favorably with the opiates for ureteric colic if used parenterally. It is given intramuscularly in a dose of 75 mg, which is repeated after 30 min if necessary.

Drugs to increase bladder activity

Drugs that increase bladder activity are sometimes used in treating patients with chronic retention of urine. These should never be used in the presence of severe obstruction, and are never used to treat acute urinary retention, which is managed by catheterization. Muscarinic agonists (e.g. bethanechol, carbachol) stimulate the detrusor muscle and are occasionally used in patients with chronic retention due to peripheral neurological damage rather than obstruction. Anticholinesterases (e.g. distigmine) are similarly used because of their parasympathomimetic action.

Drugs to decrease bladder activity

Increased frequency is often a symptom of infection. When infection is absent unstable detrusor contractions may be responsible, the consequences ranging in severity from trivial inconvenience to urge incontinence that completely ruins the quality of the patient's life. Drug treatment is usually disappointing: antimuscarinic drugs such as oxybutinin and propantheline are not very effective and have a high incidence of antimuscarinic side effects (dry mouth, dry eyes, blurred vision, constipation, confusion). Tricyclic antidepressants (e.g. amitryptyline, imipramine) are sometimes useful, perhaps in part because of their antimuscarinic effects. They are also used in nocturnal enuresis, as is desmopressin (p. 448).

Drugs for prostatic obstruction

Prostatic obstruction is usually managed surgically. Symptoms of benign prostatic hypertrophy may be improved by a 5α-reductase inhibitor (e.g. finasteride, p. 506) or by an α_1-adrenoceptor antagonist (e.g. doxazosin, p. 296). Hormonal manipulation with antiandrogens and analogs of luteinizing hormone releasing hormone (LHRH) is valuable in patients with prostatic cancer (pp. 506 and 513).

Drugs for impotence

Erectile failure has numerous organic as well as psychological causes. Drug treatment (p. 506) is generally disappointing, but intracavernosal injection of vasodilators under specialist medical supervision can be effective. The usual drug has been papaverine (7.5 mg for the initial dose, increased if necessary to 30–60 mg), to which the non-selective α-adrenoceptor antagonist phentolamine (0.25–1.25 mg) can be added if needed. Recently, prostaglandin E_1 has been licensed for this indication. It is possible that the nitrovasodilators will be used in this way in the future since NO appears to be involved in erectile function by virtue both as a vascular endothelium-derived mediator, and as a non-adrenergic non-cholinergic neurotransmitter. Adverse effects are related to the route of administration (hematoma, fibrosis), as well as to local (persistent erection necessitating emergency aspiration of the corpora cavernosa) and systemic (e.g. hypotension, headache, flushing and syncope) drug actions.

The Endocrine System VIII

(with Anne Dornhorst)

Diabetes Mellitus

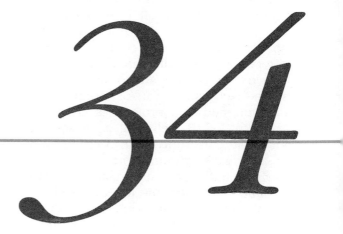

34

Pathophysiology **458**

Principles of management **459**

Diet in diabetes mellitus **460**

Drugs used to treat diabetes mellitus **461**

PATHOPHYSIOLOGY

Insulin is the most important hormone of the endocrine pancreas. It is secreted by the β cells of the islets of Langerhans. It is an anabolic hormone and controls the metabolic disposition of all three major aliments (glucose, fats and amino acids). Insulin is synthesized as a precursor (proinsulin) which is shortened by proteolysis in the Golgi complex of β cells to a double-chained molecule consisting of an A-chain connected to a B-chain (insulin). The inactive connecting C-peptide and insulin are cosecreted in equimolar proportions together with a small proportion (<10% in normals, higher in non-insulin-dependent diabetics) of proinsulin. C-peptide is useful as an index of endogenous insulin secretion: its plasma concentration is low or absent in patients with true insulin-dependent diabetes. Conversely, it is is very high in patients with functional insulinomas, but is not elevated in patients with hypoglycemia as a result of surreptitious self-injection with insulin. Its measurement, together with insulin, can therefore be helpful diagnostically.

Diabetes mellitus is caused by an absolute or relative lack of insulin. Insulin secretion is triggered by many stimuli, including carbohydrate (glucose) and some amino acids. Inhibitors of insulin secretion include insulin itself, somatostatin, adrenaline and other α-adrenergic agonists, β-adrenoceptor antagonists and diazoxide. The control of insulin secretion has recently become much more clearly understood. The problem is the linkage between secretion of a hormone on the one hand and metabolic demand on the other. Hormone secretion frequently involves exocytosis of vesicles containing preformed hormone or transmitter in response to increased cytoplasmic calcium concentration. In pancreatic β cells the membrane potential is apparently largely determined by an adenosine triphosphate (ATP)-sensitive potassium channel. Following a meal blood glucose increases, cytoplasmic ATP in β cells increases and this metabolic signal turns off the potassium channels hence depolarizing these cells and activating voltage-sensitive calcium channels. The resulting influx of calcium ions causes secretion of the insulin-containing vesicles as well as increased synthesis of new hormone.

In insulin-dependent diabetes (IDDM, sometimes called type I or juvenile onset diabetes) there is an absolute deficiency of insulin, and unless insulin treatment is given the patient will ultimately (and usually sooner rather than later) die with diabetic ketoacidosis. Such patients are usually (but not invariably) young and non-obese at presentation. There is an inherited predisposition to the disease with a ten-fold increase in first degree relatives of an index case and a strong positive association with particular human leukocyte antigen (HLA) types and a negative ('protective') association with others. Twin studies have shown, however, that genetically predisposed individuals must also be exposed to an environmental factor to express this tendency (concordance in identical twins is somewhat less than 50%). Viruses (including Coxsackie and Echo viruses) are one such environmental factor, and may cause direct damage to islet cells which results in exposure of antigens and initiation of an autoallergic process that is then self-perpetuating and which results, after a variable period, in eventual destruction of the islets. More than 90% of islets have to be destroyed before the individual becomes frankly diabetic.

By contrast, in non-insulin-dependent diabetes (NIDDM, sometimes called type II or maturity onset diabetes) there is a relative lack of insulin secretion coupled with marked resistance to its action. The circulating concentration of immunoreactive insulin measured by standard assays (which do not discriminate well between insulin and proinsulin) may be normal or even increased, but more discriminating assays indicate that there is an increase in proinsulin and that true insulin concentration is reduced. Non-insulin-dependent diabetes is always associated with reduced sensitivity of tissues to the action of insulin. Such patients are usually (though not invariably) middle aged or elderly at presentation, and are usually obese. Twin studies show that concordance of this form of diabetes in identical twins is nearly 100%. Non-insulin-dependent diabetes is not associated with diabetic ketoacidosis, although it can be complicated by non-ketotic hyperosmolar coma or, rarely (and then usually in association with treatment with a biguanide), with lactic acidosis. In both kinds of diabetes mellitus the increased concentration of glucose in the circulating blood gives rise to osmotic effects: diuresis (polyuria) with consequent volume reduction and thirst, leading to polydipsia; altered refraction due to the altered refractive index of a sugary solution in the aqueous and lens leads to blurred vision (or occasionally and paradoxically to improved vision, in individuals where the change in refraction is fortuitously beneficial). In addition, glycosuria predisposes to *Candida* infection, especially in women. The loss of calories in the urine is coupled with inability to store energy in glycogen or fat, or to lay down protein in muscle, and weight loss with loss of fat and muscle ('amyotrophy') is common in uncontrolled diabetics.

Both kinds of diabetes mellitus are complicated by both microvascular and macrovascular complications. Microvascular complications include retinopathy, which consists of so-called background retinopathy (dot and blot hemorrhages and hard exudates which do not of themselves threaten vision) and proliferative retinopathy in which new vessels form, probably because of growth factors secreted in ischemic areas of retina, and can bleed and cause blindness. Cataracts are also more common in diabetics, perhaps because of the accumulation of sorbitol in the lens. A similar explanation may be important in diabetic neuropathy, which typically causes a stocking distribution of loss of sensation (especially to vibration sense) with associated painful paresthesiae. Microangiopathy of vasa nervorum and glycosylation of membrane proteins are additional pathophysiological factors. The other form of microvascular complication of special importance is glomerulopathy: only approximately one-third of diabetic patients ultimately develop diabetic nephropathy, which leads to renal failure, and it is not known what renders certain individuals susceptible to this complication. Microalbuminuria is prognostically useful as it is a forerunner of overt diabetic nephropathy. There is evidence that an inherited abnormality of red blood cell cation transport detected as an increased rate of sodium–lithium ion countertransport predicts individuals who are predisposed to develop this complication but this is a research rather than a routine investigation.

Macrovascular disease is the result of accelerated atheroma, and results in an increased incidence of myocardial infarction, peripheral vascular disease (manifested as claudication and amputation) and stroke. The pathophysiologic connection between diabetes mellitus and atheroma is imperfectly understood, but factors of probable relevance include a strong association (pointed out by Reaven) between diabetes and obesity, hypertension and hyperlipidemia (especially hypertriglyceridemia).

PRINCIPLES OF MANAGEMENT

It is important to define ambitious but realistic goals for each patient. In the case of young insulin-dependent patients there is good evidence that improved diabetic control reduces the incidence of microvascular complications. It is well worth trying hard to minimize the metabolic derangement associated with diabetes mellitus in order to reduce the development of such complications. Education and support are essential to motivate the patient to learn how to adjust insulin dose to optimize control. This can only be achieved by the patient performing blood glucose monitoring at home and learning to adjust their insulin dose accordingly. The treatment regimen must be individualized and usually requires either twice daily or four times daily subcutaneous injections. Follow-up must include structured care with regular screening for evidence of microvascular disease. This is especially important in the case of proliferative retinopathy (and also of maculopathy), because prophylactic laser therapy in patients with early disease has been shown (in controlled trials in which therapy was given only to one eye) to reduce the incidence of blindness from proliferative retinopathy.

By contrast striving for tight control of blood sugar in NIDDM patients is only appropriate in selected cases. Evidence that tight control reduces macrovascular complications in NIDDM is less convincing than in the effect on development of microvascular disease in IDDM patients, perhaps because metabolic abnormality may precede diagnosis by many years, so much damage will already have been done before treatment is started. In older NIDDM patients (aged >65 years) treatment should aim to minimize symptoms of polyuria, polydipsia or recurrent candidal infection, and to avoid the patient slipping into non-ketotic hyperosmolar coma. Aggressive therapy of the elderly increases the risk of hypoglycemia without proven clinical benefit. In the younger IDDM patient (especially those aged less than 50 years at presentation) vigorous efforts to achieve optimal glycemic control are believed to be justified in the reasonable if unproved hope of reducing future development of vascular disease.

Maintaining glucose as close as possible to normal throughout the day without producing hypoglycemia or severely restricting the patient's life is achieved by one or more of the following interventions:

1. Diet.
2. Diet plus insulin.
3. Diet plus oral hypoglycemic drugs.

By maintaining blood glucose levels below 8 mmol/l and limiting glycosuria to less than 20 g daily, polyuria, polydipsia, dehydration and weight loss can usually be avoided. Glycosylated hemoglobin (HbA_{1c}) provides a convenient measure of integrated control of hyperglycemia over the life of the red cell (120 days) and should be <7%. In older diabetics even these modest goals may not be achieved without considerable sacrifice and difficulty for the patient and it may be necessary to accept some glycosuria and moderate hyperglycemia.

*D*IET IN DIABETES MELLITUS

The aim for patients with either IDDM or NIDDM is to achieve ideal weight and to maintain it. If the patient is obese, calorie intake should be restricted so that weight is gradually (not more than 1 kg/week) lost. The emphasis of the diet for the NIDDM patient is to provide a healthy diet identical to that recommended to other individuals to reduce the risk of developing atheromatous disease (p. 267), together with attention to coexistent risk factors such as smoking, hypertension and physical inactivity. This means a diet high in vegetable fiber (fruit and fresh vegetables) and low in saturated fat and refined sugar. A relative increase in polyunsaturated or monounsaturated fat is appropriate. Excessive protein intake is undesirable especially in the setting of potentially progressive renal impairment. Tissue insensitivity to insulin in NIDDM patients is associated with a reduction in the number of insulin receptors on the surface of fat and muscle cells. Weight loss (by caloric restriction) and increased exercise, result in an increase in the number of insulin receptors, and hence in greater insulin sensitivity and a fall in blood glucose.

The diet for patients with IDDM should also be a healthy one as regards atherogenic potential, but additional constraints are imposed by the necessity of matching caloric intake with insulin injections. Healthy people have considerable latitude in the timing and caloric value of individual meals, but in IDDM patients caloric intake must be distributed so as to match the pattern of insulin activity. One gram of carbohydrate yields 4 calories, 1 g of protein 4 calories and 1 g of fat 9 calories. A common way to distribute daily calories is to give 2/7th at each of three meals and the remaining 1/7th at bedtime. This may need modification for individual patients; for example, a snack mid-afternoon may relieve the hypoglycemia that often occurs at this time in patients taking intermediate-acting insulins. The carbohydrate content of a healthy diabetic diet approximates that of normal persons, i.e. 45–55% of total calories. Simple sugars should be restricted, because they are rapidly absorbed causing postprandial hyperglycemia, and be replaced by polysaccharides (complex sugars) that are broken down to simple sugars by digestion and absorbed more slowly. A fiber-rich diet reduces peak plasma glucose after meals and reduces the dose of insulin required. Pulses such as beans and lentils have the property of flattening the glucose absorption curve. Protein calories should constitute around 20% of total. Protein sources containing little fat (and that mainly unsaturated rather than saturated), for example low fat milk, poultry, fish and vegetable proteins, should be recommended in view of the long-term risk of atheromatous disease. Saturated fat and cholesterol should be minimized. There is no place for commercially promoted 'special diabetic foods' which are expensive and are often high in fat and calories at the expense of complex carbohydrate.

DRUGS USED TO TREAT DIABETES MELLITUS

INSULIN

Use

Insulin is indicated in all patients with type I diabetes mellitus (although it is not strictly necessary during the early 'honeymoon' period before islet cell destruction is complete) and in some patients with type II diabetes mellitus. Indeed, some authorities avoid the terms type I, type II, preferring an empirical classification based on insulin requirement (IDDM and NIDDM). Insulin is usually administered by subcutaneous injection. Many insulin preparations are available that differ in their pharmacokinetics of absorption and thus duration of action. Insulin can be extracted from either ox or pig pancreas, but such animal insulins have been almost entirely replaced by recombinant human insulin. The main advantage of human insulin is that production by bacterial culture can be standardized. In addition there are rather fewer allergic side effects although this advantage is modest. The effective dose of human insulin is usually rather less than of animal insulins because of the lack of blocking antibodies. Consequently some patients have become hypoglycemic when changed from an animal insulin to the same number of units of human insulin. Awareness of hypoglycemia and counterregulatory hormone release tends to diminish as diabetic patients age, and there was initially considerable concern that human insulin might differ qualitatively from animal insulins in causing less awareness of hypoglycemia. Double blind cross-over comparisons of human and animal insulins in which hypoglycemia was deliberately induced under controlled conditions have not borne out these fears, and it appears that there is no difference between the symptoms of hypoglycemia caused by human and by animal insulins.

Soluble insulin is a simple solution and is the only type suitable for intravenous use in the treatment of ketoacidosis and other emergencies. Its short action makes it unsuitable for use as a single daily dose in the long-term management of diabetes since hyperglycemia recurs before the next injection is due, but it is useful given before meals. When the effect wanes before the next dose is due a longer acting insulin with a later onset such as isophane insulin, can be added. Unlike protamine zinc insulin (PZI) this does not contain excess protamine and can thus be coinjected with soluble insulin without unpredictable results. Formulations of human insulins are available in various ratios of short and longer lasting (e.g. 30:70, commonly used twice daily). Some of these are marketed in prefilled injection devices ('pens') which are extremely convenient for patients. Injections are often given twice daily so that insulin reaches its peak activity at 3–4 pm and 3–4 am. The small dose of soluble insulin controls hyperglycemia just after the injection. The chief danger is of a hypoglycemic reaction in the early hours of the morning. When starting a diabetic on a two-dose regime it is therefore helpful to divide the daily dose into two-thirds to be given before breakfast and one-third to be given before the evening meal. If the patient is engaged in hard physical work the morning dose of insulin is reduced somewhat to prevent exercise-induced hypoglycemia. The dose is determined by monitoring blood sugar level when insulin is expected to be maximally active. If this is done it is usually possible to increase the dose to improve hyperglycemia without causing hypoglycemia at other times.

Diabetics with absolute insulin deficiency must be treated with exogenous insulin. Insulin is also required for symptomatic maturity onset diabetics in whom diet or oral hypoglycemic drugs fail. Approximately one-third of NIDDM patients require insulin treatment within 15 years of diagnosis. Unfortunately insulin makes weight loss considerably more difficult because of the appetite stimulating effect of lowering blood sugar, but the anabolic effects of insulin are extremely valuable in some wasted patients, especially those with diabetic amyotrophy. Insulin is needed in acute diabetic emergencies such as ketoacidosis, during pregnancy, perioperatively and with severe intercurrent disease (infections, myocardial infarction, burns etc.).

Insulin requirements are increased by up to a third by intercurrent viral infection, and patients must be instructed to intensify home blood sugar monitoring when they have a cold or other infection (even if they are eating less than usual) and increase the insulin dose if necessary. The dose will subsequently need to be reduced when the infection has cleared. Vomiting which precludes taking the normal diet often causes patients to stop insulin for fear of hypoglycemia. Since vomiting rapidly produces ketosis there is little danger of hypoglycemia but it may result in ketoacidosis. Patients having elective surgery should be admitted to hospital 48 hours before operation and if they are on long-acting insulins, should be changed to a regime of three times daily soluble insulin. Patients receiving oral hypoglycemic agents should be changed to insulin if they have proved difficult to control with oral agents. During surgery it is easiest to infuse 1–3 units of soluble insulin hourly together with a glucose infusion. The infusion rates are adjusted to produce a blood glucose concentration of 6–8 mmol/l. This is continued until oral feeding and intermittent soluble insulin control can be resumed. A similar regime is suitable for emergency operations but frequent measurements of blood glucose are required. Patients with very mild diabetes can be managed without insulin but the blood glucose must be regularly checked in the postoperative period.

Ketoacidosis

The following factors may prevent successful diabetic control:

1. Failure to adhere to diet.
2. Infection, e.g. urinary tract infection, tonsillitis, pneumonia.
3. Chronic renal failure provoking hypoglycemic reactions.
4. Violent exercise.
5. Insulin resistance.
6. Pregnancy.
7. Drugs, e.g. oral contraceptives, corticosteroids, thiazide diuretics.
8. Endocrine disorder: thyrotoxicosis, Cushing's syndrome.
9. Alcohol.

The metabolic changes in ketoacidosis resemble those of starvation since despite the increased concentrations of glucose and ketones in the plasma, these substrates are not available to the metabolizing enzymes within cells ('starving amidst plenty'). Increased glycogenolysis and gluconeogenesis in the liver result in hyperglycemia, which in turn leads to osmotic diuresis, electrolyte depletion and desalination. A total body deficit of potassium ion is inevitable since in the face of acidosis and an osmotic diuresis conservation of potassium is even less efficient than that of sodium. Plasma potassium concentration can however be increased due to a shift from intracellular to extracellular compartment, so large amounts of potassium chloride should not be administered empirically until blood results are available and urine output established. Increased breakdown of muscle releases glucogenic amino acids that are taken up by the liver and converted to glucose. Fat is mobilized from adipose tissue releasing glycerol (which is converted to glucose by the liver) and free fatty acids that are metabolized by β-oxidation to acetyl coenzyme A (CoA). In the absence of glucose breakdown acetyl CoA is converted to acetoacetate with a consequent excessive production of ketone bodies: acetone, acetoacetate and β-hydroxybutyrate. Increased release of ketogenic amino acids from proteolysis also contributes to formation of ketone bodies. These are neutralized by plasma bicarbonate leading to a fall in bicarbonate, the formation of excess carbon dioxide, acidosis and hyperventilation ('Küssmaul' breathing). Hyperglycemia gives rise to an osmotic diuresis with loss of electrolytes and water which, coupled with intracellular dehydration, produces shock. There are therefore a number of abnormalities that require correction:

1. **Desalination and potassium deficit** A generous volume of physiological saline (0.9%), given intravenously, is crucial to restore extracellular fluid volume. An approximate guide is 1.5–2 litres over the first 2 hours, 2 litres over the next 4 hours and 2 litres over the next 6 hours; monitoring of central venous pressure and urine output (following bladder catheterization) are useful guides to the rate of volume replacement. When blood glucose falls below 17 mmol/l, 5% glucose is given in place of saline. Potassium must be replaced, and if the urinary output is satisfactory and plasma potassium concentration low, 20 mmol/hour can be given, the rate of replacement being judged by frequent measurements of plasma potassium concentration and egg monitoring.
2. **Hyperglycemia** Intravenous insulin is infused at a rate of up to 0.1 unit/kg/hour with a syringe pump until there is no ketosis (judged by blood pH, standard bicarbonate and blood ketones) and until the blood glucose is below 15 mmol/l. If ketones have not cleared at this blood glucose level the infusion is slowed to 0.05 units/kg/hour and 4 g of glucose/unit of insulin added to prevent hypoglycemia, thus allowing continuation of the insulin until metabolic normality is restored. Intramuscular injection, although less satisfactory than intravenous infusion, is an acceptable alternative route of administration when facilities for intravenous infusion are not available using a 10 unit starting dose followed by 5 units hourly depending on blood glucose. Subcutaneous injections are absorbed slowly, particularly in shocked patients, and should not be used in this situation.

3. **Metabolic acidosis** This usually resolves with adequate treatment with saline and insulin. Bicarbonate treatment to reverse the extracellular acidosis is controversial, and may paradoxically worsen intracellular and cerebrospinal fluid acidosis. We do not advocate its routine use. If arterial pH is <7.0 the patient should be managed on the intensive care unit if possible, and may need inotropic support.
4. Other measures include aspiration of the stomach since **gastric stasis** is common and **inhalation of vomit** can be fatal, and treatment of the precipitating cause of **coma** (e.g. antibiotics for bacterial infection).

Hyperosmolar non-ketotic coma

Less insulin is required in this situation since the blood pH is normal and insulin sensitivity is retained. Fluid loss is restored using physiological saline (there is sometimes a place for half strength, 0.45% saline) and large amounts of intravenous potassium are often required. Magnesium deficiency is common and contributes to the difficulty of correcting the potassium deficit; it should be treated. There is a case for prophylactic heparin, since the incidence of thrombotic episodes is high.

Mechanism of action

Insulin acts via receptors that are transmembrane glycoproteins that recycle between the plasma membrane and an intracellular pool. Each receptor has two insulin binding sites, but occupancy of one results in marked reduction in affinity of the other. Insulin is internalized with the receptor and passed to lysosomes leaving the receptor to be recycled to the plasma membrane. Receptor occupancy results in:

1. Activation of insulin-dependent glucose transport processes (in adipose tissue and muscle).
2. Inhibition of adenylyl cyclase-dependent processes (lipolysis, proteolysis, glycogenolysis).
3. Intracellular accumulation of potassium and phosphate which are linked to glucose transport in some tissues.

Secondary effects include increased cellular amino acid uptake, increased DNA and RNA synthesis and increased oxidative phosphorylation.

Adverse reactions

1. Hypoglycemia is the most important complication of insulin treatment. It is treated with an intravenous injection of 50% glucose in unconscious patients but sugar may be given orally in those with milder symptoms. Glucagon (1 mg intramuscularly, repeated after a few minutes if necessary) is useful if the patient is unconscious and intravenous access is not available (e.g. to ambulance personnel during transfer to hospital, or to a partner or family member at home). The patient usually regains consciousness within 5 min, and must be given a sweet drink when he/she does.
2. Insulin-induced posthypoglycemic hyperglycemia (Somogyi effect) occurs when the patient develops mild hypoglycemia which induces an overshoot of regulatory mechanisms (adrenaline, growth hormone, corticosteroids, glucagon) that elevate blood sugar. This sometimes occurs during twice daily insulin therapy when nocturnal hypoglycemia coincides with the peak effect of intermediate-acting insulin. Ketonuria may result and the unsuspecting physician may misinterpret the situation as requiring increased insulin, thus producing further hypoglycemia. The syndrome is appropriately managed by slowly decreasing insulin dosage and dietary adjustment.
3. Local or systemic allergic reactions to insulin. Skin sensitivity with itching, redness and swelling at the injection site is the commonest reaction.
4. Lipodystrophy is the disappearance of subcutaneous fat at or near injection sites. Atrophy is now less common with better education regarding rotation of injection sites and wider use of pure insulins. Fatty tumors occur if repeated injections are made at the same site and these still occur with pure insulins. Injections should therefore be made in unexposed areas.

5. Insulin resistance, defined arbitrarily as a daily requirement of more than 200 units, due to antibodies, is relatively unusual. Changing the patient to a highly purified insulin preparation is often successful. A small dose should be used initially to avoid hypoglycemia.

Pharmacokinetics

Insulin is broken down in the gut and by the liver and is given by injection. The half-life ($t_{1/2}$) is 3–5 min. It is metabolized to inactive A and B peptide chains largely by hepatic insulinase (insulin glutathione transhydrogenase) which breaks the disulfide bridges between A and B chains. Insulin from the pancreas is mainly released into the portal circulation and passes to the liver where up to 60% is degraded before reaching the systemic circulation (presystemic metabolism). There is, however, no evidence that diabetes ever results from increased hepatic destruction of insulin. In severe cirrhosis the liver fails to inactivate insulin with consequent increased plasma insulin levels and consequent hypoglycemia.

Oral hypoglycemic drugs

Oral hypoglycemic drugs are useful only as adjuncts to (and not in place of) continued dietary restraint. They should be prescribed only if an adequate trial of diet alone for at least 1 month has been unsuccessful. They fall into two major groups:

1. Sulfonylureas.
2. Biguanides.

Most symptomatic NIDDM patients usually initially achieve satisfactory control with diet alone or combined with one of these agents. The small proportion who cannot be controlled with drugs at this stage (primary failure) require insulin. Subsequent failure, after initially adequate control (secondary

failure) occurs in around one-third of patients after 15 years.

The results of the University Groups Diabetes Program (UGDP) performed in the USA and published in the 1970s have contributed to the controversy surrounding the use of these drugs. The objectives of this study were to evaluate the efficacy of treatment in the prevention of vascular complications by a long-term multicenter trial. After 8 years follow-up the study concluded that the combination of diet and a sulfonamide (tolbutamide) was no more effective than diet and placebo in prolonging life. There was excess cardiovascular mortality in groups treated with hypoglycemic drugs (both sulfonylureas and biguanide). The results of this large study were generally ignored in the UK. Perhaps the most important message is the importance of diet and the potential value of measures designed to limit progression of atheromatous disease (i.e. diet and other lifestyle changes) and in the futility of putting exclusive faith in the value of oral agents beyond their ability to control symptoms such as polyuria.

SULFONYLUREAS

Use

These drugs (e.g. tolbutamide, chlorpropamide, glibenclamide, gliclazide) are used for non-insulin-dependent diabetics who have not responded to diet alone and who show no tendency to ketosis. They improve symptoms of polyuria and polydipsia, but have not been shown to reduce vascular complications or increase longevity (see above), and make weight loss more difficult to achieve by stimulating appetite. Whenever oral hypoglycemic agents are used it is necessary to stress to a patient that such drugs are prescribed in addition to dietary treatment and not in its place. Chlorpropamide is associated with a greater incidence of adverse effects (hypoglycemia due to its long half-life, and flushing with alcohol, see below) than other drugs of this class, and is now used less often for this reason. Tolbutamide and gliclazide are shorter acting than glibenclamide so the risk of hypoglycemia is reduced; they are preferred in the elderly for this reason. Glibenclamide is given once daily with breakfast, the usual starting dose being 5 mg (or less if it is used despite the risk of hypoglycemia in elderly patients) increased according to response to a maximum of 15 mg daily. Tolbutamide is started in a dose of 250 mg twice daily increasing to a maximum of 1 g twice daily according to response. Gliclazide is usually started as a single daily dose of 40 mg increased to a maximum single dose of 160 mg with breakfast; the dose can be further increased if necessary to a maximum of 160 mg twice daily.

Mechanism of action

The hypoglycemic effect of these drugs depends upon the presence of functioning β cells and *in vitro* they stimulate insulin release from isolated islets of Langerhans. Sulfonylureas, like glucose, depolarize β cells which results in insulin release. They do this by blocking ATP-dependent potassium channels in the cell membrane, thereby causing depolarization even when ATP levels in the cell are low. Depolarization causes Ca^{2+} ion entry and insulin secretion. Consequently, acute administration results in a fall in blood sugar accompanied by a rise in plasma insulin. Thus, even in normal subjects, these drugs produce hypoglycemia. Sulfonylureas differ in their effects on water excretion. Chlorpropamide has been employed as an antidiuretic agent in the treatment of patients with diabetes insipidus who have some residual antidiuretic hormone (see chapter 33). It may cause dilutional hyponatremia in some diabetics. It probably acts both by stimulating antidiuretic hormone release and by potentiating its action on the kidney. Tolbutamide has similar but less marked activity, whereas glibenclamide is mildly diuretic.

Adverse effects

The chief danger of these drugs is hypoglycemia, which can result in coma and irreversible neurological damage. Chlorpropamide, the longest acting agent, was responsible for many cases and also causes flushing in susceptible individuals when alcohol is consumed; it has now largely been superseded for these reasons. Tolbutamide and other sulfonylureas are associated with adverse reactions in about 3% of patients, chiefly allergic skin reactions ranging from mild maculopapular to severe generalized photosensitivity reactions occurring from within the first 6 months to up to 2 years of treatment (previous sensitization to sulfonamides is believed to be a factor), drug fever, gastrointestinal upsets, transient jaundice (usually cholestatic), hematopoietic changes including thrombocytopenia, neutropenia and pancytopenia. Serious effects other than hypoglycemia are extremely uncommon.

Pharmacokinetics

Sulfonylureas are all well absorbed from the gastrointestinal tract without presystemic metabolism and the chief differences between them lie in their relative potencies and rates of elimination. Glibenclamide is almost completely metabolized by the liver. Glibencamide is converted to weakly active metabolites before excretion in bile and urine. The activity of these metabolites is only clinically important in patients with renal failure, in whom they accumulate and can cause hypoglycemia. Plasma $t_{1/2}$ in later phases of elimination after oral administration is 6–12 hours, but it has a more prolonged duration of action that may persist for over 16 hours presumably due to a delay in its elimination from pancreatic islet tissue, although tissue accumulation with repeated dosing has not been demonstrated. Tolbutamide is converted to inactive metabolites in the liver which are excreted in urine. The $t_{1/2}$ shows considerable individual variability, but is usually 4–8 hours. Gliclazide is extensively metabolized, although up to 20% is excreted unchanged in urine. Plasma $t_{1/2}$ ranges from 6 to 14 hours (mean 10 hours).

Drug interactions

Useful interactions include the concurrent use of sulfonylurea and metformin to achieve glycemic control in patients who remain symptomatic on either agent alone.

Oral hypoglycemic drugs are, as a group, prone to produce adverse effects due to interaction with other drugs. Monoamine oxidase inhibitors, although they do not alter the $t_{1/2}$ of sulfonylureas, potentiate their activity by an unknown mechanism. Drugs that are highly protein bound, for example clofibrate, aspirin, coumarin anticoagulants and sulfonamides, displace sulfonylureas from protein binding, and may potentiate their action due to the transient increase in free drug concentration that they cause, although inhibition of metabolism has usually proved to be responsible when such interactions have been re-valuated with modern methods. Several drugs (e.g. corticosteroids, thiazide diuretics, frusemide, oral contraceptives, large doses of thyroxine and nicotinic acid) antagonize the hypoglycemic effects of sulfonylureas by virtue of actions on insulin release or glucose tolerance.

BIGUANIDES: METFORMIN

Use

Metformin is used in non-insulin-dependent diabetics without a tendency to ketosis in whom dietary carbohydrate restriction has not controlled hyperglycemia and who remain symptomatic. Its main use is in the overweight patient because its anorectic effect aids weight reduction (in contrast to sulfonylureas and insulin which stimulate appetite powerfully). Metformin also exerts a useful additive effect in patients uncontrolled by sulfonylureas alone. The usual dose is 500 mg every 8 hours, or 850 mg twice daily with or after meals; the usual maximum daily dose is 2 g (occasionally up to 3 g). Metformin should be withdrawn and insulin substituted if necessary when patients suffer serious intercurrent illness, especially myocardial infarction and conditions associated with hypotension or reduced renal function, and also before major elective surgery. Its use is contraindicated in patients with renal failure (it is eliminated in urine, see below) and in patients at increased risk of developing lactic acidosis (e.g. alcoholics and patients with cirrhosis or poor tissue

perfusion due to cardiac failure). Plasma creatinine and liver function tests should be monitored before and during its use, and vitamin B_{12} determined annually during long-term use.

Mechanism of action

The mechanism whereby biguanides produce hypoglycemia remains uncertain, but is quite different from that of the sulfonylureas. They have no effect in normal individuals (i.e. they do not cause hypoglycemia) and, unlike sulfonylureas, do not depend upon insulin release for their actions since they are effective in pancreatectomized animals. Effects of metformin of potential relevance to the mechanism of its hypoglycemic action include: (1) reduced glucose absorption from the gut (metformin improves oral glucose tolerance test more than intravenous glucose tolerance); (2) facilitation of glucose entry into tissues by a non-insulin responsive mechanism thus increasing glucose uptake by peripheral tissues; and (3) inhibition of gluconeogenesis in the liver. There is some evidence to suggest that metformin suppresses oxidative glucose metabolism and enhances anaerobic glycolysis, producing increased plasma lactate and pyruvate levels which may be of relevance to the mechanism whereby it predisposes to lactic acidosis.

Adverse effects

Metformin affects the gastrointestinal tract causing nausea, a metallic taste, anorexia, vomiting and intermittent diarrhea which occur upon initial drug administration. About 3% of patients cannot tolerate this drug even in small doses because of these effects. An extremely uncommon, but severe and potentially life-threatening, toxic effect is the occurrence of lactic acidosis which has a mortality in excess of 60%. This presents with the features of a metabolic acidosis (drowsiness or coma, abdominal pain, vomiting and hyperventilation) often with shock. Treatment is by reversal of hypoxia and circulatory collapse and peritoneal or hemodialysis to alleviate sodium overloading and remove the drug. Phenformin (an earlier biguanide) was more frequently associated with this problem than metformin. The occurrence of lactic acidosis cannot be predicted and has occurred as long as 4 years after beginning treatment. Patients at special risk are alcoholics and those with renal, hepatic or cardiac failure, and biguanides should be avoided for these groups. Absorption of vitamin B_{12} is reduced by metformin.

Pharmacokinetics

Oral absorption of metformin is 50–60%; it is eliminated unchanged by renal excretion, clearance being greater than glomerular filtration rate because of active secretion into tubular fluid. Metformin accumulates in patients with renal impairment. Plasma $t_{1/2}$ ranges from 1.5 to 4.5 hours but its duration of action is considerably longer (18–12 hours) presumably reflecting delayed elimination from sites of action in gut, peripheral tissues and liver.

Drug interactions

Effects of other hypoglycemic agents (sulfonylureas) are additive with the hypoglycemic effect of metformin. Alcohol predisposes to metformin-related lactic acidosis.

ACARBOSE

Acarbose has been recently introduced for the treatment of non-insulin dependent diabetes mellitus in patients inadequately controlled on diet alone or diet and oral hypoglycemic agents. Acarbose is a reversible competitive inhibitor of intestinal alpha glucoside hydrolases and delays the absorption of starch and sucrose but does not affect the absorption of ingested glucose. The postprandial glycemic rise after a meal containing complex carbohydrates is reduced and its peak is delayed. Fermentation of unabsorbed carbohydrate in the intestine leads to increased gas formation which results in flatulence, abdominal distension and occasionally diarrhea. As with any change in a diabetic's medication/diet/activities, the blood glucose must be monitored. Further experience is required before the precise role of acarbose in the management of diabetes mellitus can be defined.

Thyroid

35

Introduction **470**

Pathophysiology and principles of treatment **470**

Iodine **471**

Thyroxine and tri-iodothyronine **471**

Thyrotrophin-releasing hormone **472**

Thyroid-stimulating hormone **473**

Antithyroid drugs **473**

INTRODUCTION

The thyroid secretes thyroxine (T4) and tri-iodothyronine (T3) as well as calcitonin, which is discussed in chapter 36. The release of T3 and T4 is controlled by the pituitary hormone thyrotrophin (thyroid-stimulating hormone: TSH). Secretion of TSH by the anterior pituitary is stimulated by the hypothalamic peptide thyrotrophin-releasing hormone (TRH). Thyroid-stimulating hormone increases the vascularity, cellularity and size of the thyroid and stimulates synthesis and release of the thyroid hormones. Circulating T4 and, to a lesser extent, T3 produce negative-feedback inhibition of TSH at pituitary and hypothalamic levels.

PATHOPHYSIOLOGY AND PRINCIPLES OF TREATMENT

Thyroid disease is commoner in women than in men, and is manifest as either goiter or as under- or overactivity of the gland (with or without goiter). Hypothyroidism is common, especially in the elderly. It is usually caused by autoimmune destruction of the gland, and if untreated causes the clinical picture of myxoedema. Treatment is by life-long replacement with thyroxine.

Hyperthyroidism is also common. In older individuals the commonest cause of hyper-thyroidism is a multinodular toxic goiter. In young women it is usually caused by autoimmune disease, an immunoglobulin being formed that binds to and stimulates the TSH receptor, thereby promoting synthesis and release of T3 and T4 independent of TSH. This results in a smooth vascular goiter and often in deposition of mucopolysaccharide in several tissues, most notably in the extrinsic eye muscles which become thickened and cause proptosis. This clinical picture is known as Graves' disease. Graves' disease has a remitting/relapsing course, and often leads finally to hypothyroidism. Eye signs usually occur within 18 months of onset and commonly resolve over 1–2 years irrespective of the state of the thyroid, but excessively aggressive treatment of hyperthyroidism in patients with eye signs must be avoided because of a strong clinical impression that iatrogenic hypothyoidism can exacerbate eye disease. Reduction of periorbital edema can be achieved by sleeping with the head of the bed elevated. Simple moisturizing eye drops (e.g. hypromellose) may be useful. Five per cent guanethidine eye drops may improve the appearance of the eyes and diuretics are sometimes prescribed in the hope of reducing orbital edema. Tarsoroplasty is indicated to prevent corneal abrasion in severe cases. Radiotherapy is useful in moderate Graves' ophthalmopathy, provided this is not threatening vision. Severe and distressing exophthalmos warrants a trial of prednisolone 60 mg daily. Urgent surgical decompression is required if such treatment is not successful and visual acuity deteriorates due to optic nerve compression. Other etiologies of hyperthyroidism include acute viral or autoimmune thyroiditis (which usually resolve spontaneously), iatrogenic iodine excess (e.g. thyroid storm following iodine-containing contrast media, and hyperthyroidism in patients treated with amiodarone, see chapter 29), and acute *postpartum* hyperthyroidism.

Treatment options include surgery, which is most appropriate when there are mechanical problems such as tracheal compression, radiotherapy with radioactive iodine which is

THYROXINE AND TRI-IODOTHYRONINE **471**

well tolerated and free of surgical complications such as laryngeal nerve damage, and antithyroid drugs that enable a euthyroid state to be maintained until the disease remits or definitive treatment with radioiodine is undertaken. This is usually followed by hypothyroidism, and such patients usually need life-long thyroxine treatment.

I ODINE

The thyroid gland selectively concentrates iodine from plasma. Dietary iodide normally amounts to 100–200 µg/day and is absorbed from the stomach and small intestine by an active process. Following uptake into the thyroid, iodide is oxidized to iodine from which a series of iodinated tyrosine compounds including T3 and T4 are made. Amongst its actions TSH stimulates concentration of iodine in the thyroid and iodination of tyrosine residues. Iodine is used therapeutically to treat those cases of simple non-toxic goiter due to iodine deficiency. In this condition administration of oral potassium iodide, 3 mg, daily will prevent further enlargement of the gland but does not usually cause a reduction in size. Iodized salt is used to prevent this type of endemic goiter in areas where the diet is iodine deficient according to a defined World Health Organization (WHO) policy.

For a patient with thyrotoxicosis about to undergo subtotal thyroidectomy, preoperative treatment with iodide (60 mg potassium iodide orally per day in divided doses) in combination with carbimazole or propylthiouracil reduces the vascularity of the gland and prevents thyroid crisis by reducing the release of T3 and T4 by the gland. This action of iodine in inhibiting thyroid hormone release is maintained for only 1–2 weeks, following which thyroid hormone release is markedly *increased* if the cause of the hyperthyroidism has not been dealt with.

T HYROXINE AND TRI-IODOTHYRONINE

Use

L-Thyroxine is used in the treatment of uncomplicated hypothyroidism. The usual starting dose for an adult is 50 µg daily (25 µg in patients with ischemic heart disease), increasing the dose by 50 µg (25 µg in patients with ischemic heart disease) every 4 weeks until the patient has responded clinically and the TSH level has fallen within the normal range. The optimal maintenance dose is usually 100–200 µg L-thyroxine daily. Excessive dosage or too rapid an increase in dose may precipitate cardiac complications, particularly in patients with overt ischemic heart disease. If angina pectoris limits the dose of thyroxine, the addition of a β-blocker (e.g. atenolol) will allow further increments in thyroxine dosage. Long-term overdosage is highly undesirable and causes osteoporosis as well as predisposing to cardiac arrhythmias.

Cretinism is treated similarly and thyroxine must be given as early as possible; in the UK the adoption of the Guthrie test has greatly facilitated the early detection of hypothyroidism. The rapid action of tri-iodothyronine is useful in treating myxedema coma. It is given in doses of up to 100 μg 12 hourly intramuscularly and at the same time maintenance therapy is commenced with thyroxine 50 μg given orally (or if necessary by a gastric tube). Hypothyroidism sometimes coexists with Addison's disease which is another autoimmune disorder, and hydrocortisone is also given empirically to patients with myxedema coma. Apart from primary thyroid hypofunction, hypothyroidism may result from hypopituitarism. This is also treated with oral thyroxine in the usual doses. Corticosteroid replacement must be started first, otherwise acute adrenal insufficiency will be precipitated.

Mechanism of action

Thyroxine is a prohormone; after entering cells it is converted to T3 which binds to receptor protein which interacts with DNA in the cell nuleus and causes the synthesis of new messenger RNA and hence of new proteins. The main actions of thyroid hormones are:

1. Stimulation of metabolism resulting in a raised basal metabolic rate.
2. Promotion of normal growth and maturation, particularly of the central nervous system and skeleton.
3. Possibly sensitization to the effects of catecholamines. This could explain many of the features of thyrotoxicosis, for example tachycardia and hyperactive reflexes, but the case is unproven.

Adverse effects

Adverse effects of the thyroid hormones relate to their physiological functions. Rapid increases in thyroxine dose in hypothyroidism can lead to sudden death due to ventricular fibrillation. Angina, myocardial infarction, tachycardia and congestive cardiac failure can be precipitated. Diarrhea is a common symptom of excessive thyroxine. Tremor, restlessness, heat intolerance and other features of hyperthyroidism are dose-dependent toxic effects of these hormones.

Pharmacokinetics

The normal range of serum T4 concentration is 50-100 μg/l and the usual range of serum T3 is 1–1.6 μg/l; 99.95% of T4 is bound to thyroid-binding globulin (TBG) whilst only 99.5% of T3 is bound. Drugs such as phenytoin, salicylates and phenylbutazone may reduce TBG binding capacity, thereby interfering with the results of diagnostic tests based upon this function.

Thyroid hormones are absorbed from the gut. The effects of T4 are not usually detectable before 24 hours and maximal activity is not attained for many days during regular daily dosing, depending on the half-life ($t_{1/2}$), which is itself variable. Tri-iodothyronine produces effects within 6 hours and peak activity is reached within 24 hours. It is therefore often preferred for the urgent treatment of myxedema coma. The $t_{1/2}$ of T4 is 6–7 days in euthyroid individuals, but may be much greater than this in hypothyroidism, and that for T3 is 2 days or less. It is therefore unnecessary to administer thyroid hormone more frequently than once a day.

The liver conjugates thyroid hormones and they undergo an enterohepatic circulation.

THYROTROPHIN-RELEASING HORMONE

Thyrotrophin-releasing hormone is a simple tripeptide (glu–his–pro) which is produced in the hypothalamus and is responsible for TSH release. It was useful in diagnosis of hypothyroidism before the development of sensitive TSH assays. It is given intravenously. When it is given to normal people there is a dose-related release of TSH and prolactin. In primary hypothyroidism (i.e. caused by disease in the thyroid gland itself) an exaggerated and prolonged TSH release occurs without change in T4 or T3 concentrations. In cases of hypothyroidism secondary to hypopituitarism there is a greatly attenuated TSH response, and TRH is used to indicate pituitary TSH reserve in pituitary disease.

THYROID-STIMULATING HORMONE

This is the most important physiological regulator of thyroid function. It binds to receptors on thyroid follicular cells and activates adenylyl cyclase resulting in increased cyclic 3',5'-adenosine monophosphate (AMP) formation. This stimulates iodine trapping, iodothyronine synthesis and release of thyroid hormones. Thyroid-stimulating hormone is secreted by basophil cells in the adenohypophysis. It comprises two conjoined polypeptide chains: the α-chain is identical to the α-chain of luteinizing hormone (LH) and follicle-stimulating hormone (FSH), and the β-chain confers specificity for the thyroid TSH receptor. Like TRH it may be used to distinguish primary and secondary hypothyroidism: injection of TSH (10 IU) causes a rise in radioiodine or technetium (^{99m}Tc) uptake by the thyroid in patients with hypopituitarism, but no rise in those with primary thyroid failure.

ANTITHYROID DRUGS

CARBIMAZOLE

Use

Carbimazole is used to treat hyperthyroidism, particularly in children under 18 years and in women of child-bearing potential in whom radioiodine treatment has in the past been a cause of concern, and during pregnancy when radioiodine remains contraindicated. A single daily dose of 30–60 mg in adults (15 mg in children) is used until the patient is euthyroid, usually in 4–6 weeks. Patients are warned to report any evidence of infection, especially sore throat, immediately, and indeed some centers use written advice leaflets and consent forms to underline the importance of this. The dose of carbimazole is then reduced to a maintenance regime of 5–15 mg daily. Treatment is maintained for 1–2 years and the drug is then gradually withdrawn. If relapse occurs during drug withdrawal, the dose is again raised until clinical improvement is restored. If dosage adjustment proves difficult, smoother control may be obtained by giving thyroxine, 100 μg/day, together with a blocking dose of carbimazole, 60 mg/day.

Mechanism of action

Carbimazole is hydrolyzed to methimazole in plasma and it is not possible to demonstrate the presence of carbimazole in the thyroid, although methimazole is present. Thus carbimazole acts by way of its active metabolite methimazole which acts as a substrate for peroxidase and is itself iodinated and degraded within the thyroid thus diverting oxidized iodine away from thyroglobulin thereby decreasing thyroid hormone biosynthesis. Methimazole is concentrated by cells with a peroxidase system (salivary gland, neutrophil, macrophage/monocytes in addition to thyroid follicular cells). It has an immunosuppressive action within the thyroid, and interferes with generation of oxygen radicals by macrophages thereby interfering with the presentation of antigen to lymphocytes. Methimazole also prevents T3 and T4 synthesis by interfering with tyrosine iodination and the coupling of iodotyrosines, but does not affect hormone secretion. Thus hormone release diminishes after a latent period during which time the thyroid becomes depleted of hormone.

Adverse effects

In therapeutic use carbimazole is a relatively non-toxic drug. Pruritus and rashes are common, and usually respond to changing to propylthiouracil as an alternative agent. Nausea and hair loss occur occasionally. Drug fever, leukopenia and arthralgia are rare, but neutropenia is potentially fatal if the drug is continued: if the patient reports sore throat or other evidence of infection an **urgent** white cell count must be obtained, and the drug stopped if there is neutropenia.

Pharmacokinetics

Carbimazole is rapidly absorbed after oral administration and hydrolyzed to its active metabolite methimazole which is rapidly concentrated in the thyroid within minutes of administration. Methimazole has an apparent volume of distribution equivalent to body water and the half-life varies according to thyroid status, being 9.3, 6.9 and 13.6 hours in euthyroid, hyperthyroid and hypothyroid subjects, respectively. It is metabolized in the liver and thyroid.

PROPYLTHIOURACIL

Use

Propylthiouracil has similar actions, uses and toxic effects to carbimazole, but has an additional action in inhibiting the peripheral conversion of T4 to the more active T3. As with carbimazole, dangerous leukopenia may develop but is very rare. The initial total daily dose is 300–600 mg and the maintenance dose is 50–150 mg. The scheme of attaining a euthyroid state with a large dose of drug and then reducing the dose to maintain this is carried out as with carbimazole. Propylthiouracil is absorbed rapidly from the intestine. The plasma $t_{1/2}$ is short, but the duration of action within the thyroid is prolonged, and as with carbimazole phenylthiouracil can be given once daily, although many endocrinologists still prefer to give the drug in three divided doses. Antithyroid drugs cross the placenta and are found in milk so that the child of an affected mother may be born with a goiter which may persist during suckling. Overtreatment must therefore be avoided especially in treating pregnant women. Thyroxine does *not* cross the placenta, so blocking doses of antithyroid drugs with added T4 must *never* be used in pregnancy since this will inevitably result in a severely hypothyroid infant. Propylthiouracil is less likely than carbimazole to produce effects in the infant since it is more highly protein bound and is ionized at pH 7.4. This reduces its passage across the placenta and into milk. Fetal heart rate must be monitored during treatment with propylthiouracil and the dose increased if this exceeds 150/min to avoid hyperthyroidism in the infant.

POTASSIUM PERCHLORATE

Potassium perchlorate prevents the trapping and concentration of iodine in the thyroid. It rarely produces aplastic anemia and is no longer used in the UK.

β-ADRENOCEPTOR ANTAGONISTS

β-Blockers reduce the resting tachycardia, relieve the subjective feelings of anxiety and sweating, reduce tremor and prolong the hyperactive reflexes of thyrotoxic patients. They also have an action in blocking the conversion of T4 to T3 in the tissues. This effect seems to be a general property of β-blockade and is irrespective of β-specificity or intrinsic sympathomimetic activity. These drugs are useful to control symptoms while awaiting laboratory confirmation of the diagnosis in uncertain cases and during initiation of therapy with antithyroid drugs, and in thyroid crisis. They are also used with iodine as a rapid preparation for surgery when the patient may be operated upon after only 10–14 days of β-blockade. The gland is said to be less friable, firmer and less likely to tear than after conventional preparation with antithyroid drugs. It must be recognized that patients treated with β-blockers are not euthyroid and therefore inadequate treatment or omission of a dose may provoke a thyroid crisis in the postoperative period. β-Blockers do not affect uptake of radioactive iodine as do conventional antithyroid drugs and have also been used as adjunctive therapy to radioiodine. Accurate assessment of the effects of the radioactive therapy may be made via thyroid function tests without the confounding effects of concurrent antithyroid drug therapy. β-Blockers are also useful in the short-term treatment of neonatal hyperthyroidism due to thyroid-stimulating immunoglobulin from the mother, because this remits within around 6 weeks as maternal-derived immunoglobulin is cleared by the infant.

Thyroid crisis

Thyroid crisis is a severe, and usually sudden, exacerbation of hyperthyroidism with hyperpyrexia, tachycardia, vomiting, dehydration, hyperkinesis and shock which may arise postoperatively, following radioiodine therapy or with intercurrent infection; rarely it arises spontaneously in a previously undiagnosed/untreated patient. Mortality is substantial and urgent treatment is required with:

1. β-Blockers to control tachycardia and tremor.
2. Fluids and cooling to combat dehydration and hyperthermia.
3. Antithyroid drugs to reduce hormone synthesis followed by iodides to slow secretion (200 mg propylthiouracil every 4 hours by nasogastric tube).

4. Glucocorticoids (which antagonize conversion of T4 to T3).

In addition:

5. Fast atrial fibrillation can be especially difficult to treat because of resistance to digoxin, and DC cardioversion is often indicated.
6. Salicylates must be avoided, because of their uncoupling effect on oxidative phosphorylation which renders the metabolic state even more severe.

RADIOACTIVE IODINE

Radioactive iodine is an effective oral treatment for thyrotoxicosis (other than patients with thyroiditis or iodine excess in whom iodine uptake by the thyroid is reduced). It is safe and causes no discomfort to the patient. Within the past decade it has become first-line treatment and has largely replaced surgery. Dosing has been a subject of controversy. It is now standard practice in many units to give an ablative dose followed by replacement therapy with thyroxine, so late onset undiagnosed hypothyroidism is avoided. The usually employed isotope is ^{131}I with a $t_{1/2}$ of 8 days. Thyroxine replacement is started after 4–6 weeks and continued for life. There is no increased incidence of leukemia, thyroid or other malignancy after therapeutic use of ^{131}I, but concern remains regarding its use in children or young women. However, the dose of radiation to the gonads is less than many radiological procedures such as barium enema, and there is no evidence that therapeutic doses of radioactive iodine damage the germ cells or reduce fertility. It is contraindicated during pregnancy because it damages the fetus, causing congenital hypothyroidism and consequently possible mental retardation ('cretinism'). Patients are usually treated as outpatients in the first 10 days of the menstrual cycle and after a negative pregnancy test. Pregnancy should be avoided for at least 4 months and a woman should not breast feed for at least 2 months after treatment. High-dose ^{131}I is used to treat patients with well-differentiated thyroid carcinoma to ablate residual tumor after surgery. Thyroxine is stopped at least a month before treatment to allow TSH to increase thereby stimulating uptake of isotope by the gland. Patients are isolated in hospital for several days as a protection for potential contacts.

Calcium Metabolism

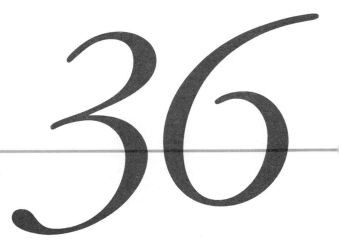

36

Introduction   **478**

Principles of treatment of hypercalcemia   **478**

Vitamin D   **479**

Calcium   **481**

Calcitonin   **481**

Bisphosphonates   **482**

INTRODUCTION

Plasma calcium is maintained within a narrow physiological range by parathyroid hormone (PTH), vitamin D and calcitonin. Parathyroid hormone is rapidly metabolized by liver and kidney so that a heterogeneous mixture of inactive PTH fragments is present in plasma. Plasma calcium concentration is the major factor controlling PTH secretion, a reduction in calcium concentration stimulating PTH release. Acute hypomagnesemia elevates plasma PTH but prolonged magnesium depletion impairs secretion. This may result from a requirement for magnesium ion by parathyroid adenylyl cyclase, since PTH release by hypocalcemia is mediated by cyclic adenosine monophosphate (AMP). Parathyroid hormone raises blood calcium and lowers phosphate concentration.

Parathyroid hormone acts on kidney and bone. Both effects are mediated by stimulation of tissue adenylyl cyclase with elevation of cyclic AMP. Parathyroid hormone causes phosphaturia and increased renal tubular reabsorption of calcium, which in association with mobilization of calcium from bone, increases plasma calcium concentration. Parathyroid hormone actions on bone include stimulation of osteoclast activity, formation of new osteoclasts from progenitor cells and transient depression of osteoblast activity.

Parathyroid hormone also plays a role in the regulation of vitamin D metabolism. Increased gut absorption of calcium previously attributed to PTH is in fact an indirect effect via increased production of 1,25-dihydroxycholecalciferol.

Parathyroid hormone replacement has no place in long-term management of hypoparathyroidism. Parathyroid hormone is administered as a single test dose (200 units intravenously) in the diagnosis of pseudohypoparathyroidism. In this condition there is end-organ resistance to the hormone, so plasma calcium does not rise and there is no increase in urinary phosphate or cyclic AMP excretion.

Several important metabolic diseases affect the bones, notably hyperparathyroidism (treatment of which is surgical), osteomalacia and rickets, Paget's disease of bone and osteoporosis. Some of these (e.g. osteomalacia) are associated with normal or low plasma calcium concentration, some (e.g. hyperparathyroidism) with hypercalcemia, and some (e.g. osteoporosis) with normal calcium concentration. The most important drug used in the prevention and treatment of postmenopausal osteoporosis is estrogen (as hormone replacement therapy), and this is described in chapter 38. Other drugs used (calcium, vitamin D and etidronate) are described below.

PRINCIPLES OF TREATMENT OF HYPERCALCEMIA

Hypercalcemia may be a life-threatening emergency and is produced by numerous pathological processes ranging from bony destruction by tumor to hyperparathyroidism. In patients with known disseminated untreatable malignancy correction of hypercalcemia may not be in the patient's best interest, as hypercalcemia is a kinder mode of death than many others. When treatment is indicated it is important to use the time provided by whatever measure is effective in lowering plasma calcium to treat the cause of the hypercalcemia since the effect of other therapy is short-lived. Management divides into the general and specific.

General management

1. Maintenance of hydration with physiological saline, and avoidance of thiazide diuretics.
2. Avoidance of excessive dietary vitamin D.
3. Avoidance of immobilization.

Specific management

INCREASING CALCIUM EXCRETION

Physiological normal saline is infused intravenously as rapidly as the patient's cardiovascular state permits. This restores blood volume and causes increased urinary elimination of calcium. Once extravascular volume has been restored, frusemide, 100 mg, orally increases urinary calcium loss further.

DECREASING BONE RESORPTION

1. Plicamycin given intravenously in a dose of 15 µg/kg over half an hour on 4 successive days is often effective, and used to be a mainstay of treatment. It has now largely been replaced by the bisphonates. Its main action is to decrease osteoclast activity. Nausea and vomiting are common complications and rarely a bleeding disorder and disturbance of liver function occurs.
2. Calcitonin (see below).
3. Bisphosphonates (see below).

GLUCOCORTICOIDS

Glucocorticoids are useful in treating the hypercalcemia associated with sarcoidosis.

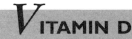

VITAMIN D

The term 'vitamin D' is used to cover a range of related substances that share the ability to prevent or cure rickets. These include ergocalciferol (vitamin D_2), cholecalciferol (vitamin D_3), α calcidol (1-α-hydroxycholecalciferol) and calcitriol (1,25-α-dihydrocholecalciferol). The metabolic pathway of vitamin D is diagrammatically shown in Fig. 36.1. Vitamin D_3 is synthesized in skin by the action of ultraviolet light on 7-dehydrocholesterol, or absorbed from food in the upper gut. It is fat soluble so bile is necessary for its absorption. Renal 1-α-hydroxylase is activated by PTH and inhibited by phosphate, thus controlling the amount of active 1,25-dihydroxycholecalciferol (1,25-DHCC) produced. This enzyme is also suppressed by 1,25-DHCC itself. 1,25-Dihydroxycholecalciferol is effectively a hormone in that it is synthesized in the kidney and acts on the intestine to increase formation of a calcium-binding protein which augments intestinal calcium absorption. Vitamin D itself is the biologically inactive precursor of 1,25-DHCC. Enzyme induction, particularly due to antiepileptic drugs, causes metabolic inactivation of calciferol causing osteomalacia and rickets. 1,25-Dihydroxycholecalciferol mobilizes calcium from bone; presumably this provides calcium for synthesis of new bone mineral. Its action on the kidney is to stimulate calcium reabsorption, although this is a minor effect. The maximum antirachitic effect of cholecalciferol is delayed for several weeks and plasma calcium similarly increases only slowly. Storage of the vitamin occurs so that the plasma half-life ($t_{1/2}$) does not determine the duration of its action and a single large dose may be effective for several weeks.

Use

Dietary deficiency of vitamin D in the UK occurs where there is poverty and poor diet

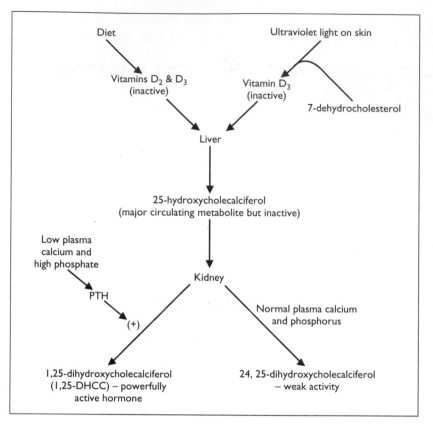

Fig. 36.1 Metabolic pathway of vitamin D. PTH = parathormone.

accentuated by lack of sunlight, and is particularly common in Asian communities living in the north (chapatis and other unleavened breads reduce absorption of vitamin D), and in elderly people living alone. It results in rickets and osteomalacia. A daily dose of 10 μg cholecalciferol is recommended in infants and children up to their seventh birthday and 2.5 μg thereafter. Pregnant and lactating women should take about 20 μg daily. Several different vitamin D preparations are listed in the *British National Formulary* which have different concentrations and purposes:

1. Calcium and ergocalciferol tablets provide a physiological dose of vitamin D: ergocalciferol (vitamin D) 10 μg with 300 mg calcium lactate and 150 mg calcium phosphate. These are chewed or crushed before being taken and are used in the prophylaxis and treatment of rickets and osteomalacia. The small dose of calcium (2.4 mmol) is unnecessary, but a preparation of vitamin D alone is not available.

2. Calciferol tablets 250 μg or 1.25 mg provide a pharmacological dose of vitamin D and are used for treatment of hypoparathyroidism and in cases of vitamin D-resistant rickets due to intestinal malabsorption or chronic liver disease.

3. 1-α-Hydroxycholecalciferol (1-α-HCC). This metabolite is available for oral administration. It rapidly undergoes hepatic hydroxylation to 1,25-DHCC. It is used in:

   (a) Renal rickets, where chronic renal failure leads to impaired 1,25-DHCC synthesis resulting in calcium malabsorption and hypocalcemia with phosphate retention leading to secondary elevation of PTH levels. Bony changes of osteomalacia and hyperparathyroidism ensue. 1-α-Hydroxycholecalciferol is given in a dose of 1 μg daily (together with a phosphate-binding agent such as aluminum hydroxide).

(b) Hypoparathyroidism, which is usually treated with vitamin D in large doses but the response is slow, and unpredictable episodes of hypercalcemia occur. This relative resistance to vitamin D is due to deficient 1,25-DHCC production secondary to PTH deficiency or hyperphosphatemia. 1-α-Hydroxycholecalciferol, 1–2 μg, plus calcium supplements correct plasma calcium levels within a matter of days and normocalcemia may be maintained with smaller doses within a relatively narrow dosage range.

(c) Vitamin D-resistant rickets.

(d) Nutritional and malabsorptive rickets, which may also be treated with small doses (0.5–1 μg) of 1-α-HCC instead of conventional vitamin D.

The main adverse reaction is hypercalcemia which can in turn cause renal failure so regular plasma calcium and creatinine determinations (weekly to begin with) are essential. It is more likely to occur in renal failure than in osteomalacia. An advantage of using 1-α-HCC is that vitamin D intoxication is rapidly reversed when the drug is withdrawn, whereas reversal may take several weeks with the older vitamin D compounds.

4. Calcitriol (1,25-DHCC) is also available for the treatment of the above. Like 1-α-HCC it has a shorter biological half-life and less variable action than calciferol. Calcitriol is the treatment of choice for pseudohypoparathyroidism.

Prolonged or inappropriate use of these preparations will result in hypercalcemia with calcium deposition in the tissues, particularly in the kidney where it may cause irreversible renal failure.

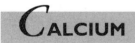 CALCIUM

Calcium lactate or gluconate is used in conjunction with calciferol in the treatment of rickets and osteomalacia and in hypocalcemic tetany. It is also lifesaving in the emergency treatment of cardiac arrhythmia due to hyperkalemia (p. 369). In emergency it is given as calcium gluconate injection BP (10% solution), 10–20 ml being given intravenously over 5–10 min every 2—4 hours. It should not be given intramuscularly, at least to children, since it is painful and can cause necrosis. Given intravenously its cardiac effects (which include bradycardia and ventricular arrhythmias) mimic and potentiate those of digoxin. The place of routine calcium supplements in the prevention and treatment of osteoporosis is not firmly established but it is certainly justified to supplement the diet if intake is below 1 g of elemental calcium daily. Effervescent or chewable preparations of calcium carbonate are available that are easy to take and can be taken with each meal thereby delivering 200–300 mg into an acid-secreting stomach.

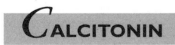 CALCITONIN

This hormone is a polypeptide secreted by thyroid parafollicular C-cells. Acting via cyclic AMP it lowers plasma calcium and phosphate levels and antagonizes the effects of parathormone on bone. These effects are produced by:

1. A major effect on bone via a slowing of osteoclastic resorption, leading to a reduced release of calcium, phosphorus and hydroxyproline. The magnitude of the fall in plasma calcium levels depends upon the initial bone turnover and where this is high as in Paget's disease or thyrotoxicosis, the fall may be large. In normal adults the fall in plasma calcium is often unimpressive.
2. A minor renal effect promoting phosphate, calcium and sodium excretion.
3. Calcitonin inhibits 1-α-hydroxylase, thereby blocking the activation of vitamin D and reducing intestinal absorption of calcium.

Use

Synthetic calcitonin (porcine, human and, especially, salmon) is used therapeutically to lower plasma calcium concentration in some patients with hypercalcemia, and in the treatment of pain and some of the neurological complications (e.g. deafness due to VIII nerve compression) of severe Paget's disease. Calcitonin is given by subcutaneous or intramuscular injection. Recently it has been found that sufficient absorption occurs across the nasal mucosa to enable this route to be employed clinically, opening up the possibility of widening its indications to include the prevention and/or treatment of osteoporosis in women at risk, especially those in whom estrogen replacement is contraindicated. Calcitonin may induce antibody formation, salmon being less immunogenic than pork, but this rarely interferes with treatment (cf. insulin antibodies, p. 461).

The two main indications for calcitonin treatment in patients with Paget's disease are bone pain and hypercalcemia, although calcitonin has been partly supplanted by bisphosphonates in treating hypercalcemia in this setting. Patients vary in their response, but pain relief usually occurs within 2 months of beginning treatment (80 units thrice weekly usually results in a fall in plasma calcium, phosphate and alkaline phosphatase with reduced urinary hydroxyproline excretion). In patients with nerve compression or severe pain higher doses (e.g. 80–160 units daily for 3–6 months) may be used. It is not known whether prolonged therapy prevents the development of deformity.

Hypercalcemia due to malignancy, vitamin D intoxication, infantile hypercalcemia or immobilization of patients with Paget's disease all respond to calcitonin. Doses of 4 units/kg/day are used and in emergencies higher doses of 8 units/kg/6 hours have been given intravenously without problem. Calcitonin is useful in the preparation of patients with severe hyperparathyroidism for surgery but has no place in the long-term management of this condition.

In postmenopausal osteoporosis it is given with dietary calcium and vitamin D supplements if the diet is inadequate in these.

Adverse effects

1. Pain at the injection site.
2. Nausea (countered by giving the injection with an antiemetic before going to bed) and diarrhea.
3. Flushing of the face (20–30%).

*B*ISPHOSPHONATES

Bisphosphonates structurally resemble pyrophosphate except that the two phosphorus atoms are linked by carbon rather than oxygen. This renders such compounds very stable: no enzyme is known that degrades them. Several bisphosphonates (e.g. disodium pamidronate, sodium clodronate) have been used to treat hypercalcemia of malignancy. Disodium etidronate is currently used widely.

DISODIUM ETIDRONATE

Use

Etidronate is active when given by mouth, making it more convenient to use than calcitonin. It is also cheaper. Like calcitonin it is indicated in Paget's disease and in hypercalcemia of malignancy (alternative diphosphonates for this indication include pamidronate and sodium clodronate). Etidronate is also used with calcium carbonate in patients with established vertebral osteoporosis. It is started at low dosage (5 mg/kg/day as a single dose) over 6 months when many patients achieve remission for 3–24 months; a further course may be given on relapse. Use for longer than 6 months at a time does not prolong remission. Higher doses (up to 20 mg/kg/day) should be used only if lower doses fail or if rapid control of disease is needed. Etidronate is effective when calcitonin has failed (and *vice versa*) and they may be used in conjunction. It is indicated for treatment of patients with bone pain (which responds well) or if there is extensive involvement of the skull or spine with possible danger of irreversible neurological damage or when a weight-bearing bone is involved. Stress fractures in long bones contraindicate its use, because of the reduction in new bone formation that it causes. When used to treat hypercalcemia of malignancy it is given by intravenous infusion (7.5 mg/kg/day for 3 days) followed by 20 mg/kg by mouth daily for 30 days. It is not recommended for more than 3 months for this indication. For vertebral osteoporosis 400 mg is given by mouth for 14 days followed by calcium carbonate 1.25 g daily for 76 days, this 3-month cycle then being repeated and treatment continuing in this way for 3 years.

Mechanism of action

Etidronate modifies the crystal growth of calcium hydroxyapatite by chemical adsorption to the crystal surface. This high affinity for calcium phosphate has been exploited in its use for nuclear bone scanning as a complex of ^{99m}Tc (a γ-emitter) with ethane hydroxydiphosphonic acid. This is used to identify areas of increased skeletal turnover, particularly Paget's disease and bony metastases. Etidronate inhibits bone resorption and formation thereby reducing the accelerated bone turnover of Paget's disease, returns the histological bone pattern towards normal, lowers the associated elevated biochemical indices of the disease and relieves symptoms.

Adverse effects

Etidronate is well tolerated and at low doses there is only a low incidence of gastrointestinal complaints (diarrhea, nausea, abdominal pain, constipation, transient loss of taste). High doses can cause hyperphosphatemia, but this is probably harmless. Hypocalcemia is usualy mild and asymptomatic. A few patients with Paget's disease (approximately 5%) experience exacerbation of bone pain during treatment with high doses, and there is reduced healing of fractures.

Pharmacokinetics

Etidronate is given orally but is poorly (1–5%) absorbed; food and antacids further reduce absorption. It disappears from the blood extremely rapidly into bone where its effects persist. Within 24 hours about 50% of the absorbed dose is excreted unchanged in the urine, the remainder is excreted over many weeks. There are no known drug interactions apart from reduction of its absorption by antacids.

Adrenal Hormones

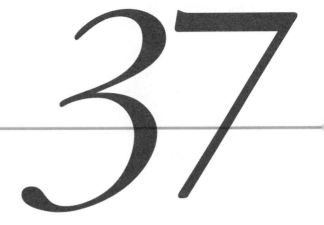

Adrenal cortex **486**

Adrenal medulla: pheochromocytoma **492**

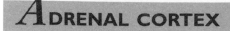

ADRENAL CORTEX

The adrenal cortex secretes:

1. **Glucocorticoids** principally cortisol (hydrocortisone) and small amounts of corticosterone. The rate of secretion of cortisol is not constant during the day, the maximum concentration in the blood (170–720 nmol/l) being reached at about 8.00 am under usual diurnal conditions and the minimum (< 220 nmol/l) around midnight.
2. **Mineralocorticoids** principally aldosterone and small amounts of desoxycorticosterone;
3. **Androgens** (e.g. testosterone, androsterone) in relatively small amounts.

Glucocorticoids

The actions of glucocorticoids and the effects of their oversecretion (Cushing's syndrome) and undersecretion (Addison's disease) are summarized in Table 37.1. Physiologically glucocorticoids influence carbohydrate, protein and, to a lesser extent, lipid metabolism, and their increased secretion plays a vital part in the response to stress. Glucocorticoids stimulate the mobilization of amino acids from skeletal muscle, bone and skin, promoting their transport to the liver where they are converted into glucose and stored as glycogen (gluconeogenesis). Fat mobilization by catecholamines is enhanced by glucocorticoids. Pharmacologically the main therapeutic actions of the glucocorticoids stem from anti-inflammatory and immunosuppressive effects. They reduce circulating numbers of eosinophils, basophils and T lymphocytes while increasing neutrophils. Glucocorticoids interact with a cytoplasmic receptor causing the dissociation of a phosphorylated heat shock protein and subsequent derepression of nuclear DNA and new protein synthesis. One such protein that has been characterized is lipocortin; this inhibits phospholipase A_2 thus inhibiting formation of several proinflammatory mediators including eicosanoids of both cyclo-oxygenase (e.g. prostaglandin E_2, thromboxane A_2) and lipoxygenase (e.g. leukotriene B_4) pathways, as well as of platelet-activating factor (PAF). When potent steroids are applied topically to skin or mucous membranes they cause local vasoconstriction, and indeed when given systemically in massive doses (e.g. >1 g hydrocortisone) they cause generalized vasoconstriction.

Adverse effects

Adverse effects of glucocorticoids tend to be common to the group of drugs as a whole, whereas different drugs of this group tend to be used for somewhat different indications. Adverse effects of the group as a whole are therefore considered first, before describing uses of individual drugs.

1. Rapid withdrawal after prolonged steroid administration can cause acute adrenal insufficiency. Gradual withdrawal is less hazardous, but even in patients who have been successfully weaned from chronic treatment with steroids, for 1–2 years afterwards a stressful situation (such as trauma, surgery, infection, emotional crisis or status asthmaticus) may precipitate an acute adrenal crisis and necessitate administration of large amounts of steroids, electrolytes, glucose and water. Other features of corticosteroid withdrawal can include malaise, fever, arthralgia, myalgia and pseudotumor cerebri (raised intracranial pressure and papilloedema without space-occupying lesion).

    Suppression of the adrenal cortex is unusual if the daily dose of prednisolone is less than 5 mg or its equivalent. The rate at which patients can be weaned off their steroids depends in part on their under-

Table 37.1 Actions of cortisol and consequences of under- and oversecretion.

	Actions	Deficiency	Excess
Carbohydrate, protein and fat metabolism	Enhances gluconeogenesis; antagonizes insulin; hyperglycemia ± diabetes mellitus; centripetal fat deposition; hypertriglyceridemia; hypercholesterolemia; decreased protein synthesis, e.g. diminished skin collagen	Hypoglycemia, loss of weight	Cushing's syndrome: weight gain, increase in trunk fat, moon face, skin striae, bruising, atrophy, wasting of limb muscles
Water and salt metabolism	Inhibits fluid shift from extracellular to intracellular compartment; antagonizes vasopressin action on kidney; increases vasopressin destruction and decreases its production. Sodium and water retention, potassium loss	Loss of weight, hypovolemia, hyponatremia	Edema, thirst, polyuria; hypertension; muscular weakness
Hematological	Lowers lymphocyte and eosinophil counts; increases red blood cells, platelets and clotting tendency		Florid complexion and polycythemia
Alimentary	Increases production of gastric acid and pepsin	Anorexia and nausea	Dyspepsia; aggravation of peptic ulcer
Cardiovascular system	Sensitizes arterioles to catecholamines; enhances production of angiotensinogen Fall in high-density lipoprotein with increased total cholesterol	Hypotension, fainting	Hypertension, atherosclerosis
Skeletal	Decreased production of cartilage and bone; osteoporosis; antivitamin D; increased renal loss of calcium; renal calculi formation		Backache due to osteoporosis, renal calculi, dwarfing in children (also anti-GH effect)
Nervous system	Altered neuronal excitability. Inhibition of uptake of catecholamines		Depression and other psychiatric changes
Anti-inflammatory	Reduces formation of fluid and cellular exudate; reduces fibrous tissue repair		Increased spread of and proneness to infections
Immunological	Large doses lyse lymphocytes and plasma cells (transient release of immunoglobulin)		Reduced lymphocyte mass, diminished immunoglobulin production
Feedback	Inhibits release of ACTH and MSH	Pigmentation of skin and mucosa	

ACTH = adrenocorticotropic hormone. MSH = melanocyte-stimulating hormone. GH = growth hormone.

lying condition and also on the dose and duration of therapy. Provided there is no exacerbation of disease the daily dose may be reduced by 2.5–5.0 mg weekly down to a dose of 5 mg prednisolone per day. This is then reduced by 1 mg at a time depending upon symptoms and, if very prolonged therapy has been employed, plasma cortisol concentrations measured. These should reach 270 nmol/l in an early morning sample before steroid treatment is finally discontinued, followed by an adrenocorticotropic hormone (ACTH) stimulation test ('synacthen' test) or in special circumstances an insulin stress test to test adrenal reserve. After long-term

Table 37.2 Relative potencies of corticosteroids and mineralcorticoids.

Compound	Relative potency		Equivalent doses for anti-inflammatory effect (mg)
	Anti-inflammatory	Mineralocorticoid	
Cortisol (hydrocortisone)	1	1	80
Cortisone	0.8	1	100
Prednisolone and prednisone	4	0.8	20
Methylprednisolone	5	0.5	16
Triamcinolone	4	0	20
Dexamethasone	25	0	2
Betamethasone	25	0	2
Aldosterone	0	1000*	–
Fludrocortisone	15	500	–

* Injected – other preparations as oral doses.

steroids are discontinued the patient should continue to carry a steroid card for at least a year.

2. Intercurrent illness in patients receiving corticosteroids increases dose requirements and can cause acute adrenal failure. With moderate illness it is sufficient to double the dose of whichever steroid is being used. It is not usually necessary to give more than 40 mg prednisolone or its equivalent daily. In severely ill patients, particularly when vomiting or electrolyte loss is a problem, parenteral hydrocortisone hemisuccinate, 100 mg, 6 hourly is preferred.

3. Complications due to chronic administration of steroids consist of iatrogenic Cushing's syndrome (see Table 37.1). These usually only develop when exogenous glucocorticoid therapy is greater than physiological production, i.e. 7.5 mg prednisolone or more per day or its equivalent.

(a) General appearance: Cushingoid.

(b) Effects on inflammation: Glucocorticoids decrease the inflammatory and immune responses and resistance to infection is reduced. Symptoms and signs of acute infection are suppressed, although the spread of infection is enhanced. It follows that patients on steroids who develop an infection require vigorous treatment with the appropriate antibiotic.

Steroids also increase susceptibility to opportunistic infection with fungi and other organisms. Old tuberculous lesions may reactivate and such lesions should be carefully watched in patients on chronic steroid treatment: occasionally it may be necessary to give antituberculous cover with isoniazid and rifampicin.

(c) Electrolyte balance may be altered and some salt and water retention is usual. Potassium loss and hypokalemia can be severe especially if steroids are combined with a diuretic.

(d) Hypertension often accompanies glucocorticoid usage.

(e) Diabetes mellitus is exacerbated and its control made more difficult by steroids, often necessitating increased doses of insulin or oral hypoglycemic drugs. Glucocorticoids may also precipitate diabetes in predisposed individuals.

(f) Osteoporosis is a particular problem with long-term use, particularly with high dosage. Vertebral crush fractures are common and can occur even after short courses of high-dose glucocorticoid treatment.

(g) Peptic ulceration: A link between glucocorticoid therapy and peptic ulceration remains controversial, and the data are limited. On balance it seems probable that glucocorticoid therapy is weakly linked with peptic ulceration. It can mask symptoms and signs of perforation.

(h) Mental changes: Anxiety, elation, sleeplessness and depression may develop. Occasionally a psychotic episode is precipitated. Special care is therefore required in patients with a history of mental illness.

(i) Posterior capsular cataracts have been reported. Local application of steroids to the eye encourage the spread of infection and for this reason they should never be used in active herpes simplex infections (dendritic ulcer). The pharmacogenetically controlled response of intraocular pressure to steroids is discussed in chapter 13 (p. 124).

(j) Proximal myopathy.

(k) Linear growth: Prolonged use of pharmacological doses in childhood (e.g. in Still's disease) leads to stunting of growth. This must be offset against the stunting effect of chronic disease itself: steroid treatment that is sufficient to suppress disease activity in children with inflammatory bowel disease but not excessive actually *increases* the rate of growth.

(l) Teratogenesis: There is evidence in animals that glucocorticoids taken by the mother affect the fetus; evidence in humans is inevitably less clear cut, but use of pharmacologic (suprareplacement) doses early in pregnancy probably increases the incidence of abnormalities such as cleft lip.

(m) Necrosis of bone.

HYDROCORTISONE (CORTISOL)

Use

Hydrocortisone is predominantly glucocorticoid but also has significant mineralocorticoid activity (Table 37.2). At physiological concentrations it plays little if any part in controlling blood glucose, but it does cause hyperglycemia (and can precipitate frank diabetes mellitus) when administered in pharmacological doses. This is caused by enhanced gluconeogenesis combined with reduced insulin sensitivity increasing overall insulin demand. Hydrocortisone is given (usually with fludrocortisone to replace mineralocorticoid) as replacement therapy in patients with adrenocortical insufficiency (due to autoimmune, tuberculous or other disease of the adrenal cortex, to abrupt discontinuation of long-term corticosteroid treatment or for adrenocortical insufficiency secondary to anterior pituitary disorder): clinically stable patients usually need 20 mg in the morning and 10 mg in the evening by mouth, but there is considerable interindividual variation and plasma concentration profiling throughout the day is useful to individualize doses. Stressful events (e.g. intercurrent surgery or infection) necessitate increased dosage, and emergency treatment of acute adrenal failure requires intravenous hydrocortisone succinate in high doses (e.g. 100 mg 8 hourly) in addition to large volumes of physiological saline to correct hypovolemia and glucose if hypoglycemic. Hydrocortisone is also used as replacement treatment in children with congenital adrenal hyperplasia due to 21-hydroxylase deficiency; this suppresses endogenous ACTH which otherwise stimulates overproduction of adrenal androgens.

Intravenous hydrocortisone, 100–200 mg, 6 hourly is also used in status asthmaticus, followed by oral prednisolone once improvement occurs, and even larger doses (up to 500 mg) are used in anaphylaxis and other severe allergic reactions. Large doses of hydrocortisone (0.5–1 g 8 hourly) or other corticosteroids (e.g. prednisolone, methylprednisolone) are commonly employed to treat acute graft rejection following organ transplantation, although there is no definite evidence that these drugs are effective for this indication, and there is no good evidence that any one of these drugs is superior to another. Oral hydrocortisone is used to treat several connective tissue diseases, and frequently has dramatic effects on symptoms although evidence that corticosteroids influence longer term outcome is generally lacking. Systemic treatment should generally be reserved for severe and/or life-threatening phases of such diseases, for example fulminating systemic lupus erythematosus with renal or cerebral involvement. Several forms of vasculitis are responsive to systemic steroid treatment (e.g. giant cell arteritis) but these are usually conventionally treated with prednisolone (see below), as also are several steroid responsive malignancies. Hydrocortisone acetate is an insoluble suspension which can be injected into joints (5–50 mg intra- or periarticular) or inflamed bursae for localized anti-inflammatory effect in rheumatoid or in osteo- or other seronegative arthritis. Local treatment using hydrocortisone acetate foam enemas is also effective in patients with ulcerative proctocolitis, but systemic absorption is substantial and prednisolone enemas are preferred for this reason. Aphthous ulcers are treated with hydrocortisone tablets (2.5 mg) which are allowed to dissolve slowly in the mouth in contact with the ulcer. Severe dermatological disorders (e.g. Stevens–Johnson syndrome) are treated with systemic steroids, and many common skin disease including atopic eczema and selected cases of psoriasis are benefited by topical corticosteroid treatment, including hydrocortisone cream which is relatively mild and hence of particular use on the face where more potent steroids are contraindicated (p. 656). Hydrocortisone is still sometimes used to treat hypercalcemia caused by sarcoidosis, vitamin D intoxication or malignancy.

Pharmacokinetics

Hydrocortisone is rapidly absorbed from the gastrointestinal tract, but there is considerable interindividual variation in bioavailability due to variable presystemic metabolism. The plasma $t_{1/2}$ is approximately 90 min, but the biological $t_{1/2}$ in terms of anti-inflammatory and other effects is longer. It is extensively and rapidly metabolized in the liver and other tissues to tetrahydro metabolites that are conjugated with glucuronide before being excreted in urine.

CORTISONE ACETATE

Cortisone acetate is a prodrug being rapidly converted to hydrocortisone in the liver. Thus cortisone is unsuitable for topical use, but parenterally it has been given as replacement therapy for patients with Addison's disease or congenital adrenal hyperplasia instead of hydrocortisone. However, it has little to commend it over hydrocortisone and its absorption from the intestine can be unreliable and some patients with liver disease fail to convert it to the active metabolite, so its use is not recommended.

PREDNISOLONE AND PREDNISONE

Use

Prednisolone and prednisone are analogs of hydrocortisone that are more potent than the natural hormone as regards anti-inflammatory and metabolic actions, and involution of lymphoid tissue, but less potent as regards mineralocorticoid effects. Prednisone is converted almost completely into the biologically more active prednisolone in the liver, and so should not be used in patients with liver disease. There are no situations in which prednisone is preferred over its more active metabolite, and the rest of this account refers to prednisolone.

Prednisolone can be used as replacement therapy in patients with adrenal insufficiency, but current practice is generally to use hydrocortisone (the natural hormone) for this indication. The anti-inflammatory effect of prednisolone can bring dramatically rapid and profound relief of inflammatory symptoms of connective tissue and vasculitic diseases (p. 252), but whether this benefits the underlying course of the disease is often obscure, and if used for prolonged periods in high dose adverse Cushingoid effects are potentially appalling. Treatment must therefore be re-evaluated regularly and if long-term use is deemed essential the dose reduced to the lowest effective maintenance dose, if possible not more than 5 mg daily, given as a single dose first thing in the morning. Alternate day dosing produces less suppression of the pituitary adrenal axis, but not all diseases are adequately treated in this way (e.g. giant cell arteritis). Prednisolone therapy is considered in progressive rheumatoid arthritis when other forms of treatment have failed, or as an interim measure while a slowly acting drug such as penicillamine or chloroquine has time to act. Intra-articular injection of 20 mg prednisolone or an equivalent dose of longer acting steroid may be useful, but repeated use carries a substantial risk of damage to the joint. Low doses of prednisolone (5–10 mg daily) may be symptomatically useful in the short-term management of patients with severe articular symptoms from systemic lupus erythematosus, and larger doses (e.g. 60 mg daily) may be appropriate for limited periods in such patients with steroid responsive forms of glomerulonephritis or still larger doses (e.g. 150 mg daily) in those with active progression of central nervous system involvement.

Prednisolone is used for the short-term treatment of severe exacerbations of asthma (p. 385), before stabilizing the patient on long-term inhaled steroids, and, together with antibiotics, in treating severe acute exacerbations of chronic obstructive airways disease. Prednisolone is also used to treat interstitial lung disease (e.g. intrinsic or extrinsic forms of fibrosing alveolitis, and some patients with sarcoidosis) during active inflammatory (as opposed to end-stage fibrotic) stages of illness.

Several hepatic disorders (chapter 31) are improved by prednisolone, including some forms of acute hepatitis (viral as well as alcoholic) and chronic active hepatitis. Prednisolone is also used to treat inflammatory bowel disease, and is available formulated as suppositories and enemas to minimize systemic effects.

Some forms of nephrotic syndrome, notably that caused by minimal change glomerulonephritis, are markedly steroid responsive, whereas many others are not.

The immunosuppressant effect of prednisolone is utilized in treating patients who have received organ transplants, usually in combination with other immunosuppressant drugs such as cyclosporin or azathioprine in order to prevent rejection (chapter 45). Several hematologic malignancies as well as some benign hematologic disorders are responsive to glucocorticoids, and prednisolone is commonly used. These include Hodgkin's disease, other lymphomas, and acute leukemias (for which uses prednisolone is combined with other antineoplastic drugs, see chapter 45). Some combined regimens for the palliation of solid tumors also include prednisolone. Benign disorders for which prednisolone is indicated include autoimmune hemolytic anemia and idiopathic thrombocytopenic purpura.

DEXAMETHASONE

Use

Dexamethasone (9-α-fluoro-16-α-methyl prednisolone) is powerfully anti-inflammatory, but is reserved for a few distinct indications: as a diagnostic agent in the investigation of suspected Cushing's syndrome (low- and high-dose dexamethasone suppression tests) since it does not cross-react with endogenous cortisol in conventional radioimmunoassays; in the symptomatic treatment of cerebral edema associated with primary or secondary brain tumor; in the prevention of respiratory distress syndrome and intraventricular hemorrhage in premature neonates by administration to mothers at high risk of premature delivery; and in combination with antiemetics such as metoclopramide to prevent vomiting in patients about to receive cytotoxic chemotherapy. Dexamethasone has also been widely used in treating patients with various kinds of shock; evidence of its efficacy in these settings is unconvincing however.

Mineralocorticoids

ALDOSTERONE

Aldosterone is the main mineralocorticoid secreted by the adrenal cortex. It has no glucocorticoid activity but is about 1000 times more active than hydrocortisone as a mineralocorticoid. Adrenocorticotrophic hormone (ACTH) has minor stimulatory action on aldosterone production, but the main factors that control its release are plasma sodium and potassium and angiotensin II. Pituitary failure, producing a total absence of ACTH, allows aldosterone production by the zona glomerulosa to continue even though hydrocortisone is no longer released from the zona fasciculata.

Aldosterone acts on the distal nephron to increase sodium/potassium exchange thereby conserving sodium and causing urinary loss of potassium and hydrogen ions. Absence of aldosterone contributes importantly to the clinical picture of Addison's disease due to adrenal cortical destruction and results in sodium loss, potassium retention and reduction in the volume of extracellular fluid. Primary hyperaldosteronism (Conn's syndrome) is due to either a tumor or hyperplasia of the zona glomerulosa of the adrenal cortex. Clinical features include:

1. Nocturia, due to the lack of urinary concentrating ability caused by hypokalemia.
2. Weakness (persistent or episodic), flaccid paralysis, paresthesia and tetany from the combination of hypokalemia and hypomagnesemia.
3. Hypertension.

4. Sodium retention but with a normal or mildly raised plasma sodium concentration and minimal or absent edema, potassium loss with hypokalemia.

Spironolactone competes with aldosterone for its receptors and is sometimes used to treat primary or secondary hyperaldosteronism. It is discussed in chapter 33, p. 443.

Aldosterone undergoes substantial presystemic metabolism in the liver and cannot therefore usefully be given orally.

FLUDROCORTISONE

Fludrocortisone (9-α-fluorohydrocortisone) is a very potent synthetic mineralocorticoid, being approximately 500 times more powerful than hydrocortisone. It is active by mouth, the adult dose as replacement therapy in adrenocortical insufficiency being 50–300 μg/day. It is sometimes used in patients with symptomatic postural hypotension due to autonomic neuropathy in conjunction with support stockings and other drugs such as partial agonists at the β-adrenoceptor.

*A*DRENAL MEDULLA: PHEOCHROMOCYTOMA

Adrenaline is the main hormone of the adrenal medulla; its main clinical use is in the emergency management of anaphylactic shock and other life-threatening disorders. This is described elsewhere (pp. 368 and 643). In this section the diagnosis and management of pheochromocytoma, a functional neuroendocrine tumor arising from the adrenal medulla or other chromaffin tissue of neuroectodermal origin that secretes adrenaline, noradrenaline or dopamine, is described. These depend to a large extent on a rational use of drugs.

Diagnosis

Biochemical diagnosis of pheochromocytoma is usually made by measuring the urinary excretion of vanillyl mandelic acid (VMA) or some other catecholamine metabolite. Occasionally additional evidence is needed from combined biochemical/pharmacological tests. These are of two kinds: suppression tests, which are useful when there is a modest elevation in VMA excretion that could be a 'false positive' due to anxiety or other physiological cause of increased catecholamine secretion rather than to a catecholamine-secreting tumor; and provocation tests that are very seldom useful but can be of help when there is concern that normal VMA excretion is a 'false negative' perhaps because of intermittent secretion from a tumor that remained quiescent during the period of the urine collection.

SUPPRESSION TESTS

A substantial number of patients presenting with hypertension and symptoms suggestive of pheochromocytoma have borderline elevations of both plasma catecholamines and urinary metabolites thereof. Diagnostic accuracy has been greatly improved in such cases by the development of tests designed to suppress catecholamine secretion in patients without pheochromocytoma. Two such tests are available, based on suppression by pentolinium or clonidine. Either of these provides useful information; clonidine has the advantage of more general availability.

Clonidine suppression test

Clonidine is an α_2-receptor agonist which acts centrally to decrease sympathetic outflow. It therefore suppresses sympathetic activity, without influencing catecholamine secretion by an autonomous tumor. Patients rest supine for 30 min and are then given 300 µg clonidine orally; blood pressure and heart rate are measured half hourly and blood is sampled for plasma catecholamine determination at hourly intervals for 3 hours. Clonidine lowers blood pressure both in essential hypertensives and in patients with pheochromocytomas, but if the test works perfectly it will decrease plasma noradrenaline only in non-tumor patients. In practice, the test performs well, although individual responses to clonidine are variable.

Pentolinium suppression test

Pentolinium, 2.5 mg, is administered intravenously to recumbent subjects with an indwelling line for venous blood sampling for plasma catecholamine determination at 0, 10, 20 and 30 min. Blood pressure is measured regularly and the patient allowed home if there is no significant postural hypotension at 1 hour. Patients exhibiting a fall in plasma catecholamines but not into the normal range are given a higher dose of pentolinium (5 mg) on a subsequent occasion, following which they may need to be admitted overnight to allow the resulting postural hypotension to resolve. Failure of high-dose pentolinium to suppress catecholamines to within the normal range is strongly suggestive of pheochromocytoma and requires further investigation. Pentolinium blocks cholinergic transmission at autonomic ganglia and at nicotinic receptors in the adrenal medulla, thereby suppressing noradrenaline and adrenaline release caused by sympathetic nervous overactivity. It does not suppress catecholamine secretion by pheochromocytomas.

PROVOCATION TESTS

Provocative tests are seldom indicated, and their use should largely be confined to those rare situations where there is a high clinical suspicion of an intermittently secreting tumor in a patient who is normotensive. They should only be carried out in centers with appropriate facilities to deal with adverse events such as hypertensive crises, cardiac arrhythmias or severe hypotension. Even so this approach is not without danger and some investigators have advocated performing provocation tests with concurrent α-blockade to minimize risk. If this method is used changes in catecholamine levels are measured without reliance on blood pressure responses. Several drugs, including histamine, have been recommended as provocative agents; we prefer glucagon in this situation, as it is not *itself* hazardous unlike several of the other drugs proposed, although it may of course provoke a dangerous release of catecholamines from a tumor if one is present.

Glucagon test

Glucagon stimulates release of catecholamines from the adrenal medulla by a mechanism that is not understood. Patients with pheochromocytoma may experience exaggerated increases in circulating catecholamines following glucagon. Following determination of response to a cold pressor stimulus glucagon is administered as an intravenous bolus (1–2 mg). A positive test requires at least a three-fold increase in plasma catecholamines, 1–3 min following drug administration and a simultaneous rise in blood pressure of 20/15 mmHg greater than the cold pressor response. Compared to histamine provocation glucagon is safer, has fewer side effects, and produces fewer false positive results.

Preoperative management

α-Adrenoceptor blockade is the cornerstone of preoperative management. The drug of choice is the irreversible α-antagonist phenoxybenzamine. This alkylating agent forms a stable covalent bond with the α-receptors. It is introduced at low doses (10 mg b.d.) and increased until the blood pressure is controlled. During this titration phase additional doses of a reversible α-blocker (intravenous phentolamine or oral prazocin, depending on the degree of urgency) may be used to control spikes of pressure. Phenoxybenzamine causes postural hypotension, dry mouth and sedation. The patient who is adequately α-blocked is inevitably symptomatic and is best managed in bed in hospital until surgery. It is important that surgical intervention is not attempted until adequate α-blockade is established, and any intravascular volume deficit has been corrected. This is not easy to judge clinically since the main physical sign of both α-blockade and of hypovolemia is postural hypotension. Daily weighing is helpful and in practice it is best to err on the side of caution and to delay surgery if there is any doubt as to volume status.

Once α-blockade is established a β-adrenoceptor antagonist such as atenolol is commenced to reduce the risk of life-threatening tachyarrhythmias, which are otherwise especially likely during induction of anesthesia. This also controls the reflex tachycardia that otherwise accompanies non-specific α-blockade. β-Blockers should not be given before adequate α-blockade is established as unopposed α stimulation produces marked vasoconstriction and may precipitate a hypertensive crisis.

There is considerable theoretical advantage in using an irreversible α-blocker in patients with pheochromocytoma, because of the risk of sudden massive increases in circulating concentrations of vasoconstrictor agonist. Reversible α-blockers such as prazosin are displaced from the receptors by large concentrations of agonist, and the α-blockade they produce is therefore surmountable. The antagonism caused by such reversible competitive blockers results in a rightward parallel shift of the log dose–response curve with preservation of the maximum attainable response (Fig. 2.4a, p. 15). Preoperative α-blockade with prazosin is consequently surmountable. Labetalol (a combined α- and β-blocker) has also been advocated in pheochromocytoma. It is a reversible drug and its potency as an α-antagonist is weaker than its effect on β-receptors. Thus, not only is it inadequate to prevent a severe hypertensive crisis, but like other β-blockers it can exacerbate hypertension in pheochromocytoma. By contrast irreversible antagonists such as phenoxybenzamine cause flattening of the log dose–response curve of noradrenaline with reduction in the maximum response attainable (Fig. 2.4b p. 15). The advantage of this in a condition where sudden marked elevations of catecholamine concentration occur is evident.

Intraoperative medication

The risk of tachyarrhythmias at the time of induction of anesthesia has already been mentioned. It is greatly reduced if the patient is adequately β-blocked, but an intravenous β-blocker (e.g. propranolol) must be available for emergency use. Hypertensive crisis may occur intraoperatively, especially when the tumor is manipulated, if α-blockade is inadequate. Intravenous vasodilators should be ready for this eventuality. Phentolamine has been used but currently sodium nitroprusside is the most acceptable vasodilator for rapid correction of hypertensive surges.

Following removal of the tumor the concern is for sudden and severe hypotension. As described above, the risk of this is minimized by an adequate duration of α-blockade preoperatively and normovolemia.

If hypotension occurs, volume replacement should be instituted taking care that this is not excessive. If the arterial pressure fails to respond rapidly, a pressor agent is required. Drugs acting on catecholamine receptors (adrenaline, noradrenaline, dopamine, dobutamine) are unlikely to be effective because of α-blockade and also possibly receptor down-regulation due to the high circulating concentrations of catecholamines before the tumor was removed. Angiotensin II is therefore the preferred pressor agent in this context, and is given by intravenous infusion at a rate of 1–2 ng/kg/min increasing as necessary to 10 ng/kg/min.

Reproductive Endocrinology

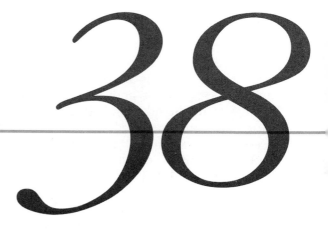

Female reproductive endocrinology **498**

Male reproductive endocrinology **504**

*F*EMALE REPRODUCTIVE ENDOCRINOLOGY

Introduction

Three main hormones are secreted by the ovary: estradiol-17β, estrone and progesterone. The ovary is also a source of androgens although most androgen production in women is by the adrenal. Estrogens are physiologically concerned with the development of secondary sex characteristics in the female including breast development and female distribution of fat. Progesterone acts on the endometrium to render it receptive to the fertilized zygote and thus allow implantation to take place. It also causes the mid-cycle rise in basal body temperature. The pituitary gonadotrophins, follicle-stimulating hormone (FSH) and luteinizing hormone (LH) control ovarian steroid secretion. Estrogens exert negative feedback control on both LH and FSH, whereas progesterone has less effect on gonadotrophin secretion. The hypothalamus secretes gonadotrophin-releasing hormone (GnRH) which stimulates the anterior pituitary to release LH or FSH. Follicle-stimulating hormone stimulates maturation of the ovarian follicle and release of estrogens, whilst LH stimulates progesterone release from the corpus luteum, and in mid-cycle the sudden rise in LH causes ovulation.

ESTROGENS

Use

1. Oral contraception (see below).
2. Replacement hormone therapy at the menopause is effective in preventing menopausal symptoms of flushing and vaginal dryness. It also reduces osteoporosis, slowing or eliminating bone loss at all sites (including the vertebral bodies and femoral neck) in the early years following the menopause. Estrogen replacement therapy also reduces the risk of cardiovascular disease (stroke and heart attack). There is an increased risk of endometrial cancer, so in women with a uterus a progestagen must be used in combination with the estrogen during the latter part of the cycle as this obviates this excess risk, albeit at the expense of side effects from the progestagen. To date an effect of estrogen replacement therapy on the risk of breast cancer has not been proven, but there is concern based on the known biological features of breast cancer that a small increase is likely, and present negative studies lack the statistical power to demonstrate an increase of a few per cent. Calendar packs of estrogen and progestagen are available and are convenient: 625 μg or 1.25 mg of conjugated estrogen is given daily, with the addition of norgestrel, 150 μg, daily for 12 days from day 16 of the cycle. Transdermal patches are also available, but are expensive and around 15% of women develop local irritation due to the vehicle. There are theoretical advantages in a route of administration that avoids presenting the liver with a high concentration of estrogen (e.g. there may be less effect on hepatic synthesis of coagulation factors and other proteins), but currently such patches are not justified for routine use, although they are useful for women who do not tolerate an oral preparation.
3. Estrogens are no longer used to suppress lactation because of the risk of thromboembolism. Bromocriptine (p. 511) is used instead.
4. Neoplastic disease: stilbestrol is less used for prostate cancer than in the past because of the risks of fluid retention and thrombosis, and because GnRH analogs (p. 513) provide a safer and better tolerated alternative.
5. Ethinylestradiol, 0.5–1 mg daily, is used under specialist supervision in the treatment of patients with hereditary hemorrhagic telangiectasia.

Adverse effects

Estrogens commonly cause nausea and headaches. Gynecomastia and impotence are predictable dose-dependent effects in men. Withdrawal uterine hemorrhage occurs 2–3 days after stopping estrogen treatment. Salt and water retention with edema, hypertension and exacerbation of heart failure can occur with pharmacological doses. The risk of thromboembolism is increased. Estrogens are carcinogenic in some animals and there is an increased incidence of endometrial carcinoma in women following uninterrupted treatment with exogenous estrogen unopposed by progestagen. Some decades ago treatment with stilbestrol during pregnancy was commonly employed in women with threatened miscarriage, without evidence of efficacy. An increased incidence of an otherwise extremely rare tumor, namely adenocarcinoma of the vagina, occurred in the daughters of those so treated during their teens and twenties (p. 76).

Pharmacokinetics

Absorption of estrogens via skin or mucous membranes is rapid. Synthetic derivatives such as ethinyl estradiol and diethylstilbestrol are also well absorbed when given by mouth. The most potent natural estrogen is estradiol-17β. It is largely oxidized to estrone and then hydrated to produce estriol. These three estrogens are metabolized in the liver and excreted as glucuronide and sulfate conjugates in bile and urine. Estimation of urinary estrogen excretion provides a measure of ovarian function. The synthetic estrogen diethylstilbestrol is as potent as estradiol but has a longer action because it is metabolized more slowly. Ethinyl estradiol is more potent still and also has a prolonged action because of slow hepatic metabolism, the half-life ($t_{1/2}$) being about 25 hours.

ESTROGEN ANTAGONISTS

Tamoxifen competes with estrogen for its high-affinity receptors in target tissues; it is of great value in the treatment of carcinoma of breast (see chapter 45). Clomiphene inhibits estrogen binding to its receptors in the hypothalamus and anterior pituitary, thereby blocking feedback inhibition and increasing secretion of GnRH, FSH and LH. It is used as first-line treatment of infertility in anovulatory women in a proportion of whom the increase in FSH/LH caused by clomiphene induces ovulation; there is an increased likelihood of multiple pregnancies.

PROGESTERONE AND PROGESTAGENS

Use

Progestagens act on tissues primed by estrogens, whose effects they modify. There are two main groups of progestagens: the naturally occurring hormone progesterone and its analogs; and testosterone analogs such as norethisterone. The main therapeutic uses of progestagens are in the oral contraceptive (either alone or in combination with estrogen, see below); in combination with estrogen when this is used as hormone replacement therapy in women with an intact uterus in order to prevent the increased risk of endometrial cancer caused by unopposed estrogen action; for endometriosis; and, with limited evidence of efficacy, in a variety of menstrual disorders including premenstrual tension, dysmenorrhea and menorrhagia. Progestagens in common use include norethisterone, desogestrel, levonorgestrel (which is the active isomer of racemic norgestrel), norgestimate and gestodene. These differ considerably in potency (e.g. norgestimate is one-third to one-quarter as potent as gestodene). The newer progestagens (e.g. desogestrel, gestodene, norgestimate) produce good cycle control, gestodene being particularly effective, and have a less marked adverse effect on plasma lipids than the older progestagens.

Mechanism of action

Progestagens act on cytoplasmic receptors and initiate new protein formation. Their main contraceptive effect is via an action on cervical mucus which renders it impenetrable to sperm. Nortestosterone derivatives are metabolized to a small extent to estrogenic metabolites which may account for an additional antiovulatory effect in some women. In addition, a pseudodecidual (pseudopregnant) change in the endometrium discourages implantation. Pharmacological effects of large doses of progestagens include inhibition of uterine contractility, sodium retention and negative nitrogen balance.

Adverse and metabolic effects

Progestagens cause or contribute to many of the symptoms of the contraceptive pill or hormone replacement therapy, including bloating with fluid retention and weight gain, acne, breast discomfort, altered libido, gastrointestinal and premenstrual symptoms. Testosterone-related progestagens (e.g. norethistrone) cause masculinization of a female fetus if used during pregnancy. Several of the earlier progestagens had adverse effects on lipid metabolism: levonorgestrel used continuously reduces circulating concentrations of high density lipoprotein (HDL) and is therefore no longer recommended when given in this way for women with risk factors for cardiovascular disease. Norethisterone has little effect on circulating lipoproteins, and desogestrel, gestodene and norgestimate cause small increases in HDL, although whether these potentially beneficial effects are clinically important is not known.

Newer progestagens do not cause clinically important changes in blood glucose. Desogestrel, norgestimate and gestodene increase serum concentrations of sex hormone binding globulin and reduce free testosterone concentration. (These antiandrogenic effects can be clinically useful in adolescent females, in reducing acne.)

Pharmacokinetics

Progesterone is subject to presystemic hepatic metabolism. It is more effective when injected intramuscularly or administered sublingually. It is excreted in the urine as pregnanediol and pregnanelone. Norethisterone, a synthetic progestagen component of many oral contraceptives, is rapidly absorbed orally, is subject to little presystemic metabolism and has a $t_{1/2}$ of 7.5–8 hours.

THE COMBINED ORAL CONTRACEPTIVE

Since the original pilot trials in Puerto Rico proved that steroid oral contraception was feasible, this method has become the leading method of contraception worldwide. Nearly half of all women in their twenties in the UK use this form of contraception. It is the most consistently effective contraceptive method and allows sexual relations to proceed without interruption, but lacks the advantage of protection against sexually transmitted disease afforded by condoms. The estrogen most commonly used is ethinylestradiol in a dose of 35 µg/day or less. The main contraceptive action of the combined oral contraceptive is to suppress ovulation by interfering with gonadotrophin release by the pituitary via negative feedback on the hypothalamus. This prevents the mid-cycle rise in LH which triggers ovulation. Whereas other estrogens like stilbestrol also suppress ovulation for a few cycles they may fail to do so when used over a long time. Ethinylestradiol differs in that no such pituitary 'break-through' occurs.

Progestagens currently used in combined oral contraceptives include desogestrel, gestodene and norgestimate. These 'third generation' progestagens are only weak antiestrogens, have less androgenic activity than their predecessors and are associated with less disturbance of lipoprotein metabolism.

Endocrine effects of the combined oral contraceptive include:

1. Prevention of the normal premenstrual rise and mid-cycle peaks of LH and FSH and of the rise of progesterone during the luteal phase.
2. Increased hepatic synthesis of proteins including thyroid-binding globulin, ceruloplasmin, transferrin, coagulation factors and renin substrate; increased fibrinogen synthesis can raise erythrocyte sedimentation rate.
3. Reduced carbohydrate tolerance.
4. Decreased albumin and haptoglobulin synthesis.

Use

The combined estrogen–progestagen pill is taken daily for 21 consecutive days, the initial cycle being commenced on the first day of the menstrual cycle. Medication is either stopped for 7 days after the 3 week treatment or dummy tablets taken, and withdrawal of estrogen produces uterine bleeding some 2–3 days after the last active dose. The pill is restarted after 7 drug-free days and bleeding ceases. If a dose is forgotten the woman should take it as soon as she remembers, and the next one at the usual time. If she is more than 12 hours late she should be advised to use additonal contraception (e.g. a barrier method) for the next 7 days and if this period extends beyond the current cycle, to start the next packet of pills immediately without a 7 day break and without taking dummy pills.

The combined contraceptive pill should be stopped 4 weeks before major elective surgery, because of the increased risk of venous thrombosis. Alternative contraception (e.g. a barrier method) is used. Oral contraception can be restarted any time after 3–4 weeks following childbirth, but a progesterone only preparation may be preferred by women who are breast feeding because progestagen, unlike estrogen, does not affect lactation.

Postcoital contraception (the 'morning-after' pill) consists of two doses each of ethinylestradiol, 100 µg, and levonorgestrel, 500 µg, given 12 hours apart within 72 hours of unprotected intercourse. The failure rate of this method is 0–3% but up to 50% of women experience nausea and vomiting (if one of the doses is vomited within 3 hours of ingestion it should be repeated). A single dose of mifepristone, 600 mg, is highly effective as a postcoital contraceptive (p. 503). Abortion statistics suggest that postcoital contraception is underutilized in the UK.

Adverse effects

The overall acceptability of the combined pill is around 80%: minor side effects can often be controlled by a change in preparation. Users have an increased risk of venous thromboembolic disease, this risk being greatest in women over 35 years of age, especially if they smoke cigarettes and have used oral contraceptives for 5 years or more continuously. (This increased risk must not be confused with the decreased risk of stroke and myocardial infarction that is conferred by low doses of natural conjugated estrogen given to menopausal women as hormone replacement.) The increased risk of thromboembolism made it desirable to reduce estrogen dose as low as possible. Deep vein thrombosis is uncommon with 35 µg or less of ethinylestradiol, lower doses or progestagen only pills are appropriate in women at higher risk of thrombotic disease. Increased blood pressure is common with the pill and is clinically significant in about 5% of patients. When medication is stopped the blood pressure usually falls to normal levels. In normotensive non-smoking women without other risk factors for vascular disease there is no upper age limit on using the combined oral contraceptive, but it is prudent to use the lowest effective dose of estrogen, especially in women aged 35 or over. Mesenteric artery thrombosis and small bowel ischemia, and hepatic vein thrombosis and Budd–Chiari syndrome are rare but serious adverse events linked to use of oral contraception. These cardiovascular adverse effects are related to estrogen. Jaundice similar to that of pregnancy cholestasis can occur, usually in the first few cycles. Recovery is rapid on drug withdrawal. Oral contraceptives may affect migraine in a number of ways:

1. Precipitation of attacks in the previously unaffected.
2. Exacerbation of previously existing migraine.
3. Alter the pattern of attacks, in particular, focal neurological features may appear.
4. Occasionally the incidence of attacks may decrease or they may even be abolished whilst the patient is on the pill.

Other important adverse effects include an increased incidence of gallstones. Early use of the pill for prolonged periods may increase the risk of breast cancer, although this remains uncertain, and there is no evidence of increased mortality from this cause in users of the contraceptive pill. There is an epidemiological association with increased risk of liver cancer, but a reduced risk of endometrial and ovarian cancer. The incidence of vascular adenoma is increased by the combined oral contraceptive, but remains rare. There is a decreased incidence of benign breast lesions and functional ovarian cysts. Diabetes mellitus may be precipitated by the pill. Amenorrhea after stopping combined oral contraception is not unusual (about 5%) but is rarely prolonged, and although there may be temporary impairment of fertility permanent sterility is very uncommon.

Contraindications

Absolute contraindications to combined oral contraception include phlebitis and thromboembolism, severe liver disease, arterial disease, cancer of breast or uterus, melanoma, meningioma, porphyria and pregnancy. Relative contraindications include migraine (especially if associated with focal neurological symptoms), cholelithiasis, depression, hypertension, hyperlipidemia and diabetes mellitus.

Drug interactions

- Oral anticoagulants: estrogens increase plasma levels of factor VII and reduce the efficacy of oral anticoagulants. This is not a contraindication to their continued use in patients to be started on warfarin (in whom pregnancy is highly undesirable, see p. 79), but is a reason for increased frequency of monitoring of the International Normalized Ratio (INR) if oral contraception is started after a patient has been stabilized on warfarin (chapter 27).
- Antihypertensive therapy is adversely affected by oral contraceptives, partly at least because of increased circulating renin substrate.

Enzyme inducers (e.g. rifampicin, carbamazepine, phenytoin and griseofulvin) decrease the plasma levels of contraceptive estrogen, thus decreasing the effectiveness of the combined contraceptive pill. Breakthrough bleeding and/or unwanted pregnancy have been described. Oral contraceptive steroids undergo enterohepatic circulation and conjugated steroid in bile is broken down in the gut by bacteria to the parent steroid, and subsequently reabsorbed. Broad-spectrum antibiotics (e.g. ampicillin, tetracycline) alter colonic bacteria, increase fecal excretion of contraceptive estrogen and decrease plasma concentrations resulting in possible contraceptive failure; this does not appear to be a problem with progestagen only pills.

PROGESTAGEN ONLY CONTRACEPTIVE

Use

Progestagen only contraceptive pills (e.g. norethisterone, 350 µg, norgestrel, 75 µg) are associated with a high incidence of menstrual disturbances but are useful if estrogen-containing pills are poorly tolerated or contraindicated (e.g. in women with risk factors for vascular disease such as older smokers, diabetics) or during breast feeding. Contraceptive effectiveness is less than with the combined pill since ovulation is suppressed in only approximately 40% of women and the major contraceptive effect is on the cervical mucus and endometrium. This effect is maximal 3–4 hours after ingestion and declines over the next 16–20 hours, so the pill should be taken at the same time each day, preferably 3–4 hours before the usual time of intercourse. Pregnancy rates are of the same order as with the intrauterine contraceptive device or barrier methods (approximately 1.5–2 per 100 women per year compared with 0.3 per 100 women per year for the combined preparation). Progestagen only pills are taken continuously throughout the menstrual cycle which is convenient for some patients.

Depot progesterone injections are more effective than oral preparations: a single intramuscular injection of 150 mg medroxyprogesterone acetate provides contraception for 10 weeks with a failure rate of 0.25 per 100 women per year. It is mainly used as a temporary method (e.g. while waiting for vasectomy to become effective), but is occasionally indicated for long-term use in women for whom other methods are unacceptable. The side effects are essentially similar to those of oral progestagen only preparations. After 2 years' treatment up to 40% of women develop amenorrhea and infertility so that pregnancy is unlikely for 9–12 months after the last injection. Treatment with depot progestagen injections should not be undertaken without full counselling of the patient.

Adverse effects

There is no evidence of serious adverse effects from progestagen only contraceptive pills and the main problems are irregular menstrual bleeding, which can be heavy but usually settles down after a few cycles, and occasionally breast tenderness.

ANTIPROGESTAGENS

Mifepristone is a competitive antagonist of progesterone. It is used as a medical alternative to surgical termination of early pregnancy (currently up to 63 days' gestation, although it is also effective during the second trimester). The dose is 600 mg by mouth followed by gemeprost (a prostaglandin that ripens and softens the cervix), 1 mg, as a vaginal pessary unless abortion is already complete. Gemeprost can cause hypotension, so the blood pressure must be monitored for 6 hours after it is administered. The patient is followed up at 8–12 days, and surgical termination is essential if complete abortion has not occurred. Contraindications include ectopic pregnancy. Many women do not find this method as quick and trouble free as they anticipated; nevertheless a large fraction of women who have had both surgical abortion and medical abortion by this method prefer the medical option.

Oxytocic drugs

OXYTOCIN

Oxytocin has rather little antidiuretic activity, although large doses can cause fluid retention. It produces contractions of the smooth muscle of the fundus of the pregnant uterus at term and of mammary gland ducts. It is reflexly released from the pituitary following suckling and by emotional stimuli. Any role in the initiation of labor is not established. There is no known disease state of over- or underproduction. Synthetic oxytocin is effective by any parenteral route and is usually given as a constant rate intravenous infusion to initiate or augment labor, often following artificial rupture of membranes. A low dose is used to initiate treatment (e.g. 1 milliunit/min) titrated upward if needed. Oxytocin is also sometimes given as an intramuscular or intravenous bolus after delivery of the shoulders (usually with ergometrine which acts more rapidly) to prevent or control *postpartum* hemorrhage. Like vasopressin, oxytocin has a short plasma $t_{1/2}$ (5–10 min), mainly because of tissue inactivation, but a small amount is excreted via the kidney.

ERGOMETRINE

Ergometrine (an alkaloid derived from ergot, a fungus that infects rye) is a powerful oxytocic. The uterus is sensitive at all times but especially so in late pregnancy. Ergometrine is used in the third stage of labor to decrease *postpartum* hemorrhage. It is given intramuscularly (200–500 µg: onset about 5 min, duration about 45 min), or intravenously in emergency (100–500 µg: onset within 1 min). It is often given with oxytocin (ergometrine, 500 µg, plus oxytocin, 5 IU), the actions of which it complements: oxytocin produces slow contractions with full relaxations in between, whilst ergometrine produces faster contractions superimposed on a tonic persistent contraction. (It is for this reason that ergometrine is unsuitable for induction of labor.) Given intramuscularly oxytocin acts in 1–2 min, although the contraction is brief, but ergometrine takes 5 min to act.

Ergometrine can cause hypertension, particularly in toxemic patients, in whom it should be used with care if at all.

PROSTAGLANDINS

Prostaglandins are naturally occurring lipid-derived mediators. They are 20-carbon unsaturated fatty acids containing a 5-carbon (cyclopentane) ring. Prostaglandins are involved in a wide range of physiological and pathological processes including inflammation (see chapter 23) and hemostasis and thrombosis (see chapter 27). Prostaglandin E_2 has potent contractile activity on the human uterus, and also softens and ripens the cervix. It also has many other actions including inhibition of acid secretion by the stomach, increased mucus secretion within the gastrointestinal tract, contraction of gastrointestinal smooth muscle, relaxation of vascular smooth muscle and increase in body temperature. Synthetic prostaglandin E_2 (dinoprostone) is used for the induction of late (second trimester) therapeutic abortion, because the uterus is sensitive to its actions at this stage, whereas oxytocin only reliably causes uterine contraction later in pregnancy. Prostaglandin E_2 has also been used to induce or augment labor, but oxytocin is preferred for this, because it lacks the many side effects of prostaglandin E_2 that relate to its actions on extrauterine tissues. These include nausea, vomiting, diarrhea, flushing, headache, hypotension and fever. Dinoprostone may be given by extra-amniotic instillation, or by vaginal tablets, 3 mg, that are dipped in water or saline before insertion, followed by a second dose 6–8 hours later if necessary. Carboprost is used for *postpartum* hemorrhage in patients with an atonic uterus unresponsive to ergometrine and oxytocin.

Other specialized uses of prostaglandins in the perinatal period include the use of prostaglandin E_1 (alprostadil) in neonates with congenital heart defects that are 'ductus-dependent'. It preserves the patency of the ductus arteriosus until surgical correction is feasible. Conversely, in infants with inappropriately patent ductus arteriosus, indomethacin given intravenously can cause closure of the ductus by inhibiting the endogenous biosynthesis of prostaglandins involved in preserving ductal patency.

MALE REPRODUCTIVE ENDOCRINOLOGY

Introduction

The principal hormone of the testis is testosterone which is secreted by the interstitial (Leydig) cells. Testosterone circulates in blood 95% bound to a plasma globulin. The plasma concentration is variable but should exceed 10 nmol/l in adult males. Cells in target tissues convert testosterone into the more active androgen dihydrotestosterone by a 5α-reductase enzyme. An inhibitor of this enzyme (finasteride) has recently been introduced for the treatment of benign prostatic hypertrophy. Both testosterone and dihydrotestosterone are inactivated in the liver. Androgens have a wide range of activities, the most important of which include actions on:

- Development of male secondary sex characteristics (including male distribution of body hair, breaking of the voice, enlargement of the penis, sebum secretion and male pattern balding).
- Protein anabolic effects influencing growth, maturation of bone and muscle development.
- Spermatogenesis and seminal fluid formation.

Testicular function is controlled by the anterior pituitary:

1. Follicle-stimulating hormone acts on the seminiferous tubules and promotes spermatogenesis.
2. Luteinizing hormone stimulates testosterone production.

The release of FSH and LH by the pituitary is in turn mediated by the hypothalamus via gonadotrophin-releasing hormone.

Androgens and anabolic steroids

Use

Many cases of impotence are psychological in origin, in which case treatment with androgens is inappropriate. In impotent patients with low concentrations of circulating testosterone replacement therapy improves secondary sex characteristics and may restore erectile function and libido but does not restore fertility. (Treatment of patients with hypogonadism secondary to hypothalamic or pituitary dysfunction who wish to become fertile includes gonadotrophins or pulsatile gonadotrophin-releasing hormone.) Replacement therapy is most reliably achieved by intramuscular injection of testosterone esters in oil, of which various preparations are available. They must usually be given at 2–3 week intervals to control symptoms. Alternatively testosterone undecanoate or mesterolone can be taken by mouth; these are formulated in oil, favoring lymphatic absorption from the gastrointestinal tract. The dose of mesterolone is 25 mg three or four times a day for the first several months, which may subsequently be reduced for maintenance according to response. Delayed puberty, due to gonadal deficiency (primary or secondary) or severe constitutional delay, can be treated by testosterone esters or gonadotrophins. Care is needed because premature fusion of epiphyses may occur, resulting in short stature, and such treatment is best supervised by specialist clinics. Occasional patients with disseminated breast cancer derive considerable symptomatic benefit from androgen treatment.

Anabolic steroids (e.g. nandrolone, stanozolol, danazol) have proportionately greater anabolic and less virilizing effects than other androgens. They have generally been disappointing in therapeutics, and have been widely abused by athletes and body builders. Legitimate uses are few, but include the treatment of some aplastic anemias, the vascular manifestations of Behçet's disease and in the prophylaxis of recurrent attacks of hereditary angioneurotic edema. They dramatically reduce circulating concentrations of lipoprotein (a), which is a strong independent cardiovascular risk factor; the biological meaning (if any) of this intriguing effect is unknown.

Mechanism of action

Testosterone and dihydrotestosterone interact with cytoplasmic receptors in responsive cells that derepress DNA transcription, leading to synthesis of RNA and new proteins.

Adverse effects

Virilization in women and increased libido in men are predictable effects. In women, acne, growth of facial hair and deepening of the voice are common undesirable features produced by androgens. Other masculinizing effects and menstrual irregularities can also develop. In the male, excessive masculinization can result in frequent erections or priapism and aggressive behavior. Young children may undergo premature fusion of epiphyses or other abnormal growth phenomena. Other adverse effects include jaundice, particularly of cholestatic type; because of this complication methyltestosterone is no longer prescribed. Azoospermia occurs due to inhibition of gonadotrophin secretion. In patients treated for malignant disease with androgens, hypercalcemia, which may be severe, is produced by an unknown mechanism. Salt and water retention is unusual with androgens compared with estrogens. Oral testosterone preparations in oil cause various gastrointestinal symptoms including anorexia, vomiting, flatus, diarrhea and oily stools.

Pharmacokinetics

Although testosterone is readily absorbed orally considerable presystemic metabolism occurs in the liver. It can be administered sublingually, although this route is seldom used. Testosterone in oil is well absorbed from intramuscular injection sites but is also rapidly metabolized. Esters of testosterone are much less polar and are more slowly released from oily depot injections and are used for prolonged effect. Inactivation of testosterone takes place in the liver. The chief metabolites are androsterone and etiocholanolone which are mainly excreted in the urine. About 6% of administered testosterone appears in the feces having undergone enterohepatic circulation.

Antiandrogens

CYPROTERONE

Use

Cyproterone acetate is used in men with inoperable prostatic carcinoma, before initiating treatment with gonadotrophin-releasing hormone analogs to prevent the flare of disease activity induced by the initial increase in sex hormone release. It has also been used to reduce sexual drive in cases of sexual deviation and in children with precocious puberty. In women it has been used to treat hyperandrogenic effects (often seen in polycystic ovary disease) including acne, hirsutism and male pattern baldness. Early fears raised by the occurrence of tumors in animal studies (pituitary and liver adenomas and mammary adenocarcinomas) have not been realized in humans, but its potentially adverse effects on HDL and LDL caution against long-term use, and the risk/benefit ratio should be considered carefully before embarking on treatment for relatively minor indications. The usual dose is 25–100 mg daily for 10 days of each cycle, and it is given with ethinylestradiol to prevent pregnancy; lower doses (2 mg/day) are used cyclically to suppress sebum production in combination with an estrogen (ethinylestradiol) in treating women with severe refractory acne.

Mechanism of action

Cyproterone acts by competing with testosterone for its high affinity receptors, thereby inhibiting prostatic growth, spermatogenesis and masculinization. It also has strong progestational activity and a very weak glucocorticoid effect.

Adverse effects

Side effects include gynecomastia in approximately 20% of patients (occasionally with benign nodules and galactorrhea), inhibition of spermatogenesis (which usually returns to normal 6 months after cessation of treatment) and tiredness and lassitude (which can be so marked as to make driving dangerous).

Finasteride

Use

Finasteride is a 5α-reductase inhibitor used for benign prostatic hypertrophy. Previously the only alternative to surgery in this condition has been the use of an α-receptor antagonist (e.g. prazosin, doxazosin). Prostate specific antigen should be measured before starting treatment with finasteride as there is concern that the diagnosis of prostate cancer might be delayed. The dose is 5 mg daily. Unwanted effects include impotence and reduced libido.

Drugs affecting male sexual performance

The complex interplay between physiological and psychological factors that determines sexual desire and performance makes it difficult to assess the influence of drugs on sexual function. In randomized placebo-controlled blinded studies a small but significant fraction of men receiving placebo discontinue their participation in the study because of the occurrence of impotence that they attribute to therapy. Drugs that affect the autonomic supply to the sex organs are not alone in interfering with sexual function. Indeed bendrofluazide, a thiazide diuretic, caused significantly more impotence in the Medical Research Council (MRC) trial of mild hypertension than did propranolol, a β-receptor antagonist. Drugs that do interfere with autonomic function and can also cause erectile dysfunction include phenothiazines, butyrophenones and tricyclic antidepressants. Pelvic non-adrenergic non-cholinergic nerves are involved in erectile function and utilize nitric oxide as their neurotransmitter. Nitric oxide release from endothelium in the corpus cavernosum is also believed to be abnormal in some cases of organic impotence, including that caused by diabetes mellitus. Replacement therapy with nitrates is being explored. Some cases of organic erectile failure (including some diabetics) can be treated successfully with intracavernosal injections of papaverine, a vascular smooth muscle relaxant, the starting dose being 7.5 mg, increasing if necessary to 30–60 mg. Phentolamine, an α-adrenoceptor antagonist, can be added in a dose of 0.25–1.25 mg if response is not adequate. Recently intracavernosal prostaglandlin E_1 has been licensed for this indication. Adverse effects comprise local changes due to the injection including hematoma, priapism (which may necessitate emergency decompression by aspiration and metaraminol injection), fibrotic changes resembling Peyronie's disease, and systemic effects including hypotension and syncope. The initial doses must be given under close supervision.

The existence of aphrodisiac drugs that increase libido is probably a myth, although there is a market for such agents. The use of cocaine, amphetamine or yohimbine as sexual stimulants, as well as more traditional mixtures, has its devotees, but their medical use in the treatment of impotence is disappointing. Cannabis enjoys a reputation for enhancing sexual enjoyment and desire. The reason for this is not clear but it may be due to a general release of inhibition. Continual smoking of cannabis increases prolactin secretion and lowers male serum testosterone levels. A few cases of reduced libido and impotence in males and females are associated with idiopathic hyperprolactinemia and in such cases bromocriptine, 5-10 mg/day, may restore potency. Androgens play a role in both male and female arousal, but their use is not appropriate except in patients with reduced circulating concentrations of testosterone.

Pituitary

39

Anterior pituitary hormones and related drugs **510**

Posterior pituitary hormones **514**

ANTERIOR PITUITARY HORMONES AND RELATED DRUGS

GROWTH HORMONE (SOMATOTROPIN)

Somatotropin is a protein of molecular weight 27 000 which consists of 191 amino acids. The rate of secretion varies during the day. The normal output over 24 hours is approximately 1.4 mg. Secretion is stimulated by hypoglycemia, fasting and stress, α- and β-adrenoceptor and dopamine and serotonin agonists. The serotoninergic pathway is involved in the stimulation of somatotropin release during slow wave sleep. Secretion is inhibited by glucose, protein and corticosteroid administration. The hypothalamus also secretes a growth hormone (GH) release inhibiting hormone (somatostatin). Somatostatin, a tetradecapeptide, has been synthesized and also inhibits insulin, glucagon and gastrin secretion. Somatotropin is an anabolic hormone that promotes protein synthesis and synergizes with insulin causing amino acid uptake by cells. Its effect on skeletal growth is mediated by somatomedin (a small peptide synthesized in the liver, secretion of which depends upon GH).

Somatotropin is used to treat children with dwarfism due to isolated growth hormone deficiency or deficiency due to hypothalamic or pituitary disease. This is often difficult to diagnose, and requires accurate sequential measurements of height together with biochemical measurements of somatotropin during pharmacological (e.g. insulin, clonidine, glucagon, arginine or L-dopa) or physiological (e.g. sleep, exercise) stimulation. Somatotropin deficiency is an important cause of growth retardation. Somatotropin treatment also increases height in children with Turner's syndrome. Somatotropin derived from pooled human pituitary glands (obtained from victims of road traffic accidents) was associated with transmission of Jakob–Creutzfeldt disease. It has been replaced by genetically engineered human somatotropin made in a bacterial system. Injections should begin early, before puberty, and continue until growth ceases. The optimal dose is not yet defined, but 0.1 mg/kg/day subcutaneously has been recommended, and this should probably be increased during puberty. Its use in children with growth hormone deficiency after epiphyseal fusion is currently being investigated. Replacement therapy with gonadotrophin or sex hormones is delayed until maximum growth has been achieved in such patients. The availability of unlimited supplies of pure and safe human growth hormone from recombinant technology has stimulated considerable research into potential new indications including its use in adults with hypopituitarism, to promote healing of wounds and as an anabolic hormone in osteoporosis associated with aging.

Somatotropin oversecretion produces gigantism and acromegaly. This is usually associated with a functional adenoma of the acidophil cells of the adenohypophysis, and treatment is neurosurgical whenever possible. A drug that selectively inhibits somatotropin secretion and is fully satisfactory for clinical use has yet to be found. Somatostatin is effective in lowering somatropin levels in acromegalics but has to be given by continuous intravenous infusion and has widespread effects on other hormones. Octreotide is a long-acting analog of somatostatin and is useful for the short-term treatment of acromegaly before surgery. It is also valuable in functioning gastroenteropancreatic tumors. Bromocriptine is an alternative: it suppresses prolactin and somatotropin in a minority of patients with acromegaly (approximately 15–20% are responsive). It has little effect on other pituitary functions. The visual fields and size of the pituitary fossa must be assessed repeatedly in order to detect further growth of the tumor if it is used for a prolonged period.

OCTREOTIDE

Use

Octreotide is a synthetic octapeptide analog of somatostatin which inhibits peptide release from endocrine-secreting tumors of the pituitary or gastrointesinal tract. It is used to treat patients with symptoms from the release of pharmacologically active substances from gastroenteropancreatic tumors including patients with carcinoid syndrome, insulinoma, VIPoma or glucagonoma. It reduces secretion of mediators such as serotonin, vasoactive intestine peptide (VIP) and glucagon from such tumors, thereby reducing symptoms of flushing, diarrhea or skin rash, but does not reduce the size of the tumor. It is more effective than bromocriptine in lowering somatotropin in patients with acromegaly but is not generally an acceptable alternative to surgery. It is less convenient to use than bromocriptine because it must be administered parenterally. It may be effective in those very rare patients with thyrotoxicosis secondary to excessive secretion of thyroid-stimulating hormone (TSH). It has been reported to reduce portal pressure in portal hypertension secondary to cirrhosis, and to reduce ileostomy diarrhea. The usual starting dose is 50 µg twice daily subcutaneously, increased gradually according to response to a maximum of 200 µg three times daily. The drug is given between meals to minimize gastrointestinal side effects. Ultrasound examination of the gallbladder is recommended before treatment and then 6 monthly.

Adverse effects

Side effects are mainly gastrointestinal upsets including anorexia, nausea, vomiting, abdominal pain, diarrhea and steatorrhea; in addition it causes impaired glucose tolerance by reducing insulin secretion, and an increased incidence of gallstones and/or biliary sludge after only a few months' treatment, especially at high dose.

Pharmacokinetics

Octreotide is subject to extensive hepatic metabolism, little of the drug being excreted unchanged in the urine. The plasma half-life ($t_{1/2}$) is 90–120 min, compared with only 2–3 min for somatostatin. Its effects in suppressing hormone secretion last up to 8 hours, enabling two to three times daily dosing.

BROMOCRIPTINE

Use

1. Lactation can be suppressed by giving bromocriptine in a single dose of 2.5 mg initially followed by 2.5 mg twice daily for 2 weeks. Breast tenderness and engorgement after stopping treatment is treated with bromocriptine 2.5 mg daily for 1 week. Bromocriptine is more effective than estrogen and can be given even when suckling has commenced.

2. Hyperprolactinemia is an important factor in male and female hypogonadism and accounts for about 10% of cases of secondary amenorrhea. Milder degrees of hyperprolactinemia may present as infertility with normal menstruation. Galactorrhea occurs in only 30% of these patients: galactorrhea on its own is rarely due to hyperprolactinemia. In men hyperprolactinemia most commonly presents late with symptoms related to the underlying pituitary tumor, although a history of impotence with or without decreased volume of seminal ejaculate is often obtained on direct enquiry. Galactorrhea and gynecomastia are uncommon. The influence of prolactin on gonadal function is not understood, but bromocriptine is often successful in the treatment of impaired sexual function with hyperprolactinemia. The dose needed is usually 2.5–7.5 mg twice daily. Pituitary lactotroph adenomas usually decrease in size during treatment with bromocriptine. Visual fields are measured and the pituitary imaged at diagnosis, and if a macroadenoma is present they are repeated during treatment. Fertility and cyclical ovarian function is usually restored in 2–6 months. Fetal malformation has not been reported. Nevertheless, if pregnancy occurs the drug should be stopped. Multiple ovulations (as

occur with gonadotrophins and clomiphene) have not been reported. If a pituitary tumor (usually a lactotroph adenoma) is the primary cause of hyperprolactinemia, the tumor may enlarge during pregnancy necessitating restarting bromocriptine or surgical intervention. Thus visual fields should be carefully measured during bromocriptine therapy for infertility.

3. Hyperprolactinemia may also be associated with hypothyroidism and with drugs (cannabis, phenothiazines). In hypothyroidism, thyroid replacement therapy corrects hyperprolactinemia. Drug therapy (in particular phenothiazines, butyrophenones, metoclopramide, oral contraceptives and methyldopa) may produce galactorrhea, which usually ceases when the drug is stopped. If the condition persists, bromocriptine may reverse it, but a pituitary tumor should also be looked for. When a neuroleptic drug cannot be withdrawn, concurrent administration of bromocriptine may suppress galactorrhea, but the use of a dopamine agonist in psychiatric patients treated with dopamine antagonist is seldom rational.

4. Bromocriptine provides an effective medical treatment for a few patients with acromegaly but surgery is generally preferred. It not only suppresses secretion of somatotropin and prolactin, but may also suppress somatomedin production by the liver.

5. Bromocriptine is effective in Parkinsonism, although large doses may be needed (up to 100 mg daily in divided doses), and it seldom produces additional benefit in patients on full doses of levodopa.

Adverse effects

With low doses of bromocriptine (2.5–12.5 mg daily) the only toxic effects commonly encountered are constipation and nausea. Postural hypotension occurs with initial doses of bromocriptine, which is therefore begun in low dose (2.5 mg) last thing at night and the dose increased gradually (2.5 mg every 3 days to the required level). High doses (over 20 mg daily) cause nasal congestion, dry mouth, metallic taste, vascular spasm, cramps in the legs, dystonic reactions, visual hallucinations and cardiac arrhythmias.

Mechanism of action

Bromocriptine is a semisynthetic ergot derivative with dopamine D_2 receptor agonist properties and additional actions on 5-hydroxytryptamine receptors ($5HT_{1A}$, $5HT_2$) and adrenoceptors. Bromocriptine stimulates inhibitory dopamine receptors in the anterior pituitary, thus inhibiting prolactin secretion. In normal subjects it produces a small increase in somatotropin secretion, but in acromegaly it suppresses somatotropin release accounting for its clinical usefulness in this disorder.

Pharmacokinetics

Bromocriptine is administered orally and 90% is absorbed via the small intestine. It is metabolized in the liver and excretion is predominantly via the bile. Mean $t_{1/2}$ is 66 hours. Raised prolactin and somatotropin levels fall within a few hours of starting treatment, but the length of this action appears to vary with the original level of the circulating hormone.

GONADOTROPINS

The human pituitary secretes follicle-stimulating hormone (FSH) and luteinizing hormone (LH). Follicle-stimulating hormone is a glycoprotein (molecular weight 30 000) which in females controls development of the primary ovarian follicle, stimulates granulosa cell proliferation and increases estrogen production whilst in males it increases spermatogenesis. Luteinizing hormone is also a glycoprotein (molecular weight 30 000) which induces ovulation, stimulates thecal estrogen production and initiates and maintains the corpus luteum in females. In males LH stimulates androgen synthesis by Leydig cells thus having a role in the maturation of spermatocytes and the development of secondary sex characteristics.

Human menopausal urinary gonadotrophin (HMG), human chorionic gonadotrophin (HCG) and synthetic LH are prepared commercially. They are used to induce ovulation in anovulatory women whose problem is secondary ovarian failure and who have failed in treatment with clomiphene. Treatment must be carefully monitored with repeated pelvic ultrasound by specialists experienced in their use to avoid ovarian hyperstimulation and multiple pregnancies. They are also successful in treating men with oligospermia due to secondary testicular failure. They are, of course, ineffective in primary gonadal failure.

CLOMIPHENE

Use

Clomiphene (see also chapter 38) is used to treat anovulatory infertility by inducing ovulation, but multiple ovulation may occur resulting in multiple births. It has replaced partial or wedge resection of the ovary in treating infertility caused by polycystic ovary syndrome, but must be used with caution in this condition because of the risk of increasing the size of the cysts. For this indication it is given as a course of 50 mg daily for 5 days starting on the second to fifth day of a cycle (or on any day if cycling has stopped). A second course of 100 mg/day for 5 days can be tried if this is not effective. Three courses constitutes an adequate therapeutic trial.

Mechanism of action

Clomiphene is an antiestrogen which blocks estrogen receptors in the hypothalamus. Thus feedback inhibition by estrogen is blocked and gonadotropin secretion is stimulated.

Adverse effects

Adverse effects, in addition to multiple pregnancy, include visual disturbance, hot flushes, abdominal discomfort and other gastrointestinal symptoms, breast tenderness, weight gain, rashes, acute psychotic reactions and alopecia.

DANAZOL

Use

Danazol (see chapter 38) is used to treat endometriosis, and has also been used in menorrhagia and in gynecomastia. It is also effective in preventing attacks of angioedema in some patients with hereditary angioneurotic edema. It is given starting on the first day of the menstrual cycle in a dose of 100 mg four times a day, adjusted according to response up to 200 mg four times daily, usually for 6 months. Its use is contraindicated in pregnancy and during breast feeding.

Mechanism of action

Danazol inhibits gonadotropin secretion, and combines androgenic activity with antiestrogen and antiprogestagen effects.

Adverse effects

Danazol causes fluid retention and hence weight gain. Nausea and several effects related to its androgenic action including acne, hirsutism, deepening of the voice, male pattern balding, cholestatic jaundice and, rarely, clitoral hypertrophy have been described. Benign intracranial hypertension, neutropenia and thrombocytopenia have also been reported. It adversely affects serum lipids and glucose sensitivity, and long term use should be avoided if possible.

GONADORELIN ANALOGS

Gonadorelin (gonadotrophin-releasing hormone) is a FSH/LH releasing factor, produced in the hypothalamus. It is used in a single intravenous dose to assess anterior pituitary reserve in patients with suspected impairment. Gonadorelin analogs (e.g. buserelin, goserelin) initially stimulate the release of FSH/LH, but then down-regulate this response and thereby reduce pituitary stimulation of male or female gonads leading effectively to medical orchidectomy/ovariectomy. This has therapeutic applications in, respectively, prostate cancer (see chapter 45) and endometriosis, fibroids, or breast cancer. The initial stimulation phase is managed in the case of patients with prostate cancer by initiating treatment only after starting therapy with an antiandrogen (cyproterone acetate, chapter 38). Buserelin is given intranasally (300 μg three times daily); goserelin is given by subcutaneous injection into the anterior abdominal wall (3.6 mg once monthly for up to 6 months). Side effects are predictable from the effective ovariectomy and include menopausal symptoms of hot flushes, vaginal dryness, reduced libido and reduced breast size in addition to local symptoms from irritation of the nasal mucosa. Reduced estrogen secretion causes a decrease in trabecular bone density, so long-term use is not recommended for benign disease. One rational strategy is to combine a gonadorelin with a small estrogen replacement dose for indications such as endometriosis.

ADRENOCORTICOTROPHIC HORMONE

Adrenocorticotrophic hormone (ACTH) is no longer commercially available in the UK. A synthetic analog of ACTH containing only the first 24 amino acids is available as tetracosactrin. This possesses full biological activity, the remaining 15 amino acids of ACTH being species specific and associated with antigenic activity. The $t_{1/2}$ of tetracosactrin (15 min) is slightly longer than that of ACTH, but otherwise its properties are identical. Tetracosactrin is used as a diagnostic test in the evaluation of patients in whom Addison's disease is suspected. A single intravenous or intramuscular dose of 250 μg is administered, followed by venous blood sampling for cortisol determination. There is a small but real risk of anaphylaxis. Tetracosactrin and ACTH used to be used in chronic disease such as asthma and Crohn's disease as alternatives to corticosteroid treatment, but their effects were unpredictable and tetracosactrin is no longer recommended for use in this way.

POSTERIOR PITUITARY HORMONES

Vasopressin (antidiuretic hormone; ADH) and oxytocin are peptide hormones synthesized in the supraoptic and paraventricular hypothalamic nuclei and transported along nerve fibers to the posterior lobe of the pituitary for storage and subsequent release (neurosecretion).

Vasopressin and desmopressin (DDAVP) are discussed in chapter 33 on fluid and electrolyte balance in relation to diabetes insipidus. Oxytocin has a related octapeptide structure to that of vasopressin, and is discussed in chapter 38 on reproductive endocrinology.

Selective Toxicity

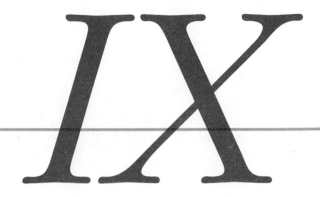
IX

Antibacterial Drugs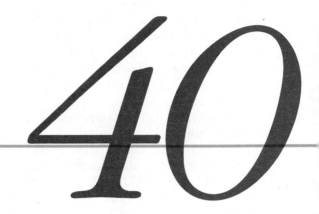

Principles of antibacterial chemotherapy   **518**

Bacterial resistance   **524**

Drug combinations   **525**

Prophylactic use of antibacterial drugs   **525**

Hazards of inappropriate antibacterial drug use   **530**

Commonly prescribed antibacterial drugs   **530**

PRINCIPLES OF ANTIBACTERIAL CHEMOTHERAPY

Bacteria are a common cause of disease but produce beneficial as well as harmful effects. For example, the gastrointestinal bacterial flora of the healthy human assists in preventing colonization by pathogens. Consequently, antibacterial therapy should not be used indiscriminately.

A distinction is conventionally drawn between bactericidal drugs that kill bacteria and bacteriostatic drugs that prevent their reproduction, elimination depending on host defense (Table 40.1). This difference is relative as bacteriostatic drugs are often bactericidal at high concentrations and in the presence of host defense mechanisms. In clinical practice the distinction is seldom important unless the body's defense mechanisms are depressed. Antibacterial drugs can be further classified into four main groups according to their mechanism of action (Table 40.1).

The choice of an appropriate antibacterial drug depends on:

1. **Diagnosis of infection** This is usually made on history and clinical examination supported by appropiate investigations, for

example chest X-ray, lumbar puncture and bacteriological culture and sensitivities. The site and severity of infection are important factors. The clinical features sometimes necessitate initiating drug treatment before bacteriological results are available (e.g. if the patient is hypotensive or shocked, or if there is neutropenia) and hence the initial drug choice is based on knowledge of likely causative bacteria in a particular clinical setting (e.g. cellulitis is usually the result of streptococcal or staphylococcal infection). An up-to-date knowledge of prevalent organisms and their sensitivities can be invaluable in settings such as oncology wards where patients are undergoing cancer chemotherapy.

2. **Patient factors** This includes age, sex (pregnant, lactating), weight, allergies, genetic factors, renal and hepatic function, immune status and concurrent medication that may cause drug interactions.

3. **Drug factors** These include antibacterial spectrum, pharmacokinetics, adverse effects, drug interactions, convenience and cost.

Table 40.1 Classification of antibacterial agents.

Bactericidal	Bacteriostatic	Mechanism of action	Antibacterial agent
Penicillins Cephalosporins Aminoglycosides Co-trimoxazole	Erythromycin Tetracyclines Chloramphenicol Sulfonamides	Inhibition of cell wall synthesis	Penicillins Cephalosporins Monobactams Vancomycin
	Trimethoprim	Inhibition of: DNA gyrase / RNA polymerase	Quinolones Rifampicin
		Inhibition of protein synthesis	Aminoglycosides Tetracyclines Erythromycin Chloramphenicol
		Inhibition of folic acid metabolism	Trimethoprim Sulfonamides

The dose and route of administration also depend on the infection (e.g. anatomical site, severity) and patient factors (e.g. age, weight, renal function). The dose may also be guided by plasma concentration measurements of drugs with a narrow therapeutic index (e.g. aminoglycosides). The duration of therapy depends on the nature of the infection and response to treatment.

Table 40.2 outlines recommended initial treatment for common bacterial infections.

Close liaison with the local microbiology laboratory not only provides the physician with information on local prevalence of organisms and sensitivities but also allows feedback on quality of diagnostic specimens.

The MIC is often quoted by laboratories and in promotional literature. It is the minimal inhibitory concentration of a particular agent below which bacterial growth is not prevented. Although the MIC provides useful information in comparing the susceptibility of organisms to antibacterial drugs it is an *in vitro* test in a homogenous culture system whilst *in vivo* the concentration at the site of infection may be considerably lower than the plasma concentration which one might predict to be bactericidal, for example, drug penetration and concentration in an abscess cavity is very poor.

Table 40.2 Summary of antibacterial therapy. All treaments are *oral* and for *adults* unless otherwise stated.

Clinical conditions	Likely causative organism(s)	Suggested treatment
Respiratory tract infections		
Pharyngitis Tonsillitis Scarlet fever	Viruses Group A streptococci	Most infections are viral and require symptomatic treatment only If treatment is required: *1st choice* Penicillin V, 250–500 mg, 6 hourly or benzylpenicillin, 600 mg, i.v. or i.m. 6 hourly if seriously ill or vomiting *Alternative* Erythromycin, 500 mg, 6 hourly
Acute otitis media Sinusitis	Group A streptococci Hemophilus influenzae Strep. pneumoniae	*1st choice* Amoxycillin, 250 mg, 8 hourly *Alternative* Erythromycin, 500 mg, 6 hourly
Acute bronchitis in healthy adults	Viruses H. influenzae Strep. pneumoniae	Mild cases, usually viral, require symptomatic treatment only. Severe cases with purulent sputum: *1st choice* Amoxycillin, 250 mg, 8 hourly *Alternative* Trimethoprim, 200 mg, 12 hourly
Acute or chronic bronchitis	H. influenzae Strep. pneumoniae	*1st choice* Amoxycillin, 250 mg, 8 hourly or trimethoprim, 200 mg, 12 hourly *Alternative* Tetracycline, 500 mg, 6 hourly (if impaired renal function doxycycline, initially 200 mg, then 100 mg, daily) or erythromycin, 500 mg, 6 hourly
Acute epiglottitis in children	H. influenzae	Chloramphenicol or cefotaxime Initially i.v. treatment is required

Table 40.2 (contd)

Clinical conditions	Likely causative organism(s)	Suggested treatment
Pneumonia		
Pneumonia – classical lobar	Strep. pneumoniae	1st choice Benzylpenicillin, 1.2 g, i.v. 6 hourly Alternative Erythromycin, 500 mg, 6 hourly (i.v. for the first 48 hours)
Severe pneumonia Cause unknown (community acquired)	Strep. pneumoniae Staphylococcus aureus H. influenzae (sometimes resistant) Legionella pneumophila Mycoplasma pneumoniae	Initially ampicillin, 500 mg, i.v. 6 hourly plus erythromycin, 1 g, oral or i.v. 6 hourly. Revise treatment when causative organism/sensitivities are known
Other pneumonias –'bronchopneumonia', e.g. in patients with chronic bronchitis	Strep. pneumoniae H. influenzae Staph. aureus and others	Many possible regimes Usually start treatment with amoxycillin, 500 mg, 8 hourly plus flucoxacillin, 500 mg, 6 hourly if Staphylococcus is a possibility. Co-amoxiclav is an alternative. Add gentamicin i.v. in severely ill patients
Pneumonia – post-influenza	Beware Staph. aureus Strep. pneumoniae H. influenzae	If definitely staphylococcal: flucloxacillin, 1 g, i.v. 6 hourly plus sodium fusidate, 500 mg, i.v. 8 hourly. Otherwise flucloxacillin, 500 mg, i.v. 6 hourly plus gentamicin i.v. plus ampicillin, 500 mg, i.v. 6 hourly
Legionnaires' disease	Legionella pneumophila	1st choice Erythromycin up to 1 g i.v. 6 hourly plus, initially for up to 3 days, rifampicin, 300 mg, i.v. 8 hourly
Pneumonia – primary atypical	Mycoplasma pneumoniae Chlamydia psittaci Coxiella burnetti	1st choice Erythromycin, 500 mg, 6 hourly Alternative Tetracycline, 500 mg, 6 hourly (if renal function is impaired doxycycline initially 200 mg, then 100 mg daily)
Pneumonia in the immunosuppressed	Wide variety of organisms, Gram-negative organisms, anaerobes and fungi	Broad-spectrum penicillin + aminoglycoside or 'third generation' cephalosporin alone. Pneumocystis carinii and Cytomegalovirus pneumonia must be considered (see Chapter 43)
Aspiration pneumonia	Mouth organisms including anaerobes	Ampicillin, 500 mg, i.v. 6 hourly plus metronidazole, 400 mg, orally 8 hourly (or 1 g rectally 8 hourly for 3 days then every 12 hours)
Genitourinary infections		
Acute cystitis arising outside hospital in adults	E. coli Staph. saprophyticus Strep. faecalis Other organisms (uncommon)	1st choice Trimethoprim, 200 mg, 12 hourly Alternative Amoxycillin, 250 mg, 8 hourly or a 4-quinolone In pregnancy amoxycillin or cefadroxil, 500 mg, 12 hourly should be used. Avoid trimethoprim in the first 3 months of pregnancy
Acute pyelonephritis	As above	In mild cases and not vomiting, as above. In severely ill patients and/or vomiting patients, gentamicin i.v. plus cefuroxime, 750 mg, i.v. 8 hourly

Table 40.2 (contd)

Clinical conditions	Likely causative organism(s)	Suggested treatment
Prophylaxis against urinary tract infection	As above	*1st choice* Trimethroprim, 100 mg, at night *Alternative* Nitrofurantoin, 100 mg, at night Avoid nitrofurantoin in impaired renal function
Hospital acquired and chronic urinary tract infection	Variety of organisms, often multiple resistant	Often difficult to eradicate. With indwelling catheters use chlorhexidine 0.9% bladder washout 12 hourly
Initial and recurrent genital herpes	Herpes simplex	Treatment should start within 7 days of infection. Topical acyclovir is of no benefit. Sexual partner may also need treatment. Acyclovir, 200 mg, five times daily for 5 days. For severe infections consider i.v. therapy

Severe systemic infections (septicemia)

Clinical conditions	Likely causative organism(s)	Suggested treatment
Severe systemic infection – causative organism unknown	Many possibilities	Initial choice of antibiotics depends on the clinical conditions and the pathogen background of the hospital
Immunocompetent or immunosuppressed but no recent antibiotic treatment	Many possibilities	Gentamicin i.v. plus ampicillin, 500 mg, 6 hourly (erythromycin if penicillin sensitive) plus metronidazole, 400 mg, orally 8 hourly for 3 days then 12 hourly) *Add* flucloxacillin, 500 mg, i.v. 6 hourly if *Staphylococcus* is suspected
Immunosuppressed and seriously ill for whom the above treatment has failed or for those patients who have recently relapsed	Many possibilities	Antibiotic regimes should include an aminoglycoside plus a ureidopenicillin, e.g. piperacillin (or a cephalosporin) plus metronidazole (as above)
Severe infection with Gram-negative organisms	E. coli Proteus Klebsiella	*1st choice* Ampicillin, 500 mg, i.v. 6 hourly plus gentamicin i.v. *Alternative* For gentamicin-resistant *Klebsiella* cefuroxime, 1.5 g, i.v. 8 hourly plus amikacin i.v.
	Pseudomonas	Piperacillin plus or minus amikacin
Severe infection with Gram-positive organisms	*Staph. aureus*	Flucloxacillin, 500 mg, i.v. 6 hourly plus sodium fusidate, 500 mg, i.v. 8 hourly (vancomycin or teichoplanin may be substituted for flucloxacillin in penicillin-sensitive patients)
	Staph. epidermidis	Multiple resistance is common Treatment depends on sensitivities
	Group A streptococci	*1st choice* Benzylpenicillin, 1.2 g, i.v. 6 hourly *Alternative* Erythromycin, 500 mg, i.v. 6 hourly
	Clostridium perfringens	*1st choice* Benzylpenicillin, 1.2 g, i.v. 4 hourly *Alternative* Metronidazole, 500 mg, 8 hourly in penicillin allergy

Table 40.2   (contd)

Clinical conditions	Likely causative organism(s)	Suggested treatment

Infective endocarditis

Bacteriological diagnosis is impossible once antibiotics have been given. Three sets of blood cultures must be taken by separate venepuncture **before** treatment is started. The management of endocarditis requires *expert laboratory advice* as detailed sensitivity tests and serum assays are necessary.

Treatment (a) No penicillin allergy	Penicillin-sensitive streptococci	Benzylpenicillin, 1.2 g, i.v. 4 hourly, gentamicin i.v. for 14 days; then amoxycillin, 500 mg to 1 g, 8 hourly for 14 days
	Streptococci with reduced sensitivity to penicillin	Benzylpenicillin, 1.2 g, i.v. 4 hourly, gentamicin i.v. for not less than 4 weeks
(b) In penicillin allergy	Streptococci	Replace benzylpenicillin with vancomycin
(c) No penicillin allergy	Staphylococci	*1st choice* Flucloxacillin, 2 g, i.v. 4 hourly plus sodium fusidate, 500 mg, 8 hourly for not less than 4 weeks *Alternative* Replace sodium fusidate with gentamicin i.v. for 14 days maximum
(d) In penincillin allergy	Staphylococci	Teicoplanin or vancomycin
	Other organisms	Depends on sensitivities

Bacterial meningitis

Bacterial meningitis in adults	*N. meningitidis*	Benzylpenicillin, 1.2 g, i.v. 4 hourly
	Strep. pneumoniae	Benzylpenicillin, 1.2 g, i.v. 2 hourly
	H. influenzae	*1st choice* Cefotaxime, 2 g, 8 hourly i.m. or i.v. *Alternative* Chloramphenicol, 500 mg to 1 g, 6 hourly initially i.v. then 500 mg orally 6 hourly
	Before culture or smear results are known	*1st choice* Cefotaxime, 2 g 8 hourly i.m. or i.v. *Alternative* In penicillin-sensitive patients chloramphenicol alone
Bacterial meningitis in neonates	Coliforms Group B streptococci enterococci, *Salmonella*, *Listeria* etc.	Infants up to 3 weeks: seek advice of microbiologist

Osteomyelitis

Osteomyelitis	*Staph. aureus*	Prolonged treatment necessary, seek expert advice *1st choice* Initially flucloxacillin, 500 mg, i.v. 6 hourly plus sodium fusidate, 500 mg, i.v. 8 hourly, then oral therapy *Alternative* Initially erythromycin, 500 mg, i.v. 6 hourly plus sodium fusidate, 500 mg, i.v. 8 hourly
Osteomyelitis in children under 5 years	May be *H. influenzae* *Staph. aureus*	Amoxycillin plus flucloxacillin

Table 40.2 (contd)

Clinical conditions	Likely causative organism(s)	Suggested treatment
Oropharyngeal infections		
Actinomycosis – cervicofacial	*Actinomyces israelii*	Benzylpenicillin, 6–12 g (10–20 megaunits) i.v. daily in divided doses for 4–6 weeks followed by penicillin V, 500 mg, 6 hourly. May need treatment for 6 months. Seek advice of the microbiologist
Sialadenitis (suppurative parotitis)	*Staph. aureus* Group A streptococci Pneumococci	Flucloxacillin, 500 mg, 6 hourly or penicillin V, 500 mg, 6 hourly according to sensitivities
Angular cheilitis	*Candida albicans* Group A streptococci *Staph. aureus*	Nystatin, 500 000 unit, tablets sucked 6 hourly or miconazole oral gel, 5 ml, 6 hourly to deal with oral candidosis. Apply chlorhexidine antiseptic cream 6 hourly if necessary
Wound, soft tissue, skin and superficial infections		
Serious wound infection	Many possibilities including *Staph. aureus* Group A streptococci, anaerobic organisms etc.	Before culture results are available *1st choice* Flucloxacillin, 500 mg, 6 hourly plus metronidazole, 400 mg, 8 hourly if anaerobes are suspected *Alternative* In penicillin-sensitive patients erythromycin can be substituted for flucloxacillin, ampicillin and benzylpenicillin Superficial wounds may require local antiseptic treatment only
Erysipelas	Group A streptococci	*1st choice* Benzylpenicillin, 1200 mg, i.m. or i.v. 6 hourly *Alternative* In penicillin-sensitive patients erythromycin, 500 mg, 6 hourly i.v.
Cellulitis	*Staph. aureus* or group A streptococci	Mild infection – oral amoxiclav Serious infection – parenteral benzylpenicillin flucloxacillin
Impetigo	*Staph. aureus* and/or group A streptococci	*1st choice* Flucloxacillin, 500 mg, 6 hourly *Alternative* Erythromycin, 500 mg, 6 hourly. Remove crust with antiseptic. Avoid local antibiotics due to risk of sensitization
Severe boils	*Staph. aureus*	*1st choice* Flucloxacillin, 500 mg, 6 hourly *Alternative* Erythromycin, 500 mg, 6 hourly
Gastrointestinal infections and enteric fever		
Gastroenteritis	*Salmonella* *Shigella*	No antibacterial treatment unless evidence of systemic spread or the patient is severely ill. Antibacterials prolong duration of carrier state in *Salmonella* infections
	Campylobacter	Erythromycin, 500 mg, 6 hourly for 5 days (only with prolonged symptoms)
Pseudomembranous colitis (antibiotic associated)	Toxin of *C. difficile*	Metronidazone 500 mg 6 cl. p. 0; in severe infections vancomycin, 125 mg, orally 6 hourly for 5 days. Stop other antibiotics. A repeat course may be necessary
Spontaneous colitis of the elderly (can be antibiotic associated)	*C. perfringens*	Metronidazole, 400 mg, orally 8 hourly

Table 40.2 (contd)

Clinical conditions	Likely causative organism(s)	Suggested treatment
Esophageal *Candida*		Fluconazole, 50–400 mg, orally daily or amphotericin i.v.
Enteric fever	*Salmonella typhi, S. paratyphi* a, b and c	*1st choice* Ciprofloxacin, 500–750 mg, orally 12 hourly *Alternative* Chloramphenicol, 500 mg, 6 hourly. Cotrimoxazole 2 tablets 12 hourly or amoxycillin, 1 g, 8 hourly. *Do not* treat carriers with chloramphenicol
Acute cholecystitis	Coliforms *Strep. faecalis*	*1st choice* Ampicillin, 500 mg, i.v. 6 hourly plus gentamicin i.v. Metronidazole may be added if anaerobic infection is suspected

*B*ACTERIAL RESISTANCE

The resistance of bacterial populations to antimicrobial agents is constantly changing and can become a serious clinical problem, particularly if the resistant strain supplants the sensitive, thus rendering a previously useful drug inactive. The evolution of drug resistance arises either by:

1. Selection of naturally resistant strains (which have arisen by spontaneous mutation) existing within the bacterial population by elimination of the sensitive strain by therapy or environmental contamination. Thus the incidence of drug resistance is related to the prescription of that drug. The hospital environment with intensive and widespread use of broad-spectrum antibacterials is particularly likely to promote the selection of resistant organisms.
2. Transfer of resistance between organisms can occur either by transfer of naked DNA (transformation), by conjugation with direct cell to cell transfer of extrachromosomal DNA (plasmids), or by passage of the information by bacteriophage (transduction). In this way transfer of genetic information concerning drug resistance (frequently to a group of several antibiotics simultaneously) may occur between species.

Mechanisms of drug resistance can broadly be divided into:

1. Inactivation of the antimicrobial agent either by disruption of its chemical structure (e.g. penicillinase) or by addition of a modifying group that inactivates the drug (e.g. chloramphenicol, inactivated by acetylation).
2. Restriction of entry of the drug into the bacterium by altered permeability, for example sulfonamides, tetracycline.
3. Modification of the bacterial target. This may take the form of an enzyme with reduced affinity for an inhibitor (e.g. sulfonamide), or an altered organelle with reduced drug-binding properties (e.g. erythromycin and bacterial ribosomes).

The prescriber can minimize bacterial resistance by:

1. Avoidance of unnecessary prescription of antimicrobial drugs.
2. Use of adequate dose for adequate duration.
3. Restriction of certain drugs, for example amikacin, for specific clinical and bacteriological indications.
4. Use of drug combinations in selected circumstances (especially tuberculosis, chapter 41).

DRUG COMBINATIONS

Most infections can be treated with a single agent; however, there are four main situations in which more than one antibacterial drug is prescribed concurrently:

1. To achieve broad antimicrobial activity in critically ill patients with an undefined infection (e.g. aminoglycoside plus a penicillin to treat septicemia).

2. To treat mixed bacterial infections (e.g. following perforation of bowel) where no single agent would affect all the bacteria present.
3. To prevent emergence of resistance (e.g. in treating tuberculosis, chapter 41).
4. To achieve an additive or synergistic effect (e.g. co-trimoxazole in the treatment of *Pneumocystis carinii* pneumonia).

PROPHYLACTIC USE OF ANTIBACTERIAL DRUGS

There are a limited number of occasions when it is appropriate to use antibacterial drugs prophylactically. Where possible a suitable specific narrow spectrum drug should be used. A summary of the common indications and drugs used for prophylactic therapy follows.

Antibiotic prophylaxis of infective endocarditis

These guidelines are based on the Working Party Report of the British Society for Antimicrobial Chemotherapy (*Lancet* 1990; **i**: 88–89).

PATIENTS AT RISK

Patients at risk are those with congenital or acquired cardiac defects causing turbulent flow from high to low pressure chambers, for example small ventricular septal defect (VSD), but not atrial septal defect (ASD), those with prosthetic heart valves, pacemakers or prosthetic joint replacements, those with a past history of infective endocarditis, drug addicts and alcoholics. Patients with a

history of coronary thrombosis or cardiac surgery of the coronary artery graft type do not normally require cover.

PROCEDURES TO BE COVERED
Dental treatment
Dental extractions, deep scaling and periodontal surgery (Fig. 40.1). Plan the dental treatment carefully to reduce the need for antibiotic cover. A patient at risk should normally be advised to have dubious teeth extracted, and to maintain meticulous dental hygiene. As much treatment as possible is done under the same antibiotic cover.

Other procedures
See Table 40.3.

Special risk patients
Special risk patients are those who:

1. Need a general anesthetic and have received a penicillin more than once in the previous month or have a prosthetic valve or are allergic to penicillin.
2. All patients who have previously had endocarditis. Warning/information cards are available from most microbiology departments for those patients at risk.

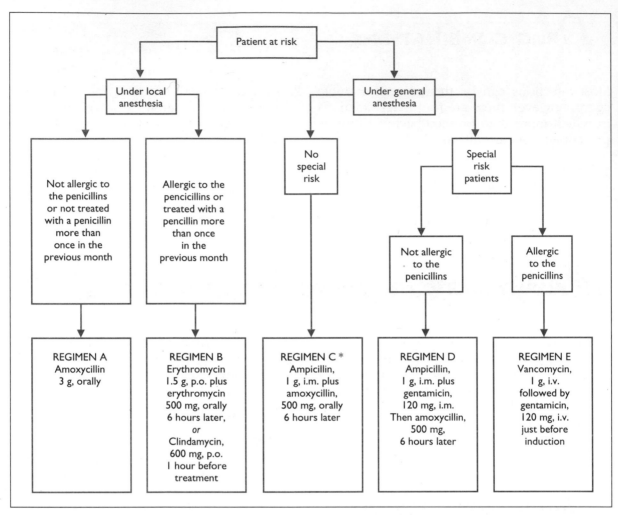

Fig. 40.1 British Society for Antimicrobial Chemotherapy antibiotic prophylactic regimens recommended for dental treatment.

*Alternatives for adults requiring regimen C for dental surgery are as follows: *either* (a) amoxycillin, 3 g, orally 4 hours before anesthesia plus a further 3 g orally as soon as possible after the operation; *or* (b) amoxycillin, 3 g, plus probenecid, 1 g, orally 4 hours before anesthesia.

Table 40.3 British Society for Antimicrobial Therapy recommendations regarding antibiotic prophylaxis for other procedures.

Procedure	Valve	Regimen (as in Fig. 40.1)
Genitourinary instrumentation	Damaged original or prosthetic valve	No penicillin allergy: regimen D Penicillin allergy: regimen E
Obstetric/gynecological procedures (including intrauterine device insertion)	Prosthetic valves only	As above
Gastrointestinal endoscopy, barium enema	Prosthetic valves only	As above
Tonsillectomy/adenoidectomy	(a) Damaged original valves	No penicillin allergy: regimen C Penicillin allergy: regimen E
	(b) Prosthetic valves	No penicillin allergy: regimen E Penicillin allergy: regimen E

Administration and timing of antibiotics

1. Oral amoxycillin should be given under supervision 1 hour before the procedure and 6 hours after the procedure, unless otherwise stated.
2. Oral erythromycin should be given 1–2 hours before and 6 hours after the procedure.
3. Give intramuscular and intravenous antibiotics immediately before the procedure (vancomycin should be infused over 1 hour and followed by gentamicin).

Prophylactic preoperative antibiotics

GENERAL PRINCIPLES

1. Prophylaxis should be used where the procedure commonly leads to infection, or if infection, although rare, would be expected to have devasting results.
2. The antimicrobial should be bactericidal and directed against the likely pathogen.

3. The aim is to provide high plasma and tissue concentrations of an appropriate drug at the time of bacterial contamination. Intramuscular injections can usually be given with the premedication or intravenous injections at the time of induction. Treatment should be short: usually not more than 48 hours. Most problems in this area arise because of failure to discontinue 'prophylactic' antibiotics, a mistake that is easily made by a busy junior house surgeon who does not want to take responsibility for changing a prescription for a patient who is apparently doing well postoperatively. Local hospital drug and therapeutics committees can help considerably by instituting sensible guidelines regarding duration of prophylactic antibiotics.
4. Change to oral therapy as soon as possible postoperatively.
5. Administer metronidazole rectally when possible instead of using the more expensive intravenous formulation, which is no more effective.

Table 40.4 summarizes the use of antibacterial drugs preoperatively.

Table 40.4 Prophylactic preoperative antibiotics.

Indications	Common pathogens	Recommendation (adult dose)
1. Acute appendicitis	Non-sporing anaerobes Streptococci of Lancefield groups F, C and G	Metronidazole, 1 g, suppository with premedication and repeated 8 hourly until oral medication (200–400 mg 8 hourly) can be started
		Cefuroxime, 750 mg, i.v. at induction, repeated 8 hourly until cefadroxil, 500 mg to 1 g, twice daily can be started
2. Amputations, lower limb for ischemia	*Clostridium perfringens*	Benzylpenicillin, 1.2 g, i.v. at induction, continue 6 hourly for 3 days *Or* (if allergic to penicillin) metronidazole, 1 g, suppository with premedication, then 400 mg tablets 8 hourly for 4 days
3. Biliary tract surgery	Coliforms, streptococci (usually *Strep. faecalis*) Anaerobes are rarely involved	Not usually justified, but if complicated cefuroxime, 750 mg, i.v. at induction followed by two doses at 8 and 16 hours postoperatively. *Strep. faecalis* may not be sensitive to cefuroxime. For improved cover: ampicillin, 500 mg, i.v. at induction and repeat 6 hourly for 24–48 hours *Plus* gentamicin i.v. at induction and for 24–48 hours, adjusting dose according to renal function
4. Cardiac surgery and vascular prosthetic surgery	*Staphylococcus epidermidis* *Staph. aureus*, coliforms, fungi	'Clean' surgical field. Cefuroxime, 750 mg, i.v. at induction repeated 8 hourly for 48 hours

Table 40.4 (contd).

Indications	Common pathogens	Recommendation (adult dose)
5. Colorectal surgery	Anaerobes, coliforms, *Strep. faecalis*	Cefuroxime, 750 mg, i.v. at induction plus two doses at 8 and 16 hours postoperatively *Plus* metronidazole, 1 g, suppository* premedication plus two doses at 8 and 16 hours postoperatively NB For *Strep. faecalis* not sensitive to cefuroxime, replace with ampicillin plus gentamicin (see biliary tract surgery)
6. Gastric surgery	Streptococci, anaerobes	Not usually justified unless low production of gastric acid, e.g. carcinoma, H_2 antagonist therapy. Cefuroxime, 750 mg, i.v. at induction plus two doses at 8 and 16 hours postoperatively *Plus* metronidazole, 1 g, suppository premedication plus two doses at 8 and 16 hours postoperatively
7. Gynecology and obstetrics	Fecal anaerobes	Prophylaxis mainly indicated for vaginal hysterectomy: Metronidazole, 1 g, suppository at premedication and repeated 8 hourly until oral medication (200–400 mg 8 hourly) can be started Cesarean section in the presence of sepsis: add cefuroxime, 750 mg, i.v. at induction, repeated 8 hourly until cefadroxil, 500 mg, twice daily can be started. Continue for 24–48 hours
8. Head and neck surgery	*Staph. aureus*, streptococci, anaerobes	Cefuroxime, 750 mg, i.v. at induction and repeated 8 hourly until cefadroxil, 500 mg to 1 g, twice daily can be started. Continue for 24–48 hours *Plus* metronidazole, 1 g suppository at premedication and repeated 8 hourly for 24–48 hours
9. Orthopedic implants	*Staph. aureus* *Staph. epidermidis*	Cefuroxime, 750 mg, i.v. at induction and repeated 8 hourly for 24–48 hours *Alternative* Flucloxacillin, 500 mg, i.v. at induction and repeated 6 hourly for 24–48 hours. If penicillin allergic, erythromycin, 500 mg, i.v. at induction and repeated 6 hourly for 24–48 hours. Change to oral therapy when possible *Plus* gentamicin i.v. at induction, adjusting dose according to renal function. Continue for 24–48 hours.
10. Urological procedures – inserting stents, cystoscopy removing catheters etc. Only in the presence of bacteriuria	Coliforms and other urinary pathogens (includes fecal anaerobes)	Ampicillin, 500 mg, just prior to procedure *Plus* gentamicin as a single dose (2 mg/kg) *Alternative* An appropriate antibiotic according to sensitivities
11. Plastic surgery, skin grafting	*Staph. aureus* *Staph. epidermidis*	(a) Minor skin grafting – not recommended (b) Skin grafting of extensive burns – depends on results of sensitivities, usually ampicillin, 500 mg, i.v. at induction then oral therapy (250–500 mg qds). Continue for 48 hours *Plus* gentamicin i.v. at induction adjusting dose according to renal function. Continue for 48 hours

*For left-sided surgery use metronidazole i.v.

Prophylactic antibiotics in medicine

GENERAL PRINCIPLES

There are various clinical situations in which prophylactic therapy may be appropriate although the advantages and disadvantages of antimicrobial therapy and the severity of the patient's condition must be carefully assessed:

1. To prevent colonization by a small number of virulent microorganisms.
2. To prevent an increase of organisms already present to a number sufficient to produce clinical infection.
3. To prevent latent infection becoming clinically established.

Table 40.5 summarizes the prophylactic use of antibacterial drugs in medicine.

Table 40.5 Prophylactic antibiotics in medicine.

Indications	Common pathogens	Recommendation (adult dose)
1. Neutropenic patients	Gram-negative organisms of patient's gastrointestinal tract	Broad-spectrum penicillin + aminoglycoside or 'third generation' cephalosporin
2. Human and animal bites	Streptococcus, Staphylococcus, anaerobes, sepsis	Co-amoxiclav, two tablets 8 hourly for 2 days
3. Recurrences of rheumatic fever	Group A streptococci	Penicillin V until child is 18 years old, or for at least 5 years, whichever is the longer Dose: 1 month to 12 years: 25 mg/kg per day in two divided doses; over 12 years: 250 mg twice daily Or (if allergic to penicillin): erythromycin
4. Meningoccocal disease: close domestic contacts or very close medical contacts	Neisseria meningitidis	Adults: Ciprofloxacin, 500 mg, single dose Children: Rifampicin 1–12 years 10 mg/kg twice daily; under 1 year 5 mg/kg twice daily for 2 days
5. Prevention of a secondary case of diphtheria	Corynebacterium diphtheriae	Erythromycin, 500 mg, four times daily for 5 days
6. Whooping cough: contact in an unvaccinated child under 1 year old	Bordetella pertussis	Erythromycin, 500 mg, four times daily for 5 days
7. Infants of mothers with sputum-positive tuberculosis	Mycobacterium tuberculosis	Seek urgent expert advice with respect to assessment for isoniazid chemoprophylaxis
8. Recurrent cystitis	Escherichia coli, occasionally other coliforms	Depends on culture and sensitivities. Trimethoprim is commonly effective
9. Tetanus prone wound	Prevention of tetanus and secondary infection	1. Immunized patients: booster dose of toxoid (unless this has been already given in the last 5 years). Extensive or dirty wounds will require a local infusion of human tetanus immunoglobulin (HTIG) plus antibiotics as below

Table 40.5 (contd)

Indications	Common pathogens	Recommendation (adult dose)
		2. Non-immunized patients: human tetanus immunoglobulin (HTIG) 500 units (increase the dose in the event of a 24-hour delay) and a course of absorbed tetanus toxoid *Plus* single injection of Bicillin™ *Or* phenoxymethylpenicillin, 500 mg, four times daily or amoxycillin, 500 mg, three times daily for 7–10 days (in event of delay or sepsis). In patients who are allergic to penicillin use erythromycin, 250 mg, four times daily for 5 days *Plus* metronidazole, 400 mg, 8 hourly for 7–10 days
10. Cerebrospinal fluid (CSF) leakage	*Strep. pneumoniae*	1. Traumatic CSF leakage (e.g. skull base fracture): Penicillin V, 500 mg, five times daily. Continue for 10 days after cessation of closure of the fistula 2. Postoperative (e.g. lumbar) ciprofloxacin, 500 mg, twice daily plus flucloxacillin, 500 mg, four times daily after cessation or closure of fistula
11. Sickle cell or splenectomy patients	Pneumococci	Vaccination plus penicillin V, 250 mg, twice daily in selected patients

HAZARDS OF INAPPROPRIATE ANTIBACTERIAL DRUG USE

1. Development of resistant organisms.
2. Superinfections, for example, broad-spectrum antibiotics leading to *Clostridium difficile* superinfection with subsequent life-threatening pseudomembranous colitis.
3. Adverse drug effects.
4. Obscuring the correct diagnosis.
5. Cost.

It should be remembered that the commonest cause of pyrexia is a viral infection, and that antibiotics, not uncommonly, cause fever as an adverse effect.

COMMONLY PRESCRIBED ANTIBACTERIAL DRUGS

β-Lactam antibiotics

This group is so named because each member contains a β-lactam ring. This can be broken down by β-lactamase enzymes produced by bacteria, notably by many strains of *Staphylococcus* and by *Hemophilus influenzae* which are thereby resistant. β-Lactam antibiotics kill bacteria by inhibiting bacterial cell wall synthesis. Antibiotics in this group include the penicillins, monobactams, carbapenems and cephalosporins.

PENICILLINS

Use

Benzylpenicillin (penicillin G) is the drug of choice for streptococcal, pneumococcal, gonococcal and meningococcal infections and also for anthrax, diphtheria, gas gangrene, leptospirosis, syphilis, tetanus, yaws, and the treatment of Lyme disease in children. Benzylpenicillin is inactivated by gastric acid.

Adverse effects

1. Anaphylaxis can occur (1 in 100 000 injections), therefore always enquire about previous reactions before administration.
2. Skin rashes, usually morbilliform, occur in 3–5% of patients, and are rarely severe but Stevens–Johnson syndrome can occur.
3. Serum sickness – type III hypersensitivity.
4. In renal failure, accumulation of the drug can, rarely, cause encephalopathy and fits, hemolytic anemia and thrombocytopenia.

The main shortcomings of benzylpenicillin are:

1. It is acid labile and so must be given parenterally (inactivated in gastric acid).
2. It has a short half-life so frequent injections are required.
3. Development of resistant β-lactamase-producing strains.
4. It has a narrow antibacterial spectrum.

Two preparations with similar antibacterial spectra are used to overcome the acid lability/frequent injection problems:

1. Procaine penicillin. This complex releases penicillin slowly from an intramuscular site so twice daily dosage only is required. Bicillin™ is a combination of benzyl penicillin and procaine penicillin for intramuscular administration.
2. Phenoxymethylpenicillin. This is acid stable and so is effective when given orally (40–60% absorption). While useful for mild infections blood concentrations are variable so it is not used in serious infections or with poorly sensitive bacteria. Tablets are given on an empty stomach to improve absorption.

Flucloxacillin was developed to overcome β-lactamase-producing strains. It has a similar antibacterial spectrum to benzylpenicillin but is less potent. However, the lactam ring is not exposed and it is effective against β-lactamase-producing organisms. It is used for the treatment of staphylococcal infections (90% of hospital staphylococci are resistant to benzylpenicillin and 5–10% are resistant to flucloxacillin).

EXTENDED RANGE PENICILLINS

Ampicillin/amoxycillin

Use

These have a similar antibacterial spectrum to benzylpenicillin but in addition are effective against most strains of *H. influenzae*, *E. coli*, *Strep. faecalis* and *Salmonella*. They are used for a variety of chest infections (bronchitis, pneumonia), otitis media, urinary tract infections, biliary infections and the prevention of bacterial endocarditis (amoxycillin). Amoxycillin is somewhat more potent than ampicillin, penetrates tissues better and is given three rather than four times daily. Both are susceptible to β-lactamases.

Adverse effects

Rashes are common, and may appear after dosing has stopped. There is an especially high incidence in patients with infectious mononucleosis or lymphatic leukemia.

Pharmacokinetics

The half-life of each drug is about 1.5 hours and they are predominantly renally excreted.

Co-amoxiclav

Use

Co-amoxiclav is a combination of amoxycillin with clavulanic acid, a β-lactamase inhibitor. In addition to those bacteria susceptible to amoxycillin, most *Staph. aureus*, 50% of *E. coli*, some *H. influenzae* strains as well as many *Bacteroides* and

Klebsiella are susceptible to co-amoxiclav. Adverse effects are similar to amoxycillin but abdominal discomfort is more common. Ampicillin has been combined with another β-lactamase inhibitor, sulbactam, which is available for oral or parenteral use.

Antipseudomonal penicillins

Regular penicillins are not effective against *Pseudomonas*. This is not usually a problem, since these organisms seldom cause disease in otherwise healthy people. They are, however, important in neutropenic patients (e.g. those undergoing cancer chemotherapy) and in patient with cystic fibrosis. Penicillins with activity against *Pseudomonas* have been developed, and are particularly useful in these circumstances. These include carbenicillin (the first member of this group) and piperacillin (the most potent, and currently most popular).

Use

These expensive intravenous penicillins are not used routinely. Their efficacy against Gram-positive organisms is variable and poor. They are useful against Gram-negative infections, particularly with *Pseudomonas,* and are also effective against many anaerobes. Timestin is a combination of ticarcillin and clavulanic acid (a β-lactamse inhibitor) designed to overcome the problem of β-lactamase formation by *Pseudomonas.*

Adverse effects

These drugs have a fairly broad spectrum of activity and predispose to superinfection. Rashes, sodium overload (especially with carbenicillin, which is a sodium salt and is given in doses of many grams daily) and thrombocytopenia or non-thrombocytopenic platelet dysfunction occur.

Pharmacokinetics

Absorption of these drugs from the gut is inadequate in the life-threatening infections for which they are mainly indicated. They are given intravenously every 4–6 hours. Their half-lives vary from 1 to 1.5 hours. They are renally excreted.

CEPHALOSPORINS

This group of antibiotics is derived from a strain of micro-organism found near a sewage outlet in the Mediterranean off the coast of Sardinia.

First generation cephalosporins

So-called first generation cephalosporins (e.g. cephalexin, cefaclor, cefadroxil) are effective against *Strep. pyogenes* and *Strep. pneumoniae*, *E. coli* and some staphylococci. They have few *absolute* (i.e. uniquely advantageous) indications. Their pharmacology is similar to the penicillins and they are principally renally eliminated.

Second and third generation cephalosporins

Efficacy of second and third generation cephalosporins has been increased to include *H. influenzae* and in some instances *Pseudomonas* and anaerobes. This has only been achieved with some loss of efficacy against Gram-positive organisms. β-Lactamase stability has been increased. Arguably the most generally useful of the group is cefuroxime, which combines lactamase stability with activity against streptococci, staphylococci, *H. influenzae* and *E. coli*. It is given by injection 8 hourly (an oral preparation is also available). It is expensive, although when used against Gram-negative organisms that would otherwise necessitate use of an aminoglycoside, this is at least partly offset by savings from the lack of need for plasma concentration determinations.

Of the third generation cephalosporins, ceftazidime, ceftriaxone and cefotaxime are useful in severe sepsis especially because, unlike earlier cephalosporins, they penetrate the blood–brain barrier well and are effective in meningitis.

Adverse effects

About 10% of patients allergic to penicillins are allergic to cephalosporins. Some first generation cephalosporins are nephrotoxic, particularly if used with frusemide, aminoglycosides or other nephrotoxic agents. Some of the third generation drugs are associated with bleeding due to increased prothrombin times that is reversible with vitamin K.

MONOBACTAMS

Monobactams (e.g. aztreonam) contain a 5-monobactam ring and are resistant to β-lactamase degradation.

Aztreonam

Use

Aztreonam is primarily active against aerobic Gram-negative organisms and is an alternative to an aminoglycoside. It is used in severe sepsis, often hospital acquired, especially infections of the respiratory, urinary, biliary, gastrointestinal and female genital tracts. It has a narrow spectrum of activity and cannot be used alone unless the organism's sensitivity to aztreonam is known.

Mechanism of action

The 5-monobactam ring binds to bacterial wall transpeptidases and inhibits bacterial cell wall synthesis in a similar way to the penicillins.

Adverse effects

Rashes occur but there appears to be no cross-allergenicity with penicillins.

Pharmacokinetics

Aztreonam is poorly absorbed after oral administration so it is given parenterally. It is widely distributed to all body compartments including cerebrospinal fluid. Excretion is renal and usual half-life (1–2 h) is increased in renal failure.

IMIPENEM–CILASTATIN

Use

This antibacterial agent combines a carbapenem (thienamycin), imipenem, with cilastatin which is an inhibitor of the enzyme dehydropeptidase I found in the brush border of the proximal renal tubule. This enzyme breaks down imipenem in the kidney. Imipenem has a very broad spectrum of activity against Gram-positive, Gram-negative and anaerobic organisms. It is β-lactamase stable. It is used for treating severe infections in the lung, abdomen and in patients with septicemia, where the source of the organism is unknown.

Adverse effects

Imipenem is generally well tolerated but seizures, myoclonus, confusion, nausea and vomiting, hypersensitivity, positive Coombs' test, taste disturbances and thrombophlebitis have all been reported.

Pharmacokinetics

Imipenem is both renally filtered and metabolized in the kidney by dehydropeptidase I; this is inhibited by cilastin in the combination. The half-life is 1 hour. It is given intravenously as an infusion in three or four divided doses daily.

Aminoglycosides

Use

Aminoglycosides are highly polar, sugar-containing derivatives of bacterial proteins. They are all powerful bacteriocidal agents, active against many Gram-negative organisms and some Gram-positive organisms, with activity against staphylococci and *Enterococcus fecalis*, but not (when used alone) against other streptococci. They synergize with penicillins in killing *Strep. feacalis* in endocarditis. Aminoglycosides are used in serious infections including septicemia, either singly but usually in combination with other antibiotics (penicillins or cephalosporins). Gentamicin is the most widely used and has a broad spectrum but is ineffective against anaerobes, many streptococci and pneumococci.

Netilmicin is similar to gentamicin but is probably less ototoxic, and is therefore preferred in patients in whom prolonged treatment is envisaged, especially those with hearing or visual impairment and patients with impaired renal function, including the elderly. Tobramycin is probably somewhat less nephrotoxic than gentamicin. Amikacin is more effective than gentamicin for pseudomonal infections and is occasionally effective against organisms resistant to gentamicin; it is often reserved for neutropenic patients undergoing cancer chemotherapy. Topical gentamicin and tobramycin eye drops are used for treating eye infections.

Mechanism of action

These drugs are transported into cells and block bacterial protein synthesis by binding to the 30S ribosome. They are bactericidal.

Adverse effects

These are important and related to duration of therapy and trough plasma concentrations. Therapeutic monitoring is performed by measuring plasma concentrations before dosing (trough) and at 'peak' levels (at an arbitary 1 hour after dosing). Twice-weekly therapeutic monitoring is adequate for most patients with normal renal function during maintenance, but especially if the patient is severely ill and if acute tubular necrosis is a clinical possibility more frequent monitoring initially is essential. Eighth nerve damage – cochlear (deafness) and vestibular (dizziness – seen especially with streptomycin treatment for tuberculosis) – is potentially catastrophic and is usually irreversible. Acute tubular necrosis and renal failure is usually reversible if diagnosed promptly and the drug stopped or the dose reduced. Hypersensitivity rashes occur in patients and in those drawing up the drug, but are uncommon. Bone marrow suppression is rare. Exacerbation of myasthenia gravis is predictable in patients with this disease.

Pharmacokinetics

Aminoglycosides are poorly absorbed from the gut, and are given by intramuscular or intravenous injections. They are poorly protein bound (30%) and are excreted renally. Half-lives are short, usually 2 hours. Three times daily administration is usually adequate. In patients with renal dysfunction dose reduction and/or increased dose interval is required. Cerebrospinal fluid (CSF) penetration is poor, and neurosurgeons sometimes insert a reservoir with direct access to a lateral ventricle in patients with Gram-negative

meningitis resistant to other antibiotics that penetrate CSF better (e.g. chloramphenicol).

Drug interactions

Aminoglycosides enhance neuromuscular blockade of non-depolarizing neuromuscular antagonists. Loop diuretics potentiate their nephrotoxicity and ototoxicity.

Chloramphenicol

Use

Chloramphenicol has a broad spectrum of activity and penetrates tissues exceptionally well. It is bacteriostatic but is extremely effective against streptococci, staphylococci, H. influenzae, salmonellae and others. Uncommonly it causes aplastic anemia so its use is largely confined to H. influenzae epiglottitis, meningitis, typhoid fever and topical use as eye drops.

It was previously used widely in chronic respiratory disease, and retains a place in patients with life-threatening pulmonary infections in whom other antibiotics are contraindicated or likely to be ineffective.

Mechanism of action

Chloramphenicol inhibits bacterial ribosome function by inhibiting the 50S ribosomal peptidyl transferase, preventing peptide elongation.

Adverse effects

1. **Hematologic** Dose-related erythroid suppression is common and predictable, but in addition aplastic anemia occurs unpredictably with an incidence of approximately 1:40 000. This is irreversible in 50% of cases. It is only extremely rarely, if ever, related to topical eye drops. It provides a strong reason for not using the drug for trivial infections, but should not preclude its use in life-threatening situations: fatal anaphylactic reactions have been reported.
2. **Gray baby syndrome** (See p. 84.) The gray color is due to shock (hypotension

and tissue hypoperfusion). Chloramphenicol accumulates in neonates (especially if premature) due to reduced glucuronidation in the immature liver. The syndrome usually occurs at plasma concentrations greater than 50 μg/ml.

3. **Other effects** Chloramphenicol can also cause sore mouth, diarrhea, encephalopathy and optic neuritis.

Pharmacokinetics

Chloramphenicol is well absorbed following oral administration and can also be given by the intramuscular and intravenous routes. It is widely distributed and CSF penetration is excellent. It mainly undergoes hepatic glucuronidation. The half-life is 6 hours. In neonates this is prolonged due to the immaturity of the glucuronidation enzymes.

Drug interactions

Chloramphenicol inhibits metabolism of alcohol, warfarin, phenytoin and theophylline. This can cause clinically important toxicity if effects and/or plasma concentrations of these drugs are not monitored closely and their dose modified accordingly.

Macrolides

Macrolide antibiotics (e.g. erythromycin, clarithromycin, azithromycin) have an antibacterial spectrum similar, but not identical, to that of penicillin. Distinctively, they are effective against several unusual organisms including *Chlamydia, Legionella* and *Mycoplasma*. There is most experience with erythromycin. Characteristics of drugs of this group are compared in Table 40.6.

ERYTHROMYCIN

Use

Uses of erythromycin include respiratory infections (including *Mycoplasma pneumoniae*, psittacosis and Legionnaires' disease), whooping cough, *Campylobacter enteritis*, and non-specific urethritis. Erythromycin is a useful alternative to penicillin in penicillin-allergic patients (with the notable exception of meningitis, because it does not penetrate CSF adequately). It is useful for skin infections such as low-grade cellulitis and infected acne, and is an acceptable drug for patients with an infective exacerbation of chronic bronchitis. It is most commonly administered by mouth four times daily, although when necessary it may be given by intravenous infusion.

Mechanism of action

Macrolides binds to bacterial 50S ribosomes, inhibiting the ribosomal translocation enzyme.

Pharmacokinetics

Erythromycin is well absorbed orally. Food delays its absorption but may reduce gastrointestinal side effects. Erythromycin is distributed adequately to most sites except brain and CSF. It is inactivated by hepatic N-demethylation, less than 15% being eliminated unchanged in the urine.

Table 40.6 Comparison of macrolides.

	Erythromycin	Azithromycin	Clarithromycin
Experience	Extensive	Limited	Limited
Oral dose frequency	Usually qds	od	bd
$t_{1/2}$	1–1.5 hours	40–60 hours	5 hours approx.
Intravenous preparation available	Yes	No	Yes
Gastrointestinal adverse effects	Common	Less common	Less common
Tissue penetration	Reasonable	Extremely high	High

Adverse effects

Erythromycin is a remarkably safe antibiotic, and may be used in pregnancy and children. Nausea, vomiting, diarrhea and abdominal cramps are the most common adverse effects reported, and may be related to direct pharmacological action on vasoactive intestinal peptide (VIP) receptors. Cholestatic jaundice has been reported following prolonged use. Intravenous use frequently causes local pain and phlebitis.

Drug interactions

Erythromycin inhibits cytochrome P_{450} and causes accumulation of theophylline, warfarin and terfenadine. This can result in clinically important adverse effects.

AZITHROMYCIN AND CLARITHROMYCIN

These macrolides have somewhat different *in vitro* activities than erythromycin. Each has greater activity against *H. influenzae*. Azithromycin is less effective against Gram-positive bacteria than erythromycin but has a wider spectrum of activity against Gram-negative organisms. The long half-life of azithromycin is probably related to its extensive tissue penetration and subsequent slow release from peripheral compartments. A single dose of azithromycin is as effective as 7 days' tetracycline in the management of non-specific urethritis due to *Chlamydia*.

Azithrombin and clarithromycin are approximately four times more expensive than erythromycin.

Tetracyclines

Use

Tetracyclines (e.g. tetracycline, chlortetracycline, oxytetracycline, doxycycline, minocycline) are molecular modifications of a four-ringed nucleus (hence the name). They have a broad range of antibacterial activity covering both Gram-positive and -negative organisms, and in addition organisms such as *Rickettsia, Chlamydia* and *Mycoplasma*. They are used in atypical pneumonias, chlamydial and rickettsial infections, and remain useful in treating exacerbations of chronic bronchitis. They are not used routinely for staphylococcal or streptococcal infections because of the development of resistance. Minocycline is used to eliminate carriage of *Neisseria meningitidis* from the nasopharynx. Tetracyclines are used in the long-term treatment of acne (chapter 48).

Mechanism of action

Tetracyclines bind to the 30S subunit of bacterial ribosomes and prevent binding of the aminoacyl-tRNA to the ribosome acceptor site, thereby inhibiting protein synthesis.

Adverse effects

1. Nausea and diarrhea.
2. Fungal superinfection, and pseudomembranous colitis due to *Clostridium difficile*.
3. Worsening of prerenal and renal failure.
4. Discoloration and damage of teeth and bones of the fetus if the mother takes tetracyclines after the fifth month of pregnancy and in children.
5. Minocycline causes reversible and dose-related ataxia.

Pharmacokinetics

Tetracyclines are well absorbed orally when fasting, but their absorption is reduced by food and antacids. They undergo elimination by both the liver and the kidney. The half-life varies with the different members of the group, from 6 to 12 hours. The shorter acting drugs are given four times daily, the longer ones once daily. Doxycycline is given once daily, can be taken with food and is not contraindicated in renal impairment, but is more expensive than other members of this group.

Drug interactions

Tetracyclines chelate with calcium salts in the stomach and their absorption is reduced with antacids or food.

Sodium fusidate

Use

Fusidic acid is a steroid derivative used for the treatment of staphylococcal infections, including strains which are penicillin resistant. It penetrates tissues including bone well. It is usually used in conjunction with flucloxacillin for serious staphylococcal infections. It is also available as eye drops for bacterial conjunctivitis.

Mechanism of action

Fucidin inhibits bacterial protein synthesis.

Adverse effects

Adverse effects are rare, but include cholestatic jaundice.

Pharmacokinetics

Fucidin is administered either orally or intravenously. Its half-life is 4–6 hours. It is excreted primarily via the liver.

Vancomycin

Uses and antibacterial spectrum

Vancomycin is valuable in resistant infections due to *Staph. pyogenes*. It is also rarely used for treating other infections, for example *Staph. epidermidis* endocarditis, and is given orally for the treatment of pseudomembranous colitis caused by *Clostridium difficile*.

Mechanism of action

Vancomycin inhibits bacterial cell wall synthesis.

Adverse effects

1. Hearing loss.
2. Venous thrombosis at infusion site.
3. 'Red man' syndrome due to cytokine/histamine release following excessively rapid intravenous administration.

4. Hypersensitivity: rashes etc.
5. Nephrotoxicity.

Pharmacokinetics

Vancomycin is not absorbed from the gut, and is usually given as an intravenous infusion. It is eliminated by the kidneys. Because of its concentration-related toxicity the dose is adjusted according to plasma concentration monitoring.

Teicoplanin

Teicoplanin has a longer duration of action but is otherwise similar to vancomycin.

Metronidazole

Use

Metronidazole is a synthetic drug with high activity against anaerobic bacteria, including *C. welchii* and *Bacteroides fragilis*. It is also active against several medically important protozoa and parasites (chapter 44). It is used to treat trichomonal infections, amebic dysentry, giardiasis, gas gangrene, pseudomembranous colitis and various abdominal infections, lung abscess and dental sepsis. It is widely used prophylactically before abdominal surgery.

Mechanism of action

Metronidazole binds to DNA and causes strand breakage; in addition it acts as an electron acceptor for flavoproteins and ferredoxins.

Adverse effects

1. Nausea and vomiting.
2. Peripheral neuropathy.
3. Convulsions, headaches.
4. Hepatitis.

Pharmacokinetics

Metronidazole is well absorbed after oral or rectal administration, but is too often administered by the relatively expensive intravenous route. The half-life is approximately 6 hours. It is eliminated by a combination of hepatic metabolism and renal excretion. Dose reduction is required in renal impairment.

Drug interactions

Metronidazole interacts with alcohol because it inhibits aldehyde dehydrogenase and consequently causes a disulfiram-like reaction. It is a weak inhibitor of cytochrome P$_{450}$.

Sulfonamides and trimethoprim

Sulfonamides and trimethoprim inhibit the production of folic acid at different sites of its synthetic pathway, and are synergistic *in vitro*. There is now widespread resistance to sulfonamides and they have largely been replaced by more active and less toxic antibacterial agents. Sulfonamides, for example sulfadimidine, alone are occasionally used to treat urinary tract infections. The sulfamethoxazole–trimethoprim combination (co-trimoxazole) is effective in urinary tract infections, prostatitis, exacerbations of chronic bronchitis and invasive *Salmonella* infections but with the exception of *Pneumocystis carinii* infections (when high doses are used), trimethoprim alone is generally preferred as it avoids sulfonamide side effects whilst having similar efficacy *in vivo*.

SULFONAMIDES

Adverse effects

Sulfonamides frequently cause unwanted effects including hypersensitivity reactions such as rashes, fever and serum sickness-like syndrome and Stevens–Johnson syndrome. The latter is much more common with long-acting preparations. Rarely, agranulocytosis, megaloblastic, aplastic, hemolytic anemia and thrombocytopenia occur. Sulfonamides are

oxidants and can precipitate hemolytic anemia in glucose-6-phosphate dehydrogenase (G6PD)-deficient individuals.

Pharmacokinetics

Sulfonamides are generally well absorbed after oral administration and widely distributed to body compartments. Acetylation and glucuronidation are the most important metabolic pathways. Some of the older sulfonamides precipitate in acid urine. The half-life of sulfamethoxazole is 11 hours and sulfadoxine 120–200 hours.

Drug interactions

Sulfonamides potentiate the action of sulfonylureas, oral anticoagulants, phenytoin and methotrexate due to inhibition of metabolism.

TRIMETHOPRIM

Use

Trimethoprim is a broad-spectrum antibacterial drug and has largely taken the place of co-trimoxazole in the treatment of urinary tract infections, acute and chronic bronchitis.

Adverse effects

Trimethoprim is generally well tolerated but occasionally causes gastrointestinal disturbances, skin reactions and, rarely, bone marrow depression.

Pharmacokinetics

Trimethoprim is well absorbed, highly lipid soluble and widely distributed in the body. At least 65% is eliminated unchanged in the urine. Trimethoprim competes for the same renal clearance pathway as creatinine.

Adverse effects

In addition to those associated with trimethoprim and sulfonamides, the high doses used in the management of *Pneumocystis* pneumonia in immunosuppressed patients cause vomiting (helped by prophylactic antiemetics), a higher incidence of serious skin reactions, hepatitis and thrombocytopenia.

Quinolones

Nalidixic acid has been available for over 20 years but low activity, poor tissue distribution and adverse effects limited its use to being a second- or third-line treatment for urinary tract infection. Changes to the basic quinolone structure such as the addition of fluorine and a piperazine ring have dramatically increased antibacterial potency, particularly against *Pseudomonas aeruginosa*. Oral bioavailability is good and thus the 4-fluoroquinolones offer an oral alternative to parenteral aminoglycosides and antipseudomonal penicillins for treatment of *Pseudomonas* urinary and chest infections. Although the 4-fluoroquinolones have a very broad spectrum of activity, all those presently available have very limited activity against streptococci. There is most experience with ciprofloxacin which has the additional advantage of being available for intravenous use. The quinolones inhibit bacterial DNA gyrase.

Use

Ciprofloxacin is used for respiratory (**but not pneumococcal**), urinary, gastrointestinal and genital infections, septicemia and meningococcal meningitis contacts. In addition to *Pseudomonas* it is particularly active against infection with *Salmonella, Shigella, Campylobacter, Neisseria* and *Chlamydia*. The licensed indications for the other quinolones are more limited. The indiscriminate use of these expensive agents is likely to lead to unnecessary bacterial resistance: the 4-fluoroquinolones have some unique attributes amongst antibacterial agents and their widespread prescription when equally effective and safe agents are available is to be deplored.

Adverse effects

Ciprofloxacin is generally well tolerated but should be avoided by epileptics (rarely causes convulsions), children (causes arthritis in growing animals) and those with G6PD deficiency. Anaphylaxis, nephritis, vasculitis, dizziness, hepatic and renal damage have all been reported. An excessively alkaline urine and dehydration can cause crystallization.

Pharmacokinetics

Approximately 80% of an oral dose of ciprofloxacin is systemically available. It is widely distributed entering all body compartments including the eye and CSF. Ciprofloxacin is removed primarily by glomerular filtration and tubular secretion. The half-life is 4 hours.

Drug interactions

Coadministration of ciprofloxacin and theophylline causes elevated blood theophylline concentrations due to inhibition of cytochrome P_{450}. As both drugs are epileptogenic this is particularly significant.

Mycobacterial Infections

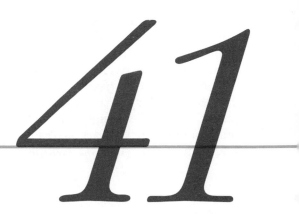

Introduction **542**

Principles of management of tuberculosis **542**

First-line drugs in tuberculosis therapy **543**

Treatment of tuberculous meningitis **546**

Chemoprophylaxis **547**

Acquired immune deficiency syndrome (AIDS) and tuberculosis **547**

Role of corticosteroids in tuberculosis therapy **547**

Second-line drugs for the treatment of resistant tuberculosis **547**

Mycobacterium leprae *infection* **548**

INTRODUCTION

Tuberculosis ('consumption') was the commonest cause of death in Victorian England, but its prevalence fell with the great improvements in living standards that occurred in the twentieth century. However, the incidence of *Mycobacterium tuberculosis* infection in the UK is once again increasing particularly in immigrants and in human immunodeficiency virus (HIV)-related cases. Infection with *Mycobacterium tuberculosis* usually occurs in the lungs, but can affect any organ, especially lymph nodes, gut, meninges, bone, adrenals or urogenital tract. Other atypical (non-tuberculous) mycobacterial infections are less common, but are occurring with increasing frequency in HIV-1 infected individuals. *Mycobacterium tuberculosis* is an intracellular organism, an obligate aerobe, in keeping with its predilection for the well-ventilated apical segments of the lung.

PRINCIPLES OF MANAGEMENT OF TUBERCULOSIS

The treatment of tuberculosis requires combination therapy with more than one (initially three or four) drugs. The rationale for this is that by using several drugs one is less likely to encounter a bacterium resistant to all agents, and therefore it is more likely to achieve a cure, with a low relapse rate (<2%). Development of resistance is thereby avoided.

Following several Medical Research Council (MRC) clinical trials in Hong Kong and East Africa, the British Thoracic Society now recommends standard therapy for pulmonary tuberculosis for 6 months (longer regimes were used previously). A combination of isoniazid, rifampicin, pyrazinamide and ethambutol (or streptomycin) is administered for the first 2 months, followed by rifampicin and isoniazid for a further 4 months. Ethambutol and/or streptomycin may be omitted in patients who are at a relatively low risk of carrying bacilli resistant to isoniazid, which includes 99% of the UK born population. The initial use, however, of four drugs is advisable in immigrants from countries where bacterial resistance to isoniazid is more frequent. In such patients initial use of three drugs might lead to a higher incidence of treatment failures, because the organism would only be sensitive to rifampicin and pyrazinamide – not the most effective antituberculous combination. Initial four-drug combination therapy should also be used in all patients with non-tuberculous mycobacterial infection, which often involves organisms that are resistant to both isoniazid and pyrazinamide. Patients with open active tuberculosis are initially isolated on the ward to reduce the risk of spread, but may usually be taken out of isolation after 5–7 days' therapy.

In cases where compliance with a daily regimen is a problem, the initial 2 months of triple or quadruple chemotherapy can be given on an intermittent supervised basis twice or three times a week. At the end of the 2-month period the precise identification and sensitivities of the organism will be available. If they are fully sensitive treatment will continue with daily or intermittent rifampicin and isoniazid for a further 4 months. After 6 months, treatment can usually be discontinued unless the sputum remains positive, or the patient is immunocompromised or poorly compliant. If the initial drug sensitivities reveal isoniazid resistance, treatment with ethambutol plus rifampicin must be continued for a total of 12 months. The duration of chemotherapy will also need to be extended if either isoniazid, rifampicin or pyrazinamide have to be discontinued because of side effects.

The usual drug doses for daily and intermittent treatment are shown in Table 41.1.

The regimens described are applicable to patients infected with bacilli either fully sensitive or resistant to only isoniazid and/or streptomycin. The treatment of tuberculosis which is resistant to multiple drugs is more difficult, regimens having to be individualized according to the drug resistance pattern.

Table 41.1 Dose of commonly used antituberculous drugs (mg).

	Daily dosing mg		Twice weekly dosing mg		Thrice weekly dosing mg	
	Weight <50 kg	Weight >50 kg	Weight <50 kg	Weight >50 kg	Weight <50 kg	Weight >50 kg
Isoniazid	300	300	15 mg/kg	15 mg/kg	15 mg/kg	15 mg/kg
Rifampicin	450	600	600	600–900	600	600–900
Pyrazinamide	1500	2000	3000	3500	2000	2500
Ethambutol	15 mg/kg	15 mg/kg	45 mg/kg	45 mg/kg	30 mg/kg	30 mg/kg
Streptomycin	750*	1000†	750*	1000†	750*	1000*

* Reduced to 500 mg in patients 40–60 years old.
† Reduced to 750 mg in patients 40–60 years old.

*F*IRST-LINE DRUGS IN TUBERCULOSIS THERAPY

ISONIAZID (ISONICOTINIC ACID HYDRAZIDE)

Use

This is one of the most important agents for the treatment of tuberculosis. It is bactericidal only to *Mycobacterium tuberculosis* with a minimal inhibitory concentration (MIC) of about 0.2 μg/ml. In tuberculosis a daily dose of 5 mg/kg (Table 41.1) for adults and 6 mg/kg for children is usually employed. High doses are used in tuberculous meningitis, where an injectable preparation is available for patients unable to take oral drugs. Isoniazid is often given in combination with ethambutol or rifampicin. When using high dose isoniazid (e.g. treating tuberculous meningitis) or in patients with special risk factors (e.g. diabetes, alcoholism) pyridoxine, 20 mg, daily is given to prevent peripheral neuropathy (chapter 32).

Mechanism of action

Isoniazid acts only on growing bacteria, possibly by interference with the synthesis of mycolic acid, a constituent of the bacterial wall.

Adverse effects

Toxic effects are uncommon with the usual dose of 300 mg/day.

1. Restlessness, insomnia and muscle twitching.
2. Peripheral neuropathy, which is commoner in patients who are slow acetylators, and which may be prevented by pyridoxine administration of 10–20 mg daily.
3. Hepatitis, clinically significant in 1% of patients; rarely hepatic necrosis. It is possible that acetylisoniazid is responsible for this effect, since enzyme inducers such as

rifampicin result in higher binding of the acetyl metabolite in the liver and are associated with increased toxicity.

4. Drug-induced systemic lupus erythematosus.

Pharmacokinetics

Isoniazid is readily absorbed from the gut, diffuses well into the body tissues, including the cerebrospinal fluid (CSF), and penetrates into macrophages so that it is effective against intracellular tubercle bacilli. It undergoes genetically controlled polymorphic acetylation in the liver (chapter 13). The proportion of a given population characterized as fast or slow acetylators depends upon the group's ethnic make-up, a high percentage of fast acetylators being found in Japanese and Eskimo populations. In European populations 40–45% are rapid acetylators. The half-life ($t_{1/2}$) of isoniazid is less than 80 min in fast acetylators and greater than 140 min in slow acetylators. Fifty to seventy per cent of a dose is excreted in the urine within 24 hours as metabolite or free drug. Impaired renal function is not usually a problem, but abnormally high and potentially toxic levels may be reached in slow acetylators with renal impairment.

Drug interactions

Isoniazid is partly metabolized by hepatic cytochrome P_{450}, and inhibits metabolism of certain drugs, for example, phenytoin and carbamazepine, thereby causing toxicity in some patients. Prednisolone causes a significant decrease in the plasma concentrations of isoniazid because of enhanced metabolism and renal clearance. Isoniazid antagonizes the hypoglycemic effect of insulin.

RIFAMPICIN

Use

Rifampicin is a derivative of rifamycin which is produced by *Streptomyces mediterranei*. Tubercle bacilli are inhibited at concentrations well below 0.5 µg/ml. Rifampicin is given as 450–600 mg once daily before meals (Table 41.1). It is also used in the treatment of nasopharyngeal meningococcal carriers since it is present in saliva, the dose being 600 mg twice daily for 2 days or 2400 mg once daily. It is also used in other severe infections such as Legionnaires' disease (600 mg daily by intravenous infusion).

Mechanism of action

Rifampicin acts by inhibiting bacterial RNA polymerase and because of its high lipid solubility it diffuses easily through cell membranes to kill intracellular bacteria.

Adverse effects

The use of large doses (as in intermittent therapy) produces toxic effects in about one-third of patients:

1. After a few hours influenza-like symptoms, flushing and rashes occur.
2. Abdominal pain.
3. Hepatotoxicity: hepatitis and cholestatic jaundice occur and it is important to measure pre- and intratreatment serum aminotransferases. Serious liver damage is uncommon but minor histological changes and rises in aminotransferase are common and in the absence of jaundice are not an indication for stopping treatment.
4. Thrombocytopenia is rare.
5. Urine and tears become pink/red which may be a useful guide to compliance with therapy.

Pharmacokinetics

Absorption from the gut is almost complete but is delayed by food. Peak plasma levels of about 10 µg/ml are reached 3 hours after a single oral dose of 600 mg and significant levels persist for 12 hours. The $t_{1/2}$ is 1–5 hours. Renal insufficiency does not significantly raise plasma concentrations of rifampicin. Eighty-five to ninety per cent of the drug is protein bound in plasma but rifampicin penetrates well into most tissues, cavities and exudates, although relatively little enters the brain and CSF. It is metabolized by deacetylation and is excreted mainly in the bile. The drug and its metabolite undergo prolonged enterohepatic circulation. Higher plasma levels and a longer $t_{1/2}$ follow administration of probenecid. Toxicity is increased by biliary obstruction or impaired liver function. Less than 10% appears unchanged in the urine.

Drug interactions

Rifampicin markedly induces hepatic microsomal cytochrome P_{450} activity thereby accelerating the metabolism of several commonly used drugs:

- Corticosteroids.
- Warfarin.
- Estrogens. In women using the contraceptive pill an alternative method of contraception should be provided.

ETHAMBUTOL

This is the D-isomer of ethylenediimino dibutanol. It inhibits about 75% of strains of *M. tuberculosis* at a concentration of 1 µg/ml. Other organisms are completely resistant. Resistance to ethambutol develops slowly and the drug inhibits strains that are resistant to isoniazid or streptomycin. The daily dose is 15–25 mg/kg (Table 41.1).

Mechanism of action

The cellular mechanism of action of ethambutol is not clear. It inhibits bacterial cell wall synthesis and is bacteriostatic.

Adverse effects

1. Retrobulbar neuritis with scotomata and loss of visual acuity occurs in 10% of patients on the higher dose. The first signs are loss of red-green perception. Prompt withdrawal of the drug may be followed by recovery. Testing of color vision and visual fields should precede treatment and the patient should be regularly examined for visual disturbances.
2. Rashes, pruritus, joint pains.
3. Nausea, abdominal pain.
4. Confusion, hallucinations.
5. Peripheral neuropathy.

Pharmacokinetics

Ethambutol is well absorbed (75–80%) from the intestine, and a single dose of 25 mg/kg gives a peak plasma level of 5 µg/ml at 2-4 hours. The plasma $t_{1/2}$ is 5–6 hours. The drug is concentrated in red cells and this provides a depot for entry into the plasma. About 80% is excreted unchanged in the urine. Ethambutol is contraindicated in renal failure.

PYRAZINAMIDE

Use

This is a powerful drug which is well tolerated in a oral dose of 20–35 mg/kg (maximum 3.0 g, Table 41.1). Because of its ability to kill bacteria in the acid intracellular environment of a macrophage it exerts its main effects in the first 2–3 months of therapy, and is most active against slowly or intermittently metabolizing organisms. It is inactive against atypical mycobacteria. Resistance to pyrazinamide develops quickly if used alone.

Mechanism of action

The enzyme pyrazinamidase in mycobacteria cleaves off the amide portion of the molecule producing pyrazinoic acid which is bacteriocidal by unknown mechanisms.

Adverse effects

1. Hyperuricemia which may precipitate gout.
2. Pretreatment hepatic enzymes must be measured, as about 5–15% of patients develop hepatotoxicity. Measurements must be repeated during treatment. It should be avoided if there is a history of alcohol abuse and treatment should not be continued for more than 2 months.
3. Rashes and photosensitivity.
4. Sideroblastic anemia.
5. Hypoglycemia, probably due to increased glucose uptake by adipose tissue.

Pharmacokinetics

Pyrazinamide is converted in the liver by an amidase to pyrazinoic acid and this undergoes further metabolism to hydroxypyrazinoic acid by xanthine oxidase. Peak concentrations of the metabolites occur 6 hours after oral administration. Pyrazinamide is almost completely absorbed and $t_{1/2}$ is 11–24 hours. Pyrazinamide and its metabolites are excreted via the kidney, and renal failure necessitates dose reduction. It crosses the blood–brain barrier to achieve therapeutic CSF concentrations almost equal to those in the plasma and is therefore a drug of first choice in tuberculous meningitis.

STREPTOMYCIN

Use

This is an aminoglycoside antibiotic. It has a wide spectrum of antibacterial activity but is primarily used to treat mycobacterial infections. It is only given parenterally (intramuscularly). Once daily dosing of 0.75–1.0 g is adequate. Therapeutic drug monitoring of trough plasma concentrations may be performed to minimize the risk of toxicity.

Mechanism of action

As with other aminoglycosides it is actively transported across the bacterial cell wall and its antibacterial activity is due to it binding to the 30S subunit of the bacterial ribosome and inhibiting protein synthesis.

Adverse effects

These are the same as for other aminoglycosides (chapter 40). The main problems are eighth nerve toxicity (vestibulotoxicity more than deafness), nephrotoxicty and, less commonly, allergic reactions.

Contraindications

Streptomycin is contraindicated in patients with eighth nerve dysfunction, pregnancy, and those with myasthenia gravis as it has weak neuromuscular blocking activity.

Pharmacokinetics

Oral absorption is minimal. Streptomycin is mainly excreted via the kidney and dosage requires adjustment in renal impairment. The $t_{1/2}$ of streptomycin varies from 2 to 9 hours. It crosses the blood–brain barrier when the meninges are inflamed.

TREATMENT OF TUBERCULOUS MENINGITIS

Many of the problems in treating tuberculous meningitis arise from the poor penetration of most antimicrobials into the CSF. Pyrazinamide and isoniazid are the most useful drugs. They are highly effective and achieve concentrations in the CSF that are inhibitory to tubercle bacilli. Streptomycin penetrates well only when the meninges are inflamed and therefore is only effective in the early stages of treatment. Ethambutol is also used with satisfactory penetration in the acute stage of the disease, particularly with higher dosage levels. Rifampicin penetrates poorly into the CSF presumably because of the high protein-bound fraction in the plasma and the concentration in the CSF only just reaches the MIC for tubercle bacilli.

The optimal regimen for treating tuberculous meningeal infection is yet to be defined. The following is often satisfactory: isoniazid, 10 mg/kg, with pyridoxine, 20 mg, daily; rifampicin, 10mg/kg, daily; pyrazinamide, 30 mg/kg, daily and either ethambutol, 15 mg/kg, daily or streptomycin, 0.75-1.0 g, daily. After 2 months the regimen should be modified to the first three anti-tuberculous drugs. After 6 months treatment should be continued with isoniazid and rifampicin for at least a further 12 months. Corticosteroids are used in the initial stages of treatment in the hope of reducing the risk of meningeal adhesions and obstructive hydrocephalus.

CHEMOPROPHYLAXIS

Contacts of patients with tuberculosis who are under 16 years of age with a positive reaction to tuberculin but no other evidence of disease should be considered for chemoprophylaxis. The usual regimen is isoniazid, 300 mg, daily for 6 months, but with the increasing resistance of the mycobacterium to isoniazid, the use of daily rifampicin, 450–600 mg, combined with isoniazid is being evaluated.

ACQUIRED IMMUNE DEFICIENCY SYNDROME (AIDS) AND TUBERCULOSIS THERAPY

The immunocompromised state in HIV infection increases the difficulty of eradicating the tubercle bacillus. The absence of normal immune defenses necessitates prolonged courses of therapy. Treatment is continued for 9 months or for 6 months after the time of documented culture conversion, whichever is longer.

ROLE OF CORTICOSTEROIDS IN TUBERCULOSIS THERAPY

Corticosteroids are not often necessary in tuberculosis therapy but may assist in the resolution of large lymph nodes; suppression of severe drug allergy; advanced pleural effusions; patients likely to die before chemotherapy can be effective; and tuberculous meningitis to reduce the formation of meningeal adhesions which could result in permanent neurological deficit. The only absolute indication for glucocorticoid treatment in patients with tuberculosis is adrenal failure (Addison's disease), which must not be forgotten since tuberculous adrenal disease is again increasing.

SECOND-LINE DRUGS FOR THE TREATMENT OF RESISTANT TUBERCULOSIS

The commonest cause of treatment failure or relapse is non-compliance with therapy. The previous drugs used should be known and current bacterial sensitivity found. If the organisms are still sensitive to the original drugs, then more fully supervised and prolonged therapy with these drugs should be prescribed. If bacterial resistance has arisen then alternative drugs are used, supervised by a clinician with experience in the use of such agents.

CAPREOMYCIN

This is an effective drug but, like other aminoglycosides, it can produce nephrotoxicity and ototoxicity. A daily intramuscular dose of 15 mg/kg does not usually produce toxic effects. Nevertheless blood concentrations should be monitored. Hypokalemia, hypocalcemia and hypomagnesemia can complicate capreomycin therapy and may require treatment.

ETHIONAMIDE AND PROTHIONAMIDE

Ethionamide and prothionamide both produce nausea after oral administration. They are given as a single daily dose in the late evening with a sedative. Other toxic effects include liver damage, neuropathy and mental disturbance.

CYCLOSERINE

Cycloserine is the most toxic of the second-line drugs. Epilepsy and toxic psychosis may occur even with therapeutic doses (1 g orally daily).

MYCOBACTERIUM LEPRAE INFECTION

This organism causes leprosy, an infection with two expressions: lepromatoid (the organism being localized to skin or nerve) or lepromatous (a generalized bacteremic disease affecting many organs, analogous to miliary tuberculosis). The main drugs used in therapy are dapsone and rifampicin. Dapsone is 4,4'-diaminodiphenyl sulfone, and is given as 100 mg (1–2 mg/kg/day) once daily. Rifampicin is a more expensive alternative, and as resistance develops quickly it must be given with a second agent. It is usually given as a single daily dose (450–600 mg orally). Other agents used in leprosy therapy are ethionamide, prothionamide and clofazimine. The advised World Health Organization (WHO) regimen for multibacillary leprosy is:

1. Rifampicin, 600 mg, orally once monthly.
2. Clofazimine, 50 mg, daily unsupervised plus 300 mg supervised every 4 weeks (chapter 43).
3. Dapsone, 100 mg, daily unsupervised given for 24 months.

DAPSONE

Use

Dapsone is a sulfonamide derivative and is a bacteriostatic sulfone. It has been the standard drug for treating all forms of leprosy, but irregular and inadequate duration of treatment as a single agent has produced resistance. Dapsone is used to treat leprosy, *Pneumocystis* infection, dermatitis herpetiformis and in a combined preparation with pyrimethamine for malaria. It is given as a once daily oral dose of 100 mg for leprosy.

Mechanism of action

Dapsone is a competitive inhibitor of dihydrofolate synthane, thereby blocking the production of dihydrofolic acid.

Adverse effects

1. Anemia and agranulocytosis.
2. Gastrointestinal disturbances and rarely hepatitis.
3. Allergy and rashes, including Stevens–Johnson syndrome.

4. Peripheral neuropathy.
5. Methemoglobinemia.
6. Hemolytic anemia, especially in glucose-6-phosphate dehydrogenase (G6PD) deficient patients in whom it is contraindicated.

Pharmacokinetics

Dapsone is well absorbed from the gastrointestinal tract (>90%) and widely distributed. The $t_{1/2}$ is long (average 27 hours). It is extensively metabolized in the liver partly by N-acetylation. There is some enterohepatic circulation, 10–20% of the drug being excreted unchanged in the urine.

Drug interactions

The metabolism of dapsone is increased by hepatic enzyme inducers such as rifampicin, so that the half-life is reduced to 12–15 hours.

Fungal and Viral Infections

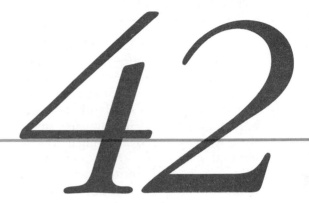

Antifungal drug therapy   **552**

Antiviral drug therapy   **557**

Interferons   **561**

Immunoglobulins   **563**

ANTIFUNGAL DRUG THERAPY

Introduction

Fungi, like mammalian cells but unlike bacteria, are eukaryotic and possess nuclei, mitochondria and cell membranes. Their membranes are unusual in containing distinctive sterols. The similarity between fungal and mammalian cells mitigates against selective toxicity and antifungal drugs are in general more toxic than antibacterial agents. The very success of antibacterial therapy has created ecological situations in which opportunistic fungal infections can flourish. In addition, potent immunosuppressive and cytotoxic therapies have produced patients with seriously impaired immune defenses, in whom fungi that are non-pathogenic to healthy individuals become pathogenic and cause disease. Table 42.1 summarizes an approach to antifungal therapy in the immunocompromised host.

Polyenes

AMPHOTERICIN B

Use

Amphotericin is uniquely valuable in treating life-threatening systemic fungal infections, but has considerable toxicity. It is an antibiotic derived from *Streptomyces nodosus* which was isolated from soil collected in the Orinoco basin in Venezuela. It is a polyene macrolide with a hydroxylated hydrophilic surface on one side of the molecule and an unsaturated conjugated lipophilic surface on the other. It is insoluble in water but can be complexed to bile salts to give an unstable colloid which can be given intravenously. Micellar preparations have recently been introduced. These are more stable and appear to cause less toxicity; they are, however, expensive and are often reserved

Table 42.1 Antifungal drug therapy in the immunocompromised host.

Fungal infection	Drug therapy for superficial infection	Drug therapy for deep-seated infection
Candida	Nystatin – topical Clotrimazole – topical Miconazole – topical Fluconazole – oral	Amphotericin B ± flucytosine Fluconazole – oral or i.v. Itraconazole – oral
Aspergillus		Amphotericin B i.v. Itraconazole
Cryptococcus		Amphortericin B i.v. ± flucytosine Itraconazole Fluconazole – oral or i.v.
Disseminated histoplasmosis		Amphotericin B i.v. Ketoconazole Itraconazole
Disseminated coccidiomycosis		Amphotericin B i.v. ?Itraconazole
Blastomycosis		Ketoconazole ?Itraconazole Amphotericin B i.v. for severe infection

for patients who experience unacceptable adverse effects from the regular formulation. Amphotericin B is given as an intravenous infusion freshly prepared in 5% dextrose over 4–6 hours. A test dose of 1 mg is given at least 6 hours before starting treatment. The initial dose is 5 mg daily in 500 ml of 5% dextrose which is increased daily by 5 mg to a dose of 0.5–1 mg/kg daily and continued for 6–12 weeks. Treatment on alternate days at 1–1.5 mg/kg may reduce toxicity. Amphotericin is also given topically as lozenges (10 mg 3 hourly) or suspension for oral or esophageal and gastrointestinal moniliasis, respectively. There is some evidence that effective therapy may be achieved by reduced doses and therefore lower toxicity if amphotericin is combined with 5-fluorocytosine. The dose of amphotericin should then be 0.3 mg/kg/day. The antifungal spectrum of amphotericin B is broad and includes: *Candida* spp. (local and systemic infections), *Blastomyces dermatitidis* (causes North American blastomycosis), *Histoplasma capsulatum* (causes histoplasmosis), *Cryptococcus neoformans* (causes cryptococcosis), *Coccidioides immitis* (causes coccidioidomycosis), *Sporotrichum schenckii* (causes local and systemic sporotrichosis). *Aspergillus* spp. are usually resistant. Resistance is seldom acquired during treatment.

Mechanism of action

Amphotericin binds to a sterol in fungal cell membranes and increases their permeability, allowing leakage and loss of small molecules such as glucose and potassium ions. Amphotericin has a higher affinity for the ergosterol of fungal membranes than for the cholesterol of mammalian membranes, resulting in clinically useful selectivity, although many of the adverse effects of amphotericin are due to similar toxic effects on mammalian membranes.

Adverse effects

1. Fever, chills, headache, nausea and vomiting, and hypotension during intravenous infusion. Pulse and temperature should be monitored every 30 min and the infusion can be halted if necessary.
2. Nephrotoxicity is almost invariable and results from vasoconstriction, tubular damage resulting in renal tubular acidosis, and acute renal failure. Fortunately most of these effects are reversible if detected early and the drug discontinued or the dose reduced.
3. Hypokalemia.
4. Normochromic normocytic anemia due to temporary marrow suppression is common.

Amphotericin B should not be withheld in serious progressive infection caused by a sensitive fungus despite toxic effects. Dose reduction may be appropriate.

Pharmacokinetics

Amphotericin is poorly absorbed following oral administration; therefore for systemic mycoses it must be given by intravenous infusion. Liposomal delivery systems deliver adequate plasma concentrations, with a lower incidence of toxicity. Given intravenously it distributes very unevenly throughout the body: concentrations in the CSF are only one-fortieth of the plasma concentration. It is concentrated in the reticuloendothelial system. The $t_{1/2}$ is 18–24 hours. Amphotericin B is over 90% protein bound. Only 5% is excreted in the urine and elimination is unaffected by renal failure.

NYSTATIN

Nystatin is another polyene antifungal antibiotic isolated from *Streptomyces* with an identical mode of action to amphotericin B, but its greater toxicity precludes systemic use. Nystatin has a broad antifungal spectrum. Its indications are limited to cutaneous and mucocutaneous infections, especially those caused by *Candida* spp. which do not gain resistance to nystatin during therapy. Epidermophytes are not sensitive. Preparations of nystatin include tablets, pastilles, lozenges or suspension, given in doses of 100 000–500 000 units three times daily for oral or intestinal *Candida* infections. Patients often prefer amphotericin B because nystatin has an intensely bitter taste. Cutaneous infections are treated with ointment, vaginitis by suppositories and aerosol has been used for bronchopulmonary fungal colonization.

Adverse effects

1. Adverse effects seldom result from the topical use of nystatin.
2. Large oral doses cause nausea and diarrhea.

Pharmacokinetics

Very little nystatin is absorbed from the gastrointestinal tract.

Griseofulvin

Use

Griseofulvin was isolated from *Penicillium griseofulvium*. It is systemically active, but unlike amphotericin is useful only for mild infections since its spectrum is limited to dermatophytes (ringworm fungi). Resistance is not a problem. Treatment is given orally (0.5–1 g daily in two divided doses) with meals. Treatment should be for 6 weeks in skin infections and up to 12 months for nail infections.

Mechanism of action

Griseofulvin is actively taken up by fungi. Its mode of action is obscure, but it binds to the microtubules that form the mitotic spindle and blocks polymerization of the microtubule. It also interferes with fungal DNA replication, resulting in distorted hyphal growth.

Adverse effects

1. Headaches and mental dullness or inattention (uncommon).
2. Diarrhea or nausea (uncommon).
3. Rashes.
4. Griseofulvin can precipitate attacks of acute intermittent porphyria.

Pharmacokinetics

Griseofulvin is nearly insoluble in water and is formulated as micronized particles. Its absorption is facilitated by a fatty meal. It has a slow onset of action because it must first be taken up into slow growing keratinized structures to reach the site of infection. Cell turnover time thus determines efficacy of treatment so that palmar and plantar skin requires at least 8 weeks' treatment, fingernails 6 months and toenails up to 1 year for eradicative treatment. Griseofulvin is metabolized by the liver to inactive 6-demethylgriseofulvin, which is excreted in the urine. Less than 1% free griseofulvin is renally excreted, so that it is used in usual doses in renal failure.

Drug interactions

Griseofulvin induces hepatic cytochrome P_{450} enzyme activity and consequently interacts with warfarin reducing its anticoagulant effect. Other inducing agents (e.g. rifampicin, barbiturates) enhance griseofulvin metabolism.

Flucytosine (5-fluorocytosine)

Use

Flucytosine is used for systemic candidiasis and cryptococcosis, providing the strain is sensitive. The optimal oral dose is 200 mg/kg/day in 6-hourly divided doses. For very ill patients an intravenous preparation is available. It is used in combination therapy with amphotericin. Topical use is unacceptable because of the danger of widespread emergence of resistant *Candida* spp.

Its spectrum is relatively restricted to *Cryptococcus neoformans, Candida albicans* and some other *Candida* spp., *Torulopsis* spp. and *Cladosporum* spp. There are big differences in sensitivity between strains: 5–15% have innate resistance, and resistance is relatively easily acquired during therapy. Filamentous fungi, especially *Aspergillus,* are resistant.

Mechanism of action

Flucytosine enters the fungus by active transport. Its precise mode of action is unknown. It is deaminated to 5-fluorouracil, a known antimetabolite that inhibits thymidylate synthetase thereby depressing DNA synthesis. Its relative specificity is due to the presence of cytosine deaminase in fungi but not in mammalian cells.

Adverse effects

Flucytosine is less toxic than amphotericin B.

1. Gastrointestinal upsets.
2. Leukopenia.
3. Hepatitis may occur so liver function tests should be monitored.

At plasma concentrations below 100 µg/ml there is little danger of toxicity. Depression of bone marrow and hepatotoxicity are associated with higher concentrations. Plasma drug assays are useful in patients with impaired renal function.

Pharmacokinetics

Flucytosine is well absorbed from the gut, peak concentrations of 75–90 µg/ml being attained on a dose of 50 mg/kg 6 hourly. It penetrates adequately into CSF, in contrast to amphotericin B, and is consequently particularly useful when combined with amphotericin in treating cryptococcal meningitis. It is largely excreted unchanged by glomerular filtration with less than 10% of the dose undergoing metabolism. The $t_{1/2}$ is 6 hours and this is increased in renal failure.

Drug interactions

The effect of flucytosine is antagonized by concurrent administration of cytosine arabinoside. Amphotericin acts additively or synergistically with flucytosine, and flucytosine should always be used with amphotericin. This combination is useful because amphotericin is more effective but more toxic than flucytosine which also penetrates the blood–brain barrier better than amphotericin. Concurrent use of amphotericin reduces the likelihood of resistance to flucytosine emerging during therapy.

Imidazoles

Imidazole antifungal drugs are fungistatic at low concentrations and fungicidal at higher concentrations. They are used topically and are active against both dermatophytes and yeasts such as *Candida*. Some imidazoles are also used systemically although they have limited efficacy and significant toxicity, limiting systemic use. They act similarly to one another by inhibiting fungal ergosterol synthesis. Ergosterol is an important constituent of fungal membranes. Imidazoles inhibit lanosterol 14α-demethylase (which is a fungal cytochrome P_{450} enzyme) and have considerable specificity for fungal cytochromes. Membrane leakage and dysfunction of membrane adenosine triphosphatase (ATPase) ensue.

KETOCONAZOLE

Use

Ketoconazole is used as oral or topical therapy for dermatophytic infections and some phycomycetes. It is active against systemic infection with *Candida, Blastomyces, Histoplasma capsulatum* and *Cryptococcus neoformans. Aspergillus* and *Mucor* spp. are resistant. It is given orally (200–400 mg once daily). Its systemic use has waned because of the high incidence of hepatic and endocrine side effects.

Adverse effects

1. Nausea and vomiting, reduced by giving the drug with food.
2. Transient liver function abnormalities in 5–10% of patients; fulminant hepatic damage, jaundice and fever are rare.
3. Gynecomastia (by blocking testosterone synthesis).
4. Impotence and azoospermia.
5. Adrenal insufficency (by inhibiting cortisol biosynthesis).

Pharmacokinetics

Ketoconazole is given orally and achieves maximum plasma concentrations in 1–2 hours. It is approximately 90% protein bound but is nevertheless still relatively widely distributed in the tissues. Cerebrospinal fluid concentrations, however, are only 5% of that in the plasma. It is extensively metabolized by hydroxylation and oxidative N-dealkylation by the liver, and only 2–4% of the dose is found in the urine as parent drug. The mean elimination $t_{1/2}$ is 8 hours.

Drug interactions

- Antacids and H_2-blockers reduce ketoconazole absorption.
- Ketoconazole reduces the metabolism of cyclosporin, enhancing its nephrotoxcity.
- Warfarin metabolism is unaffected.
- Rifampicin increases the metabolism of ketoconazole.
- Ketoconazole should not be used with amphotericin B because it reduces its effectiveness.

CLOTRIMAZOLE

This imidazole is only used for topical treatment of *Candida* or dermatophyte infections as a 1% cream, solution or powder. It is poorly absorbed from the gastrointestinal tract and induces its own metabolism, therefore it is not used systemically.

MICONAZOLE

Miconazole (2% cream or powder applied twice daily) is used topically to treat cutaneous *Candida*, ringworm and pityriasis rosea. It is only used intravenously to treat *Pseudoallecheria boydii*. It is poorly absorbed, and extensively metabolized by the liver; only 3% of a dose is found in the urine. It has a short plasma elimination $t_{1/2}$ of 30 min. If given intravenously it can cause nausea, vomiting, fevers, chills and fits.

Triazoles

This group of drugs (e.g. fluconazole) is derived from the imidazoles. They are nitroimidazoles and have a wider antifungal spectrum. Their mechanism of action is identical to that of other imidazoles (e.g. ketoconazole), by inhibition of lanosterol α-demethylase. Fluconazole is however far more specific for this fungal cytochrome P_{450} enzyme and consequently less liable to cause adverse effects due to inhibition of human steroid biosynthetic enzymes for testosterone or cortisol.

FLUCONAZOLE

Use

Fluconazole is a potent and broad-spectrum antifungal agent. It is active against *Candida* spp., *Cryptococcus neoformans*, *Histoplasma capsulatum. Cryptococcus cruseii* and *Aspergillus* spp are resistant however. It is used clinically to treat superficial *Candida* infections and esophageal *Candida*, for the acute therapy of disseminated *Candida*, systemic therapy for blastomycosis and histoplasmosis, for dermatophytic fungal infections and prophylaxis in neutropenic patients. It may be given orally or intravenously as a once daily dose. For superficial infections it is given as 50–100 mg/day. In systemic or meningitic infections 200–400 mg intravenously daily is required for 4–6 weeks, followed by a daily maintenance dose. For prophylaxis in cytotoxic immunosuppressed patients 50–100 mg is adequate.

Adverse effects

Unlike ketoconazole, fluconazole does not reduce the synthesis of testosterone or cortisol.

1. Gastrointestinal upsets with nausea, abdominal distension, diarrhea and flatulence.
2. Skin rashes – erythema multiforme.
3. Hepatitis – raised liver enzymes.

Contraindications

Fluconazole is contraindicated in pregnancy because of fetal defects in rodents. Breast milk concentrations are similar to those in plasma, and fluconazole should not be used in nursing mothers.

Pharmacokinetics

Fluconazole is absorbed rapidly after oral administration with maximum plasma concentrations achieved within 1–2 hours.

Absorption is virtually complete and is unaffected by food or gastric pH. There is no presystemic metabolism. Mean $t_{1/2}$ is 30 hours. Fluconazole is only 11% bound to plasma proteins and is widely distributed throughout the body penetrating the CSF well. It is excreted 80% by the kidney, and dose reduction is needed in renal failure. Fluconazole is a weak inhibitor of human hepatic cytochrome P_{450}.

Drug interactions

Fluconazole reduces the metabolism of phenytoin, and possibly cyclosporin. Plasma concentrations of these drugs should be monitored during concomitant treatment with fluconazole. Rifampicin enhances the metabolism of fluconazole.

ITRACONAZOLE

Itraconazole is similar to fluconazole in its antifungal spectrum and mechanism of action. It is given orally once daily as a 100 mg dose to treat dermatophyte infections, superficial oropharyngeal candidiasis and pityriasis versicolor. It is 85% absorbed from the gastrointestinal tract and undergoes 45% presystemic metabolism and is almost totally excreted by hepatic metabolism. It is highly protein bound (99 %) with a plasma $t_{1/2}$ of 20 hours. Its major side effects are gastrointestinal disturbances. It causes several adverse drug interactions, increasing cyclosporin and warfarin plasma concentrations. Rifampicin, phenobarbitone and phenytoin increase itraconazole metabolism. It does not cause the endocrine problems of ketoconazole.

TIACONAZAOLE

Tiaconazole is a broad-spectrum antifungal triazole, marketed only as a solution for topical administration to treat nail infections with dermatophytes and yeasts. No other topical imidazole preparations are effective in fungal nail infections. The recommended duration of therapy is 6–12 months. Systemic absorption after topical application is negligible, local irritation is the only reported side effect.

Terbinafine

Terbinafine is an allylamine, and is fungicidal. It can be given orally and is used to treat ringworm (tinea pedis, cruris or corporis) or dermatophyte infections of the nails if oral therapy is considered appropriate. It is given 250 mg once daily for 2–6 weeks or longer in infections of the nailbed as an alternative to griseofulvin. It acts by inhibiting sterol synthesis by the fungal enzyme squalene epoxidase. It does not interfere with human cytochrome P_{450}. It is well absorbed, strongly bound to plasma proteins and concentrated in the stratum corneum. It is eliminated by hepatic metabolism and the mean elimination $t_{1/2}$ is 17 hours. Its major side effects are nausea, abdominal discomfort, anorexia, diarrhea and rashes (including urticaria). Dose reduction is needed in hepatic failure and if cimetidine is given concurrently. Rifampicin increases its metabolism.

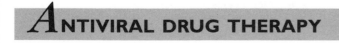

ANTIVIRAL DRUG THERAPY

Introduction

Many viral illnesses are mild and/or self-limiting, but a few are inherently deadly (witness the now extinct smallpox, and the all too prevalent AIDS). Patients who are immunocompromised, especially by AIDS, are also at risk of serious illness from viruses that are seldom serious in otherwise healthy hosts.

Antiviral drug therapy is therefore increasingly important, and is considered in this section apart from human immunodeficiency virus (HIV), which is considered separately in chapter 43. Antiviral chemotherapy is intrinsically more difficult than antibacterial therapy because:

1. Viral replication is essentially intracellular so that drugs must penetrate cells to be effective.
2. Viral replication, although under the control of the viral genome, involves metabolic processes of the host cells.
3. Although viral replication begins almost immediately the host cell is penetrated, the clinical signs and symptoms of infection often appear after peak replication is over. Clinical manifestations often result from inflammatory and other processes mounted by the host in response to viral damage to tissues.
4. Few viral infections can be routinely rapidly and specifically diagnosed with certainty using present techniques.

There are some events in viral colonization which might be susceptible to drug action:

1. When the virus is outside cells it is susceptible to antibody attack, but it has proved difficult to find drugs that are non-toxic yet can destroy viruses in this situation.
2. Viral attachment to the cell surface probably involves a specific chemical reaction between the virus coat and the cell surface. Neuraminidase, an enzyme that destroys myxovirus receptors, including those on cell surfaces, has an effect on experimental infections in animals.
3. Penetration of the cell membrane can be prevented (e.g. by amantadine for influenza A).
4. Uncoating of the virus with release of viral nucleic acid intracellularly.
5. Viral nucleic acid acts as a template for new strands of nucleic acid that in turn direct the production of new viral components utilizing the host cell's synthetic mechanisms. Most antiviral drugs in current use act at this stage of viral growth.
6. Release of new viral particles.

ACYCLOVIR

Use

Acyclovir is a potent and selective inhibitor of herpes viruses (particularly herpes simplex). It is also effective against herpes zoster but much less active against cytomegalovirus (which also belongs to the group of herpes viruses).

1. Three per cent acylovir ointment applied five times daily for up to 14 days accelerates healing in herpetic keratitis.
2. The efficacy of local application of acylovir in genital and labial herpes simplex has been unimpressive. In spite of its low bioavailability, 200 mg five times daily orally accelerates healing in genital herpes. It is much less effective in secondary than primary infection. It does not eliminate vaginal carriage, so Cesarian section is indicated to avoid neonatal herpes.
3. Treatment of shingles (herpes zoster) should be started within 72 hours of the onset, and is useful for patients with severe pain, although it shortens the illness by only a short time and is expensive. Acyclovir, 800 mg, five times a day is given for 7 days.
4. In generalized herpes simplex or herpetic meningoencephalitis acyclovir can be given intravenously in doses of 5 mg/kg infused intravenously over 1 hour three times daily for 5 days. The acyclovir dose in immunocompromised hosts with herpes simplex, shingles or herpes simplex encephalitis is 10 mg/kg intravenously three times daily for at least 10 days. Reduced dosage is required for patients with impaired renal function.

Mechanism of action

Acyclovir is a cyclic analog of the purine guanosine. Its selective action results from metabolic activation to its monophosphate, solely in infected cells, via a specific thymidine kinase coded for by the virus but not by the host genome. Acyclovir monophosphate is converted to the di- and triphosphates and the triphosphate inhibits viral DNA synthesis.

Adverse effects

1. Reversible rise in plasma urea and creatinine.
2. Neurological disturbances.
3. Rashes.
4. Nausea and vomiting.
5. Increase in liver enzymes.

Contraindications

Acyclovir is contraindicated in pregnancy as it is an analog of guanosine and so potentially teratogenic.

Pharmacokinetics

Bioavailability in humans is only 20% after 200 mg orally and may be dose dependent. The mean $t_{1/2}$ is 3 hours. Acyclovir crosses the blood–brain barrier to give a CSF concentration of approximately 50% of the plasma concentration. Plasma protein binding is approximately 20%. Clearance is largely renal and includes an element of tubular secretion; renal impairment reduces clearance.

Drug interactions

Probenecid prolongs the half-life of acyclovir by 20%, by inhibiting renal tubular secretion.

AMANTADINE

Amantadine has a prophylactic action in preventing the spread of influenza A, and also has an unrelated action in Parkinson's disease (chapter 18). Its usefulness as an antiviral agent is limited to influenza A: it is inactive on influenza B and only weakly active on influenza C and rubella. These are all RNA viruses. Its mode of action is unknown. Prophylaxis with amantadine (200 mg daily) has an advantage over immunization in that the latter can be ineffective when a new antigenic variant arises in the community and spreads too rapidly for a killed virus vaccine to be prepared and administered. Prophylaxis by amantadine during an epidemic should be considered for persons at special risk, for example with severe lung or cardiac disease. Amantadine is less effective during periods of antigenic variation than during periods of relative antigenic stability. The effectiveness of amantadine as treatment rather than prophy-

laxis when given during the first 48 hours of illness is slight: fever is shortened by 24–30 hours and headache and respiratory symptoms are reduced. The mean $t_{1/2}$ is approximately 12 hours. Amantadine is eliminated by renal excretion and precautions are needed when it is given to patients with renal failure.

Adverse effects

1. Dizziness, nervousness and headaches with short-term use.
2. Livedo reticularis.

FOSCARNET (TRISODIUM PHOSPHONOFORMATE)

Use

Foscarnet was originally found to have activity against the influenza virus and more recently has been found to be active against several other important viruses, notably HIV-1 and all human herpes viruses including acyclovir-resistant herpes viruses and cytomegalovirus (CMV). It is used to treat CMV infections (retinitis, pneumonitis, colitis and esophagitis) and acyclovir-resistant herpes simplex virus (HSV) infections in immunocompetent and immunosuppressed hosts. Foscarnet is given as a loading dose of 30 mg/kg intravenously over half an hour followed by 60–90 mg/kg as a 1 hour infusion 8 hourly. After 2–3 weeks treatment doses are reduced to 20–30 mg/kg/day. Dose reduction is required in patients with renal failure.

Mechanism of action

Foscarnet is a nucleotide analog that inhibits viral DNA synthesis. It acts as a non-competitive inhibitor of viral DNA polymerase and inhibits reverse transcriptase from several retroviruses. It is inactive against eukaryotic DNA polymerases at concentrations that inhibit viral replication.

Adverse effects

1. Nephrotoxicity is reduced by adequate hydration and dose reduction if the creatinine rises. Monitoring of renal function is mandatory.
2. Central nervous system effects include irritability, anxiety and fits.

3. Nausea, vomiting and headache.
4. Thrombophlebitis.
5. Hypocalcemia and hypomagnesemia.
6. Hypoglycemia (rare).

Pharmacokinetics

Foscarnet is poorly absorbed after oral administration. It does not undergo presystemic metabolism, is only 14–17% protein bound and is widely distributed. Plasma concentrations decay in a triphasic manner, the half-lives being 0.5, 3 and 18 hours. Foscarnet is excreted renally by glomerular filtration and tubular excretion. Approximately 20% remains in the body bound in bone.

Drug interactions

The nephrotoxicity of foscarnet is potentiated by other nephrotoxins, including pentamidine, gentamicin, cyclosporin and amphotericin B. Administration with pentamidine can also cause marked hypocalcemia.

GANCICLOVIR (DIHYDROXYPROPOXY-METHYLGUANINE)

Use

Ganciclovir is the first antiviral drug to be licensed for sight or life-threatening CMV infections (retinitis, pneumonitis, colitis and esophagitis) in immunocompromised hosts. It also has potent activity against herpes virus 1 and 2. It is an analog of guanine. It is administered at an induction dose of 5 mg/kg every 12 hours for 14–21 days as an intravenous infusion over 1 hour, followed by a maintenance dose of 6 mg/kg for 5 days every week or 5 mg/kg for 7 days a week, continuously.

Mechanism of action

Ganciclovir inhibits viral replication. It is metabolized intracellularly in herpes-infected cells by virally encoded thymidine kinase to its monophosphate. It undergoes further phosphorylation by host kinases to the triphosphate, which competitively inhibits the DNA polymerase of CMV and, if incorporated into nascent viral DNA, causes chain termination. Ganciclovir is concentrated ten times in infected cells compared to uninfected cells.

Adverse effects

1. Neutropenia and bone marrow suppression (thrombocytopenia and less often anemia), cell counts usually return to normal within 2–5 days of discontinuing the drug.
2. Temporary or possibly permanent inhibition of spermatogenesis or oogenesis.
3. Phlebitis and pain at the infusion site.
4. Rashes and fever.
5. Gastrointestinal upsets.
6. Transient increases in liver enzymes and creatinine in underhydrated patients.

Contraindications

Ganciclovir is contraindicated in pregnancy (it is teratogenic in animals) and in breast-feeding women.

Pharmacokinetics

Absorption of ganciclovir is poor following oral administration, necessitating intravenous administration. It is <2 % protein bound and is widely distributed. Mean elimination $t_{1/2}$ is 2–5 hours. Ganciclovir is virtually totally excreted by the kidney, and dose reduction is needed in renal failure.

Drug interactions

Probenecid reduces renal clearance of ganciclovir. Antineoplastic drugs, co-trimoxazole and amphoteriicin B increase its toxic effects on rapidly dividing tissues including bone marrow, skin and gut epithelium. Zidovudine should not be given concomitantly with ganciclovir because of the potentiation of bone marrow suppression.

IDOXURIDINE (5-IODO-2-DEOXYURIDINE)

Idoxuridine is an analog of the DNA nucleotide thymidine and inhibits replication of some DNA viruses, particularly herpes viruses. Probable mechanisms of action include incorporation into DNA and/or competitive inhibition of enzymes involved in nucleic acid synthesis. It is only relatively selective for viral nucleic acid synthesis and causes toxic effects on mammalian bone marrow resulting in leukopenia and thrombocytopenia.

Use

Viral resistance to idoxuridine develops readily and to be effective the drug must be started early after the onset of infection. It is too toxic for systemic use, but has several indications for topical use:

1. **Herpetic keratitis** Hourly drops of 0.1% idoxuridine in saline encourage resolution of corneal ulcers providing a deep stromal reaction has not occurred. Prolonged use however may cause blepharitis, conjunctivitis and punctate lesions of the corneal epithelium.
2. **Herpes labialis** Recurrent lesions may be aborted by treating the affected area with 5.0% idoxuridine solution at the first sign of recurrence (usually a burning sensation in the affected skin precedes vesicle formation).
3. **Herpes zoster** Applied topically as a 5% idoxuridine solution in dimethyl sulfoxide idoxuridine hastens healing of shingles and may reduce the occurrence of postherpetic neuralgia. Dimethyl sulfoxide enhances skin penetration but is an irritant and must never be applied to the eye. It is important to begin treatment as early as possible, preferably as lesions are developing, and is especially valuable in the elderly (in whom postherpetic neuralgia is common) and those with immunological impairment (e.g. steroid or cytotoxic treatment).

TRIBAVIRIN (RIBAVIRIN)

Use

Tribavirin is active against a number of RNA and DNA (HSV-1 and -2, influenza) viruses.

Its major indication is for the treatment of bronchiolitis secondary to respiratory syncytial virus infection in infants and children. It is also effective, given systemically, in Lassa fever. Administration for bronchiolitis is via aerosol inhalation or nebulizer, of a solution of 20 mg/ml for 12–18 hours (dose – 6 g/day) for at least 3 days and up to a maximum of 7 days.

Mechanism of action

Tribavirin is taken up into cells and phosphorylated to tribavirin 5'-monophosphate by adenosine kinase and then rapidly phosphorylated to the di- and triphosphates by other cellular kinases. Tribavirin 5'-monophosphate is a powerful inhibitor of inosine monophosphate dehydrogenase which affects the pool size of intracellular ribonucleotides and deoxynucleotides. What effect this has on viral replication is presently unclear. Tribavirin 5'-triphosphate inhibits the guanylation reaction in formation of the 5' cap of mRNA and inhibits viral RNA methyltransferase. It has little or no effect on mammalian RNA methyltransferase.

Adverse effects

No sytemic adverse effects of tribavirin have been reported following aerosol or nebulizer administration.

1. Worsening respiration and bacterial pneumonia.
2. Pneumothorax.

Pharmacokinetics

Following nebulized administration negligible amounts of tribavirin are absorbed systemically.

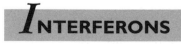

INTERFERONS

Interferons are cytokines (mediators of cell growth and function). They are glycoproteins secreted by cells infected with viruses or foreign double-stranded DNA. They are non-antigenic and are active against a wide range of viruses, but unfortunately are relatively species specific. Thus it is necessary to produce human interferon to act on human cells. Interferon production is triggered not only by viruses but also by tumor cells or previously encountered foreign antigens. Some interferons are important in immune cell regulation.

Four main types of interferon with different structures, derivation and properties are recognized:

1. **Interferon-α** known previously as leukocyte or lymphoblastoid interferon. Subspecies of the human α gene produce variants designated by the addition of a number, e.g. interferon-α_2, or in the case of a mixture of proteins, by Nl, N2 etc. Two methods of commercial production have been developed and these are indicated by: rbe – produced from bacteria (*Escherichia coli*) genetically modified by recombinant DNA technology, and lns – produced from cultured lymphoblasts stimulated by Sendai virus.

   Interferon-α_2 may also differ in the amino acids at positions 23 and 24 and these are shown by the addition of a letter. Thus α2a has lys–his at these sites whilst α2b has arg–his. At present it is not certain whether these different molecules have different therapeutic properties.
2. **Interferon-β** from fibroblasts.
3. **Interferon-ω** 60% homology to interferon-α and not yet clinically available.
4. **Interferon-γ** formerly called 'immune' interferon as it is produced by lymphocytes in response to antigens and mitogens.

Commercial production of pure interferon by cloning of interferon genes into bacterial and yeast plasmids is now available to facilitate large scale production.

Use

Interferon-α is of benefit in chronic hepatitis B and chronic hepatitis C infection (chapter 31), and is given thrice weekly by subcutaneous injections of 1–5 million units, for 6–12 months. Interferon-β is undergoing phase III clinical studies in multiple sclerosis. Interferon-β_{2B} is used to treat condylomata acuminata by intralesional injection. All three interferons are used to treat hairy cell leukemia. Interferon-α2a and -α2b are used to treat Kaposi's sarcoma in AIDS patients, and interferon-α_{N1} is licensed for recurrent or metastatic renal cell carcinoma (chapter 45). Recombinant interferon-γ_{1B} has been used for the treatment of chronic granulomatous disease and is under investigation for the treatment of mesothelioma and carcinoma of the ovary. Interferon therapy is beneficial in chronic myelogenous leukemia, multiple myeloma and refractory lymphoma, and is being further investigated in rheumatoid arthritis and mycosis fungoides.

Mechanism of action

Interferons bind to receptors on the cell membrane. Interferon-α, -β and -ω bind to a common cell membrane receptor, but interferon-γ binds to its own receptor. Following receptor binding interferons induce adenosine triphosphate (ATP)-dependent, tyrosine kinase-stimulated phosphorylation of three proteins – interferon-stimulated gene factors (ISGF). These then bind together to form ISGF 3α, which translocates to the nucleus and binds to DNA regulating RNA transcription of certain proteins. Consequently a number of enzymes with antiviral activity are increased, namely, 2',5' oligoadenylate synthetase (which activates ribonuclease L which preferentially cuts viral RNA), and protein kinase activity. The onset of these effects takes several hours but may persist for days even after plasma interferon concentrations have been completely cleared. Interferon also increases presentation of viral antigens in infected cells and up-regulates macrophage activation and T and natural killer cell cytotoxicity, thereby increasing viral elimination.

Adverse effects

1. Fever, malaise, chills – an influenza-like syndrome, and neuropsychiatric symptoms similar to a postviral syndrome.
2. Lymphocytopenia and thrombocytopenia are reversible and tolerance may occur after a week or so.
3. Anorexia and weight loss.
4. Alopecia.

5. Confusion, tremor and fits.
6. Transient hypotension or cardiac arrhythmias.
7. Hypothyroidism.

Pharmacokinetics

Most clinical experience is with interferon-α, which has been given intravenously, intramuscularly, subcutaneously and topically (nasal, vaginal, mucosal and eye). More than 80% of an intramuscular dose is absorbed. After subcutaneous administration, peak plasma concentrations occur after 4–8 hours and decline over 1–2 days. Cerebrospinal fluid concentrations are 1–5% of those in the plasma. Mean half-life is 3–5 hours. Elimination of interferons is complex, inactivation occurring in liver, lung, kidney, heart and striated muscle.

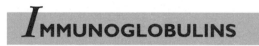

IMMUNOGLOBULINS

Some pooled human immunoglobulins have high titers against specific viruses such as cytomegalovirus, hepatitis A, hepatitis B, varicella and measles. Immunoglobulin is given intramuscularly as near as possible to the time of exposure and may be used prophylactically (chapter 47). Parenterally administered immunoglobulins reach peak serum concentrations in 4–6 days then decline with a half-life of 20–30 days.

HIV and AIDS

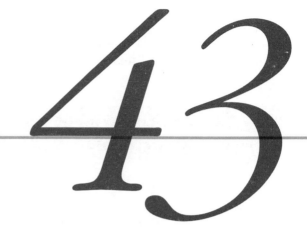

43

Introduction   **566**

Pathophysiology and immunopathogenesis of HIV-1 infection   **566**

General guidelines for the treatment of HIV-1-infected individuals   **567**

Antiretroviral drugs   **568**

Infective complications of HIV infection   **571**

Mycobacterium tuberculosis *therapy*   **573**

Mycobacterium avium-intracellulare *complex therapy*   **574**

Antifungal therapy   **574**

Herpes virus therapy   **575**

*I*NTRODUCTION

It was estimated that at January 1992 there were 11.8 million people infected with human immunodeficiency virus-1 (HIV-1) worldwide. This is expected to rise to 17.5 million in 1995, and this epidemic is likely to exterminate a considerable proportion of the human population, particularly in third world countries. This represents an enormous burden on the health-care facilities and resources of all countries.

*P*ATHOPHYSIOLOGY AND IMMUNOPATHOGENESIS OF HIV-1 INFECTION

Following inoculation of a naive host with biological fluid (blood, blood products or sexual secretions) containing HIV-1, the virus adheres to cells expressing the CD4 receptor (lymphocytes, macrophages and dendritic cells in the blood, lymphoid organs and central nervous system) and enters the cell, the viral envelope being absorbed into the

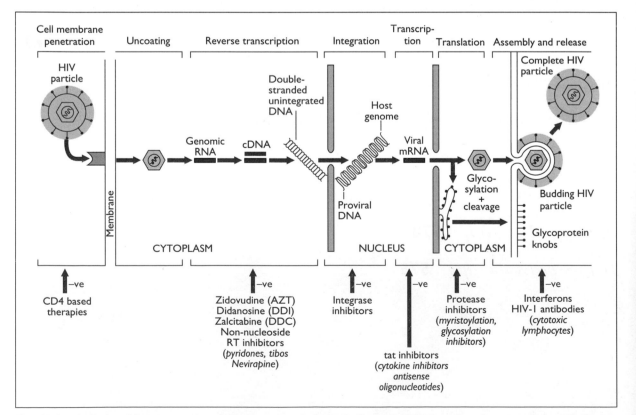

Fig. 43.1 Life-cycle of human immunodeficiency virus-1 (HIV-1) illustrating the actual and potential (in italics) sites of action of antiviral agents. RT = reverse transcriptase. cDNA = complementary DNA. mRNA = messenger RNA.

host membrane. After uncoating, the viral genome is released into the host cell, where viral reverse transcriptase produces complimentary DNA (cDNA), using the viral RNA as a template. This viral DNA is then integrated by a viral integrase enzyme into the host genome. Viral cDNA is then transcribed by the host, producing messenger RNA (mRNA) that yields viral proteins after translation. These peptides are then cleaved by the viral protease enzyme to form the structural viral proteins that eventually make up the new virion containing viral RNA. Figure 43.1 summarizes the life-cycle of the virus and shows potential points of therapeutic attack.

Several points in the HIV life-cycle are potentially vulnerable to therapeutic attack:

1. Entry of virus into the cell.
2. Viral DNA polymerase (reverse transcriptase).
3. The integrase enzyme.
4. The transactivator of transcription (tat) protein that accelerates replication of viral RNA.
5. Viral protease.

Newly formed HIV-1 virions infect previously uninfected CD4-positive cells and subsequently impair the host immune response by killing or inhibiting CD4-positive cells, thus rendering the host immunosuppressed and consequently at high risk of infections by commensal and opportunistic organisms. At present the diagnosis of HIV-1 infection is based on enzyme-linked immunosorbent assay (ELISA) techniques

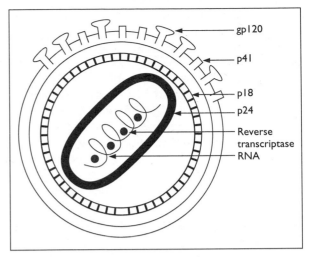

Fig. 43.2 HIV structure consisting of membrane glycoprotein gp120 and peptide protein p41 plus an outer membrane of p18 and a nuclear membrane of p24 protein containing viral RNA and reverse transcriptase enzyme.

identifying HIV-1 antibodies and/or structural proteins in blood (see Fig. 43.2 for the structure of the virus). Patients who are infected with HIV-1 will, after a latent period (5–10 years) of good health, begin to have a reduced CD4 lymphocyte count which, as it falls, predisposes the individual to opportunistic infections and certain malignancies (Kaposi's sarcoma and lymphoma). Ultimately it is these infections and malignancies that define the later stages of HIV-1 infection, known as the acquired immune deficiency syndrome (AIDS).

$\mathcal{G}$ENERAL GUIDELINES FOR TREATMENT OF HIV-I-INFECTED INDIVIDUALS

Patients who have developed AIDS (as defined by World Health Organization and the Centers for Disease Control, Atlanta criteria) should be treated with antiretroviral therapy. These agents have been shown to prolong survival. They may also reduce the rate of progression to AIDS in HIV-1-infected individuals. Treatment is with oral azidothymidine (zidovudine; AZT), 100 mg, five times a day or dideoxyinosine (didanosine; DDI), 200 mg, twice daily (weight adjusted) if the patient is AZT intolerant. Many patients who have been taking AZT for 4 months or more appear to fare better if switched to DDI. Dideoxycytidine (DDC) is restricted to patients who are intolerant of AZT and DDI. Patients who progress (in terms of viral load) on AZT may benefit from a switch to DDI or the addition of DDC. The recommended dose of DDC is 0.75 mg 8 hourly. Present opinion is divided as to whether HIV-1-infected individuals who are asymptomatic with a CD4 count of 500/mm³ or below should be treated routinely with anti-HIV nucleoside therapy. Studies in the USA (based on surrogate endpoints) suggest a benefit in treating such individuals, whereas the larger European Concorde study did not reveal a clear clinical benefit with AZT.

HIV-1-infected patients who develop infections with *Pneumocytsis carinii* and who recover require secondary prophylaxis with oral co-trimoxazole (two tablets twice daily). Similarly, patients who have recovered following esophageal candidiasis or crytococcal meningitis require prophylactic therapy with fluconazole, 200 mg, once daily. A number of other opportunistic infections in HIV-1-infected individuals once treated acutely similarly require maintenance prophylaxis.

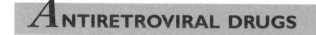

ANTIRETROVIRAL DRUGS

Nucleoside reverse transcriptase inhibitors

Of these agents only zidovudine (AZT) has been shown in clinical studies to reduce mortality in late stage AIDS, reduce the incidence of opportunistic infections and possibly to reduce the rate of progression of HIV-1 infection to AIDS. Didanosine and DDC appear to reduce HIV-1 viral replication, at least as indicated by surrogate markers.

ZIDOVUDINE (AZIDOTHYMIDINE; AZT)

This was originally synthesized as an anticancer nucleoside analog in 1964, but had little antineoplastic activity. It was the first nucleoside analog licensed for the treatment of HIV-1 infection. It is an analog of thymidine in which the 3'-hydroxyl has been replaced by an azido (N_3) group.

Use

AZT is licensed only for the treatment of HIV-1 infection. It is given orally as 100 mg five times daily (or 200 mg three times a day to aid compliance) to patients who have developed AIDS. Lower doses have been investigated but evidence that 300 mg/day is effective is inconclusive.

Mechanism of action

The parent drug AZT enters the cells by diffusion and undergoes anabolic phosphorylation firstly to the monophosphate (AZT-MP), then the diphosphate (AZT-DP) (the rate-limiting step) and finally the triphosphate (AZT-TP). The intracellular half-life of AZT-TP is 2–3 hours. AZT-TP is a competitive inhibitor of viral reverse transcriptase (RT) (competing with endogenous thymidine triphosphate) and when incorporated into nascent viral DNA causes chain termination, because the incoming nucleotide triphosphate cannot make a phosphate bond with the 3' carbon which lacks a hydroxyl group, (Fig. 43.3). Host nuclear DNA polymerases are much less sensitive (at least 100-fold) to inhibition by AZT-TP, thus producing a selective effect on viral replication.

Adverse effects

1. Bone marrow suppression causing anemia with reticulocytopenia and granulocytopenia, which are dose dependent. This

occurred in 15% of patients in the original studies with high-dose AZT. At the currently recommended lower dose (100 mg five times daily) it occurs in 1–2% of patients.
2. Nausea and vomiting.
3. Fatigue and headache.
4. Melanonychia (blue-gray nail discoloration).
5. Insomnia.
6. Myopathy – rare.
7. It is mutagenic and carcinogenic in animals. AZT may be used with caution in pregnancy to reduce fetal-HIV-1 infection.

Pharmacokinetics

Zidovudine is almost totally absorbed (>90%) from the gut. The plasma elimination half-life is 1–2 hours. It is widely distributed achieving cerebrospinal fluid (CSF) concentrations of 50% that in plasma. Plasma protein binding is 30–40%. About 25–40% of a dose undergoes presystemic metabolism in the liver. The major metabolite (80%) is the glucuronide and approximately 20% appears unchanged in the urine. Plasma concentrations after a single oral dose of 100–300 mg achieve the concentration that inhibits 90% growth (IC_{90}) for cells acutely infected with HIV-1.

Drug interactions

- Probenecid inhibits the glucuronidation and renal excretion of AZT. However, the combination of AZT and probenecid produces fevers, rashes and constitutional symptoms in patients and it is not widely used to reduce the dose of AZT.
- AZT and antituberculous chemotherapy cause a high incidence of anemia.
- Ganciclovir and AZT combined therapy produces profound bone marrow suppression and should be avoided.
- Paracetamol increases AZT clearance and does not produce a higher incidence of anemia: early concerns in this regard have been allayed.
- *In vitro* evidence suggests that AZT/DDI or AZT/DDC combinations may be synergistic. Such combination therapy is currently being studied.

DIDEOXYINOSINE (DIDANOSINE; DDI)

This drug is an analog of deoxyadenosine (Fig. 43.3). It is used in AZT-intolerant patients. Dideoxyinosine is metabolized intracellularly via DDI-monophosphate to dideoxyadenosine-monophosphate (DDA-MP) and then ultimately

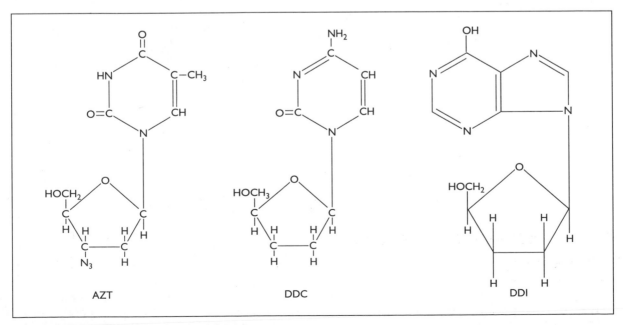

Fig. 43.3 Structures of AZT, DDC and DDI.

to dideoxyadenosinetriphosphate (DDA-TP), which inhibits RT as does AZT-TP. The intracellular half-life of DDA-TP (12 hours) allows the drug to be given twice daily. Dideoxyinosine is acid labile and its absorption is affected by gastric pH, so it is administered orally as a buffered solution or capsule. The bioavailablity is 30–45%, with a plasma half-life of 0.5–1.5 hours. DDI is both renally excreted and hepatically metabolized to hypoxanthine, xanthine and uric acid. The major side effects are peripheral neuropathy, nausea and vomiting, pancreatitis (which can be fatal), rashes, hyperuricemia and myositis. Anemia and granulocytopenia do occur but much less frequently than with AZT. The buffered solution in which DDI is administered reduces ketoconazole and dapsone absorption.

DIDEOXYCYTIDINE (DDC)

This nucleoside analog is reserved for patients with HIV-1 infection who are intolerant of AZT and DDI (Fig. 43.3). Perhaps its best use will prove to be in combination therapy with these other agents at a low dose. Like AZT, DDC undergoes intracellular anabolic phosphorylation to DDC triphosphate, which is active against the HIV-1 RT, but is several orders of magnitude less active against host DNA polymerases (α and β). Dideoxycytidine triphosphate has an intracellular half-life of 2–3 hours. This allows 8 hourly dosing with 0.75 mg, the dose being halved in patients with neuropathy. Dideoxycytidine is well absorbed, has a mean plasma half-life of 1.5–3 hours and is primarily excreted via the kidney. Dose reduction is needed in renal failure. Major side effects are a reversible painful sensorimotor peripheral neuropathy, stomatitis, pancreatitis, rashes and malaise.

HIV-1 nucleoside analog resistance

Reduced susceptibility of HIV-1 isolates to AZT, DDI and DDC has been documented.

Resistance to AZT emerges more quickly and to a greater degree in the later stages of the disease. Progressive stepwise reductions in susceptibility of the RT correlate with the acquisition of mutations in the gene for the RT protein. There is only cross-resistance to other nucleosides with the 3'-azido side chain, therefore such isolates are at present still sensitive to DDI or DDC. However, resistance to other non-nucleoside inhibitors has been documented in patients on long-term therapy with DDI or DDC. The precise clinical significance of viral resistance to nucleoside analogs is uncertain, but the place of combined or alternating nucleoside analog regimens is being investigated.

New antiretroviral agents in phase I/II assessment

OTHER REVERSE TRANSCRIPTASE INHIBITORS

Didehydrodideoxythymidine (D4T; stavudine) is undergoing phase I/II studies. Non-nucleoside RT inhibitors include foscarnet and nevirapine.

Foscarnet (chapter 42) has to be administered parenterally and is toxic.

Neviripine is an allosteric inhibitor of HIV RT, and has entered phase II studies. It is one of several compounds that bind to the same site and inhibit reverse transcriptase *in vitro*. These compounds appear synergistic when combined with anti-HIV nucleoside analogs *in vitro*. *In vivo* resistance to nevirapine develops rapidly.

tat INHIBITOR

The HIV-1 genome contains the genes *rev, tat* and *nef,* which are potential drug targets. These genes plays an important role in regulating the replication of HIV-1 in the host cell and are necessary for pathogenic infection. The *tat* gene produces a 14 000 molecular weight protein that is essential in viral replication. It acts by transactivating the HIV-1 promoter (LTR) to amplify viral replication. A benzodiazepine compound Ro-24-7429 is a tat antagonist. In phase I/II studies in HIV-1 infected subjects it is well absorbed after oral administration with a mean plasma half-life of 4 hours. Multiple dose studies using 60–150 mg four times a day suggest that it has dose-dependent pharmacokinetics. Plasma concentrations achieved in these studies are above the ID_{90} for HIV-1 *in vitro*. Reported side effects have been mild. Studies of i*n vivo* efficacy are awaited.

VIRAL PROTEASE INHIBITOR

A retroviral protease cleaves newly translated large precursor viral polypeptides into the protein products of the *gag* and *pol* gene. Inhibitors of this viral protease inhibit maturation of viral particles to infectious virions. Compounds such as Ro-31-8959, which is an inhibitory mimetic of the viral peptide substrate (a competitive inhibitor for the protease), cause a dramatic reduction of HIV-1 replication *in vitro*. RO-31-8959 was the first drug of this class to enter clinical studies, but a problem in its development has been poor systemic bioavailability.

INTERFERONS

Interferons (chapter 42) act at many steps in the viral life-cycle, from entry to budding of new virions. Some clinical studies suggest that interferon when combined with anti-HIV-1 nucleoside analogs may provide added benefit in terms of viral suppression, although no studies have addressed the question of whether it improves survival. The need for parenteral administration and its adverse effects of myalgia, fevers and lethargy limit its acceptability. However in lower doses it may prove to be a useful adjunct to anti-HIV-1 nucleoside treatment and studies investigating this are in progress.

INFECTIVE COMPLICATIONS OF HIV INFECTION

Pneumocystis carinii

In moderate to severe cases of *Pneumocystis carinii* pneumonia (PCP) where the arterial PO_2 is less than 60 mmHg, treatment consists not only of anti-*Pneumocystis* therapy, but in addition glucocorticosteroids. Prednisolone is given as 80 mg/day for 5 days, 40 mg/day for 5 days and 20 mg/day for 11 days. This has been shown to reduce the number of patients requiring mechanical ventilation and improve survival.

CO-TRIMOXAZOLE

High-dose co-trimoxazole (chapter 40) is first-line standard therapy for PCP in patients with HIV infection. It is given intravenously at the equivalent of 20 mg/kg/day trimetho-prim in two divided doses for a total of 21 days. If the patient improves after 5–7 days, oral therapy may be substituted for the remainder of the course. The major adverse effects of this therapy are nausea and vomiting (which is reduced by the prior administration of an antiemetic intravenously), rashes, hepatitis, bone marrow suppression and hyperkalemia. Treatment may have to be discontinued in 20–55% of cases because of side effects and one of the alternative therapies listed below subistituted. After recovery from an episode of PCP, secondary prophylaxis with oral co-trimoxazole (one double strength tablet twice or thrice daily) is preferred to nebulized pentamidine as it reduces the risk of extrapulmonary as well as pulmonary relapse. Dapsone 100 mg orally once daily is also effective for secondary prophylaxis.

PENTAMIDINE

Use

This is an aromatic amidine and is supplied for parenteral use as pentamidine isethionate. It has activity against a range of pathogenic protozoa. In addition to *Pneumocystis carinii* it is also effective against African trypanosomiasis (*Trypanosoma rhodesiense* and *T. congolese*) and kala-azar (*Leishmania donovani*). It is effective in 70–80% of PCP episodes, and is administered as a slow intravenous infusion over 2 hours at 4 mg/kg/day for 21 days. Parenteral administration via the intramuscular route has been used but sterile injection site abscesses occur commonly. Pentamidine has also been given via the nebulized route to treat PCP (4 mg/kg/day, up to 600 mg/day) but the recurrence rate is higher than with systemic therapy.

Mechanism of action

Pentamidine has a number of actions on protozoan cells. It damages cellular DNA especially extranuclear (mitochondrial) DNA and prevents its replication; it inhibits RNA polymerase and at high concentrations it damages mitochondria. Polyamine uptake into protozoa is also inhibited by pentamidine. *Pneumocystis carinii* is killed even in the non-replicating state.

Adverse effects

Nebulized route
Cough and bronchospasm occur which are reduced by preadministration of nebulized β_2-agonist.

Intravenous route
1. Hypotension and acidosis (due to cardiotoxicity) if given too rapidly.
2. Dizziness and syncope.
3. Hypoglycemia due to toxicity to the pancreatic β-cells producing hyperinsulinemia.
4. Nephrotoxicity (rarely irreversible).
5. Pancreatitis.
6. Reversible neutropenia.

Intramuscular route
The above problems occur plus pain at the injection site and sterile abscesses.

Pharmacokinetics

Pentamidine is not appreciably absorbed after oral administration and must be given parenterally. The half-life varies, but is approximately 6 hours after the first intravenous dose. There is drug accumulation in tissue and plasma with repeated dosing. The major route of clearance from plasma is by tissue binding and uptake. It has a large volume of distribution, but does not cross the blood–brain barrier well. Renal excretion is small (<5%), so renal failure does not necessitate dose adjustment. There are no data on pentamidine metabolism in humans. Nebulized therapy yields lung concentrations that are at least as high if not higher than those achieved after intravenous infusion.

Drug interactions

Pentamidine inhibits human cholinesterase *in vitro*. This suggests potential interactions in enhancing the effect of suxamethonium and reducing that of competitive muscle relaxants, but it is not known if this is of clinical importance.

TRIMETHOPRIM AND DAPSONE

This combination has been successfully used as an alternative therapy in treating mild to moderate PCP. The drugs are given orally – trimethoprim, 20 mg/kg/day in two divided doses and dapsone, 100 mg/day, for 21 days.

PRIMAQUINE AND CLINDAMYCIN

This combination has also been shown to be effective in mild to moderately severe PCP. The combination is given as primaquine, 30 mg/day p.o. and clindamycin, 900 mg, intravenously 8 hourly for 11 days, and 450 mg 6 hourly orally for 10 days.

ATOVAQUONE

Atovaquone is a hydroxynaphthoquinone derivative that interferes with protozoan mitochondrial respiratory chain electron transport, inhibiting *de novo* pyrimidine synthesis. It also has activity against toxoplasmosis. It is given orally, 750 mg, 6 hourly for mild to moderately severe PCP. Its major adverse effects are nausea and vomiting, rashes and hepatitis.

Toxoplasma gondii

PYRIMETHAMINE AND SULFADIAZINE

Use

This combination is the first-line therapy for cerebral and tissue toxoplasmosis. Pyrimethamine is given as an oral loading dose of 100–200 mg, then 50–100 mg/day, together with oral (or intravenous) sulfadiazine 10 mg/kg/day. Treatment should be continued for 4–6 weeks after clinical and neurological resolution, and for up to 6 months thereafter. Folinic acid is given prophylactically at 10–50 mg/day to reduce drug-induced bone marrow suppression.

Mechanism of action

Sulfadiazine acts as a competitive inhibitor of dihydrofolate synthase (competing with *p*-aminobenzoic acid) in folate synthesis. Pyrimethamine is a competitive inhibitor of dihydrofolate reductase, which converts dihydrofolate to tetrahydrofolate. Together they sequentially block the first two steps in the synthesis of folate in the parasite. Their selective toxicity is due to their greater specificity as inhibitors of these enzymes in the protozoan than in humans. Humans obtain their dihydrofolate from dietary folate circumventing the block of sulfadiazine, while adding folinic acid (which is not absorbed by these parasites) helps reduce the effects of pyrimethamine on the bone marrow.

Adverse effects

Major toxicities of the combination are:

1. Nausea and vomiting.
2. Fever and rashes which may be life threatening (Stevens–Johnson syndrome).
3. Bone marrow suppression, especially granulocytes.
4. Hepatitis.
5. Nephrotoxicity including crystalluria and obstructive nephropathy.

Pharmacokinetics

Oral absorption of pyrimethamine is good (>90%). It undergoes extensive hepatic metabolism but approximately 20% is recovered unchanged in the urine. Plasma half-life is long varying from 35 to 175 hours. Because of its high lipid solubility it has a large volume of distribution, and achieves CSF concentrations that are 10–25% of those in plasma.

Sulfadiazine is rapidly and completely absorbed after oral administration. There is, however, substantial first-pass hepatic metabolism, the major metabolite being the acetyl derivative. Mean plasma half-life is 10 hours. Cerebrospinal fluid concentrations are 70% of those in plasma. Clearance is a combination of hepatic metabolism and renal excretion with 50% of a dose being excreted in the urine, so dose reduction is needed in renal failure.

Drug interactions

These are primarily due to the sulfadiazine (chapter 40) and the combined bone marrow suppressive effect of pyrimethamine with other antifolates.

An alternative antitoxoplasmosis therapy consists of pyrimethamine in combination with clindamycin (dose 900–1200 mg, every 6–8 hours), with folinic acid as above. Newer therapies which are undergoing investigation in treating cerebral toxoplasmosis as salvage therapy include one of the newer macrolides (azithromycin, clarithromycin, chapter 40) and atovaquone (see above).

*M*YCOBACTERIUM TUBERCULOSIS THERAPY

See chapter 41.

Bacille Calmette-Guérin vaccine should *not* be given to HIV-1 infected individuals since it is a live, albeit attenuated, strain. Triple therapy with isoniazid, 300 mg/day, plus rifampicin, 600 mg/day (450 mg for patients less than

50 kg) and pyrazinamide, 20–30 mg/kg/day, is recommended. This regimen should be given orally for 2 months and then rifampicin and isoniazid continued for 9 months or for 6 months after the sputum converts to negative for bacterial growth, whichever is longer. Isoniazid may be used long term as chemoprophylaxis in patients after successful treatment. If there is isoniazid resistance, ethambutol is substituted at 25 mg/kg/day, for the first 2 months and continued thereafter at

15 mg/kg/day with rifampicin for a further 10 months (12 months total). Response rates in HIV patients are high (90%), provided there is good compliance, with a relatively low recurrence rate (10%). The incidence of adverse effects from antituberculous therapy is high in these patients and may necessitate changing medication. *Mycobacterium tuberculosis* strains that are resistant to rifampicin are beginning to emerge in this population, so *in vitro* sensitivity determination is essential.

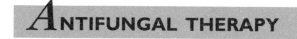

MYCOBACTERIUM AVIUM-INTRACELLULARE COMPLEX THERAPY

This infection is a systemic multiorgan system infection in HIV-1-infected patients. It has not been convincingly shown to be communicable to other individuals as has *M. tuberculosis* and some uncertainty remains as to the benefits of treating this infection in HIV-1-infected individuals. Studies are presently ongoing addressing this question with a number of combination regimens, including the use of rifabutin, azitromycin and clarithromycin which have potent anti-*M. avium-intracellulare* complex (MAC)

activity *in vitro*. The regimens used for therapy are complex combination therapies because of the resistance patterns of the organism. Successful regimens consist of rifampicin, 600 mg/day; clofazimine, 100 mg/day; ethambutol, 15–25 mg/kg/day; ciprofloxacin, 750 mg/day; and amikacin (dosage determined by plasma concentrations) intravenously or intramuscularly. If a clinical response is produced (usually 2–8 weeks) suppressive therapy with oral drugs should be given for life.

ANTIFUNGAL THERAPY

See chapter 42.

Candida

For *Candida,* if the disease is confined locally then initial therapy with nystatin is adequate. However, if infection is more extensive, treatment should be with fluconazole, 50 mg, daily for 1–2 weeks. Prophylactic fluconazole, 150 mg, weekly is under investigation. Alternatives are ketoconazole, 400 mg, daily for 1–2 weeks or itraconazole, 200 mg, daily for 1–2 weeks

Cryptococcus neoformans

First-line therapy is with amphotericin B given intravenously initially at 0.5–1 mg/kg/day (maximum 100 mg/day). The lower dose is used in combination with intravenous flucytosine; however flucytosine often causes bone marrow suppression in HIV-1-infected pateints. An effective alternative is fluconazole initially given as oral or intravenous therapy, 400 mg/day, reduced to 200–400 mg/day as maintenance therapy if the patient responds. Such combination therapy is preferred in severely ill patients. Liposomal amphotericin B has potential for reducing toxicity when used in combination with fluconazole. Itraconazole, 200–400 mg, daily is an alternative prophylactic therapy.

Histoplasmosis

Treatment is with amphotericin B, 1 mg/kg, daily intravenously for 6 weeks or itracona-zole, 400 mg, daily for 6 weeks. Prophylactic maintenance therapy with itraconazole, 400 mg/day, is recommended.

Coccidiomycosis

Treatment is with amphotericin B, 0.5–1 mg/kg, daily intravenously for 6 weeks, followed by itraconazole, 400 mg/day, as maintenance prophylaxis.

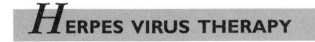

*H*ERPES VIRUS THERAPY

See chapter 42.

Herpes simplex virus 1 and 2

Acyclovir is used for treatment and in some patients it has been given orally as mainte-nance prophylaxis against recurrence (200 mg twice daily). Unfortunately, this has led to the development of acyclovir resistance of herpes virus isolates. Foscarnet is useful in acyclovir resistant strains.

Cytomegalovirus

This virus infection can be multisystem or confined to the eyes, lungs, genitourinary system or gastrointestinal tract. Successful therapeutic regimens have consisted of induction therapy with either ganciclovir or foscarnet, followed by a maintenance regimen. For ganciclovir the induction regimen is 5 mg/kg intravenously twice daily for 2 weeks followed by 5 mg/kg intravenously daily as maintenance therapy. Foscarnet is given as a total daily intra-venous dose of 60–90 mg/kg/day initially for 2 weeks and then 30 mg/kg/day. In the treatment of CMV retinitis a recent study suggested that foscarnet was superior and allowed the continued use of AZT with an improved survival time. This perhaps was due to its lack of bone marrow suppressive effects unlike ganciclovir, which with AZT causes profound marrow suppression. At present studies are ongoing with ganciclovir using granulocyte colony-stimulating factor (G-CSF) (chapter 46) to minimize the suppression of the granulocyte lineage in the bone marrow.

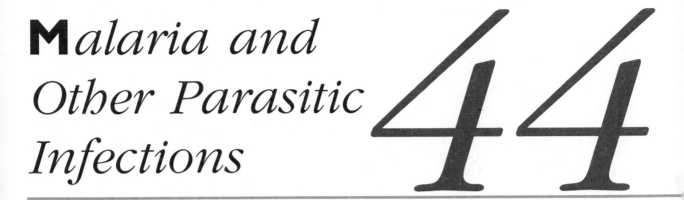

Malaria and Other Parasitic Infections

44

Malaria   **578**

Trypanosomal infection   **583**

Helminthic infection   **584**

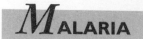MALARIA

Malaria is a protozoal disease caused by one of four forms of *Plasmodium* – *P. falciparum, P. vivax, P. ovale* or *P. malariae*. The most serious form is caused by *P. falciparum* and is transmitted by mosquito bites.

Antimalarial drug therapy involves prophylaxis and drug treatment of acute malaria. Visitors to countries where malaria is endemic should be advised about the possibility of infection and that prophylactic drug therapy should be taken, but is not 100% effective. Minimization of the risks of being bitten by mosquitos involves use of long clothing to cover extremities; mosquito repellent sprays; sleeping in properly screened rooms with mosquito nets around the bed; and burning and vaporizing synthetic pyrethroids during the night. In addition to antimalarial prophylactic drug therapy with suitable agents, travelers should be advised to carry standby malarial

drug therapy consisting of either halofantrine or quinine. Where there is doubt concerning the suitability of drug therapy for treatment or prophylaxis this may be discussed with the malaria reference laboratory at the School of Hygeine and Tropical Medicine (071-636-8636 for prophylaxis and 071-387-4411 for treatment).

Figure 44.1 illustrates the *Plasmodium* life-cycle and points of attack of various drugs.

Malaria prophylaxis

All prophylaxis is relative. Drugs used to prevent malaria are chosen mainly on the basis of local susceptibility patterns. The two

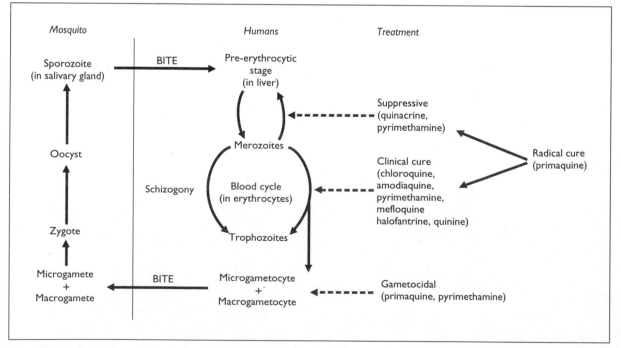

Fig. 44.1 Malaria life-cycle and type of drug treatment.

main groups of malarial prophylactic drugs are the 4-amino quinolines and dihydrofolate reductase inhibitors. Drug treatment must start at least 1 week before entering a malaria endemic region, and continue for 4 weeks afterwards.

4-AMINOQUINOLINES (CHLOROQUINE)

Chloroquine is used as a prophylactic in regions where falciparum malaria is not chloroquine resistant; the dose is 300 mg weekly. Proguanil, 200 mg, daily or amodiaquine, 400 mg, weekly are alternatives. There have been occasional reports of bone marrow suppression.

Prophylaxis of chloroquine-resistant falciparum malaria may be attempted with one of the following schemes:

1. Chloroquine, 300 mg, once weekly plus proguanil, 200 mg, daily.
2. Maloprim (12.5 mg, pyrimethamine, a dihydrohydrofolate reductase inhibitor, plus 100 mg dapsone) plus chloroquine, 300 mg, weekly for 2 weeks.
3. Mefloquine (see below) given as 250 mg weekly. This is preferably restricted to men or to women who are unlikely to become pregnant because of its as yet undetermined teratogenic potential.

PREVENTION OF MALARIA IN PREGNANCY

This is a difficult problem owing to the theoretical risk to the fetus from antimalarial drugs. Folate deficency is a known cause of birth defects; there is, however, no evidence that chloroquine, proguanil or fansidar (pyrimethamine and sulfadoxine) cause fetal damage. It would, however, appear to be a reasonable precaution to prescribe folinic acid during the first trimester if an antifolate (pyrimethamine) is used. Maloprim (pyrimethamine and dapsone) is not used in the first trimester. Chloroquine and proguanil are believed to be the safest antimalarial drugs to use in pregnancy.

Drugs used in the treatment of an acute attack of malaria

CHLOROQUINE

Use

Chloroquine is one of the most widely used antimalarial drugs, particularly against falciparum infections acquired in Africa, but even here partial resistance already exists. It is used for:

1. Malarial prophylaxis in restricted circumstances, (see above).
2. Acute malarial attack: in vivax malaria chloroquine is not radically curative because it does not eradicate hepatic forms of the parasite. It does, however, terminate an acute attack even though relapses can occur subsequently. Falciparum malaria is usually resistant to chloroquine. The routine course of chloroquine is a total dose of 1.5 g (or 30 mg/kg) orally, given in divided doses: 600 mg initially, 300 mg after 6 hours and then 300 mg daily for 2 days. Children receive a smaller dose of 20 mg/kg. In babies the dose is 5.0 mg/kg by intramuscular injection. If given intravenously it can cause encephalopathy. Following a course of chloroquine, primaquine, 15 mg, daily may be given for 14–21 days to achieve a radical cure (i.e. to eliminate hepatic forms and prevent relapse). The possibility of glucose-6-phosphate dehydrogenase (G6PDH) deficiency (chapter 13) should be borne in mind before embarking on this.
3. Use of chloroquine in connective tissue disease is described in chapter 22.
4. Chloroquine is the drug of first choice in treating infestations with *Clonorchis sinensis* and is the drug of second choice for treating *Fasciola hepatica* and *Paragonimus* infestations. Chloroquine is effective in treating extraintestinal amebiasis and in giardiasis.

Mechanism of action

Chloroquine only injures *Plasmodium* during its sojourn in the red cells. At this stage of its life-cycle the parasite lives off hemoglobin, which is taken up into a food vacuole that functions as its 'stomach' and digests the contained hemoglobin to provide energy for the parasite. The abundant iron is detoxified by heme polymerase to a pigment that is harmless to the parasite. The food vacuole is acidic and chloroquine (a weak base) is concentrated within it by diffusion trapping (chapter 6). The mechanism of action of chloroquine and other 4-aminoquinolines is believed to be due to inhibition of malarial heme polymerase within the food vacuole of the plasmodial parasite. Ferriprotoporphyrin IX accumulates in the presence of chloroquine and is toxic to the parasite, which is killed by the waste product of its own appetite (hoist with its own petard).

Adverse effects

Malarial prophylaxis
Nausea and dyspepsia occur.

Treatment of an acute malarial attack
1. Mild headache.
2. Visual disturbances.
3. Pruritus.
4. Gastrointestinal upsets.

Prolonged therapy
1. Retinopathy, characterized by loss of central visual acuity, macular pigmentation ('bull's-eye' macula) and retinal artery constriction. Visual loss is not reversible on stopping the drug, but progress is checked.
2. Lichenoid skin eruption.
3. Bleaching of hair.
4. Weight loss.
5. Ototoxicity.
6. Cochleovestibular paresis in fetal life.

Pharmacokinetics

Chloroquine is rapidly and almost completely absorbed from the intestine. Approximately 50% is bound to plasma proteins and excretion is slow. The mean half-life ($t_{1/2}$) is 120 hours, but excretion is accelerated by acidifying the urine. High concentrations (relative to plasma) are found in all tissues, especially those containing melanin, notably the retina. This presumably explains the predilection of the retina for chloroquine toxicity. Seventy per cent of a dose is excreted unchanged and the main metabolite is desethylchloroquine. Some metabolites are active antimalarial agents.

Drug interactions

Chloroquine and quinine are antagonistic and should not be used together.

QUININE

Use

Quinine is the main alkaloid of cinchona bark and is uniquely valuable for the treatment of an acute attack of chloroquine-resistant falciparum malaria. However, it has a large number of actions on a number of cell types. It is toxic to bacteria, yeasts, protozoa and some spirochetes. Its precise mechanism of action is unknown but may be similar to that of chloroquine. On animal tissues it has local anesthetic and irritant effects.

1. Quinine sulfate is the drug of choice in the treatment of an acute attack of falciparum malaria in areas where the parasite is known to be resistant to chloroquine. The usual course is 600 mg thrice daily (children 10 mg/kg) for 7 days. Initially the drug is given intravenously as a slow infusion over 4 hours, then orally when the patient improves. Mean $t_{1/2}$ is quite long and in patients with renal or hepatic dysfunction dosing should be reduced to once or twice daily. To eradicate the disease if quinine resistance is possible this should be followed by pyrimethamine, 75 mg, and sulfadoxine, 1.5 g (fansidar three tablets) given as a single dose. Mean plasma $t_{1/2}$ of both of these drugs is long: 96 hours for pyrimethamine and 200 hours for sulfadoxine. In combination they inhibit folate metabolism synergistically at two sites in the pathway. Both drugs are excreted in the urine, pyrimethamine mainly as metabolites. Fansidar occasionally causes

the Stevens–Johnson syndrome which limits its use. Pyrimethamine causes gastrointestinal upsets, megaloblastic anemia, ataxia and fits. If the organism is known or suspected to be fansidar resistant then doxycycline, 200 mg once, then 100 mg daily is substituted for 6 days (not for children under 8 or pregnant women, because of its effects on developing bones and teeth).

2. Quinine has been used in some patients with myotonia congenita and dystrophia myotoncia in doses of 300–600 mg 8 hourly.

3. Nocturnal cramps are sometimes treated by quinine 200–300 mg orally before going to bed. However, this use of a potentially toxic drug is seldom justified in such a benign condition that usually responds to simple measures such as plantar flexion of the foot against pressure, having first excluded iatrogenic causes (e.g. diuretics or β_2-agonists).

Adverse effects

1. Large therapeutic doses of quinine give rise to cinchonism which consists of tinnitus, deafness, headaches, nausea and visual disturbances.

2. Abdominal pain, diarrhea

3. Rashes, fever, delirium, stimulation followed by depression of respiration, renal failure, hemolytic anemia, thrombocytopenic purpura and hypoprothrombinemia.

4. Intravenous quinine can produce neurological toxicity:

   - Tremor of lips and limbs.
   - Delirium.
   - Fits and coma.

Pharmacokinetics

Almost complete absorption occurs in the upper part of the small intestine when quinine is given orally. Thus peak concentrations are similar following oral or intravenous administration, but are reached 1–3 hours after ingestion. Absorption from intramuscular sites is poor and local tissue necrosis can result from subcutaneous injection.

The steady-state plasma concentrations show wide interindividual variation. Mean $t_{1/2}$ is 10 hours, but is longer in severe falciparum malaria. Less than 5% is excreted unaltered in urine, the rest is metabolized in the liver, principally to hydroxy derivatives.

MEFLOQUINE

Use

Mefloquine is effective in treating acute chloroquine-resistant falciparum malaria. The dose is 20 mg/kg (maximum 1500 mg) divided into two doses given 6 hours apart. It is also used for short- or long-term (up to 3 months) prophylaxis for travelers to areas where there is multiple drug-resistant malaria. The mefloquine dose for prophylaxis is 250 mg orally, given weekly.

Mechanism of action

The mechanism of action of mefloquine is believed to be similar to the mechanism of action of chloroquine.

Adverse effects

1. Transient abdominal pain, dizziness, nausea, vomiting and weakness in about 50% of patients.

2. More uncommonly, hallucinations, psychoses and fits.

3. It is teratogenic in animals and should not be used in the first trimester of pregnancy.

Contraindications

Mefloquine is contraindicated in the first trimester of pregnancy, and if used in non-pregnant females they should be advised not to become pregnant for at least 3 months after cessation. Mefloquine is not used in patients with a history of neuropsychiatric disorders or patients with epilepsy.

Pharmacokinetics

Mefloquine is slowly absorbed from the gastrointestinal tract and mainly eliminated by hepatic metabolism with enterohepatic circulation. Mean $t_{1/2}$ is approximately 14–22 days. It should be avoided in patients with renal or hepatic impairment.

Drug interactions

Mefloquine potentiates the bradycardia caused by β-blockers and mefloquine is contraindicated in patients treated with β-adrenoceptor antagonists. Quinine also potentiates mefloquine toxicity and should not be given with this drug.

HALOFANTRINE

Use

Halofantrine is a schizonticidal antimalarial active against erythrocytic forms. It is used to treat uncomplicated chloroquine-resistant falciparum malaria, and administered orally at a dose of 500 mg 6 hourly for three doses and repeated after 1 week. Halofantrine should not be used as prophylaxis but has activity against *P. vivax*.

Mechanism of action

Halofantrine (a 4-aminoquinolone) has a mechanism of action probably similar to that of chloroquine.

Adverse effects

1. Gastrointestinal upsets and rarely mouth ulcers.
2. Pruritus.
3. Transient hepatic dysfunction.
4. Rarely neuromuscular spasms.
5. Potential proarrhythmogen as it prolongs the QTc (the corrected QT interval).

Contraindications

Halofantrine is embryotoxic but not teratogenic in animals and should not be used in pregnancy.

Pharmacokinetics

Halofantrine is poorly absorbed but does not undergo significant presystemic metabolism; absorption is improved with fatty foods. Above 500 mg given orally there is evidence that little more halofantrine is absorbed. It undergoes hepatic metabolism by the cytochrome P_{450} enzyme system to an active metabolite – desbutylhalofantrine. Mean $t_{1/2}$ of halofantrine ranges from 1 to 4 days and that of desbutylhalofantrine is 2–7 days.

Drug interactions

Unlike other antimalarial drugs no inhibitory effects on the cytochrome P_{450} mixed function oxidase system have been found at present. Fatty foods enhance its absorption six- to tenfold.

PRIMAQUINE

Use

Primaquine is used prophylactically (in conjunction with chloroquine) and to eradicate hepatic forms of *P. vivax* or *P. malariae* after standard chloroquine therapy, providing the risk of re-exposure is low. It interferes with electron transport in the mitochondria. Absorption from the gut is good. It is rapidly metabolized and the mean $t_{1/2}$ is 6 hours. Its major adverse effects are gastrointestinal upsets, methemoglobinemia and hemolytic anemia (which can be explosive and profound) in glucose-6-phosphate dehydrogenase (G6PD)-deficient individuals.

Treatment of a malaria relapse

Plasmodium falciparum does not cause a relapsing illness after treating the acute attack with such schizonticides as chloroquine, because there is no persistent liver stage of the parasite. Infections with *P. malariae* can cause recurrent attacks of fever for up to 30 years, but standard treatment with chloroquine eradicates the parasite. Following treatment of an acute attack of vivax malaria with schizonticides, or a period of protection with prophylactic drugs, febrile illness can recur due to the establishment of liver stages of the parasite. Such relapsing illness is prevented (or treated) by eradicating the parasites in the liver with primaquine, 15 mg of the base (26.3 mg of the phosphate), given daily for 2 weeks. Patients who lack G6PD in their erythrocytes can suffer an acute hemolytic episode from this drug (chapter

13). Such individuals are either treated under close inpatient supervision, or given proguanil hydrochloride continuously (100 mg daily) for 3 years. This drug is a malarial suppressant and allows time for the hepatic stages to die out naturally.

TRYPANOSOMAL INFECTION

African sleeping sickness is caused by *Trypanosoma gambiense* and *T. rhodesiense*. The insect vector is the *Glossina* (tsetse) fly. The drugs used in therapy (Table 44.1) include:

1. Drugs active in blood and peripheral tissues: suramin, pentamidine, melarsoprol and trimelarsan (also puromycin nitrofurazone).
2. Drugs active in the central nervous system: tryparsamide, melarsoprol and trimelarsan.

Scheme of treatment

1. Suramin and pentamidine are both successful in treating bloodstream infections (normal cerebrospinal fluid) of *T. gambiense*. In *T. rhodesiense* infections only suramin is effective. When central nervous system (CNS) involvement has occurred, arsenical drugs are used. Advanced CNS disease caused by either parasite may respond to melarsoprol. Trimelarsan is effective only in *T. gambiense* infections.
2. For prophylaxis a single 1 g injection of suramin protects an adult against both infections for 6–12 weeks. A single dose of pentamidine, 200–250 mg, protects for 3–6 months against *T. gambiense*.
3. Treatment against *T. cruzi* infections (South American trypanosomiasis) is unsatisfactory. Effects of 8-aminoquinolines and nitrofurazone are being investigated in this disease.

Table 44.1 gives details of the major drugs used to treat protozoal infection.

Table 44.1 Drug therapy in protozoal infection.

Protozoan species	Drug therapy	Further comment
T. cruzi (American)	Benznidazole or nifurtimox	Effective in the early stages
T. gambiense and T. rhodesiense (African)	Pentamidine and suramin are effective in the early stages	Later neurological disease – melarsoprol or eflornithine or nifurtimox
Toxoplasma gondii	Pyrimethamine/sulfadiazine	Add folinic acid to reduce risk of bone marrow suppression; see drugs and HIV infection
Pneumocystis carinii	Sulfamethoxazole/trimethoprim – high dose	Refractory cases – pentamidine; see drugs and HIV infection
Leishmania (visceral)	Sodium stibogluconate or meglumine antimoniate	Resistant cases – allopurinol + pentamidine
Leishmania (cutaneous)	Intralesional – antimonials	Usually lesions heal spontaneously
Giardia lamblia	Metronidazole, tinidazole or mepacrine	Treat family and institutional contacts

HELMINTHIC INFECTION

Table 44.2 gives details of drug treatment for
helminthic infections.

Table 44.2 Drug therapy in helminthic infection.

Helminthic species	Drug therapy	Further comment
Tapeworms		
Taenia saginata	Praziquantel or niclosamide	A single dose of praziquantel is curative
Taenia soleum Cysticercosis	Praziquantel or niclosamide	
Taenia soleum	Praziquantel	
Diphyllobothrium latum	Praziquantel or niclosamide	
Hydatid disease		
Echinococcus granulosus	Albendazole or mebendazole	Surgery for operable treated cyst
Hookworm		
Ancylostoma duodenale Necator americanus	Mebendazole/albendazole, bephenium or pyrantel	
Strongyloides stercoralis	Albendazole	
Threadworm		
Enterobius vermicularis	Mebendazole/albendazole, bephenium or pyrantel	
Whipworm		
Trichuris trichiuria	Thiabendazole	
Tissue nematodes		
Ancylostoma braziliensae	Thiabendazole	
Guinea worm		
Dracunculus medinensis	Metronidazole	Symptoms rapidly relieved
Visceral larvae/roundworms		
Toxocara canis Toxocara catis	Diethylcarbamazine	Progressive increasing dose, allergic reactions to dying larvae, need corticosteroids for ocular disease
Lymphatic filariasis		
Wuchteria bancrofti	Diethylcarbamazine	
Onchocerciasis		
Onchocerca volvulus	Ivermectin	Single dose is curative
Schistosomiasis/blood flukes		
Schistosoma mansoni Schistosoma japonicum	Praziquantel	Oxamniquine – S. mansoni Metriphonate – S. hematobium
Liver flukes/fascioliasis		
Fasciola hepatica etc.	Praziquantel	
Other gut nematodes		
Ascariasis Ascaris lumbricoides	Pyrantel or levamisole	Piperazine is effective but not well tolerated
Trichinosis		
Trichinella spiralis	Mebendazole, albendazole or pyrantel	

Cancer Chemotherapy

45

Introduction   **586**

Pathophysiology of neoplastic cell growth   **586**

General principles in the use of cytotoxic drugs   **587**

Combination chemotherapy   **591**

Resistance to cytotoxic drugs   **591**

Adjuvant chemotherapy   **592**

Complications of cancer chemotherapy   **593**

Major groups of drugs used in cancer chemotherapy   **596**

INTRODUCTION

The management of a patient with malignant disease requires a multidisciplinary approach. In addition to the three principal treatment modalities of surgery, radiotherapy and chemotherapy (including immunotherapy) the importance of attending to psychiatric and social factors is increasingly recognized. Accurate staging (i.e. determining the extent of the disease) is an essential prerequisite of successful management and in those cases where localized disease is confirmed, cure may be possible with surgery or radiotherapy. In some cases chemotherapy is also given in the knowledge that widespread microscopic dissemination almost certainly has occurred (adjuvant therapy). If disease is widespread at presentation, systemic chemotherapy is more likely to be effective although radiotherapy or surgery may be required for local disease control and to reduce tumor load before potentially curative chemotherapy. This discussion of the clinical pharmacology of the drugs used in cancer chemotherapy is not intended to be exhaustive but deals with the principles involved and the pharmacology of the more commonly used drugs.

PATHOPHYSIOLOGY OF NEOPLASTIC CELL GROWTH

The use of drugs in treating cancer is based on the premise that malignant cells differ in some way from normal cells. Although the difference in behavior between normal and malignant cells is all too obvious, and although there are quantitive differences in some metabolic processes, the basic cellular and biochemical change or changes that constitute malignancy are still not clearly defined. Both environmental and genetic factors are important in the etiology of malignant disease, and it seems highly probable that derangements of the mechanisms that control cell replication and in the synthesis of nucleotides and proteins are common features of malignant transformation. There is increasing evidence to implicate the insertion of foreign nucleic acid sequences in the host's genome (so-called oncogenes) in the genesis of malignant disease. It may be that more than one defect is required to produce malignancy, and there may be several different ways in which these defects can be produced.

Considerable progress has been made at a practical level in recent years. A number of drugs that selectively affect malignant cells have been discovered, sometimes fortuitously, sometimes as a result of a reasoned approach. Most drugs used in cytotoxic chemotherapy interfere with the synthesis of DNA and/or RNA, with the result that cell death occurs or cell multiplication ceases. These effects are not confined to malignant cells and most cytotoxic agents are also toxic to normal dividing cells, particularly those in bone marrow, the gastrointestinal tract, gonads, hair follicles and skin.

GENERAL PRINCIPLES IN THE USE OF CYTOTOXIC DRUGS

The number of cytotoxic drugs available has expanded rapidly and drugs are now available that interfere with several different stages of the cell cycle, opening the way to the rational use of drug combinations. This has been of crucial importance in achieving efficacy in several malignancies, especially lymphomas and leukemias. Originally such combinations were devised on an empirical basis: cocktails of drugs, each of which was known to have some action on a particular type of cancer, were given to the patient. By trial and error certain combinations were found to be effective and improvements in treatment were achieved. With increasing understanding of drug action it is possible that oncologists will combine these drugs logically on a sound theoretical basis, to achieve optimal drug effects. It is helpful at this stage to consider how the action of cytotoxic drugs is related to the cell cycle. Basic studies have distinguished the following phases in the cell cycle (Fig. 45.1).

In general, cytotoxic agents only affect cells in the proliferative phases since their action depends on interference with the synthesis or division of cellular material. They can be divided into two groups:

Cycle non-specific drugs

This means that they act at all stages in the proliferating cell cycle (but not in the G_0-resting phase). Because of this their dose–response curves follow first-order kinetics (cells are killed exponentially with increasing dose). The linear relationship between dose and log response (Fig. 45.2) is exploited in the use of high-dose chemotherapy. Cytotoxic drugs are given at very high doses over a short period, thus rendering the bone marrow aplastic, but at the same time achieving a very high tumor cell kill. The ensuing period of myelosuppression requires intensive support with antibiotics, red cell and platelet transfusions, growth factors, and

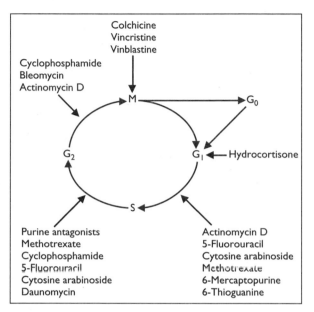

Fig. 45.1 The cell cycle and the phase specificity of some cytotoxic drugs. G_0 = resting phase. G_1 = prereplicative phase. S = DNA synthesis. G_2 = postreplicative phase. M = mitosis or cell division.

in some cases reinfusion of either previously harvested autologous or allogeneic bone marrow. Results in some hematological malignancies (e.g. leukemias, lymphomas) have been encouraging. The drugs used in such therapy are those whose predominant toxic effects are on the bone marrow, as this is the only important normal tissue that can be supported and rescued. Proven agents in this field are alkylating agents (e.g. cyclophosphamide, melphalan and nitrosoureas such as cischloroethylnitrosourea (CCNU-lomustine) and bischloroethylnitrosourea (BCNU-carmustine).

Phase-specific drugs

These drugs act only at a specific phase in the cell cycle. Therefore the more rapid the cell turnover the more effective they are. Their dose–response curve is initially exponential but at higher doses a maximum

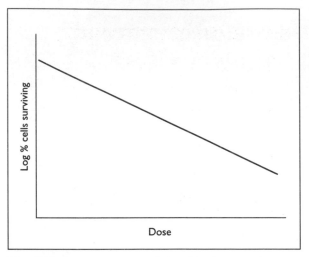

Fig. 45.2 Dose–response relationship for a cycle non-specific drug.

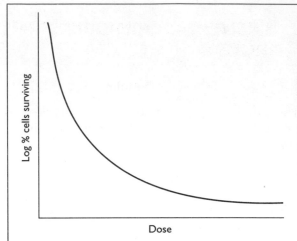

Fig. 45.3 Dose–response relationship for a phase-specific drug.

response is reached and the curve becomes asymptotic (Fig. 45.3). Table 45.1 classifies cytotoxic drugs according to their effect on the cell cycle but until the kinetic behavior of human tumors can be adequately characterized in individual patients the value of this classification is limited. The distinction between cycle non-specific and phase-specific drugs, although fairly clearcut in animal experiments, is probably oversimplified and yet to prove of practical importance in treating human cancer.

By using combinations or sequences of drugs, attempts are being made to modify the cell cycle so as to increase therapeutic efficiency. For example, one drug can be given to synchronize cells in a phase in the cycle; when a large number of cells have accumulated in this phase, a different drug is given that is highly active against this phase and a high kill of cells should be achieved. Thus vinca alkaloids block proliferating cells in mitosis where they can be killed by drugs such as bleomycin. In exper-

Table 45.1 Classification of cytotoxic drugs according to their effect on the cell cycle.

Predominantly cycle non-specific	Predominantly phase specific
Nitrogen mustard	Methotrexate
Cyclophosphamide, ifosfamide	6-Mercaptopurine
Melphalan	6-Thioguanine
Busulphan	5-Fluorouracil
Chlorambucil	Cytosine arabinoside
Lomustine (CCNU), carmustine (BCNU)	Vinca alkaloids
Dacarbazine (DTIC)	Etoposide
Actinomycin D	
Mitomycin C	
Mitozantrone	
Doxorubicin, daunomycin	

CCNU = cischloroethylnitrosourea. BCNU = bischloroethylnitrosourea.

imental systems a dose of bleomycin given 6 hours after vinblastine produces an increased cell kill. There is circumstantial evidence that this may occur in human bronchial tumors. However, most attempts at such cell kinetic scheduling have been unsuccessful in clinicial practice.

Cells in the G_0 (resting) phase present problems in treatment since they are not susceptible to cytotoxic drugs. It is therefore possible for a malignant cell to hide away and only emerge when cytotoxic treatment has been finished. This is one reason for giving prolonged courses of drugs. Cell kinetics of tumors have been studied extensively in animals, particularly in mouse leukemia. The information obtained has enabled us to deploy cytotoxic drugs more effectively. This requires extrapolation from animal tumor to humans and although this has produced considerable advances, not all the findings in animal models can be extrapolated to humans. The main conclusions from these studies are:

1. The natural history of cancer is much longer than it was once thought to be. Many tumor cells grow rapidly but this is not a uniform characteristic and their growth rates are varied and overlap with many normal tissues. Thus the length of cell cycle of a leukemic blast cell is 50–80 hours, but that of a breast carcinoma is 2–5 months. These may be compared with the 15–18 hours of a normoblast and 1–2 months for epidermal cells. It can be inferred that the course of human myelomatosis takes some 21 years from the appearance of the first malignant cell to the death of the patient. The clinical course of the disease is a relatively small proportion of the total course (Fig. 45.4). Studies in animals suggest that complete cure of cancer requires total eradication of all cancer cells. Therefore treatment will need to be prolonged beyond the point at which tumor is clinically evident if this aim is to be achieved. In animal models it is found that a given dose of a drug kills a

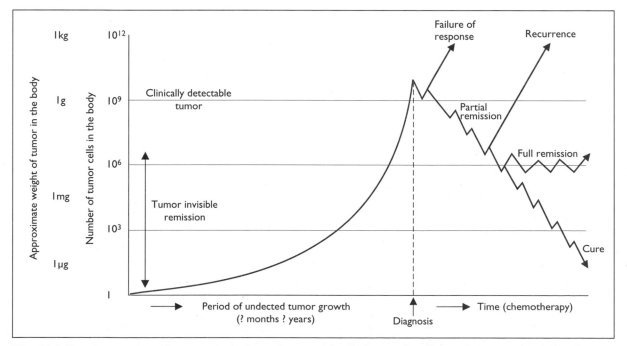

Fig. 45.4 Tumor growth and response to chemotherapy. The duration of undetected tumor growth has been shortened for diagrammatic representation: in most cases it is probably at least five times the length of the treatment phase.

constant percentage of cells in unit time and thus the number of cells present before therapy begins will determine the number of cells surviving after treatment. In lymphomas the percentage cell kill can be 90% but for solid tumors it is often only 50%. To take an extremely simplified example, and neglecting addition of cells by replication and any effect of host defense mechanisms, if 10^{11} cells are present in a clinically detectable solid tumor, approximately 40 courses of treatment with a cell kill fraction of about 50% would be necessary to eradicate the tumor. This could mean 4–5 years of therapy. Reduction of the tumor burden by preliminary surgery or radiotherapy before chemotherapy may be of value in this context.

2. The fraction of cells that are dividing in a tumor decreases as the mass of tumor increases; this is due to cells going into the G_0 (resting) phase, and means that the tumor is more susceptible to cytotoxic drugs when the mass is small, and when most cells are dividing. Tumors become less easy to treat as their size increases. Death occurs in humans when the malignant cell population reaches about 10^{12} (Fig. 45.4).

3. Cytotoxic drugs given in high doses for short repeated periods usually produce a higher kill of malignant cells than continuous low dosage schedules, because although drug toxicity is usually cumulative, the low kill of malignant cells achieved by low dosage can soon be replaced by proliferating surviving cells. Intermittent administration of large doses of cytotoxic agents allows the bone marrow to regenerate in the intervals between treatments (Fig. 45.5). Furthermore, intermittent doses are less immunosuppressant than continuous administration since immunologically competent lymphocytes are in the G_0 phase and so protected from injury during the action of the drug, but in the intervals they are able to enter the cycle to form immunoblasts should an appropriate antigenic stimulus occur.

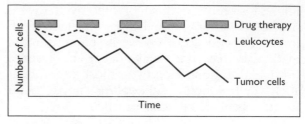

Fig. 45.5 Effect of intermittent therapy on bone marrow and tumor cells.

The superiority of intermittent dosage regimes is not absolute in human cancer and continued low dosage over long periods sometimes produces good results, perhaps because the turnover of cells in some tumors is slow.

4. Since every cancer cell has to be eliminated to produce a cure it becomes important to know when this aim has been achieved, since at that point medication can be stopped. As yet there are no practical methods for assessing very small numbers of tumor cells. Tumor markers such as myeloma protein, β-human chorionic gonadotrophin, α-fetoprotein, carcinoembryonic antigen (CEA) and CA-125, can only detect of the order of 10^5–10^6 cells, and for many tumors no reliable markers exist. It is possible that immune mechanisms may be able to cope with small numbers of malignant cells, so that it may not be necessary to kill every tumor cell with drugs. Nevertheless, the search for useful tumor marker systems continues, since by this means more rational therapy will be possible. Because of the need to eradicate all of the tumor it has become important to destroy neoplastic cells in socalled sanctuary sites. Thus it was found that relapse of acute lymphatic leukemia in children frequently occurred in the central nervous system (CNS), although blast cells had been successfully eradicated from marrow and other sites. Irradiation of the brain and spinal cord accompanied by intrathecal administration of cytotoxic agents was added to the already rigorous protocol for this disease with a consequent improvement in survival.

COMBINATION CHEMOTHERAPY

Combinations of drugs with different mechanisms of action provide greater benefit than individual agents do alone (Fig. 45.6). If the side effects of the components of the combination are different the combination may be no more difficult to tolerate than if the drugs were given singly. If they have different mechanisms of cytotoxic action there may be an increased tumor cell kill. They may also allow more rapid host recovery and better selectivity. There are now a number of well-established combination therapies for human tumors (see below). A common procedure is to employ cycle non-specific drugs followed by phase-specific agents. The first drug reduces the non-proliferating cell pool and stimulates surviving cancer cells to enter mitosis when they can be killed by the phase-specific drug. The sequence in which drugs are given has an important effect on the response in animal tumor models, but the relevance of this to human tumors is undetermined. Successful combination therapy protocols for human tumors are the result of empiricism rather than theory. Not all combinations of drugs are beneficial and some are antagonistic, or preferentially attack normal cells. Some agents are included in combination protocols because of their kinetic properties, for example lipid-soluble agents like procarbazine or nitrosoureas, which cross the blood–brain barrier, may be used to eradicate malignant cells in the CNS.

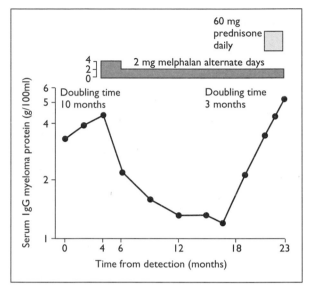

Fig. 45.6 Growth-rate relapse during treatment of myeloma as shown by the faster doubling rate of the serum paraprotein concentration. (From J.R. Hobbs. *Br Med J* 1971; **2**: 67. Reproduced by permission of the Editor.)

RESISTANCE TO CYTOTOXIC DRUGS

Resistance may be primary (i.e. a non-responsive tumor) or acquired. It resembles the acquisition of antibiotic resistance by bacterial populations in that it can result from selective killing of susceptible cells leaving primarily resistant cells or from an adaptive change by the cancer cell. Several mechanisms of resistance have been studied in human tumors and these are summarized in Table 45.2.

The ability to predict the sensitivity of bacterial pathogens to antimicrobial substances *in vitro* produced a profound change in the efficacy of treatment of infectious diseases. The development of analogous predictive tests has long been a priority in cancer research. They would be particularly desirable since in contrast to antimicrobial drugs, cytotoxic agents are administered

Table 45.2 Acquired tumor resistance to cytotoxic agents.

Mechanism	Examples
1. Reduced uptake of drug	Methotrexate; daunorubicin
2. Deletion of enzyme to activate drug	Cytosine arabinoside; 5-fluorouracil
3. Increased detoxification of drug	6-Mercaptopurine
4. Increased concentration of target enzyme	Methotrexate
5. Decreased requirement for specific metabolic product	Asparaginase
6. Increased utilization of alternative pathway	Antimetabolites
7. Rapid repair of drug-induced lesion	Alkylating agents
8. Decreased number of receptors for drug	Hormones
9. Alteration in proliferation rate. ?Underlying mechanism	Myeloma, chronic myeloid leukemia commonly terminates in a more aggressive phase

in doses that cause toxic effects in most patients. Predictive toxicity tests could provide a considerable improvement in therapy since patients with non-responsive tumors could be spared the toxic effects of these drugs. Unfortunately clinically useful tests do not yet exist. Promising results have been obtained recently using *in vitro* cultures of tumor stem cells. It is likely that with advances in cell culture techniques *in vitro* tumor colony assays will become a practical reality.

ADJUVANT CHEMOTHERAPY

About 75% of patients with solid tumors die as a result of metastases rather than of the primary tumor. These often arise in the preclinical course of a malignancy. Thus it would be unusual to detect a breast carcinoma that was smaller than 1 cm in diameter clinically (this already contains approximately 10^9 cells and has probably undergone some 30 divisions since the original malignant cell arose). Tumor cells begin to escape into the lymphatic and blood circulation when neovascularization occurs (usually when the tumor is less than 3 mm in diameter). The opportunity for systemic seeding is therefore present long before most breast tumors are clinically apparent. Adjuvant chemotherapy aims to destroy these disseminated microfoci at a time when there is no clinical evidence of residual disease. It is thought that chemotherapeutic intervention could be more successful at this stage because:

1. Total body tumor load is small and treatment is more likely to be effective with drugs possessing first-order cell kill kinetics.
2. Fewer cells in small tumors are in the G_0 phase, i.e. the cell growth fraction is higher.
3. Vascularization of small tumors is proportionately greater than in larger tumors, facilitating drug penetration.
4. Patients at this stage are less likely to be immunosuppressed and intrinsic host defenses may remain operative. There is less likelihood of extensive tumor infiltration into the marrow so chemotherapy may cause less myelosuppression than later in the disease when large volumes of marrow are replaced by malignant cells.

Against these potential benefits of eradicating early metastases must be set:

1. The possibility that in treating a group of patients with putative metastases some

patients who in fact do not have metastatic disease will be exposed to the toxic effects of chemotherapy.

2. Adjuvant chemotherapy imposes an added burden of drug toxicity on patients who may already have undergone major surgery and/or radical radiotherapy.

3. There is a danger of inducing second malignancies with cytotoxic drugs (see below), necessitating careful consideration of risk/potential benefit in patients whose primary neoplasm has a long natural history.

4. Adjuvant chemotherapy may delay but not prevent the development of metastatic disease, making this more difficult to treat when it does occur due to drug resistance. Overall survival may thus not be affected.

The balance of the arguments probably differs from tumor to tumor. Encouraging results have been reported with adjuvant therapy in some pediatric tumors (e.g. Wilms' tumor, Ewing's tumor, osteogenic sarcoma) and in breast cancer in adults. Adjuvant immunotherapy may also become important. For example, levamisole (an immunostimulant, chapter 47) with 5-fluorouracil prolongs remission following surgical treatment in Duke stage C rectal/colonic carcinoma.

COMPLICATIONS OF CANCER CHEMOTHERAPY

The chief adverse effects are summarized in Table 45.3. Chemotherapeutic drugs vary in their potential to cause adverse effects and there is considerable interindividual variation in susceptibility.

Nausea and vomiting with cytotoxic drugs

Cytotoxic drugs cause nausea and vomiting to varying degrees (Table 45.4). This is usually delayed for 1–2 hours after drug administration and often lasts for 24–48 hours. The mechanisms by which such drugs induce vomiting include stimulation of the chemoreceptor trigger zone (in the floor of the fourth ventricle, chapter 31) and stimulation of peripheral receptors mediating gastric atony and cessation of peristalsis.

If vomiting is anticipated, it is normal to use prophylactic antiemetics before treatment and to give the patient a supply of tablets to take as needed over the ensuing days. No treatment is entirely effective especially for

Table 45.3 Principal toxic effects of cytotoxic chemotherapy.

Immediate	Delayed
1. Nausea and vomiting	1. Bone marrow suppression producing infection, bleeding and anemia
2. Extravasation with tissue necrosis	2. Alopecia
	3. Infertility/teratogenicity
	4. Second malignancy
	5. Psychiatric morbidity
	6. Miscellaneous, e.g. cardiomyopathy with doxorubicin, peripheral neuropathy with vincristine (see text and Table 45.6)

Table 45.4 Emetogenic potential of commonly used cytotoxic drugs.

Severe	Moderate	Rare
Doxorubicin	BCNU, CCNU	Bleomycin
Cyclophosphamide	Mitomycin C	Cytarabine
Dacarbazine	Procarbazine	Vinca alkaloids
Mustine	Etoposide	Methotrexate
Cisplatin	Ifosfamide	5-Fluorouracil
		Chlorambucil
		Mitozantrone

CCNU and BCNU: see Table 45.1.

cisplatin-induced vomiting. Drugs used for control of vomiting are discussed in chapter 31.

Extravasation with tissue necrosis

Tissue necrosis occurs when one of the following drugs extravasates: doxorubicin, BCNU, mustine, vincristine or vinblastine. This may result in the need for skin grafting. Expert attention to vascular access is mandatory.

Bone marrow suppression

There are two patterns of bone-marrow recovery after suppression (Fig. 45.7), rapid and delayed. The usual pattern is of rapid recovery but chlorambucil, BCNU, CCNU and

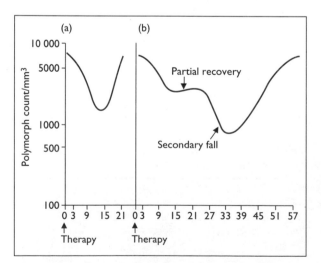

Fig. 45.7 Patterns of bone-marrow recovery following cytotoxic therapy: (a) rapid (17–21 days) and (b) delayed (initial fall 8–10 days, secondary minimum at 27–32 days, recovery 42–50 days). (After D.E. Bergasagel.)

melphalan can cause prolonged myelosuppression (up to 8 weeks). The recent advent of recombinant hematopoietic growth factors (erythropoietin, granulocyte colony-stimulating factor (G-CSF), granulocyte macrophage colony-stimulating factor (GM-CSF) and interleukin-3 (IL-3)) and their use to minimize the bone marrow suppression of various chemotherapeutic regimes holds out great promise and is discussed in chapter 46. Vincristine, bleomycin and corticosteroids seldom cause myelosuppression. The main problems in myelosuppressed patients are bleeding, infection and anemia which are all treatable. Severe thrombocytopenia (i.e. platelet count less than $20\,000 \times 10^9$/litre) is treated by platelet transfusion, which is also required in patients with milder thrombocytopenia who have active bleeding.

Infection

Infection is the commonest life-threatening complication of chemotherapy. It is often acquired from the patient's own gastrointestinal tract flora. Effective isolation is achieved in purpose-built laminar airflow units but this does not solve the problem of the patient's own bacteria. Oral non-absorbed antibiotics (e.g. neomycin) may be used to suppress the bowel flora. Classical signs of infection, other than pyrexia, are often absent in severely neutropenic patients and constant vigilance is required to detect and treat septicemia before it becomes overwhelming. Broad-spectrum antibiotic treatment must be started empirically in febrile neutropenic patients before the results of blood and other cultures are available. A parenteral aminoglycoside active against *Pseudomonas* and other Gram-negative organisms (e.g. amikacin) with a penicillin (e.g. piperacillin) or cephalosporin (e.g. cefotaxime) which is active against β-lactamase-producing organisms provide suitable initial cover in some instances, but decisions need to be informed by knowledge of local organisms and the patient's prior antimicrobial therapy and culture results (chapter 40).

Opportunistic infections are a common problem in these patients. Oral candidiasis causing pain and dysphagia is best treated with oral nystatin suspension, amphotericin lozenges or oral ketoconazole. Systemic fungal infections are life threatening and require prompt treatment with amphotericin B (chapter 42). They are difficult to diagnose, but if cultures are positive from several sites in a patient who remains febrile despite broad-spectrum antibiotic cover, empirical antifungal therapy is indicated. *Pneumocystis carinii* is an opportunistic protozoan causing severe interstitial pneumonia, it is not very common in neutropenic patients but cases tend to occur in clusters. High-dose co-trimoxazole is the most effective and generally least toxic treatment but parenteral pentamidine may be needed in patients allergic to sulfonamides, as in patients with AIDS (chapter 43). Reactivation of pre-existing tuberculosis is another unusual cause of fever in neutropenic patients. Prophylactic treatment with co-trimoxazole (two forte tablets, twice daily) and fluconazole, 100–200 mg, orally daily reduces the risk of serious infections in severely neutropenic patients and is started when the neutrophil count falls below 500×10^9/litre.

Alopecia

Doxorubicin, ifosfamide and parenteral etoposide cause alopecia. It may be alleviated in the case of doxorubicin by cooling the scalp using ice-cold gel packs or ice-cooled water caps. Some hair loss occurs with almost all cytotoxic agents.

Infertility and teratogenesis

Cytotoxic drugs predictably impair fertility and increase the incidence of fetal abnormalities. Most women develop amenorrhea if treated with cytotoxic drugs; however, many resume normal menstruation when treatment is stopped and pregnancy is then possible, especially in younger women treated with lower total doses of cytotoxic drugs. Amenorrhea is associated with low plasma estrogen and high follicle-stimulating hormone (FSH) and luteinizing hormone (LH), indicating a primary effect on the ovary. In men, a full course of cytotoxic drugs usually produces azoospermia due to direct damage to the germinal epithelium of the testis. Alkylating agents are particularly harmful. Recovery can occur but is delayed for up to several years. The re-establishment of normal spermatogenesis is most common after a short course of treatment with a single agent. Cytotoxic drugs cause testicular damage in prepubertal boys, but the long-term reproductive outcome is unknown. Prepubertal girls are probably less prone to cytotoxic-induced ovarian damage. Sperm storage before chemotherapy can be considered for males wishing to have children in the future. Both men and women must be strongly advised to use contraceptives during chemotherapy as reduction in fertility with these drugs is not universal and fetal malformations could ensue. It is best to avoid conception for at least 6 months after completion of chemotherapy.

Second malignancy

As many as 3–10% of patients treated for Hodgkin's disease (particularly those who received both chemotherapy and radiotherapy) develop a second malignancy: usually acute non-lymphocytic leukemia. This malignancy is also approximately 20 times more likely to develop in patients with ovarian carcinoma treated with alkylating agents with or without radiotherapy. This complication of treatment will probably become more commonly recognized as the number of patients surviving after successful cancer chemotherapy increases.

Summary

Cytotoxic drugs may be used in two ways in the treatment of cancer:

1. They are used when the disease has disseminated widely and is no longer amenable to eradication by surgery. If the cancer is very sensitive to drugs this may be successful, but cytotoxic drugs are not being used to maximum advantage if the tumor cell mass is large. It is conventional, although an oversimplification, to divide treatment into:

   (a) Induction of remission: treatment until the patient is clinically disease free. If no further treatment is given, however, the neoplasm will return in most patients.

   (b) Consolidation and maintenance of remission, often by the use of alternative drugs.

   (c) Late intensification: final intense form of therapy, often with phase-dependent drugs, aimed at killing the last surviving cells of the tumor.

2. Adjuvant therapy entails courses of cytotoxic drugs given when the cancer has apparently been destroyed by surgery or radiotherapy. Its object is to eradicate micrometastases.

The experimental background outlined above suggests that certain general principles should be applied when treating cancer with drugs.

1. Cytotoxic drugs should usually be used in combination.
2. Drugs should be given intermittently and in high doses.
3. Treatment usually needs to be prolonged.
4. The earlier in the disease treatment is started, the better the result.
5. The toxicity of these drugs is considerable and routine blood counts together with intensive clinical support are essential.

Major groups of drugs used in cancer chemotherapy

1. Alkylating agents.
2. Antimetabolites.
3. Vinca alkaloids.
4. Antibiotics.
5. Hormones.
6. Miscellaneous.

Alkylating agents

Alkylating agents are particularly effective when cells are dividing rapidly but they are not phase specific. They combine with DNA of both malignant and normal cells and thus damage not only malignant cells but dividing normal cells, especially those of the bone marrow and the gastrointestinal tract (Table 45.5). The alkyl groupings on these drugs are highly reactive, so that although their most important action is on DNA they also combine with susceptible groups in cells and in tissue fluids. Factors determining the selective toxicity of different alkylating agents have not been identified, although such selectivity exists. Thus, while a tumor sensitive to one alkylating agent is usually sensitive to another, cross-resistance within the group does not necessarily occur. The pharmacokinetic properties of the different drugs are probably important in this respect. Thus whilst most alkylating agents passively diffuse into cells, mustine is actively transported by some cells which may influence the selectivity of this agent.

Table 45.5 Toxicity of alkylating agents at therapeutic dosage.

Drug	Nausea and vomiting	Granulocytopenia	Thrombocytopenia	Special toxicity
Mustine	+++	+++	++++	Tissue necrosis if extravasated
Cyclophosphamide	++	+++	+	Alopecia (10–20%) Chemical cystitis (reduced by mesna) Mucosal ulceration Impaired water excretion Interstitial pulmonary fibrosis
Ifosfamide	++	++	+	Chemical cystitis (reduced by mesna) Alopecia Hypotension (if rapidly infused)
Chlorambucil	+	++	++++	Marrow suppression may be prolonged
Melphalan	0	+++	+++	Chemical cystitis (very rare)
Busulphan	0	++++	+++	Skin pigmentation Interstitial pulmonary fibrosis Amenorrhea Gynecomastia (rare)

MUSTINE AND OTHER ALKYLATING AGENTS (CHLORAMBUCIL, MELPHALAN AND BUSULPHAN)

Use

Mustine is unstable in solution and is given immediately it is made up. It is given slowly (over 2–3 min) via a rapidly running well-flushed proximal intravenous line. This minimizes the risk of local thrombosis and highly irritant extravasation into surrounding tissues. Dose and frequency depend upon the schedule being used. Mustine is usually combined with other cytotoxic drugs (e.g vinblastine, procarbazine and prednisolone (MOPP) combination) when the dose is 6.0 mg/m² body area weekly. It is used to treat Hodgkin's disease.

Mechanism of action

In solution mustine forms highly reactive ethyleneimine ions that alkylate macro-molecules, cross-linking mainly the guanine bases on opposing strands of DNA (Fig. 45.8). The tightly bound DNA strands are then unable to separate and cannot act as templates for RNA production or form new DNA. Mustine probably alkylates other cellular components such as enzymes and membranes: effects that contribute to its cytotoxicity.

Adverse effects

1. Bone marrow depression with leukopenia and thrombocytopenia. The nadir of white blood cells or platelets usually occurs at 10–14 days post-therapy and returns to normal by 3 weeks.
2. Severe nausea and vomiting.
3. If applied to the skin mustine is a vesicant and causes severe tissue necrosis if

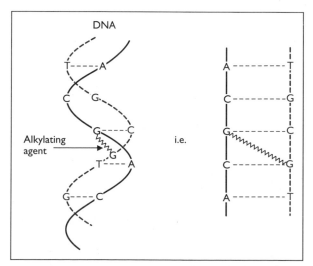

Fig. 45.8 Mechanism of intramolecular bridging of DNA by alkylating agents. A = adenine. C = cytosine. G = guanine. T = thymidine.

inadvertently injected subcutaneously (extravasated – as when an intravenous line 'tissues').
4. Increased risk of second malignancies.
5. Teratogenicity.

Pharmacokinetics

Mustine must be given intravenously. The reactive ethyleneimine ion forms spontaneously due to cyclization in solution. The plasma half-life ($t_{1/2}$) is short, probably about half an hour. The disappearance of the active compound from the plasma is largely due to combination with thiol groups of tissue protein.

CYCLOPHOSPHAMIDE

Use

Cyclophosphamide is an oxazaphosphorine alkylating agent (ifosfamide is another member in this group). It is an inactive prodrug and so can be given orally, unlike mustine, or intravenously. Large doses are nauseating and are given intravenously. Several combination regimens in current use include cyclophosphamide; rarely it may be used as sole therapeutic agent at a dose of 50–150 mg orally daily. In combinations, doses of 400–600 mg/m² are commonly used whilst in high-dose chemotherapy; for example, to prepare patients with acute leukemia and aplastic anemia for allogeneic bone marrow transplantation, doses of 45–60 mg/kg/day for 2–3 days are employed. Cyclophosphamide is most useful in the treatment of various lymphomas and leukemias and in myeloma, but it also has some effect in other malignancies. Cyclophosphamide is also used as an immunosuppressive (chapter 47).

Adverse effects

1. Nausea and vomiting.
2. Bone marrow depression; granulocytopenia is more marked than thrombocytopenia, the nadir occurring 7–10 days after administration.
3. Alopecia.
4. Stomatitis and mucositis.
5. Sterile hemorrhagic cystitis due to acrolein in the urine.
6. Chronic cyclophosphamide therapy is associated with increased risk of bladder cancer. Urotoxicity (and probably the risk of cancer) is controlled by the use of mesna (see below).
7. Impairment of water excretion may result in water intoxication.
8. Rarely myocardial damage, pulmonary fibrosis and hypoglycemia (with enhancement of the effects of sulfonylureas).

Pharmacokinetics

Cyclophosphamide is 80–90% metabolized and activated in the liver by cytochrome P_{450} with the production of a number of cytotoxic alkylating metabolites. The most potent of these is phosphoramide mustard. Cyclophosphamide can be given intravenously or orally and is almost completely absorbed from the intestine. The half-life of cyclophosphamide varies between 3 and 12 hours, When given repeatedly the $t_{1/2}$ becomes progressively shorter. It is shorter in children than in adults. The half-life of the active species (phosphoramide mustard) is probably only minutes. Cyclophosphamide and its metabolites are excreted in urine. Renal excretion of the metabolite acrolein is believed to cause the chemical hemorrhagic cystitis that often accompanies cyclophosphamide administration.

MESNA

Use

Mesna is an acronym for 2-mercaptoethane sulfonate sodium (Na) and is used to protect the urinary tract against the irritant effects of the metabolites of cyclophosphamide and ifosfamide, and in particular acrolein. Mesna is given by intravenous injection or by mouth. Because it is excreted more rapidly ($t_{1/2}$ <30 min) than cyclophosphamide and ifosfamide it is essential that mesna is given at the commencement of treatment and that the maximum interval between doses is not more than 4 hours. The dose of mesna is usually 20% of the dose of the cytotoxic given immediately; mesna dosage is repeated at 4 and 8 hours. Higher doses, for example

40%, given four times at 3-hourly intervals are used for patients at higher risk and children. Urine is monitored for output, proteinuria and hematuria.

Mechanism of action

Mesna protects the uroepithelium by supplying sulfydryl groups to form a stable thioether with acrolein. It also reduces the decomposition rate of the 4-hydroxy metabolites of these drugs to acrolein by combining to form relatively stable compounds that are not toxic to the urinary tract. This interaction with cyclophosphamide and ifosfamide metabolites occurs mainly in the kidney where dimesna (the oxidation product of mesna formed in the blood *in vivo*) is excreted and then reduced back to active mesna. Because mesna circulates in the body as dimesna and penetrates tissues minimally if at all there is no interference with the cytotoxic efficacy of cyclophosphamide and ifosfamide and their pharmacokinetics are unaltered.

Adverse effects

Somnolence and headaches occur.

Antimetabolites

Antimetabolites are structural analogs of cellular metabolites with which they compete. It was hoped that it would be possible to find and block selectively metabolic pathways that were unique to malignant cells. This hope has not been fulfilled, and the pathways blocked by antimetabolites also occur in normal cells, thus their selectivity for malignanat cells is only partial. They are usually phase specific as their action is usually confined to specific steps in the synthesis of nuclear material.

METHOTREXATE

Use

Methotrexate is a folinic acid antagonist. It is the drug of choice for choriocarcinoma (for which it is curative) and for intrathecal therapy. It is used in acute lymphatic leukemia, lymphomas and several solid tumors including osteogenic sarcoma, epidermoid carcinoma of head and neck and some bronchial carcinomas. It has also been used as an immunosuppressant (chapters 22 and 47) and to reduce the rapid cellular proliferation of severe psoriasis (chapter 48). Methotrexate is used in several different regimens:

1. **Conventional dose** Up to 50 mg/m^2/week does not require folinic acid rescue.
2. **Intermediate dose** Up to 150 mg/m^2 by intravenous bolus injection does not require folinic acid rescue unless the patient has renal impairment.
3. **High dose** 1–12 g/m^2 given intravenously over 1–6 hours always needs folinic acid rescue. This is expensive, and at present there is no evidence that it is superior to conventional doses with the possible exception of non-Hodgkin's lymphoma and osteogenic sarcoma.

Mechanism of action

Folic acid is required in the synthesis of thymidylic acid and purine nucleotides and so ultimately for the production of DNA (Fig. 45.9). Methotrexate resembles folic acid and competes with it for the active site of dihydrofolate reductase. The affinity of methotrexate for this site is 100 000 times greater than that of dihydrofolate. By blocking this step, methotrexate prevents nucleic acid synthesis and causes cell death. Folinic acid circumvents the block and thus noncompetitively antagonizes the effect of methotrexate.

Toxicity and adverse effects

Methotrexate toxicity is determined by:

1. A critical extracellular concentration for each target organ.
2. A critical duration of exposure that varies for each organ. For bone marrow and gut the critical plasma concentration is 2 x 10^{-8}M and the time factor is about 42 hours. Both factors must be exceeded for toxicity to

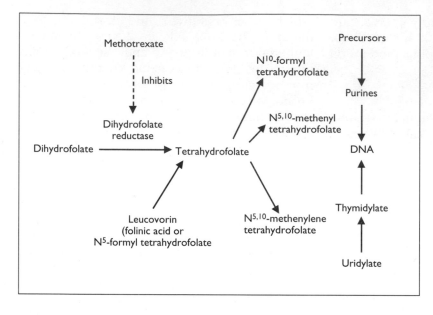

Fig. 45.9 Folate metabolism: effects of methotrexate and leucovorin.

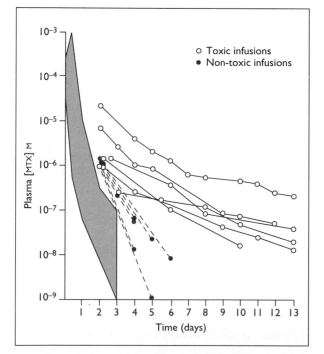

Fig. 45.10 Plasma methotrexate (MTX) disappearance curves in patients receiving 50–250 mg/kg intravenous infusions. The profile for 14 patients who had no toxicity is included within the shaded area. Patients in whom evidence of myelosuppression developed had plasma levels as shown by the open circles. Six non-toxic patients with 48 hour levels greater than 0.9 μM had the plasma levels shown by the solid circles. (From R.G. Stoller *et al.* Reprinted with permission from *N Engl J Med* 1977; **297**: 630.)

occur in these organs. The severity of toxicity is proportional to the length of time that the critical concentration is exceeded and is independent of the amount by which it is exceeded.

Folinic acid rescue bypasses the enzyme block and prevents methotrexate toxicity. Some malignant cells are less able than normal cells to take up folinate thus introducing a degree of selectivity. Rescue is commenced 24 hours after methotrexate administration with oral or intravenous doses of 10–15 mg given at 6 hourly intervals for 4–8 doses. Folinic acid administration is continued until the plasma methotrexate concentration falls below 2×10^{-8} M. Monitoring plasma methotrexate concentrations has improved the safety of using this drug and allows identification of patients at special risk of toxicity (Fig. 45.10).

Adverse effects

Several of the adverse effects of methotrexate are similar to those of radiation, and toxicity is increased in areas that have been irradiated. Effects include:

1. Myelosuppression.
2. Nausea and vomiting.
3. Stomatitis.

4. Diarrhea.
5. Cirrhosis: chronic low-dose administration (as for psoriasis) can cause chronic active hepatitis and cirrhosis, interstitial pneumonitis and osteoporosis.
6. Renal dysfunction, acute vasculitis (after high-dose treatment).
7. Seizures (especially after intrathecal administration).

Renal insufficiency poses special problems since it interferes with methotrexate elimination and plasma methotrexate concentration monitoring is essential under these circumstances. Acute renal failure can be caused by tubular obstruction by crystals of methotrexate. Diuresis (>3 l/day) with alkalinization (pH >7) of the urine by intravenous administration of sodium bicarbonate reduces the incidence of nephrotoxicity. Renal damage is caused by the precipitation of methotrexate and 7-hydroxymethotrexate in the tubules and these weak acids are more water soluble in alkaline pH because this favours their charged (anionic) form rather than the free acid. Intrathecal administration also causes special problems: convulsions, and chemical arachnoiditis leading to paraplegia, cerebellar dysfunction and cranial nerve palsies. A necrotizing demyelinating leukoencephalopathy can occur months or years after treatment.

Pharmacokinetics

Methotrexate can be given orally or by intravenous or intramuscular injection. Absorption from the gut depends on a saturable transport process. Small amounts (0.1 mg/kg) are rapidly and completely absorbed whilst larger doses of the order of 10 mg/kg are incompletely absorbed. After intravenous injection methotrexate distributes in about 75% of body weight. Disappearance from plasma is best described by a three-compartment model since a triphasic decline in plasma concentration is observed. The initial distribution phase $t_{1/2}$ is 0.75 hours; the second-phase $t_{1/2}$ is 2–3.5 hours and is largely associated with renal elimination; the final phase (which begins 6–24 hours after conventional doses and 30–48 hours after

high doses) is prolonged due to excretion via the bile and subsequent reabsorption from the gut, and is characterized by a $t_{1/2}$ of 10–12 hours. This final phase $t_{1/2}$ is important since toxicity is related to the plasma concentrations during this phase as well as to the peak concentrations achieved. The occurrence of this longer terminal phase $t_{1/2}$ may explain the high incidence of toxicity in patients receiving chronic low-dose methotrexate therapy compared to larger but more widely spaced single doses. Distribution of methotrexate into interstitial fluid spaces including cerebrospinal fluid (CSF) and pleural cavities is via passive diffusion and is slow, and it is usual to inject methotrexate directly into the CSF. When this is done methotrexate is slowly absorbed into plasma from CSF. About 50–70% of methotrexate is bound to plasma protein (principally albumin) and alterations in plasma binding affect its pharmacokinetics.

Methotrexate enters normal and malignant cells via an energy-dependent carrier-mediated transport process, as does folate. About 80–95% of the drug finally undergoes renal excretion either unchanged or as metabolites. Methotrexate is both filtered and undergoes active tubular secretion into the urine. It is partly metabolized by gut flora during enterohepatic circulation and polyglutamate derivatives may be synthesized in the liver. These metabolites account for less than 10% of an intravenous dose but if the same dose is given orally, 35% of the absorbed dose is excreted as metabolites, consistent with presystemic hepatic and gut metabolism. 7-Hydroxymethotrexate is produced in liver. It is inactive but is four times less soluble than methotrexate and contributes to renal toxicity by precipitation and crystalluria. Polyglutamate metabolites are potent inhibitors of the dihydrofolate reductase and accumulate within cells, persisting in human liver for months after methotrexate administration.

Drug interactions

- Probenecid, salicylate and other non-steroidal anti-inflammatory drugs (NSAIDs) increase methotrexate toxicity by competing for renal tubular secretion, while simultaneously displacing it from plasma albumin binding sites.

- Gentamicin and cisplatin increase toxicity by compromising renal excretion.
- Cellular uptake of methotrexate is decreased by cortisone and prednisone and enhanced by vincristine.
- Methotrexate action is antagonized by triamterene (increases intracellular dihydrofolate reductase) and allopurinol (increases purine availability).

6-MERCAPTOPURINE

Use

6-Mercaptopurine (6MP) is a purine antimetabolite. It is effective in the treatment of acute leukemias, especially in children, and as an immunosuppressant (chapter 47). The usual oral dose is 2.5 mg/kg/day; administration is continued for several weeks and if after 4 weeks there has been no response, the dose is increased to 5 mg/kg/day. It is usually given as part of a combination schedule.

Mechanism of action

6-Mercaptopurine is a sulfur analog of adenine (6-aminopurine) and hypoxanthine (6-hydroxypurine). The exact mechanism of action of 6MP, following its conversion to ribonucleoside monophosphate, is still incompletely understood. It blocks DNA synthesis, probably through inhibition of *de novo* purine synthesis, incorporation of thiopurines into nucleic acids and interference with purine interconversions.

Adverse effects

1. Bone marrow suppression; leukopenia and thrombocytopenia.
2. Nausea, vomiting and mild diarrhea are uncommon but occur with high doses.
3. Renal calculi occur rarely.

Pharmacokinetics

6-Mercaptopurine is only about 15% absorbed when given orally. Plasma $t_{1/2}$ in children is about 20 min but it is double this in adults. It is only 20% bound to plasma protein, but cerebrospinal fluid concentrations are only 20% of those in plasma. 6-Mercaptopurine is eliminated mainly by hepatic metabolism via xanthine oxidase, but approximately 20% of an intravenous dose of 6MP is excreted in the urine within 6 hours and renal impairment may therefore enhance its toxicity.

Drug interactions

Allopurinol inhibits xanthine oxidase. The dose of 6MP should be reduced to one-quarter to avoid toxicity in patients who are receiving allopurinol. This is important since allopurinol pretreatment is used to reduce the risk of acute uric acid nephropathy due to rapid tumor kill in patients with leukemia.

CYTARABINE; CYTOSINE ARABINOSIDE

Use

Cytarabine differs from naturally occurring deoxycytidine and cytidine in that arabinose replaces the deoxyribose or ribose as the sugar moiety. It is used in acute leukemia and lymphomas. The dose is 2–3 mg/kg every 24 hours for up to 7 days as a single agent or in various combination schedules.

Mechanism of action

Cytarabine is converted by anabolic phosphorylation in the cell into its triphosphate, and this is the active cytotoxic compound (Fig. 45.11). It is believed to inhibit DNA polymerase competitively and thus prevent DNA synthesis. Cytarabine is a cell cycle phase-specific drug acting mainly in the late S phase. Its effectiveness is directly proportional to the duration of exposure of cells to the drug. It is therefore necessary to use regimens that employ continuous infusion of the drug or frequent intermittent injections.

Adverse effects

1. Nausea, vomiting.
2. Stomatitis.
3. Bone marrow depression.

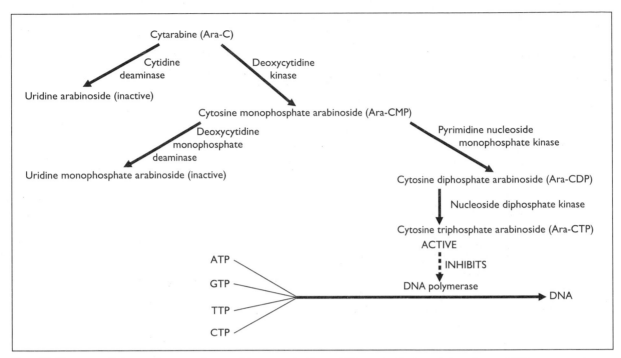

Fig. 45.11 Intracellular pathways of cytarabine metabolism. ATP = adenosine triphosphate, GTP = guanosine triphosphate, TTP = thymidine triphosphate.

Pharmacokinetics

Cytarabine is metabolized by the widely distributed enzyme cytidine deaminase so that after intravenous injection it is rapidly metabolized by the liver to uracil arabinoside. Plasma $t_{1/2}$ is 60–110 min and the kinetics are dose dependent. It is rarely given orally because less than 20% is absorbed due to intraluminal deamination in the gut. Although widely distributed in the body CSF cytarabine concentrations are only 40% of those of the plasma even when the drug is given by continuous intravenous infusion, so it is often given intrathecally if CNS activity is needed. It is excreted unchanged exclusively by the kidney and dosage modification is needed in renal impairment.

5-FLUOROURACIL

Use

5-Fluorouracil (5FU) is useful in the treatment of carcinomas of the breast, ovary, esophagus, colon and skin. It is the most effective cytotoxic agent used in treating adenocarcinoma of the gastrointestinal tract, but even so is disappointing in these notoriously unresponsive tumors. A response or partial response occurs in up to 30% of patients with cancer of the stomach, large bowel or rectum, but life is not prolonged. Similar results are obtained in carcinoma of the pancreas. Addition of other cytotoxic agents does not appear to produce a worthwhile improvement in the treatment of this type of cancer, but addition of an immunostimulant, levamisole, is somewhat encouraging in advanced colon cancers (see above and chapter 47). 5-Fluorouracil, 15 mg/kg, by intravenous injection daily for 5 days is a typical regimen, but there is a wide variety of dosage schedules. It is also given by hepatic artery infusion in patients with hepatic metastases to produce high hepatic levels without correspondingly high systemic levels. This method is partially successful but its value is offset by the complications associated with catheterization of the hepatic artery. Dose modification is required with liver dysfunction.

Mechanism of action

5-Fluorouracil is activated by anabolic phosphorylation to form:

1. 5-Fluorouridine monophosphate which is incorporated into RNA inhibiting its function.
2. 5-Fluorodeoxyuridylate which binds strongly to thymidylate synthetase and inhibits DNA synthesis.

Adverse effects

1. Oral ulceration and diarrhea occur in about 20% of patients.
2. Bone marrow suppression: megaloblastic anemia usually occurs about 14 days after beginning treatment.
3. Cerebellar ataxia (2% incidence) is attributed to fluorocitrate, a neurotoxic metabolite that inhibits the Krebs cycle by lethal synthesis.

Pharmacokinetics

5-Fluorouracil activation occurs in the target cell (and thus defines the specificity of the drug); inactivation occurs mainly in the liver (Fig. 45.12). 5-Fluorouracil is initially reduced and then cleared non-enzymatically to inactive products that are excreted in the urine. It is cleared rapidly from plasma with a $t_{1/2}$ of 10–20 min. About 20% is excreted unchanged in the urine and the remainder is metabolized. 5-Fluorouracil distributes in total body water and readily penetrates the blood–brain barrier; it is usually given by injection since it is unreliably absorbed from the gut due to high hepatic first-pass metabolism.

Vinca alkaloids

Use

Two alkaloids, vinblastine and vincristine, have been isolated from the Madagascan periwinkle plant. Vindesine is a semisynthetic modification of vinblastine. Despite their

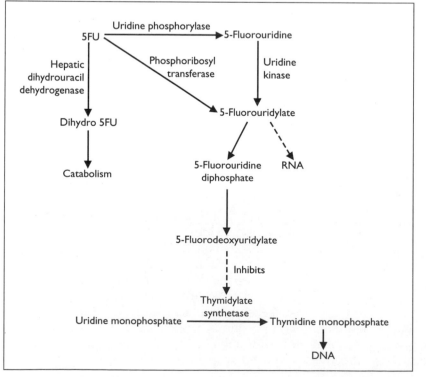

Fig. 45.12 Metabolism and activation of 5-fluorouracil (5FU).

close structural relationship they differ in their clinical spectrum and toxicity. Vinblastine is used in the treatment of testicular cancer and Hodgkin's disease. It is given in combination with other drugs (e.g. mustine, prednisolone and procarbazine) at weekly intervals. The usual dose in combination therapy is 6 mg/m² twice during each course. Vincristine is used in breast cancer, lymphomas and also in the initial treatment of acute lymphoblastic leukemia. It is usually given, in combination with other agents, in a dose of 1.4 mg/m² at monthly intervals.

Mechanism of action

Vinca alkaloids bind to tubulin, a protein that forms the microtubules that are essential for the formation of the spindle that separates the chromosomes during mitosis. They cause 'crystallization' of tubulin and dissolution of the spindle, halting mitosis. Although often called 'spindle poisons' vinca alkaloids have other actions on cell metabolism including inhibition of nucleic acid and protein synthesis. Binding to microtubules concerned with neuronal growth and axonal transport accounts for their neurotoxicity.

Adverse effects

Toxic effects of vincristine and vinblastine are strikingly different despite their structural similarity (Table 45.6).

Pharmacokinetics

Vinca alkaloids are only given intravenously: they are poorly absorbed from the gut. They are extensively metabolized by the liver to largely unknown metabolites although the principal deacetylated metabolite of vinblastine is more active than vinblastine itself. They are largely excreted in the bile and have long terminal half-lives (vincristine, 85 hours; vinblastine and vindesine, 24 hours) so they should be avoided if possible in patients with hepatic impairment. Vincristine exhibits non-linear pharmacokinetics showing a disproportionate increase in area under the plasma concentration–time curve with increasing dose. This may be because microtubules are involved in biliary secretion and their dissolution by vinca alkaloids results in the drug inhibiting its own elimination.

Podophyllin derivatives

Podophyllin is extracted from the American mandrake or May apple: it is topically effective against warts. A number of derivatives of the active principle, podophyllotoxin, have been investigated as antineoplastic drugs. One of these, etoposide, is widely used.

ETOPOSIDE

Use

Etoposide is one of the most active drugs against small cell lung cancer and is used in

Table 45.6 Comparative side effects of vinca alkaloids.

Vincristine	Vinblastine
Severe subcutaneous necrosis if extravasated	Severe subcutaneous necrosis if extravasated
Neurotoxic – high incidence of peripheral neuropathy	Neurotoxic – low incidence of peripheral neuropathy
Thrombocytosis – less often myelosuppression	Myelosuppression
Alopecia – 20–70%	Alopecia – infrequently
Gastrointestinal upset	Gastrointestinal upset
Inappropriate ADH syndrome	Inappropriate ADH syndrome

ADH = antidiuretic hormone.

combination therapy. It is also used in lymphomas, testicular teratomas and trophoblastic tumors. The usual dose is 60–120 mg/m² intravenously (orally, 120–240 mg/m²) given daily for 5 days, every 21–28 days.

Mechanism of action

Etoposide causes DNA damage similar to that seen after radiation.

Adverse effects

1. Nausea and vomiting are common, especially after oral administration.
2. Alopecia.
3. Bone marrow suppression is dose-dependent and reversible.

Pharmacokinetics

Etoposide is given by intravenous injection or orally (bioavailability 50%). It undergoes hepatic metabolism and a small amount is eliminated in the urine. The $t_{1/2}$ is approximately 12 hours.

Antibiotics

Several antibiotics (e.g. anthracyclines, mitozantrone, bleomycin) have clinically useful antineoplastic activity.

ANTHRACYCLINES

Anthracyclines are widely used for malignant disease. Daunorubicin and doxorubicin are the most widely used drugs in this group, but many new analogs (e.g. epirubicin, idarubicin), with reduced hepatic and cardiac toxicity, are undergoing clinical trial.

DOXORUBICIN

Use

Doxorubicin is a red antibiotic produced by *Streptomyces peucetius*. It is the most widely used drug of the anthracycline group with proven activity in acute leukemia,

lymphomas, sarcomas and a wide range of carcinomas. The usual dose is 30–60 mg/m² intravenously (depending on other drugs concurrently administered) every 21 or 28 days.

Mechanism of action

There are three main mechanisms of action:

1. Intercalation between adjacent base pairs in DNA, thus inhibiting further nucleic acid synthesis and leading to fragmentation of DNA and inhibition of DNA repair. This is enhanced by inhibition of DNA topoisomerase II.
2. Membrane binding alters membrane function. This alters sodium and calcium concentrations seen in the myocardium and could be involved in the development of cardiomyopathy.
3. Free-radical formation, which causes cardiotoxicity.

Adverse effects

1. Cardiotoxicity: this is the major dose-limiting factor in long-term administration. There are two forms, acute and chronic (see below).
2. Bone marrow suppression with neutropenia and thrombocytopenia.
3. Alopecia occurs almost invariably but may be mitigated by scalp cooling.
4. Nausea and vomiting.
5. 'Radiation recall' reaction: this describes the ability of anthracyclines to exacerbate or reactivate dormant radiation dermatitis or pneumonitis weeks or months after cessation of radiotherapy.
6. Extravasation causing severe tissue necrosis. Doxorubicin should never be injected into veins on the back of the hand as severe damage to nerves and tendons may result.

Anthracycline cardiotoxcity

Acute

This occurs shortly after administration, with the development of various arrhythmias that are occasionally life-threatening, e.g. ventricular tachycardia, heart block. These acute effects do not predict chronic toxicity.

Chronic

Cardiomyopathy occurs leading to death in up to 60% of those who develop signs of congestive cardiac failure. It is determined by the cumulative dose of doxorubicin administered with an incidence of less than 2% at total doses less than 400 mg/m², rising to over 20% at cumulative doses greater than 700 mg/m². Risk factors for cardiomyopathy (and that lower the cumulative dose at which this occurs) include prior mediastinal irradiation, age over 70 years, and pre-existing cardiovascular disease, including coronary artery disease and hypertension. Various drugs have been used in an effort to protect against this complication: vitamin E and N-acetylcysteine (free-radical scavengers) can protect against acute toxicity but are not effective against cardiomyopathy. Digoxin is not cardioprotective despite early claims to the contrary.

Pharmacokinetics

Doxorubicin is given intravenously as less than 5% of an oral dose is absorbed. The plasma concentration–time profile shows a triphasic decline with half-lives of 2–6 min, 0.5–2.5 hours and 15–50 hours for the three phases. The volume of distribution is large (reflecting extensive tissue uptake), most of the drug being located in cell nuclei. Hepatic extraction is high with 40% appearing in bile (40% unchanged, 20% as doxorubicinol and the remainder as other metabolites). Renal excretion accounts for less than 15%. The major metabolite, doxorubicinol has some antitumor activity. Dose reduction is recommended in liver disease. Doxorubicin does not enter the CNS.

DAUNORUBICIN

Daunorubicin is similar to doxorubicin, but its use is largely confined to the treatment of acute leukemia. It penetrates peripheral tissues less effectively than doxorubicin which may account for its narrower range of activity. Its pharmacokinetics are similar to those of doxorubicin with extensive metabolism primarily to the less active daunorubicinol. The $t_{1/2}$ of daunorubicin is about 24 hours. Adverse effects of daunorubicin are almost identical to those of doxorubicin, notably cardiotoxicity (recommended maximum cumulative dose 500–600 mg/m²).

MITOZANTRONE

This is a blue synthetic anthracenedione derivative. It is structurally similar to doxorubicin but lacks the amino sugar moiety which may account for its reduced cardiotoxicity compared to the anthracyclines. It has proven activity in advanced breast cancer and is probably effective in leukemias and lymphomas. The usual dose is 12–14 mg/m² given every 3 weeks. There is minimal cross-reactivity with doxorubicin.

BLEOMYCIN

Use

This is a mixture of several polypeptide antibiotics synthesized by *Streptomyces verticillus*. Bleomycin is used in lymphomas, testicular carcinoma and various squamous cell carcinomas. It is usually given intravenously (7.5–15 mg/m²/day by continuous infusion or 5–15 mg/m² every week) or intramuscularly, when it should be combined with lignocaine as the injection is painful.

Mechanism of action

The mode of action of bleomycin is not well understood. It prevents thymidine incorporation into DNA and can also cause fragmentation of DNA, so that cells fail to progress through the G_2 and M phases of the cell cycle. Despite these actions it has only a minimal effect on rapidly proliferating normal cells.

Adverse effects

1. Transient fever and shivering.
2. Skin hyperkeratosis, erythema and pigmentation.
3. Mouth ulceration at high doses.
4. Pulmonary diffuse interstitial fibrosis which can be fatal. It usually only occurs if the total cumulative dose exceeds 180 mg. It is also more liable to develop in the elderly and in those with pre-existing lung damage.
5. Alopecia.

Pharmacokinetics

Bleomycin disappears from plasma after intravenous injection with a half-life of approximately 9 hours. Markedly prolonged elimination occurs in renal failure and is accompanied by increased toxicity, so that caution is required when bleomycin is given concurrently with nephrotoxic agents such as aminoglycoside antibiotics or high-dose methotrexate. It is metabolized to numerous fragments that are also excreted in the urine. Distribution is correlated with the presence or absence of peptidase activity (which inactivates the drug) and in humans high drug concentrations occur in sensitive tumors in skin and lung. Selectivity of bleomycin is thus explained by the distribution of peptidases.

Hormones

Hormones cause remissions in certain types of cancer. They do not eradicate the disease, but can sometimes alleviate symptoms over a long period and do not have the disadvantage of depressing the bone marrow. Sex hormones or their antagonists (chapter 38) are most effective in tumors arising from cells that are normally hormone dependent, namely breast and prostate. They have less marked actions against hypernephroma and adenocarcinomas of the body of the uterus. There are several ways in which hormones can affect malignant cells:

1. A hormone may have a direct cytotoxic action on the malignant cell. This is likely if cancer cells that are normally dependent on a specific hormone are exposed to high concentration of a hormone with the opposite effect. For example, cells of the prostate are testosterone dependent; if a carcinoma arises from these cells, estrogens in large doses are cytotoxic to the cancer.
2. A hormone may suppress production of other hormones by a feedback mechanism. This will change the hormonal milieu surrounding the malignant cells and may suppress their activity.

In breast cancer, patients who respond to one form of endocrine therapy are more likely to respond to subsequent hormone treatment than those who fail to respond initially. Thus, sequencing one endocrine therapy after another may prolong survival and improve quality of life, often for several years.

ESTROGENS

Estrogens are now much less widely used than hitherto in the management of prostatic and breast carcinoma, because of the availability of luteinizing hormone-releasing hormone (LHRH) analogs for prostate cancer and tamoxifen for breast cancer. These are discussed in chapter 38.

AMINOGLUTETHIMIDE

Use

Aminoglutethimide was originally introduced as an anticonvulsant but was withdrawn when found to cause adrenal suppression. It is effective in about 30% of postmenopausal patients with best effects on skin and breast disease and although the response of bone metastases is higher than with tamoxifen, liver metastases seldom respond. Aminoglutethimide may be effective after tamoxifen has failed. Conventionally aminoglutethimide is given in doses of 1 g/day but doses of 250 mg/day or less are effective: at these doses the major effect is inhibition of the more sensitive aromatase.

Mechanism of action

Aminoglutethimide has two important actions:

1. Inhibition of adrenal synthesis of estrogens, glucocorticoids and mineralocorticoids by inhibition of the enzyme producing their common precursor, pregnanedione. A feedback driven rise in adrenocorticotrophic hormone (ACTH) secondary to low circulating cortisol may override adrenal blockade, so a glucocorticoid (e.g. hydrocortisone, 20 mg, twice daily) is given concurrently.

2. A second, more important effect is inhibition of tissue (fat, skin, muscle, carcinoma) aromatase, blocking conversion of androgens to estrogens. Ovarian aromatase is resistant to such inhibition, so aminoglutethimide is only useful in postmenopausal women.

Adverse effects

1. Lethargy, nausea and dizziness are common on starting treatment but decline during chronic dosing (probably due to enzyme induction).
2. Itchy erythematous rash occurs in 25% of patients after about 10 days which fades on continued treatment.

Pharmacokinetics

Aminoglutethimide is subject to polymorphic acetylation (chapter 13) to an inactive N-acetyl metabolite. Fast acetylators have a $t_{1/2}$ of around 13 hours compared to 20 hours in slow acetylators. This is not the major route of metabolism, hepatic oxidation being more important. This is self-inducible so that half-life falls during chronic dosing.

Drug interactions

Hepatic enzyme induction by aminoglutethimide can cause clinically important interactions with other drugs, e.g. warfarin.

PROGESTOGENS

Endometrial cells normally mature under the influence of progestogens and some malignant cells arising from the endometrium respond in the same way. About 30% of patients with disseminated adenocarcinoma of the body of the uterus respond to a progestogen such as megestrol, 20 mg, twice daily. Progestogens are also used in advanced breast cancer although their mechanism of action in this setting is uncertain. Progestogen bound to its receptor impairs regeneration of estrogen receptors and also stimulates 17β-estradiol dehydrogenase, the enzyme that breaks down intracellular estrogen. These actions may deprive cancer cells of estrogen effects. There is also a direct cytotoxic effect at very high doses.

Progestogens are also used in carcinoma of the kidney; a therapeutic response is rare and the explanation for it when it does occur is not known. Most experience has been with medroxyprogesterone acetate given in daily oral doses of 100–300 mg. Recent studies using larger doses (1500 mg/day) have produced responses in over 40% of patients. Other progestogens used are megestrol acetate, norethisterone acetate (SH 420) and hydroxyprogesterone. There are no important toxic effects of progestogens relevant to cancer chemotherapy.

GLUCOCORTICOSTEROIDS

Corticosteroids (chapter 37) are cytotoxic to lymphoid cells and are used in combination with other cytotoxic agents in treating lymphomas, myeloma and to induce a remission in acute lymphoblastic leukemia.

LUTEINIZING HORMONE-RELEASING HORMONE (LHRH) ANALOGS

See chapter 38.

KETOCONAZOLE

High doses of ketoconazole (chapter 42) block synthesis of testicular testosterone, adrenal androgens and other steroids. Experimentally it has produced remissions in prostate cancer.

Platinum compounds

CISPLATIN

Use

Cisplatin (*cis*-diaminedichloroplatinum) is an inorganic platinum (II) coordination complex in which two amine (NH_3) and two chlorine ligands occupy *cis* positions (the *trans* compound is inactive). Cisplatin is the most effective single agent in testicular teratomas, but is usually given in combination with various other cytotoxic drugs. When combined with high-dose bleomycin and vinblastine, a remission rate of 70% is achievable. In carcinoma of the ovary it can be combined with doxorubicin (Adriamycin) and cyclophosphamide and is more effective than a single alkylating agent. Its use has resulted in cure of many previously fatal germ cell tumors. It has been used with some success in head and neck and bladder cancers. Cisplatin is given intravenously either as a bolus or infusion in a number of cyclical regimes, often in combination with other cytotoxic agents. The usual dose is 50–100 mg/m² as a single dose or 15–20 mg/m² daily for 5 days every 3–4 weeks. Because of the efficacy of platinum compounds and the toxicity of cisplatin there has been a search for analogs yielding carboplatin and iproplatin, which are in early use and/or phase III investigation. Carboplatin has almost no renal or ototoxicity, neuropathy is rare and vomiting, although common, is less severe than after cisplatin.

Mechanism of action

Cytotoxicity results from selective inhibition of tumor DNA synthesis by formation of intra- and interstrand cross-links in the DNA molecule.

Adverse effects

1. **Severe vomiting**.
2. Nephrotoxicity is dose-related and dose limiting. It causes acute distal tubular necrosis. Prehydration and diuresis reduce the immediate effects but cumulative and permanent damage still occurs. The patient is fully hydrated and a urine flow of 200 ml/hour maintained during treatment and for 6 hours afterwards. This is achieved by intravenous infusion combined with mannitol or frusemide.
3. Clinically significant hypomagnesemia. Magnesium supplementation is usually given during the cisplatin infusion.
4. Ototoxicity develops in up to 30% of patients, mostly in the frequency range above speech tones. Tinnitus may be associated with the deafness. Cisplatin irreversibly damages the organ of Corti and this effect is related to cumulative

dose. Audiometry should be carried out before, during and after treatment.
5. Myelosuppression.
6. Peripheral neuropathy can be disabling.

Pharmacokinetics

Plasma disappearance of cisplatin is multiphasic: $t_{1/2\alpha}$ is 25–50 min and $t_{1/2\beta}$ is 60–73 hours. Although initially rapidly excreted, over 50% is retained by the body after 5 days and low urinary concentrations are found up to 1 month after treatment. No preferential accumulation occurs in tumors but high concentrations occur in ovary, testis and kidney.

Drug interactions

Because of the nephrotoxicity and ototoxicity of cisplatin, other agents such as aminoglycosides with similar toxicities should be avoided.

Miscellaneous agents

PROCARBAZINE

Use

Procarbazine is a hydrazine possessing some monoamine oxidase inhibiting properties. Its main use is in treating Hodgkin's disease. It is part of the well-established mustine, vincristine or vinblastine, procarbazine and prednisolone (MOPP or MVPP) regimens that produce complete remission in about 65% of patients. It is less effective in non-Hodgkin's lymphoma, but produces some benefit in 30–40% of such patients. Procarbazine is given daily by mouth, at a dose of 50–150 mg, usually for 2 weeks with other cytotoxic drugs.

Mechanism of action

The antitumor activity of procarbazine is believed to depend on its terminal methylhydrazine grouping which undergoes activation by microsomal enzymes, mainly in the liver, to various reactive free-radical metabolites that are cytotoxic. Its precise mode of action is unknown but it depresses DNA synthesis and combines with DNA, decreasing its viscosity and causing chromosome breaks.

Adverse effects

1. Dose-related hemopoietic suppression, leukopenia and thrombocytopenia occur after 10–14 days.
2. Nausea and vomiting occur frequently but are less prominent after repeated dosage.

Pharmacokinetics

Procarbazine is rapidly and almost completely absorbed from the intestine, peak concentrations being obtained in 30–60 min. The $t_{1/2}$ of the parent compound in plasma is about 10 min. It is metabolized to a number of compounds that are excreted by the kidneys. Some of these, particularly the hydrazines, have cytotoxic activity. Procarbazine and its metabolites penetrate the blood–brain barrier.

Drug interactions

- Procarbazine is a weak monoamine oxidase inhibitor and the usual precautions are observed to avoid interaction (chapter 12). Such interactions are rare in practice and it is doubtful whether strict dietary restriction is essential.
- Procarbazine also blocks aldehyde dehydrogenase (cf. disulfiram) and interacts with ethanol causing flushing and tachycardia.

INTERFERONS

Single agent interferon-α is licensed and effective against a number of tumor types notably hairy cell leukemia, as well as low-grade non-Hodgkin's lymphoma, cutaneous T cell lymphoma and some cases of chronic myeloid leukemia. It is also used to treat Kaposi's sarcoma in patients with AIDS. The availability of larger amounts of material and its use in combination with other drugs may improve future results. See also chapters 31, 42 and 47.

INTERLEUKIN-2

Interleukin-2 (chapter 47) has a place in renal carcinoma.

Hematology

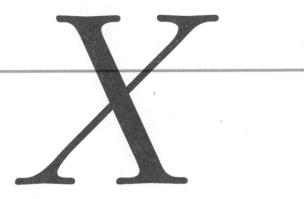

Anemia and Other Hematological Disorders

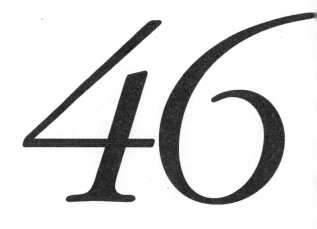

Hematinics   **616**

Aplastic anemia   **623**

Idiopathic thrombocytopenic purpura   **623**

Hematopoietic growth factors   **623**

Coagulation factors and hemophilias A and B   **627**

Hematinics

Iron

Physiology and biochemistry

Although iron is abundant in the earth's crust, anemia due to iron deficiency is prevalent throughout the world. Iron plays a vital role in the body in several transport proteins and enzymes including hemoglobin, myoglobin, cytochromes, catalase, peroxidase, guanylyl cyclase and many others. It is stored in the reticuloendothelial system and bone marrow. Total body iron is 3.5–4.5 g in an adult, of which some 70% is incorporated in hemoglobin, 5% in myoglobin and 0.2% in enzymes. Most of the remaining iron (approximately 25%) is stored as ferritin or hemosiderin. About 2% (80 mg) comprises the 'labile iron pool' and about 0.08% (3 mg) is bound to transferrin, a specific iron-binding protein.

Pharmacokinetics

Absorption is the main mechanism controlling total body iron. This remains remarkably constant in healthy individuals despite variations in diet, erythropoietic activity and iron stores. Iron absorption occurs in the small intestine and is influenced by several factors.

1. Form of iron

(a) Inorganic ferrous iron is better absorbed than ferric iron.
(b) Absorption of iron from the diet depends on the source of the iron. Most dietary iron exists as non-heme iron and is poorly absorbed (5% approximately) mainly because it is combined with phosphates and phytates (in cereals). Heme iron is well absorbed (20–40%) but is often deficient in the diet of poorer people and vegetarians.
(c) Absorption of iron from orally administered iron salts is poor, around 10%.

2. Factors increasing absorption

(a) Vitamin C (ascorbic acid) facilitates iron absorption, and iron deficiency anemia commonly accompanies vitamin C deficiency.
(b) Alcohol increases ferric but not ferrous iron absorption and there is an association between alcohol abuse and iron overload (hemosiderosis).

3. Gastrointestinal tract

Gastric acid enhances absorption of iron from food, and iron deficiency is actually commoner than vitamin B_{12} deficiency following partial gastrectomy. Iron is absorbed in the jejunum and upper ileum and malabsorption of iron can occur in celiac disease.

4. Drugs

Tetracycline chelates iron causing malabsorption of both iron and tetracycline.

Disposition of iron

Iron in the gut becomes bound to mucosal transferrin for transport across the mucosa. Iron is also transported in plasma by transferrin (a protein of molecular weight 76 000–80 000), each molecule of which binds two atoms of iron. Transferrin gives up its iron to red cell precursors in bone marrow. When red cells reach the end of their lifespan, macrophages bind the iron atoms released which are taken up again by transferrin. About four-fifths of total body iron exchange normally takes place through this cycle (Fig. 46.1). Ferritin is the main storage form of iron. It is a roughly spherical protein with deeply located iron binding sites. Ferritin is found principally in the liver. Aggregates of ferritin form hemosiderin, which accumulates when hepatic iron stores are high.

Iron deficiency

In iron-deficient states, the serum iron (normally 14–31 µmol/l in men and 11–29 µmol/l in women) falls only when stores

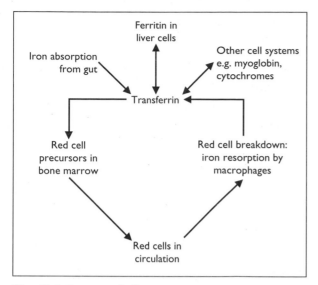

Fig. 46.1 Iron metabolism.

have become considerably depleted. The total amount of transferrin determines the total iron binding capacity (TIBC) of plasma, and is normally 54–80 μmol/l. Transferrin saturation (i.e. plasma iron divided by TIBC) is normally 20–50%, and this provides a clinically useful index of iron status. In iron-deficiency states, TIBC rises in addition to the fall in plasma iron and when transferrin saturation falls to less than 16% erythropoiesis starts to decline. Iron deficiency is the commonest cause of anemia and although commonest and most severe in third world countries, it is also prevalent in developed countries. In one study 8% of menstruating women in north-west America were found to have mild iron-deficiency anemia. The cause of iron deficiency is most often multifactorial, for example poor diet combined with excessive demands on stores (pregnancy, chronic blood loss, lactation), reduced stores (premature birth) or defective absorption (achlorhydria, surgery to the gastrointestinal tract). Although treatment of iron deficiency is straightforward, its cause should be determined so that the underlying condition can be treated. Iron deficiency anemia is seldom due to dietary deficiency alone in men or postmenopausal women and a thorough search for other causes

(notably occult gastrointestinal blood loss from a potentially curable colon cancer) should be undertaken.

Iron preparations

ORAL IRON

Most patients with iron deficiency respond to simple oral preparations. A total daily dose of 100–200 mg of elemental iron should stimulate a reticulocyte response, which begins after 5 days and lasts about 10 days. The hemoglobin concentration will start to rise at 0.1–0.2 g/dl/day. Treatment is continued for 3–6 months after hemoglobin levels have entered the normal range to replace iron stores. Failure to respond may be due to:

1. Wrong diagnosis (i.e. iron deficiency is not the primary cause of the anemia).
2. Non-compliance.
3. Continued blood loss.
4. Malabsorption (e.g. celiac disease, postgastrectomy).

There are over 70 iron-containing oral preparations but many of these are combined preparations containing vitamins as well as iron. None of these combinations carries an advantage over iron salts alone except for those containing folic acid which are used prophylactically in pregnancy. Slow-release preparations of iron are unreliably absorbed from the upper small intestine (where iron uptake is at its most efficient) and are not recommended. Treatment should start with a simple preparation such as ferrous sulfate (200 mg thrice daily), ferrous fumarate (200 mg thrice daily) or ferrous gluconate (600 mg thrice daily). These and other preparations are shown in Table 46.1.

IRON PREPARATIONS FOR CHILDREN

Liquid preparations may be preferred for infants and young children. Such preparations should be sugar free and not stain the

Table 46.1 Various iron preparations.

Iron formulation	Dose	Ferrous iron content	Approximate ratio of cost
Ferrous sulfate	200 mg	60 mg	1
Ferrous fumarate	200 mg	65 mg	2
Ferrous gluconate	300 mg	35 mg	2.6
Polysaccharide iron complex	50 mg/ml	?	11

teeth (e.g sodium iron edetate). The dose should be calculated in terms of the amount of elemental iron in the preparation. The dose for premature infants is 1.0 mg/kg daily initially or for children aged 1–5 years 7.5 ml in three divided doses (40 mg) increasing to 15 ml per day (80 mg iron) for children 6–12 years.

Adverse effects

Gastrointestinal side effects of nausea, heartburn, constipation or diarrhea are common. No preparation has been shown to be universally better tolerated than any other when equivalent doses of elemental iron are given, but individual patients often find that one salt suits them better than another. Inorganic iron as the sulfate is least expensive, but if it is not tolerated it is worth trying an organic salt such as the fumarate. Patients with ulcerative colitis and those with colostomies often suffer particularly severely from these side effects. Although iron is best absorbed in the fasting state, gastric irritation is reduced if it is taken after food.

PARENTERAL IRON

Oral iron is effective, easily administered and cheap. Parenteral iron in the form of iron dextran or iron with sorbitol and citric acid, is also effective but can cause anaphylactoid reactions and is expensive. The rate of rise in hemoglobin is the same following parenteral iron and oral iron because the rate-limiting factor is the capacity of the marrow to produce red cells (Fig. 46.2). The only advantages of parenteral iron are that the iron stores are rapidly and completely replenished; that there is no doubt about

compliance; and that it is effective in patients with malabsorption. It is usually given by a series of deep intramuscular injections.

Relative indications for parenteral iron are:

1. Malabsorption.
2. Genuine intolerance to oral iron preparations.
3. When continued blood loss is not preventable and large doses of iron cannot be readily given by mouth.
4. Failure of patient compliance.
5. When great demands are to be made on a patient's stores – as in an anemic pregnant woman just before term.

IRON DEXTRAN

Use

Dextran forms a stable complex with ferrous hydroxide with a molecular weight of 180 000. The solution for injection contains 50 mg/ml. The total dose of iron required is first calculated. Tables based on body weight and hemoglobin concentration are provided with each pack of ampules.

Pharmacokinetics

Iron dextran is usually given by deep intramuscular injections each given along a Z track into alternate buttocks. It causes a local tissue reaction with eventual formation of dense fibrous tissue. The injected iron slowly leaves the site of injection via lymphatics (50% leaves within 72 hours, and thereafter removal occurs at a much slower rate). It is ingested by macrophages and stored in ferritin in the reticuloendothelial system. From here it is released into plasma where it is transported to bone marrow by transferrin. Release of iron is so slow that transferrin does not become saturated, but concurrent oral iron therapy should be stopped.

Adverse effects

1. Gray-brown staining of the skin in relation to the injection site is common.
2. Fever, headache, sensations of heat, vomiting, arthralgia, regional lymph-node enlargement, urticaria, bronchospasm and anaphylaxis are rare.

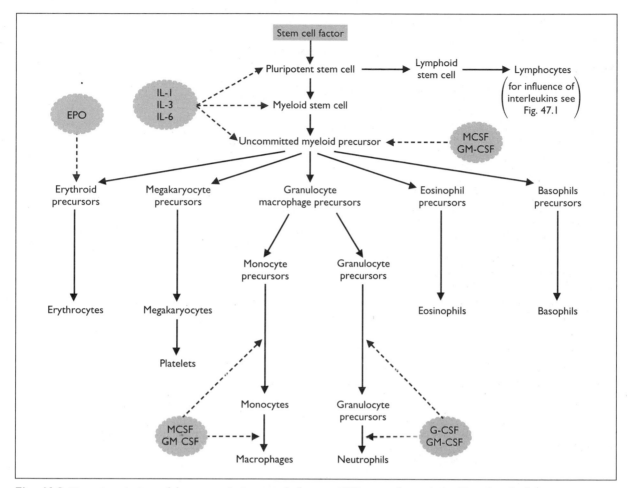

Fig. 46.2 Hematopoiesis and hematopoietic growth factors. EPO = erythropoietin. IL = interleukin. G-CSF = granulocyte colony-stimulating factor. MCSF = macrophage colony-stimulating factor. GM-CSF = granulocyte macrophage colony-stimulating factor.

Intravenous iron dextran (but not iron sorbitol citric acid, which is unsuitable for intravenous use) may be given to patients requiring parenteral iron who have a small muscle mass, a disorder of hemostasis contraindicating intramuscular injections, or who cannot tolerate intramuscular injections. Intravenous iron is contraindicated in asthmatic patients. The initial solution (50 mg/ml) is diluted in 0.9% saline or 5% dextrose to give a final concentration of 500 mg/250 ml. A small test dose is first infused (5 drops/min for 10 min). The patient is carefully observed both during and for 5–10 min after this. If this test dose is without incident, the total dose infusion is given over 6–8 hours.

IRON SORBITOL CITRIC ACID

Use

This preparation may only be given intramuscularly and, again, deep injections should be given to minimize staining of the skin. Peak concentrations, often with complete transferrin saturation, occur at 2–8 hours. Of the retained iron, 30% is immediately available for heme synthesis and the rest is stored.

Adverse effects

1. Metallic taste in the mouth.
2. A tendency to exacerbate pre-existing urinary tract infections (probably related to high levels in the urine).

3. Anaphylactoid reactions resulting in cardiovascular collapse.

VITAMIN B₁₂

Vitamin B_{12} consists of a nucleotide linked to four pyrrole rings (similar to a porphyrin) with a cobalt atom attached. Attached to the cobalt atom may be a cyanide (cyanocobalamin), hydroxyl (hydroxocobalamin), methyl (methylcobalamin) or 5'-deoxyadenoxyl group. These forms are interconvertible, cyanocobalamin spontaneously forming hydroxocobalamin on exposure to light. Liver, kidney and heart are rich sources of vitamin B_{12} and moderate amounts are found in other meats, fish and eggs. It is absorbed in the terminal ileum and absorption is dependent on the presence of 'intrinsic factor' secreted by parietal cells of the stomach. Patients with Addisonian pernicious anemia have antibodies to intrinsic factor and to parietal cells. These cause atrophic gastritis and achlorhydria with failure of intrinsic factor production and consequent malabsorption of B_{12}. Vitamin B_{12} deficiency is diagnosed by measuring serum B_{12} concentrations and assessing its absorption from the intestine by the Schilling test.

Use

Replacement therapy is required in B_{12} deficiency which may be due to:

1. Malabsorption secondary to gastric pathology (pernicious anemia, total or partial gastrectomy).
2. Intestinal malabsorption (Crohn's disease or surgical resection of the terminal ileum, irradiation damage).
3. Competition for vitamin B_{12} absorption by gut organisms (e.g blind loop syndrome due to a jejunal diverticulum or other cause of bacterial overgrowth, infestation with the fish tapeworm *Diphyllobothrium latum*).
4. Nutritional deficiency is rare and limited to strict vegans. The few such individuals who do develop megaloblastic anemia often have some coexisting deficiency of intrinsic factor.

Vitamin B_{12} replacement is given by intramuscular injection. Hydroxocobalamin is preferred as it is retained longer than cyanocobalamin, and is administered initially as five doses of 1 mg given every 2–3 days followed by 1 mg 3 monthly for maintenance. A peak in the reticulocyte response (which may be massive, 25% or more reticulocytes) occurs 5 days after starting treatment. There is an alarmingly high incidence (up to 10%) of sudden death in the early treatment phase of patients with severe pernicious anemia. This is believed to be due to the sudden fall in plasma potassium that occurs during the early hematological response. This may provoke fatal cardiac arrhythmias, and hypokalemia should be prevented. If digoxin is being administered to such patients for whatever reason, special care regarding plasma potassium is mandatory, because of the increased risk of digoxin toxicity associated with hypokalemia (chapter 28). Transfusion is seldom necessary and has a high risk of precipitating pulmonary edema. If essential packed red cells should be transfused slowly with close monitoring of fluid balance, urine output and plasma potassium.

Iron and folate deficiency are often unmasked by treatment with B_{12} of megaloblastic or mixed anemias, and iron and folate therapy can be initiated concomitantly. It is essential not to administer folate to such patients before vitamin B_{12}, because this can precipitate neurological consequences of B_{12} deficiency which may not be reversible (subacute combined degeneration of the spinal cord). Patients with vitamin B_{12} deficiency due to malabsorption (Addisonian pernicious anemia) require lifelong replacement therapy; they should be given an adequate explanation of this, as should family members in view of the forgetfulness that occurs insidiously in vitamin B_{12} deficiency. Patients should carry a card with an up-to-date record of their B_{12} therapy.

Cellular mechanism of action

Vitamin B_{12} is needed for normal erythropoiesis and for the maturation of other cell types and neuronal integrity. It is required for the isomerization of methylmalonyl coenzyme A to succinyl coenzyme A, and the conversion of homocysteine into methionine (which also utilizes 5-methyltetrahydrofolate). Vitamin B_{12} is also involved in the control of active folate metabolism, and both these vitamins are required for intracellular nucleotide synthesis.

Deficiency of vitamin B_{12} leads to a macrocytic anemia with megaloblastic erythropoiesis in the bone marrow, and may be accompanied by neurological disorders that include peripheral neuropathy, subacute combined degeneration of the spinal cord, dementia and optic neuritis.

Pharmacokinetics

Normal total body stores of vitamin B_{12} are about 3 mg. Following total gastrectomy these stores are adequate for 3–5 years following which there is an increasing incidence of vitamin B_{12} deficiency. Thus the daily B_{12} loss is 0.5–3 μg which results mainly from metabolic breakdown. Normally absorption from the diet is very efficient and the daily requirement is 3–5 μg. Absorption of vitamin B_{12} requires secretion of intrinsic factor from gastric parietal cells. Intrinsic factor is a glycoprotein of molecular weight approximately 55 000 which forms a stable complex with vitamin B_{12} in the presence of acid. The complex passes down the small intestine and is absorbed at specific receptor sites in the terminal ileum, in the presence of a neutral pH and calcium ions. Absorption is slow, starting 4 hours after ingestion, with a peak at 8–12 hours and continuing for up to 24 hours. Very small amounts (approximately 1%) of an oral dose are absorbed by passive diffusion, and although B_{12} is synthesized by colonic bacteria it is not appreciably absorbed in the colon because this is distal to the site of active absorption in the terminal ileum. Parietal cells are destroyed by an autoimmune reaction and so intrinsic factor is not produced in pernicious anemia, resulting in B_{12} deficiency.

Vitamin B_{12} is transported by two plasma proteins, transcobalamins I and II (TCI and TCII). TCII is a β-globulin and acts as a transport protein collecting B_{12} from ileal cells and transporting it to the liver. TCI is an α-globulin that carries most of the body's B_{12} and this complex is probably the storage form of the vitamin. The normal range of plasma vitamin B_{12} concentration is 170-900 ng/l. Low B_{12} plasma concentrations are found in other conditions such as pregnancy and simple atrophic gastritis, where total body B_{12} deficiency is not present. High B_{12} concentrations are found in association with hepatic necrosis (with resulting release of stores) of any etiology.

Vitamin B_{12} is secreted into bile but enterohepatic circulation results in most of this being reabsorbed via the intrinsic factor mechanism. Unbound B_{12} is excreted by glomerular filtration, but this is of minor importance.

FOLIC ACID

Use

Folic acid is given to correct or prevent deficiency states. It consists of a pteridine linked to glutamic acid via p-aminobenzoic acid (PABA). It is present in a wide variety of plant and animal tissues, the richest dietary sources being liver, yeast and green vegetables. The major dietary form is as polyglutamate conjugates with up to seven additional glutamate residues being attached to the glutamate of folic acid. These are split off by γ-carboxypeptidases in intestinal juice and serum.

Folate deficiency may be due to:

1. Poor nutritional status as may occur in children, old age or alcoholism.
2. Malabsorption caused by celiac disease, sprue or diseases of the small intestine.
3. Excessive utilization pregnancy occurs in chronic hemolytic anemias, for example sickle cell disease and leukemias.
4. Drugs such as phenytoin and phenobarbitone.

The normal requirement for folic acid is about 200 μg daily. In established folate deficiency large doses (5–15 mg p.o. daily) are given. If the patient is unable to take folate by mouth, it may be given intravenously. Patients with severe malabsorption may be deficient in both folic acid and vitamin B_{12}, and administration of folic acid alone may precipitate acute vitamin B_{12} deficiency. These patients require careful evaluation and replacement of both vitamins concurrently. Patients taking long-term anticonvulsants commonly have macrocytic red cells, but the majority have no detectable folate deficiency. A few patients, however, develop a megaloblastic anemia due to folate deficiency, the cause of which is complex but is partly due to interference with DNA synthesis and partly to induction of hepatic enzymes that increase folate breakdown. Treatment is by addition of folic acid, 5 mg, daily to the anticonvulsant regimen.

Cellular mechanism of action

Folic acid is required for normal erythropoiesis. As with vitamin B_{12} a deficiency of folic acid results in a megaloblastic anemia and abnormalities in other cell types. The role of folate in cell metabolism results from its ability to transfer groups containing single carbon atoms in biochemical reactions. These include the methylation of deoxyuridylic acid to form thymidylic acid and other reactions in purine and pyrimidine synthesis. A key reaction in folate metabolism is its reduction to various forms of tetrahydrofolate by dihydrofolate reductase. It is this enzyme that is inhibited by methotrexate (chapters 23 and 45), pyrimethamine (chapter 44) and trimethoprim (chapter 40).

Pharmacokinetics

Folate is absorbed in the proximal small intestine within 5–20 min of ingestion. There is a specific absorptive mechanism. During absorption folic acid is formylated and then methylated before entering the portal blood. About one-third of total body folate (70 mg) is stored in the liver. This is only about 4 months' supply so folate deficiency develops more rapidly than vitamin B_{12} deficiency. As

with vitamin B_{12} the feces contain folate that has been synthesized by colonic bacteria, but this occurs too low in the gut for absorption to occur. The normal range for serum folate is 4–20 µg/l but values may be falsely elevated by hemolysis and are labile, changing rapidly with alterations in dietary intake. The red cell folate concentration (normal range 140–450 µg/l) is less labile and more reliable.

IRON AND FOLIC ACID THERAPY IN PREGNANCY

Pregnancy imposes a substantial increase in demand on maternal stores of iron and folic acid. The average daily net flow of iron across the placenta from mother to fetus at term is 4.5 mg. At this stage of pregnancy 90% of maternal plasma iron turnover is directed towards the fetus, a pregnant woman during the last trimester therefore requires 5.0 mg iron daily. A net gain of around 500–600 mg of elemental iron is required for each pregnancy to accommodate the requirements of the growing fetus together with expansion of maternal red cell mass, and most women are iron-depleted by the end of the pregnancy if they do not receive supplements.

Requirements for folic acid also increase two- to three-fold and deficiency in pregnancy is associated with prematurity and infants of low birth weight for their gestational age. In the UK the usual practice is to give iron and folic acid supplements throughout pregnancy. Tablets containing 100 mg of elemental iron and 200–500 µg folic acid are available to be taken once daily, and these prevent anemia in pregnancy. Folate supplementation (400–800 µg/day) should be given before conception to women attempting to become pregnant to reduce the incidence of neural tube defects. Higher dose prophylaxis (folate, 5 mg, daily) is advised for women who have previously given birth to a child with a neural tube defect.

APLASTIC ANEMIA

Aplastic anemia is characterized by pancy-topenia associated with the replacement of normal cellular bone marrow by fat, without evidence of malignancy or proliferation of reticulin. Some cases are congenital (e.g. Fanconi's anemia) but many are acquired and in 50% of these an etiological agent (a virus, chemical or drug) can be implicated. Certain drugs have a particularly strong association with aplastic anemia, and these include phenylbutazone, oxyphenbutazone, amidopy-rine and chloramphenicol. They should be avoided for this reason unless there is a specific clinical indication, for although cases of aplastic anemia are very rare, they are frequently fatal.

TREATMENT

Support is provided with transfusions (of red cells and platelets) and appropriate antibiotics. Bone marrow transplantation from a histo-compatible donor is potentially definitive treatment, and has become the therapy of choice for young patients. For those who are unsuitable for this treatment anabolic steroids may reduce the requirement for transfusions. Two 17α-alkyl derivatives of testosterone have been used: oxymetholone and stanozolol (chapter 38). Trials of erythropoietin and other hematopoietic growth factors such as granulo-cyte colony-stimulating factor (G-CSF) and granulocyte macrophage colony-stimulating factor (GM-CSF) (see below) are presently underway and early results are promising.

IDIOPATHIC THROMBOCYTOPENIC PURPURA

It is important to exclude other causes of thrombocytopenia including cases due to drugs. Treatment options include:

1. Glucocorticosteroids: prednisolone 1 mg/kg, daily and slowly reduced; a response (rising platelet count) may take 1–2 weeks.
2. If this fails, or the disease relapses rapidly on reducing the steroid dose, splenectomy should be considered. If splenectomy is performed the patient should be immunized against pneumococcal infection several weeks preoperatively if possible, since there

is a risk of overwhelming pneumococcal sepsis following splenectomy. Gluco-corticosteroids should be continued after the operation until the platelet count rises.
3. Platelet transfusions are required to control active bleeding or to cover operations.
4. Immunosuppressive drugs (chapter 47), in particular vincristine, can be used in refractory cases. Alternative therapies include danazol, intravenous immunoglob-ulin and cyclosporin.
5. Thrombopoietin has recently been purified/cloned and is being studied.

HEMATOPOIETIC GROWTH FACTORS

Gene identification, cloning and recombinant DNA technology, have been utilized to allow the synthesis of several human hematopoietic growth factors. The place of these factors in therapy is currently being established. See Fig. 46.2 for an outline of the hematopoietic process.

RECOMBINANT HUMAN ERYTHROPOIETIN (EPOETIN)

Erythropoietin is a protein of 165 amino acids four of which are glycosylated, with a molecular weight of 34 000. Ninety per cent of endogenous erythropoietin is produced by interstitial cells of the renal cortex adjacent to the proximal tubules and ten per cent by the liver. Biosynthesis is stimulated by tissue hypoxia. The production and actions of erythropoietin are linked in a negative feedback loop that maintains red cell mass at an optimal level for oxygen transport. It is the only hematopoietic growth factor that is a hormone. Epoetin, the recombinant form of erythropoietin, is available in two forms with minor structural differences: epoetin-α as 1 ml ampoules of 2000 units and epoetin-β containing 1000, 2000, and 25 000 units as a powder to be reconstituted with water. Therapeutically the actions of the α and β forms are undistinguishable.

Use

Epoetin is used to treat the anemia of chronic renal failure. It is normally given by either intravenous or subcutaneous injection initially at a dose of 50 IU/kg three times a week (this is a convenient schedule for patients on thrice weekly hemodialysis, but is otherwise arbitrary), increasing according to response by 25 IU/kg at 4-weekly intervals. The maximum dose is 600 IU/kg in three divided doses per week. The usual maintenance dose is 100–300 IU/kg per week. Other causes of anemia – iron or folate deficiency – should be excluded. Aluminum toxicity, concurrent infection and other inflammatory diseases impair response.

Epoetin has been used with some benefit in other conditions:

1. Anemia induced by AZT, if pretreatment erythropoietin is <500 IU/l.
2. Anemia of myelodysplastic syndromes.
3. Myeloma.
4. Anemia of rheumatoid arthritis.
5. Autologous blood harvesting for transfusion during elective surgery (this hygienic practice is often impractical in countries such as the UK where an exact date for elective surgery can seldom be assured).

Mechanism of action

Epoetin binds to a membrane receptor on erythroid cell precursors in the bone marrow and is internalized. This epoetin–receptor complex increases transcription of the genes for δ-aminolevulinic acid synthetase and porphobilinogen decarboxylase, key heme biosynthetic enzymes. This increases heme biosynthesis and causes differentiation of erythroid precursors into mature erythroid cells.

Pharmacokinetics

Epoetin has a mean half-life ($t_{1/2}$) of 5 hours with a volume of distribution of 50 ml/kg. After subcutaneous injection systemic bioavailability is about 40%. Elimination occurs by catabolism in the erythroid cells in the marrow following internalization, by hepatic metabolism and urinary excretion.

Adverse effects

1. Hypertension. Blood pressure should be monitored weekly until a plateau is reached and thereafter 6 weekly. Severe hypertension with headaches and fits can occur.
2. Thrombosis, for example of shunts, or causing cardiovascular accident.
3. Influenza-like symptoms.
4. Iron deficiency may be unmasked. Many physicians start iron prophylactically with the use of epoetin.

HUMAN GRANULOCYTE COLONY-STIMULATING FACTOR (FILGRASTIM)

Granulocyte colony-stimulating factor (G-CSF) is a glycoprotein consisting of 174 amino acids variably glycosylated (molecular weight 18 000–22 000). The varying degree of glycosylation is not a factor in therapeutic efficacy, but may be important in making recombinant G-CSF more antigenic. G-CSF has been produced in both bacterial and mammalian sytems.

Use

Possible indications for G-CSF include:

1. To prevent and treat the neutropenia induced by chemotherapy.
2. Cyclical neutropenia.

Table 46.2 Comparison of the effects of granulocyte colony-stimulating factor (G-CSF) and granulocyte macrophage colony-stimulating factor (GM-CSF).

	G-CSF	GM-CSF	G-CSF and GM-CSF
Bone marrow	Marked increase in neutrophils ($\times$9.4)	Mild increase in neutrophils ($\times$1.5)	Increased cellularity and M/E ratio
Bone marrow	Increased promyelocytes	Increased eosinophils and cycling progenitors	Increased promyelocytes and myelocytes
Peripheral blood	Normal neutrophil survival	Increased neutrophil survival	Increased neutrophil count with young cells (left shift)
	Macropolycytes	Increased eosinophils and monocytes	Increased numbers of circulating immune cells
Leukocyte function	Normal surface markers and motility	Decreased motility and chemotaxis Monocytes: increased cytotoxicity	Increased stimulated superoxide production
Biochemistry	Increased urate, lysozyme and IL-2 receptor	Increased AST/ALT; decreased albumin	Increased LDH, alkaline phosphatase and cholesterol

M/E ratio = myeloid cells/erythroid cells ratio. IL-2 = interleukin-2. AST = aspartate transaminase. ALT = alanine transaminase. LDH = lactate dehydrogenase.

3. Bone marrow transplantation.
4. Aplastic anemia.
5. Human immunodeficiency virus (HIV)-related AZT-induced neutropenia.

G-CSF is usually self-administered by subcutaneous injection. If intravenous dosing is necessary, it is given as a 15–20 min infusion. The dose varies from 1 to 20 µg/kg/day (1 µg = 100 000 units) for a course of up to 14 days. Therapy is monitored by performing blood counts twice weekly. Table 46.2 compares the effects of G-CSF and granulocyte monocyte colony-stimulating factor (GM-CSF). G-CSF is primarily used to reduce neutropenia after cancer chemotherapy. G-CSF causes an immediate transient neutropenia and monocytopenia 5–15 and 30–60 min after intravenous and subcutaneous administration, respectively. This is followed by a sustained dose-dependent increase in white blood cell count in 5–6 days. Elevated neutrophil counts stabilize in the second week of a 2-week course of treatment. After cessation of therapy neutrophil counts return to baseline after 4–7 days.

Mechanism of action

G-CSF stimulates proliferation and differentiation of progenitor cells of all myelogranulo-cyte lineages. It binds to a specific receptor on myelogranulocyte precursors, enhancing cell replication and differentiation. Its action at a cellular level has not yet been defined.

Adverse effects

1. Bone pain.
2. Myalgia.
3. Fever.
4. Splenomegaly.
5. Thrombocytopenia.
6. Abnormal liver function tests (hepatitis picture).

Contraindications

G-CSF should not be given to patients with myeloid or myelomonocytic leukemia, because it increases proliferation of the malignant clone.

Pharmacokinetics

The $t_{1/2}$ of G-CSF is 1.3–7.2 hours. Subcutaneous administration produces plasma concentrations higher than 10 ng/ml for 10–16 hours. The bioavailabilty of subcutaneously administered G-CSF is 54%. There is evidence of zero-order pharmacokinetics at doses >10 µg/kg. G-CSF is extensively metabolized in the kidney, bone marrow and liver to its component amino acids and no unchanged drug is found in the urine.

GRANULOCYTE MACROPHAGE COLONY-STIMULATING FACTOR (MOLGRAMOSTIM)

GM-CSF is a glycoprotein consisting of 127 amino acids. It is variably glycosylated (molecular weight 14 000–35 000). Glycosylation is not a factor in therapeutic efficacy, but may be important in making recombinant GM-CSF more antigenic and in increasing its plasma half-life. It has been produced in yeast, bacterial and mammalian sytems.

Use

GM-CSF has been used in bone marrow transplantation, neutropenia secondary to chemotherapy, myelodysplastic syndromes, aplastic anemia and in bone marrow failure of HIV patients whether due to the virus or drug therapy (AZT/ganciclovir). There are theoretical concerns that GM-CSF could stimulate HIV replication, which at present have neither been confirmed nor refuted *in vivo*. *In vitro* it potentiates the efficacy of AZT against HIV. GM-CSF is self-administered by subcutaneous injection. The dose varies from 0.3 to 10 μg/kg/day (60 000–110 000 units/kg/day) for 7–10 days, usually starting 24 hours after chemotherapy. In bone marrow transplants therapy is given intravenously by two 2–4 hour infusions daily (110 000 units/kg/day) for a maximum of 30 days. Therapy is monitored by performing blood counts twice weekly. GM-CSF does not increase neutrophil numbers as potently as G-CSF. Each dose of GM-CSF causes a transient leukopenia (neutrophils, eosinophils and monocytes), followed by an increase in white blood cell count. Fifty-fold increases in circulating leukocytes can occur after doses of 20 μg/kg.

Mechanism of action

GM-CSF binds to specific receptors on myeloid cells and stimulates proliferation and differentiation of progenitor cells of all hematopoietic lineages and increases peripheral white blood cell numbers. GM-CSF does not shorten the time for neutrophil precursors to mature. It increases the neutrophil production rate by 50%, and the circulating half-life of neutrophils is prolonged from 8 to 48 hours.

Adverse effects

1. First dose reaction: muscle pain, hypotension, dyspnea, nausea and vomiting. These reactions are probably due to capillary leak, at high doses.
2. Fluid retention.
3. Fever, chills and anorexia.
4. Lethargy and myalgia.
5. Bone pain and arthralgia.
6. Skin eruptions: both generalized and at the injection site.
7. Pericarditis and pericardial effusion.
8. Pleural effusion.
9. Eosinophilia.
10. Abnormal liver function tests: hepatitis.

Several of these effects are mediated by cytokine release.

Pharmacokinetics

The optimal dose of GM-CSF has not been established. The $t_{1/2}$ following intravenous infusion is variable (approximately 0.5–10 hours). Difficulties with assay mean that the pharmacokinetics of GM-CSF are not yet well defined.

INTERLEUKIN-3

This is a glycoprotein of molecular weight 14 000–28 0000. T lymphocytes produce interleukin-3 (IL-3) and a recombinant protein is now available. Interleukin-3 stimulates the growth and proliferation of hematopoietic precursors. It is given by subcutaneous injection and preliminary studies show it is effective in some patients with Diamond–Blackfan anemia. Adverse effects include fever, headache, rashes, nausea, influenza-like syndrome and eosinophilia.

OTHER HEMATOPOIETIC GROWTH FACTORS

Other hematopoietic growth factors presently undergoing clinical investigation include interleukin-6 and stem cell factor. This is the growth factor that produces ongoing proliferation of hematopoietic stem cells and has synergistic effects with other growth factors on all cell lineages.

COAGULATION FACTORS AND HEMOPHILIAS A AND B

Pathophysiology

Hemophilia A is an X-linked recessive disease where there is a deficiency of factor VIII in the blood. Hemophilia B is also an X-linked recessive disorder where there is a deficiency of factor IX. Hemophilia B has an incidence one-sixth that of hemophilia A. Both types of hemophilia present with identical clinical symptoms of excessive bleeding in response to trauma, e.g. muscle hematoma, hemarthrosis, hemorrhage after minor (e.g. dental) or major surgery and intracranial bleeding following minor head injury.

Therapeutic principles

The extent of hemorrhage depends on the severity of the factor VIII or IX deficiency and the severity of the trauma. Therapy consists of reducing hemorrhage by temporarily raising the concentration of the deficient factor, appropriate supportive measures, analgesia and graded physiotherapy. In minor trauma in mild hemophilia A, infusions of a synthetic vasopressin analog (desmopressin, DDAVP, chapter 32), 0.4 µg/kg, produces a short-term two- to four-fold increase in factor VIII. Fluid overload due the antidiuretic hormone (ADH) action of DDAVP must be prevented by limiting water intake. DDAVP also stimulates release of plasminogen activator, and is therefore given with an inhibitor of fibrinolysis such as tranexamic acid. If the hemophilia and/or trauma is severe then infusions of factor VIII or IX are required. The amount required and the number of infusions depend on the severity of the trauma. For minor hemarthrosis a level of 15% of the deficient factor is targeted and is usually achieved by a single infusion. In cases with muscle bleeding or major hemarthrosis a level of 25% is targeted which may require repeated infusions for several days over a week. In patients with head injury, major trauma or surgery a minimum level of 50% is targeted and maintained by repeated infusions. Patients and their parents or other carers are taught to administer these factors at home to minimize delay in therapy.

FACTOR VIII

Factor VIII is a protein cofactor in the intrinsic pathway of blood coagulation which is deficient in patients with hemophilia A and von Willebrand disease. It used in the treatment and prophylaxis of hemorrhage in patients with factor VIII deficiency. It is a single chain protein of molecular weight 330 000. It is circulated in the blood as a procofactor bound to von Willebrand factor. It is obtained from purified pooled plasma of blood donors or more recently from microorganisms by recombinant DNA techniques. Recombinant preparations are free of all potential viral pathogens, for example hepatitis B, hepatitis C, HIV, cytomegalovirus (CMV). These are inactivated by heat or chemical treatment of pooled human plasma preparations. Factor VIII is given as an intravenous infusion over several hours and has a mean $t_{1/2}$ of 10 hours. It is highly bound to von Willebrand factor (>95%) and has a small volume of distribution and is degraded by reticuloendothelial cells in the liver. The dose of factor VIII is calculated on the basis of the severity of the injury and the required increase in plasma factor VIII concentration. The main adverse effects are due to impurities or contaminants in the pooled plasma-derived preparations; anaphylactic reactions are rare; transmission of HIV, hepatitis B and hepatitis

C viruses should not occur with present methods but recent tragedies provide a grim warning of potential future dangers. In low purity factor VIII fibrinogen can accumulate and promote abnormal hemostasis when it has initially been corrected. Transient reactions to infusions such as urticaria, flushing and headache occur but respond to antihistamines. Repeated infusions of non-recombinant factor VIII may induce antibodies to factor VIII, and to certain impurities, in the recipient.

FACTOR IX

Factor IX is a protein cofactor in the intrinsic pathway of blood coagulation which is deficient in patients with hemophilia B. It is used in the treatment and prophylaxis of hemorrhage in patients with factor IX deficiency. It acts as a cofactor for factor VIII. It is available at present as a dried fraction from pooled plasma concentrates, which also contains the other vitamin K-dependent coagulation factors (II, V and VII, see chapter 27) and is therefore sometimes used to treat life-threatening bleeding in patients overtreated with warfarin. Pure factor IX will soon be available for patients with hemophilia B which will not contain these other factors. Factor IX is given as an intravenous infusion over several hours, and has a mean plasma $t_{1/2}$ of 18 hours. Otherwise its use and adverse effects are similar to those described for factor VIII.

Immuno-pharmacology

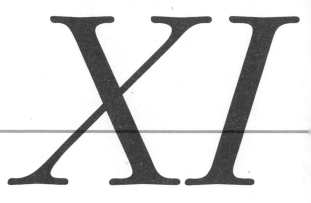

XI

Clinical Immuno- pharmacology

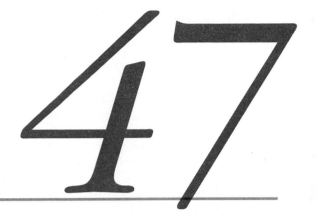

Introduction **632**

Immunosuppressive agents **634**

General adverse effects of immunosuppression **639**

Chemical mediators of the immune response and drugs that block their actions **640**

Drugs that enhance immune system function **644**

Vaccines **645**

Immunoglobulins as therapy **649**

INTRODUCTION

The introduction of a foreign antigen into the body may provoke an immune reaction. For this to occur the body must recognize the antigen as foreign. Antigens are usually large molecules with a molecular weight of over 5000. They are often multivalent and have a consistent charge and molecular profile, being proteins or large molecular weight carbohydrates. Most antigens are initially processed by macrophages before being presented to lymphocytes. The immune response is initiated by the interaction of antigen with receptors on the surface of the lymphocytes, and the response may be of two types: humoral and cellular immunity.

The immune response is an essential defense against invasion of the body by bacteria, viruses and other foreign material. However, it may be defective, disorganized or overactive and can produce a wide variety of diseases. The body has the potential to stimulate its immune system so that antibodies are produced against itself. Normally this situation is prevented by a number of suppression mechanisms. If these fail, autoimmune disease results. Deficiencies in the immune system may be congenital or result from the use of certain drugs, particularly cytotoxics and steroids.

Other important distinctions include active immunity, passive immunity and hypersensitivity.

Humoral immunity

This is the production of circulating immunoglobulin by plasma cells that are derived from B lymphocytes. In humans these lymphocytes arise largely from lymphoid tissue of the gastrointestinal tract. The humoral response occurs in two stages as follows:

1. **Primary reactions** These occur with the first exposure to the antigen. There is a small and short-lived rise in antibody titer which consists largely of IgM.
2. **Secondary reactions** These occur with subsequent exposure to the antigen. The rise in antibody is greater and persists for a long period. The antibody consists mostly of IgG. The reaction requires the intervention of helper T cells as well as B lymphocytes.

Cellular immunity

This is mediated by sensitized thymus-derived (T) lymphocytes that act directly on the antigen and produce lymphokines.

Active immunity

This consists of immunity that is developed in response either to infection or following inoculation with an attenuated strain of organism, or with a structural protein or toxic protein to which the host produces protective antibodies.

Passive immunity

This is immunity transferred by the administration of preformed antibodies (in immune globulin/serum) from another host or from recombinant techniques *in vitro*.

Hypersensitivity

Sometimes the immune response to an antigen results in damage to the tissue; this is called hypersensitivity. There are four types of hypersensitivity.

TYPE I HYPERSENSITIVITY

An antigen/antibody combination occurs on the surface of mast cells and other immune cells and releases pharmacologically active mediators. These include histamine; leukotrienes C_4, D_4 and E_4 (previously known as SRS-A); eosinophil chemotactic factor (ECF); serotonin; bradykinin and other kinins and prostaglandins. This type of reaction can cause anaphylaxis, allergic asthma, hayfever and some types of urticaria and is mediated by IgE reaginic antibodies.

TYPE II HYPERSENSITIVITY

Antibody combines with an antigen in the cell membrane. The reaction often requires complement and results in cell lysis. An example of this type of reaction is hemolytic disease which occurs in the newborn when antibodies produced by a rhesus-negative mother against the rhesus factor on the red cells of the fetus cross the placental barrier and cause hemolysis. Such reactions can be mediated by IgM or IgG antibodies.

TYPE III (ARTHUS REACTION)

This is caused by circulating complexes of antigen/antibody formed in conditions of slight antigen excess, together with complement which can cause tissue destruction directly and also by attracting polymorph neutrophils to the site. This reaction is delayed and is maximum a few hours after exposure to the antigen. Serum sickness is a result of this type of response. It is mediated by IgM or IgG antibodies.

TYPE IV (DELAYED CELL-MEDIATED HYPERSENSITIVITY)

This is due to sensitized circulating T lymphocytes reacting to antigen. Most of the manifestations of the reaction are produced via lymphokines; these are soluble factors produced by these primed lymphocytes that cause local inflammation, attract other lymphocytes and macrophages, enhance phagocytosis and increase macrophage metabolism. This type of reaction takes place 1–2 days after secondary antigen exposure and is exemplified by contact dermatitis and organ transplant rejection.

Immune responses are essential for health. Suppression of an unwanted component poses difficult problems. Ideally, immunosuppressant therapy should be highly selective and leave the rest of the immune mechanism intact. In practice two types of approach are used to try to achieve this:

1. The whole immune system can be 'damped down'. This is usually done with irradiation or drugs that are toxic to lymphocytes and thus reduce their number and interfere with their function. This has the disadvantage that suppression of immunity makes the body prone to infections, not only by bacteria but by viruses and fungi.
2. Attempts can be made to block the final chemical mediator of an unwanted immune reaction. This is most successful when the mediator is known and susceptible to blockade, for example histamine in the type I reaction that underlies hayfever, but for other types of immune response this may be impossible. It is also possible to manipulate the immune system by immunological methods and in some cases this may be the most appropriate way of obtaining selective depression of one facet of the immune response.

*I*MMUNOSUPPRESSIVE AGENTS

See Fig. 47.1.

AZATHIOPRINE

Azathioprine (see also chapter 23) is closely related to 6-mercaptopurine (6MP), to which it is metabolized, differing only in having an imidazole group added to the molecule.

Use

Azathioprine is used to prevent transplant rejection, the usual dose being 1–4 mg/kg/day orally. It has also been used with some success in the treatment of autoimmune diseases, for example systemic lupus erythematosus, rheumatoid arthritis, chronic active hepatitis and some cases of glomerulonephritis. Owing to its potential toxicity it is usually reserved for situations in which corticosteroids alone are inadequate.

Mechanism of action

Azathioprine is an antimetabolite and therefore is most effective on proliferating cells. It is metabolized to 6MP *in vivo*. Like 6MP it has little or no intrinsic activity but requires transformation by the enzyme hypoxanthine-guanine ribosyl transferase to the corresponding ribonucleotide. This interferes with all stages of purine synthesis and is incorporated into DNA. It causes immunosuppression by inhibiting lymphocytes which would normally proliferate in response to stimulation by an antigen. It inhibits delayed hypersensitivity (cell-mediated immunity) and those aspects of inflammation that depend on cell division. There is little evidence for any consistent effect on the normal humoral antibody response.

Pharmacokinetics

The drug is variably but well absorbed. It is 98% cleared by hepatic metabolism, and is partly metabolized by xanthine oxidase. It is metabolized to its active metabolite 6 MP. The mean half-life ($t_{1/2}$) of azathioprine is approximately 12 min.

Adverse effects

Bone marrow suppression occurs, particularly of granulocytes and platelets. The use of azathioprine requires regular blood counts.

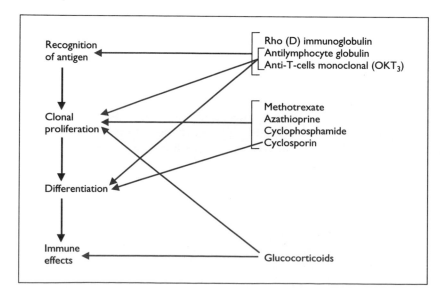

Fig. 47.1 Sites of action of immunosuppressive drugs.

Drug interactions

If azathioprine is given with a xanthine oxidase inhibitor, for example, allopurinol, accumulation and toxicity will occur, unless the dose is reduced accordingly.

METHOTREXATE

Methotrexate (chapters 23 and 45) produces immunosuppression by inhibiting the replication of rapidly dividing cells. It is used as low-dose daily oral therapy to treat rheumatoid arthritis as a second-line agent, and has also limited usefullness as adjunctive therapy in the treatment of chronic steroid-dependent asthma. The major dose-limiting toxicities when used chronically in low dose are hepatic cirrhosis and bone marrow suppression.

CYCLOPHOSPHAMIDE

Use

In addition to its use in cytotoxic chemotherapy (chapter 45) cyclophosphamide can be used to prevent graft rejection and in a variety of autoimmune disorders. Perhaps its most important role in this context is in the treatment of the nephrotic syndrome with minimal change in the glomeruli on microscopy, particularly in those patients who are resistant to corticosteroids or when steroid toxicity is troublesome. It appears to be superior to azathioprine in this type of disease. It is also used in the nephritis due to systemic lupus, Wegener's granulomatosis and, rarely, in severe rheumatoid disease. The usual dose is 3 mg/kg/day orally for 8 weeks.

Mechanism of action

Cyclophosphamide produces immunosuppression by inhibiting lymphocyte proliferation. It is most effective if given after antigenic stimulation. It reduces antibody production and depresses cell-mediated immunity and the inflammatory reaction.

GLUCOCORTICOSTEROIDS

See chapter 37.

Use

Type I reactions

Glucocorticosteroids are useful in allergic rhinitis, atopic dermatitis, acute severe asthma, chronic asthma and anaphylaxis. In allergic rhinitis and atopic dermatitis the principal benefit probably arises from non-specific anti-inflammatory effects, including vasoconstriction and decreased vascular permeability, mediated in part by decreased histamine release and facilitation of β-adrenergic stimulation. In asthma the actions are more complex, involving anti-inflammatory effects, relaxation of bronchial smooth muscle (either directly or by facilitation of β-adrenergic effects) and inhibition of histamine release and leukotriene LTC4, LTD4 and LTE4 (SRS-A) biosynthesis. Glucocorticosteroids also inhibit specific immune phenomena occurring in asthma including lymphocyte infiltration of bronchial mucosa and the deposition of immune complexes in the basement membrane. In addition glucocorticosteroids decrease serum IgE concentrations.

Type II reactions

Although glucocorticosteroids do not inhibit the normal humoral immune response, they are often effective in treating type II autoimmune diseases. They are the drugs of choice for pemphigus vulgaris and autoimmune hemolytic anemia, and are often effective in idiopathic thrombocytopenic purpura (ITP). Glucocorticoids induce remission in about 80% of cases of immune hemolytic anemia where warm-reacting antibodies are involved and about half of these will remain in long-term or permanent remission. Their mechanism of action in these conditions probably depends on several factors, including: (1) inhibition of autoantibody production in some patients; (2) inhibition of erythrophagocytosis in the absence of any alteration in antibody titer; and (3) decreased binding of autoantibody to red cells.

In pemphigus vulgaris there is a good correlation between depression of auto-antibody and clinical response, but this does not appear to be so clear in other diseases such as ITP.

Type III reactions

Glucocorticosteroids are widely used in immune complex diseases. They produce symptomatic relief without necessarily altering the fundamental disease process. Thus, in rheumatoid arthritis, although effective in controlling some features of the disease, the natural course of the disease is not improved. However, in systemic lupus erythematosus, steroid therapy is often associated with decreases in antinuclear autoantibody titer, and there is some evidence that high doses may improve renal function and prolong survival in some patients with renal involvement.

Type IV reactions

Glucocorticosteroids are potent inhibitors of these reactions, being used clinically to prevent graft rejection and in contact dermatitis.

Mechanism of action

Glucocorticosteroids are the most widely used immunosuppressive agents. They alter lymphocyte function and decrease the number of circulating T lymphocytes either by direct cell lysis or by redistributing lymphocytes throughout the body. Lymphocytopenia is dose dependent: high doses reducing lymphocyte numbers up to a maximum of 50-75%. A decrease in the absolute number of both T and B lymphocytes occurs with T cells proportionately more affected so their main action is to depress cell-mediated immunity. They do not suppress antibody formation following antigen stimulation but they may have some suppressive action on autoantibodies.

Glucocorticosteroids have a marked anti-inflammatory effect and also decrease the release of pharmacologically active substances from mast cells in type I hypersensitivity reactions. The release of lytic enzymes from the lysosomes of polymorphonuclear leukocytes is also inhibited. Glucocorticosteroids stimulate the synthesis of proteins, one of which (lipocortin) inhibits phospholipase A_2 so reducing arachidonic acid release and subsequent formation of prostaglandins, leukotrienes and thromboxane.

ANTILYMPHOCYTE GLOBULIN

Antilymphocyte globulin (ALG) is prepared by injecting human lymphocytes into animals to raise antibodies. Frequently T lymphocytes from thymus tissue are used as these play a predominant part in graft rejection. The active immunoglobulin is largely in the IgG fraction and ALG is thus a complex biological product with inherent variability from batch to batch.

Use

Antilymphocyte globulin reduces delayed hypersensitivity and prevents graft rejection and is particularly useful when rejection occurs soon after grafting. There have been no controlled trials concerning the efficacy of ALG in autoimmune disease.

Mechanism of action

Although ALG can produce cell lysis with the aid of complement, it is possible that at least some of its immunosuppressive effect is due to 'blinding' of the lymphocyte, which prevents it finding its target by blocking antigen recognition sites. Animal data suggest that ALG has no direct inhibitory effect on B cells or humoral immunity; however, in humans some evidence of response and remission with disappearance of autoantibodies has occurred in both type II and type III autoimmune disease.

Adverse effects

1. At least 50% of patients treated with ALG raised in horses develop antibodies to horse IgG. This leads to poor absorption of ALG from intramuscular injection and rapid clearance of ALG from the circulation resulting in decreased effectiveness.
2. An immune response to ALG may also result in anaphylactoid symptoms, serum sickness and rarely immune complex glomerulonephritis.
3. Another problem is specificity, since ALG frequently contains antibodies against non-lymphoid antigens such as red cells, platelets and kidney, which may produce toxic effects.

Pharmacokinetics

After injection ALG becomes attached to lymphocytes and is thus cleared from the circulation in about 6 hours. Owing to the size of the molecule free ALG is confined largely to the circulation and only low concentrations are found in tissue fluids. This means that only circulating lymphocytes are exposed to a high concentration of ALG. Antilymphocyte globulin is expensive, scarce and because of its inherent batch to batch variability difficult to assess in terms of clinical effect. Quality control is crucial.

OKT3 ANTIBODIES (ANTI-CD3 RECEPTOR ANTIBODIES)

Use

These monoclonal antibodies are used as adjuvant immunosuppressive therapy in patients with acute organ transplant rejection. They are IgG2a produced from murine hybridoma cells. After a 10-day course patients develop neutralizing antibodies to OKT3 antibodies. OKT3 are formulated in solution, filtered before use and given as an intravenous bolus. The total daily dose is 5 mg given for 10–14 days.

Mechanism of action

These antibodies are targeted at the T lymphocyte CD3 antigen and, when bound to this antigen, block T cell function. Additionally the antibody causes a decrease in CD3 (T3) positive lymphocytes in the blood. The mechanism of this depletion is not fully known but T cells are opsonized with anti-CD3 and removed by the reticuloendothelial system.

Adverse effects

1. Acute influenza-like syndrome (which may be minimized by pretreatment with glucocorticosteroids).
2. Chest pain, wheezing and dyspnea (pulmonary edema occurs after the first dose in 1% of patients).
3. Gastrointestinal disturbances.
4. Reversible meningoencephalitis.

Most of these symptoms are related to the release of cytokines from the T lymphocytes to which the antibody binds.

Pharmacokinetics

Blood concentrations decline to 10% of peak values after 24 hours with a $t_{1/2}$ of approximately 6 hours. The clearance mechanism is unknown.

CYCLOSPORIN

Cyclosporin is a cyclic hydrophobic decapeptide originally extracted from fungal cultures.

Use

Organ transplantation is the main use, for which regimens vary. A high dose of cyclosporin is given 4–12 hours before transplantation if possible. It may be given in doses of 4 mg/kg/day intravenously but this is liable to produce renal failure and it is safer to start with 14 mg/kg/day orally reducing over 3 months to a maintenance dose of around 6 mg/kg/day. Measurement of trough plasma concentrations of cyclosporin A is essential and dose adjusted to keep this between 60–200 µg/l. Opinions vary as to whether cyclosporin should be combined with steroids. Results are superior to those obtained with azathioprine.

In graft-versus-host disease and bone marrow transplantation intravenous treatment is used initially (3–5 mg/kg/day) followed by oral administration for 6–9 months. The oral maintenance dose of cyclosporin is 5–10 mg/kg, sometimes with glucocorticosteroids. A particular advantage is that unlike many other immunosuppressives it does not interfere with hematopoietic function.

Mechanism of action

Cyclosporin is a specific T lymphocyte suppressor, primarily the T helper cells, with a unique effect on the primary but not the secondary immune response. It inhibits production of interleukin-2 (IL-2) and other cytokines by activated lymphocytes. At a cellular level this is due to cyclosporin A binding to its transport protein cyclophilin. This conjugate subsequently interacts with a Ca^{2+}-calmodulin dependent calcineurin complex and inhibits its phosphorylase activity. This impairs access into the nucleus of the cytosolic component of the transcription promoter nuclear factor of activated T cells (NF ATc). This reduces transcription of messenger RNA for IL-2, for other lymphokines, and IL-2 receptor expression.

Adverse effects

1. Nephrotoxicity is a serious problem. Serum creatinine and urea are increased in patients receiving cyclosporin. Sometimes it is difficult to differentiate rejection from drug-induced renal damage. Follow-up studies suggest that the deterioration in renal function is not progressive. Nephrotoxicity is apparently minimized by calcium channel blockade (e.g. with nifedipine).
2. Hyperkalemia.
3. Nausea and gastrointestinal disturbances in up to 20% of patients.
4. Hypertension.
5. Hirsutism.
6. Gum hypertrophy that is most marked in children also treated with calcium channel blocking drugs.
7. Tremor (which can be an early sign of increasing plasma concentrations), paresthesia and fits.
8. Hepatotoxicity, but this is not dose limiting.
9. Anaphylaxis may occur with intravenous administration.
10. Although it was originally feared that the use of cyclosporin would result in a serious number of malignancies (mainly lymphoma) developing, careful control of dosage and the avoidance of undue immunosuppression has considerably reduced this risk.

Pharmacokinetics

Cyclosporin is variably absorbed after oral administration (35–45%). It undergoes some presystemic metabolism (bioavailability approximately 30%). The plasma log concentration–time relationship is biphasic with a $t_{1/2\alpha}$ of 1.2 hours and $t_{1/2\beta}$ of 27 hours. Because of its lipid solubility it has a large volume of distribution (3.5 l/kg). It is highly protein bound (90–95%). The major route of clearance is metabolism, via the hepatic cytochrome P_{450} system and up to 12 metabolites have been identified. Renal dysfunction does not affect cyclosporin clearance, but caution is needed because of its nephrotoxicity. Dose reduction is required in patients with hepatic impairment.

Therapeutic drug monitoring

Cyclosporin is assayed by radioimmunoassay (RIA) or high-performance liquid chromatography (HPLC). Radioimmunoassay is preferred for clinical monitoring despite cross-reactions with several cyclic metabolites. Trough plasma concentrations of 100–250 μg/l are satisfactory when the drug is given by intravenous infusion. Effective immunosuppresion occurs at trough concentrations of 60–200 μg/l when the drug is given orally. Careful monitoring of plasma concentrations is required for all patients but especially if there is gastrointestinal disturbance, hepatic impairment, or patients are concomitantly receiving other nephrotoxic drugs or drugs known to interact with cyclosporin. Recently the use of modelling of plasma concentrations in transplant patients appears to have reduced toxicity and improved efficacy.

Drug interactions

Ketoconazole, erythromycin, anabolic steroids and norethisterone reduce the hepatic clearance of cyclosporin by enzyme inhibition, leading to increased toxicity. Phenytoin, phenobarbitone and rifampicin increase hepatic clearance (phenytoin reduces absorption, phenobarbitone and rifampicin enzyme induce P_{450} activity), thus reducing plasma concentrations. Concomitant use of nephrotoxic agents such as aminoglycosides, vancomycin and amphotericin B may lead to cumulative nephrotoxicity with high plasma concentrations. Renal function and plasma drug concentration should be carefully monitored in patients treated with these agents. Combined use of cyclosporin and steroids in bone marrow transplant patients has led to an increase in hypertension and convulsions, perhaps due to increased fluid retention.

In view of the toxic effects of cyclosporin a number of related immunosuppressives are presently being evaluated, including staurosporin and rapamycin.

FK 506 (TACROLIMUS)

FK 506 is a macrocyclic lactone antibiotic, structurally similar to macrolides, and is derived from *Streptomyces tsukubaensis*. It is presently undergoing assessment in immuno-suppressive regimens for kidney, liver and heart transplantations. It is possibly more effective than cyclosporin in liver transplanta-tions. However, its role in immunosuppres-sion following renal transplantation is less clear and unexpected irreversible neurotoxic-ity (spastic paraparesis) has been noted. It is 50–100 times more potent than cyclosporin *in vitro* and may act intracellularly by a similar mechanism. Its mechanism of action is thought to be by suppressing the synthesis of interleukins-2, -3, and -4 and other cytokines, including granulocyte macrophage colony-stimulating factor, tumor necrosis factor-α and interferon-γ. It is initially administered intra-venously at a dose of 75 μg/kg twice daily until oral therapy (150 μg/kg twice daily) is commenced. FK 506 is mainly cleared by hepatic metabolism. The major adverse effects are neurotoxicity (headache, paresthesia, tremor and mood disturbances in addition to seizures), nephrotoxicity, hemolytic anemia, hypertension, gastrointestinal disturbances and impaired glucose tolerance. FK 506 should not be given concurrently with cyclosporin because of potential additive nephrotoxicity.

GENERAL ADVERSE EFFECTS OF IMMUNOSUPPRESSION

Prolonged use of non-specific immunosup-pressive drugs is associated with an appre-ciable incidence of adverse effects due to reduced immunity or drug-induced damage to the nuclear structure of the cell.

1. ***Increased susceptibility to infection*** Bacterial infections are common and require prompt treatment with appropri-ate antibiotics. Tuberculosis may also occur and sometimes takes unusual forms. Viral infections may be more severe than is usual and include the common herpes infection but occasionally also such rarities as multifocal leukoen-cephalopathy. Fungal infections are also common including *Candida albicans* which may be local or systemic, and protozoal infections (e.g. *Pneumocystis carinii*) also occur.

2. ***Sterility*** Azoospermia in men is particu-larly common with alkylating agents (e.g cyclophosphamide). In women hormone failure leading to amenorrhea is com-mon.

3. ***Teratogenicity*** This is less common than might be anticipated. It is, however, prudent to recommend avoiding concep-tion while on these drugs and for men to wait 12 weeks (the time required to clear abnormal sperm) after stopping treatment.

4. ***Carcinogenicity*** Immunosuppression is associated with an increased incidence of malignant disease. Large cell diffuse lymphoma can present early in treatment but with prolonged treatment other types of malignancy may arise. The incidence in transplant patients is about 1%.

Other drugs that attenuate the immune response include penicillamine, gold and chloroquine. These drugs are used in an attempt to modify disease progression in patients with severe rheumatoid arthritis (chapter 23).

CHEMICAL MEDIATORS OF THE IMMUNE RESPONSE AND DRUGS THAT BLOCK THEIR ACTIONS

An alternative method of modifying the immune response is to block the release or action of chemical mediators that play an important part in certain immune reactions, especially type I immunity. There are several pharmacologically active mediators and their relative importance differs in different species. Histamine is important, although not exclusively so.

Histamine

Histamine is widely distributed in the body and is derived from the decarboxylation of histidine. It is concentrated in mast cell and basophil granules. The highest concentrations are found in lung, nasal mucous membrane, skin, stomach and duodenum (i.e. at interfaces between the body and the outside environment). Histamine is liberated by several basic drugs, usually when given in large quantities intravenously: these include tubocurarine, morphine, codeine, pethidine and suramin. The physiological role of this potent amine is uncertain; it may function as a local controller of vascular responses, particularly in the skin, where it is concerned with response to injury. There is also evidence of its involvement in neuronal transmission in the brain. Its main functions seem to be the release of gastric acid (chapter 31) and as part mediator of the allergic response. There are two main types of histamine receptors: H_1 and H_2.

H_1-receptors

Stimulation of H_1-receptors produces the following effects on blood vessels and nerve endings in humans. Histamine causes dilatation of small arteries and capillaries, together with increased permeability, which leads to formation of edema. Histamine headache is caused by its effect on cerebral vessels. Intravenous administration causes a fall in peripheral resistance, reduction in circulating volume and fall in blood pressure. In overdose it causes shock. Intravenous histamine (or tolazoline, a histamine agonist) has been used to reduce pulmonary vascular resistance in children with pulmonary hypertension. Inhaled histamine is used to induce bronchospasm (by smooth muscle contraction) in sensitive individuals and assess the efficacy of drugs used for bronchodilatation and prophylaxis in asthmatics. Histamine causes vasoconstriction in fetal vessels (e.g. umbilical artery). Histamine injected into the skin produces the characteristic triple response which consists, in order of appearance, of:

1. A localized red spot (due to capillary dilatation).
2. A larger flush or flare (due to arteriolar dilatation via an axon-reflex mechanism).
3. A wheal (localized edema subsequent to increased vessel permeability).

Local injection of histamine causes itch and sometimes pain due to stimulation of peripheral nerves.

H_2-receptors

H_2-receptors are principally concerned with stimulation of gastric acid release (chapter 31). They make only a minor contribution to most vascular responses but some (e.g. in the pulmonary vasculature) are H_2-receptor mediated.

HYPERSENSITIVITY REACTIONS INVOLVING HISTAMINE RELEASE

Anaphylactic shock (acute anaphylaxis)

In certain circumstances injection of an antigen is followed by production of reaginic IgE antibodies. These coat mast cells and basophils and further exposure to the antigen results in rapid degranulation with release of histamine and other mediators including prostaglandin D_2 and leukotrienes. Clinically the patient presents a picture of shock and collapse with hypotension, bronchospasm and oropharyngeal and laryngeal edema often accompanied by urticaria and flushing. A similar so-called anaphylactoid reaction may occur after the non-immunological release of mediators by X-ray contrast media.

Atopy

Some individuals with a hereditary atopic diathesis have a propensity to develop local allergic reactions if exposed to appropriate antigens, causing hayfever, allergic asthma or urticaria. This is due to antigen combining with mast-cell associated IgE in the mucosa of the respiratory tract or in the skin.

Serum sickness

This is a type III hypersensitivity reaction and is due to circulating complexes of antigen/antibody and complement. These complexes can release histamine and probably other vasoactive substances from mast cells.

Use

These preparations are used in the therapy of allergic rhinitis; they are markedly effective in reducing the symptoms of sneezing, rhinorrhea, itching and nasal obstruction. They are more effective than cromoglycate.

The major drugs used via nasal insufflation to treat hayfever are:

- Beclomethasone diproprionate: dose 50–100 μg to each nostril twice daily.
- Budesonide: dose 200 μg to each nostril once daily.
- Flunisolide: dose 50 μg to each nostril t.d.s.
- Fluticasone diproprionate: 100 μg to each nostril once daily (50 μg for children).

Adverse effects

Adverse effects from all these preparations are similar: sneezing, dryness and irritation of nose and throat. Occasionally epistaxis is a problem. It is claimed that the systemic absorption of fluticasone is least and therefore the likelihood of systemic side effects lowest; this has not, however, been proven for the intranasal route.

Drugs that block effects of mediators of allergy

Possible therapeutic approaches to the management of allergic disease produced by mediators are:

(1) To block their biosynthesis.
(2) To block their release, and.
(3) To block their effects.

(a) Blockade of biosynthesis of mediators

INTRANASAL AND TOPICAL GLUCOCORTICOSTEROIDS

See chapters 30 and 37.

(b) Blockade of release of mediators

SODIUM CROMOGLYCATE AND NEDOCROMIL SODIUM

See chapter 30.

Use

Sodium cromoglycate and nedocromil are used to prevent attacks of asthma. Attempts have been made to use the drugs in other disorders where allergic factors play a part. Cromoglycate is inhaled (as a powder) in the prophylaxis of asthma or used as 2% nasal or eye drops for allergic rhinitis and conjunctivitis. Local adverse effects are occasional nasal irritation or transient stinging in the eye.

Mechanism of action

These agents were found to be effective in preventing bronchospasm when given to asthmatic subjects before challenge with an antigen. They are not bronchodilators, nor do they block the actions of histamine, 5-hydroxy-tryptamine (5HT) or leukotrienes on smooth muscle. Sodium cromoglycate was originally believed to prevent the release of pharmaco-logically active substances from mast cells when exposed to an antigen. It was believed to accomplish this by 'stabilizing' the mast cells, possibly by interfering with calcium ion entry, so that degranulation did not occur when the mast cells took part in a type I antigen/antibody reaction. However, at present it is apparent that this is not sufficient to explain their clinical effects.

In clinical studies sodium cromoglycate is not only effective in early onset asthma, in which allergic factors are important, but also to a lesser extent in late onset asthma, in which such factors are thought to play little part. Furthermore, analogs of cromoglycate that are more effective as mast cell stabilizers *in vitro* are less effective in clinical practice than cromoglycate. The clinical efficacy of cromoglycate remains unexplained.

β₂-AGONISTS

These drugs (e.g salbutamol, salmeterol, chapter 30) may also exert some of their antiasthmatic action by blocking mediator release from mast cells, but have little demonstrable effect except in asthma.

(c) Blockade of effects of mediators

ANTIHISTAMINES

There are a large number of antihistamines (H_1-receptor antagonists). Some of those in common use are shown in Table 47.1. Their antihistaminic actions are similar when used in clinically appropriate dosage but they differ in duration of effect, degree of sedation and antiemetic potential.

Use

Antihistamines are widely used to treat hyper-sensitivity reactions and are most effective in some types of urticaria and hayfever; they are less useful for anaphylactic shock. They help to reduce laryngeal edema which is occasion-ally dangerous in anaphylaxis, but are rather slow to act, so adrenaline, which is more rapidly effective, is used as the first-line drug. Antihistamines are useful if given promptly and systemically in preventing excessive reactions to bee and wasp stings which both contain histamine and trigger its release. Relief of itching is probably due to their sedative action rather than any specific effect.

Table 47.1 Properties of some H_1 antagonists.

Drug	Duration of effect (hours)	Degree of sedation	Antiemetic action	Usual dose (mg)
Promethazine	20	Marked	Some	10–25
Diphenhydramine	6	Some	Little	50
Chlorpheniramine	4–6	Moderate	Little	4
Cyclizine	6	Some	Marked	50
Clemastine	12	Some	Little	1
Triprolidine	24 (slow release)	Moderate	Little	10
Terfenadine	12	Nil	Little	60
Astemizole	24	Nil	Little	10
Cetirizine	24	Nil	Little	10
Loratidine	24	Nil	Little	10

Local application as a cream is liable to lead to contact dermatitis.

Antihistamines have not proved to be clinically useful in asthma, probably because other mediators are over-ridingly important in this disease. Antihistamines are used for their central sedative actions, particularly in the prevention of motion sickness (e.g. cyclizine). Antihistamines are also used, despite lack of evidence of efficacy, in symptomatic treatment of the common cold. They are used in various cough mixtures where their sedative action plays a role.

Sedation is often a problem with antihistamines, particularly if they are taken regularly. Several antihistamines have been introduced with little if any central effect (e.g. terfenadine, astemizole; Table 47.1). They are more expensive but are indicated in patients who find sedation a problem. These agents are available over the counter but there is concern that they cause an unusual form of ventricular tachycardia (*torsades de pointes*) in patients who are predisposed by virtue of a long QT interval. This can be inherited (Ward–Romano syndrome, a rare disorder) or acquired with the use of class III anti-arrhythmic drugs such as amiodarone or sotalol (chapter 29) and some other drugs (e.g. probucol, chapter 24).

Mechanism of action

Antihistamines are competitive antagonists of histamine at H_1-receptors. They are effective in blocking the edema and vascular response to histamine but not in improving a shocked state. Although they block bronchoconstrictor responses to histamine *in vitro*, they have little effect on bronchoconstriction in asthmatics *in vivo*. Most H_1-antagonists have some central sedative action. Use with alcohol, benzodiazepines or other central depressant drugs produces additive or synergistic depressant effects. Phenindamine is unusual in that it has excitatory properties in clinically used doses. Most of these drugs also have some antiemetic effects, which may be clinically useful (chapter 31). Additional antimuscarinic effects result in drying of secretions (cf. atropine) which contributes to their efficacy in rhinitis.

Pharmacokinetics

Antihistamines are rapidly absorbed from the intestine and are effective within about half an hour. They generally undergo hepatic metabolism and are cleared within about 6 hours. Newer agents such as cetirizine and loratidine have half-lives of 12–24 hours; astemizole has a $t_{1/2}$ of 19 hours, a slow onset of action and binds almost irreversibly to H_1-receptors. Thus it is best used in prophylaxis rather than when symptoms occur. These newer agents do not penetrate the blood–brain barrier very much and cause less psychomotor impairment than earlier antihistamines. Some, for example chlorpheniramine, are available for intravenous administration in allergic emergencies. There is no relationship between the antihistaminic potency of these compounds and their central depressant activity.

Adverse effects

1. Sedation and psychomotor impairment, especially with older agents.
2. Nausea.
3. Photosensitivity rashes.
4. Antimuscarinic effects: dry mouth, blurred vision etc.
5. Prolongation of the QT interval which may in overdose cause *torsades de pointes*; cetirizine does not prolong the QT interval.

Contraindications

Avoid in porphyria and in the Ward–Romano syndrome (congenital long QT syndrome).

ADRENALINE

Adrenaline is uniquely valuable therapeutically as an effective antagonist of the acute anaphylactic reaction. Its rapid action may be life-saving in general anaphylaxis due to insect venom allergy and reaction to drugs. The usual dose is 0.5–1.0 ml of a 1:1000 solution (0.5–1.0 mg), repeated after 10 min if necessary, given intramuscularly or if necessary intravenously. It is effective by virtue of its α-agonist activity which reverses vascular dilatation and edema and by its β_2-agonist activity producing bronchodilatation. It also reduces the release of inflammatory mediators.

Treatment of anaphylactic shock

1. Stop any drug or blood being administered intravenously and lay the patient flat.
2. Give adrenaline of 0.5–1.0 mg, intramuscularly (may have to be given intravenously, with appropriate monitoring if patient has a blood pressure <70 mmHg) and repeated after 10 min if no improvement.
3. Give intravenous colloid.
4. Administer 100% oxygen producing an inspired oxygen of 35–60%.
5. Give hydrocortisone, 100–200 mg, intravenously.
6. Give antihistamine intravenously, for example chlorpheniramine, 12.5 mg.
7. Consider nebulized salbutamol, 5 mg, or intravenous aminophylline, 250 mg over 20 min, for residual bronchospasm.

Therapy of allergic rhinitis (hayfever)

The patient presenting with symptoms of allergic rhinitis is assessed to ensure that infection is not the primary problem. If infection is the cause the presence of a foreign body is excluded and appropriate antibacterial therapy prescribed. If symptoms are due to allergy the first step in therapy is allergen avoidance and minimization of exposure (e.g. ragweed pollen). Complete avoidance is, however, difficult to achieve. For patients with mild intermittent symptoms a short-acting non-sedating antihistamine is best (e.g. terfenadine). Short-term use of a nasal decongestant such as pseudoephedrine is effective but if used longer causes rebound vasomotor rhinitis. Ipratropium bromide (20–40 μg to each nostril three times a day) is added if rhinorrhea is the predominant symptom. If symptoms are more chronic the first-line therapy is intranasal glucocorticosteroids because these are effective against all symptoms, and are more effective than cromoglycate. In children topical cromoglycate given by insufflator (10 mg into each nostril q.d.s.) or nasal spray (one spray – 2.6 mg per nostril two to four times a day) is useful. If rhinorrhea is the main problem ipratropium is added with or without a long-acting antihistamine (e.g. terfenadine, 60 mg, twice daily or astemizole, 10 mg, or cetirizine, 10 mg, daily). If these measures are ineffective consider immunotherapy or surgery if there is evidence of sinusitis.

DRUGS THAT ENHANCE IMMUNE SYSTEM FUNCTION

Adjuvants

Adjuvants non-specifically augment the immune response when mixed with antigen or injected into the same site. This is achieved in a variety of ways:

1. Release of the antigen is slowed and exposure to it prolonged.
2. Various immune cells are attracted to the site of injection and interaction between such cells is important in antibody formation.

There are a number of such substances, usually given as mixtures and often containing lipids, extracts of inactivated tubercle bacilli and various mineral salts.

Immunostimulants

Immunostimulants non-specifically enhance immune responses, examples being bacille

Calmette-Guérin (BCG) or killed *Coryne-bacterium parvum*.

LEVAMISOLE

Originally developed as an anthelminthic, levamisole stimulates immune responses. Newborn rats given a lethal number of staphylococci on the third day of life survive if treated with levamisole on the preceding 3 days. In addition, a reduction in the number of metastases in animals injected with malignant cells and a reduction in the size of established tumors suggest that immune responses to tumors are also enhanced. Clinical efficacy has not been clearly proven, however. It has been used in combination chemotherapy for some tumors, for example colonic carcinoma. It is given orally at 2.5 mg/kg daily for 3 days every 2 weeks.

Mechanism of action

Levamisole is believed to stimulate macrophages and T lymphocytes and restore depressed lymphocyte function.

Pharmacokinetics

Oral absorption is good (>95%). Plasma $t_{1/2}$ is 4–6 hours and the major route of clearance is via extensive and rapid hepatic metabolism. Levamisole undergoes 30–40% presystemic metabolism.

Adverse effects

1. Agranulocytosis (particularly if given to patients with ankylosing spondylitis, i.e. HLA-B27 genotype).
2. Rashes.
3. Taste and smell disturbances.

INTERLEUKIN-2

Interleukin-2 (IL-2) is a 15 420 molecular weight peptide with 133 amino acids that is produced primarily by T helper cells. Human recombinant IL-2 is now available. Interleukin-2 stimulates T cells and cytotoxic lymphocytes to proliferate. It was used with little success in metastatic carcinoma but has some activity against renal carcinoma. It has also been used *ex vivo* to stimulate lymphocytes into lymphokine activated killer cells that when injected back into the patient lyse tumors in a non-antigen specific manner. Interleukin-2 can be administered by intravenous bolus or continuous infusion, the latter resulting in less toxicity. It disappears from plasma in a biphasic fashion with a $t_{1/2\alpha}$ of 6–7 min during which phase most of the IL-2 is cleared and a $t_{1/2\beta}$ of approximately 70 min. The major adverse effects are fluid overload and fluid retention due to vascular leakage; this can cause life-threatening pulmonary edema (the mechanism for this may be the effect of IL-2 on activating endothelial cells), fever and chills.

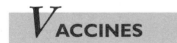

*V*ACCINES

See Table 47.2.

Immunology and general use

Vaccines stimulate the production of protective antibodies and other components of the immune response. Vaccines consist of:

1. Either an attenuated form of the infectious agent, such as the live vaccines used against some viral infections (e.g. rubella, measles, polio) or BCG used against tuberculosis.
2. Inactivated preparations of the virus (e.g influenza virus) or bacteria (e.g. typhoid vaccine).
3. Extracts of or detoxified exotoxins produced by a micro-organism (e.g. tetanus vaccine).

Table 47.2 Common vaccines, their dose regimens and major adverse effects.

Vaccine	Dose and regimen	Use	Adverse effects
BCG vaccine Live attenuated *Mycobacterium bovis*	0.1 ml intradermal injection for at-risk groups; 80% effective at providing immunity	Exposed patients: children entering school who are Heaf negative	Ulceration or subcutaneous abscess due to poor injection technique
Cholera vaccine Heat killed *Vibrio cholerae*	0.5 ml by deep i.m. or s.c. injection	Individuals due to travel in endemic countries	–
DTP vaccine Diphtheria formol toxoid, tetanus formol toxoid and live attenuated pertussis vaccine (DTP)	0.5 ml deep s.c. or i.m. at 2, 3 and 6 months	Childhood vaccination schedule	Adverse reaction to pertussis, local induration/inflammation at site. Fever, convulsions, anaphylaxis wheeze, laryngeal edema, collapse within 48 hours of injection
Hemophilus influenzae b vaccine A conjugated bacterial polysaccharide	Given as a 0.5 ml deep s.c. or i.m. injection. For primary immunity it is given as three doses at monthly intervals	Children who are less than 2 months old or 2–14 months	–
Hepatitis A vaccine Formaldehyde inactivated hepatitis virus	Two 1 ml i.m. injections 1 month apart	Vaccination should be considered for those travelling to endemic areas	Transient soreness, erythema at the injection site. Rarely an influenza-like syndrome
Hepatitis B vaccine Recombinant HB$_s$ Ag made biosynthetically	Three 1 ml doses given i.m. into the deltoid; the second dose is 1 month after the first and the third dose 3 months later	High-risk groups, e.g. health personnel, hemophiliacs	–
Influenza vaccine Inactivated influenza vaccine of surface antigen or split virion (always N and H antigens of prevalent strain)	0.5 ml deep s.c. or i.m. injection. In children repeated once in 4–6 weeks	Patients with chronic cardiac, renal and pulmonary conditions, diabetics, immunosuppressed and elderly	Contraindicated in egg allergic individuals
MMR vaccine Live mumps, measles and rubella	0.5 ml by deep s.c. or i.m. injection	All children before entry to primary school, and rubella for females <13 years if seronegative	Fever and rash, parotid swelling. Contraindicated in egg allergic patients and immunosuppressed
Meningoccal polysaccharide vaccine From groups A and C	0.5 ml by deep s.c. or i.m. injection	Adult and children ≥2 months, during epidemics and travelers going to areas of high incidence of meningococcal carriage	–

Table 47.2 (contd)

Vaccine	Dose and regimen	Use	Adverse effects
Pneumococcal vaccine 23 subtypes of pneumococcal capsule	0.5 ml s.c. or i.m. injection	Patients, e.g. splenectomized, at risk of pneumococcal infection	Hypersensitivity reactions may occur
Poliomyelitis vaccine Live attenuated virus (Sabin) or inactivated (Salk)	Live vaccine of attenuated strains 1, 2 and 3 as oral suspension. Inactivated suspension as 0.5 ml injection. Three doses are required for primary immunization	Childhood immunization schedule	Rarely (1 per 2×10^6 doses) the subject or a contact of a vaccinee develops a mild form of the disease
Smallpox vaccine Live vaccine attenuated	0.5 ml s.c.	Workers with smallpox virus. Travelers do not need it as it has been eradicated globally	–
Typhoid vaccine Whole live vaccine (killed bacteria), polysaccharide vaccine and oral attenuated vaccine	0.5 ml by deep s.c. or i.m. injection. Oral – three capsules on alternate days	Travelers and during epidemics. Oral vaccine inactivated by sulfonamides which must be avoided	Local reactions, fever, malaise, headache

Live vaccine immunization is generally achieved with a single dose, but three doses are required for oral polio (which has different strains). Live vaccine replicates while in the body and produces protracted immunity, albeit not as long as that acquired after natural infection. When two live vaccines are required (and are not in a combined preparation) they may be given at different sites simultaneously or at an interval of at least 3 weeks.

Inactivated vaccines usually require a primary series of doses of vaccine to produce an adequate antibody response. Booster injections are required at intervals. The duration of immunity acquired with the use of inactivated vaccines varies from months to years. The vaccination programmes recommended by the UK Department of Social Security (DSS in the UK), are described in detail in a memorandum 'Immunization against Infectious Disease' available to doctors from the DSS.

Adverse effects

1. Some vaccines cause little or no reactions, for example poliomyelitis.
2. Vaccines such as measles and mumps can cause a mild form of the disease.
3. Discomfort at the inoculation site.
4. Mild fever and malaise.
5. Rarely anaphylactic shock.

Contraindications

Postpone vaccination if the patient is suffering from acute illness. Ensure that the patient is not sensitive to antibiotics used in the preparation of the vaccine, for example neomycin and polymyxin. Egg sensitivity excludes the administration of influenza vaccine (also measles, mumps and rubella (MMR) and yellow fever vaccine), if evidence is obtained of previous anaphylaxis. Live vaccines should not be given to pregnant women. Live vaccines should not be given to patients who are immunosuppressed, whether due to drugs, radiotherapy or human immunodeficiency virus-1 (HIV-1) infection. Live vaccines should be postponed until at least 3 months after stopping corticosteroids and 6 months after chemotherapy. Yellow fever, BCG, or typhoid (oral) vaccines should not be administered to HIV-1-positive individuals.

IMMUNOGLOBULINS AS THERAPY

Immunoglobulin injection gives immediate passive protection for 4–6 weeks. Originally immunoglobulins of animal origin (antisera) gave a high incidence of hypersensitivity, and were abandoned for immunoglobulins from human sources. Recombinant technology will yield a greater source of antibodies of consistent quality in the future, so their importance will probably increase. Presently there are two types of immunoglobulin: normal immunoglobulin and specific immunoglobulin.

HUMAN NORMAL IMMUNOGLOBULIN

Human normal immunoglobulin (HNIG) is prepared from pooled donations of human plasma. It contains antibody to measles, mumps, varicella and hepatitis A, and other viruses.

Use

It is used to protect susceptible subjects from infection with hepatitis A, measles and to a lesser extent to protect against rubella in pregnancy. It protects against the likelihood of a clinical attack, thus reducing the risk to the fetus. It should only be used when termination is not an option. It is given intramuscularly at doses varying from 0.02 to 0.12 ml/kg for hepatitis A. For measles 0.2 ml/kg is given and for prevention of a clinical attack of rubella in pregnancy 20 ml is used (serological follow-up for rubella prophylaxis is essential). Special formulations for intravenous administration are available for replacement therapy in agammaglobulinemia, hypogammaglobulinemia, and IgG subclass deficiency (e.g. Bruton's agammaglobulin-emia; Wiskott–Aldrich syndrome) idiopathic thrombocytopenic purpura and for prophylaxis of infection in bone marrow transplant patients. Doses vary from 1 to 6 g as a course.

Adverse effects

The commonest adverse effects occur during the first infusion and are dependent upon the antigenic load (dose) given:

1. Fever, chills and rarely anaphylaxis. To minimize these reactions in immunodeficient patients the first dose should be given slowly and covered with antihistamines and glucocorticosteroids. These reactions can occur on subsequent infusions but are usually because of too fast an infusion rate or intercurrent infection.
2. Small increases in plasma viscosity merit caution in patients with ischemic heart disease.
3. Aseptic meningitis (high dose).

Contraindications

Normal immunoglobulin is contraindicated in patients with known class specific antibody to IgA.

Drug interactions

Live virus vaccinations may be rendered less effective.

SPECIFIC IMMUNOGLOBULINS

These antibodies are prepared by pooling the plasma of selected donors with high levels of the specific antibody required. The following are presently available and effective: rabies immunoglobulin; tetanus immunoglobulin (human origin – HTIG); varicella zoster immunoglobulin (ZIG) (limited supply).

ANTI-D (RHO) IMMUNOGLOBULIN

The use of this immunoglobulin is to prevent a rhesus negative mother from forming anti-bodies to fetal rhesus positive cells that enter the maternal circulation during childbirth or abortion. An intramuscular injection of 500–5000 units is given to rhesus negative mothers up to 72 hours after the birth/abortion. This prevents a subsequent child from developing hemolytic disease of the newborn.

The Skin

XII

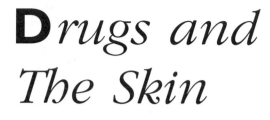

Drugs and The Skin

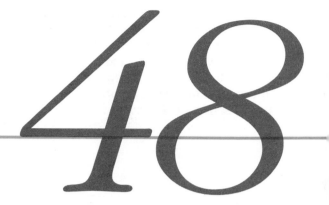

Introduction **654**

Acne **654**

Alopecia **655**

Eczema **656**

Pain and itching **657**

Psoriasis **657**

Urticaria **660**

Superficial bacterial skin infections **660**

Fungal skin and nail infections **661**

Viral skin infections **661**

Scabies **662**

Lice **662**

Adverse drug reactions involving the skin **662**

*I*NTRODUCTION

Skin diseases represent a large proportion of a community practitioner's workload. The key to therapy is correct diagnosis which is often readily confirmed by biopsy. Non-specific use of drugs such as potent topical corticosteroids, which can modify the appearance of skin lesions, should be avoided in the absence of a diagnosis.

Topical or systemic drug administration can cause a wide variety of skin lesions. There is considerable potential for topically applied drugs (notably corticosteroids) to act locally and/or to enter the systemic circulation and produce either a harmful or beneficial systemic pharmacological effect. Transdermal drug delivery is discussed in chapter 4.

*A*CNE

Incidence and pathophysiology

Acne vulgaris occurs in at least 90% of adolescents. Simple therapy is effective in most cases but severe cystic acne is a considerable therapeutic challenge. Acne is associated with *Propionibacterium* spp. infection of sebaceous glands of the skin.

Principles of treatment

The efficacy of abrasive agents is uncertain but the topical use of peeling agents such as benzoyl peroxide (2–5% solution applied twice daily) or retinoic acid (tretinoin) on a regular basis in conjunction with systemic antibiotic therapy is successful in most cases. The main side effect of peeling agents is skin irritation. Because of the powerful teratogenic effects of oral isotretinoin, there has been concern as to the safety of topical retinoic acid in the first trimester of pregnancy. However, a large study from the USA has shown that topical retinoic acid is not associated with an increased risk of major congenital abnor-

malites. Suitable antibiotics (chapter 40) include oxytetracycline (250 mg three times a day for 1–4 weeks, reducing to twice daily until improvement occurs, which may take several months), minocycline (50 mg twice daily for 6 weeks) or erythromycin (250 mg three times a day for 1–4 weeks, reducing to twice daily until improvement occurs, which may take several months). Oxytetracycline and minocycline should not be used until the secondary dentition is established. Pseudo-membranous colitis has occurred in patients on long-term tetracyclines for acne, and minocycline can cause cerebellar ataxia. Topical antibiotic preparations (e.g. tetracycline 0.22% or clindamycin, 10 mg/ml) are less effective than systemic therapy but may help those intolerant of peeling agents. Azelaic acid (20% cream apply twice daily) is a natural product of *Pityrosporum ovale*. It has antimicrobial activity and is effective topical therapy for acne. Treatment should not exceed 6 months. For patients who are refractory to these therapies the use of either low-dose antiandrogens, for example cyproterone acetate (2 mg daily, see chapter 38) or isotretinoin should be considered, under the supervision of a consultant dermatologist.

Hormonal therapy of acne

Acne depends on the actions of androgens on the sebaceous glands. Hormone manipulation is often successful in women with acne refractory to antibiotics and is useful in patients who require contraception, which is essential because of the potential for feminizing a male fetus. Cyproterone acetate, 2 mg, daily is an antiandrogen with central and peripheral activity and is combined with low-dose estrogen, ethinylestradiol, 35 μg, to provide contraception. This is effective against acne given once daily in a 21-day cycle. Newer acne therapies undergoing investigation include synthetic peptide analogs of gonadotrophin-releasing hormone, cf. goserelin (chapter 38).

Retinoid therapy in acne

The management of severe refractory acne has been dramatically changed with the advent of synthetic vitamin A analogs.

ISOTRETINOIN

Use

Isotretinoin is the D-isomer of tretinoin, another vitamin A analog. It is used for severe acne or rosacea and should be prescribed under hospital supervision. The usual dose is 0.5–1 mg/kg in one or two divided doses with food. Topical isoretinoin (0.05% gel) or tretininoin (0.025% gel or lotion) applied twice daily are alternative effective therapies. The usual course is 4 months, with 80% improvement. Benefit continues after discontinuation of therapy.

Mechanism of action

The primary action of retinoids is inhibition of sebum production, reducing the size of the sebaceous glands by 90% in the first month. They also affect keratinization of the hair follicle resulting in reduced comedones.

Adverse effects and contraindications

These are the same as for etretinate (see below).

Pharmacokinetics

Isotretinoin is well absorbed (>90%) and the bioavailabilty is increased by taking it with meals. The plasma half-life ($t_{1/2}$) is 10–20 hours. It has a large volume of distribution and is highly bound to plasma protein (99.5%). Tissue binding is very great and it is eliminated over a period of at least a month after treatment has been discontinued, which explains the persisting benefit after stopping drug therapy, but also causes a persistent risk of teratogenicity after a course of treatment. Isotretinoin is cleared from the body almost totally by hepatic metabolism.

Drug interactions

Increased incidence of raised intracranial pressure if prescribed with tetracyclines.

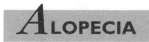

ALOPECIA

It is possible to promote hair growth by applying minoxidil sulfate (the active metabolite of minoxidil) topically as a 2% solution. This has a mitogenic effect on hair follicles. Adverse effects include local itching and dermatitis. Approximately 30% of subjects respond in 4–12 months, and the hair falls out once therapy is discontinued.

*E*CZEMA

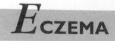

Principles of treatment

Eczema is due to epidermal inflammation and is caused by a wide variety of agents. Where possible the causal agent should be identified and exposure avoided. If the eczema is wet the topical use of drying agents such as lotions of aluminum acetate or calamine are useful. In patients where skin lesions are dry and scaly, the use of moisturizing creams (e.g. E45) combined with a keratolytic (see below) is beneficial. Topical corticosteroids are required in many cases.

CORTICOSTEROIDS

Topical corticosteroids include hydrocortisone and its fluorinated semisynthetic derivatives which have increased anti-inflammatory potency compared to hydrocortisone (see chapter 37 on glucocorticosteroids).

Use

The use of systemic corticosteroids (e.g. oral prednisolone, 60 mg, daily) for skin diseases is limited to serious disorders . such as pemphigus or refractory exfoliative dermatitis (e.g. Stevens–Johnson syndrome). Topical corticosteroids are widely used and effective in treating eczema, lichen planus, discoid lupus erythematosus, lichen simplex chronicus, palmar plantar pustulosis and occasionally in psoriasis. Corticosteroids applied topically to the skin effectively suppress inflammation, cause vasoconstriction and reduce epidermal cell proliferation. The symptoms of eczema are rapidly suppressed, but these drugs do not treat the cause and are contraindicated in the presence of infection unless combined with an appropriate antimicrobial agent. Intralesional steroid injections are often effective but should be reserved for localized lesions that are refractory to topical application.

It is wise to use the weakest corticosteroid preparation that will control the disorder. The formulation is applied thinly two to three times daily. Quantities appropriate to the area of skin involved should be prescribed. Occlusive dressings should only be used on a short-term basis (2–3 days). In resistant disease, high potency steroid should ideally be used for no more than 4 weeks to control the condition before changing to a less potent drug. Potent fluorinated corticosteroids should not be used on the face, because they cause dermatitis medicamentosa.

Many preparations are available, some of which are listed in descending order of anti-inflammatory potency in Table 48.1.

Adverse effects

1. Hypothalamic–pituitary adrenal suppression where very potent drugs are used long term on large areas of skin or when systemic absorption is increased under occlusive dressing.
2. Spread of local infection – bacterial or fungal.
3. Irreversible striae atrophicae.
4. Mild depigmentation and vellus hair formation.
5. Perioral dermatitis when applied to the face.

Table 48.1 Topical corticosteroids and their anti-inflammatory potency.

Potency	Drug and strength
Extremely potent	Clobetasol (0.05%)
	Halcinonide (0.1%)
	Diflucortolone (0.3%)
Potent	Beclomethasone (0.025%)
	Budesonide (0.025%)
	Fluclorolone (0.025%)
	Flucocinolone (0.025%)
	Fluocininide (0.05%)
Moderately potent	Clobetasone (0.05%)
	Fluandrolene (0.0125%)
Mild	Hydrocortisone (0.5–2.5%)
	Aclomethasone (0.05%)
	Methylprednisolone (0.25%)

6. Rebound exacerbation of disease, e.g. pustular psoriasis.
7. Exacerbation of glaucoma if applied to the eyelids.
8. Contact dermatitis (rare).
9. Hirsutism and acne if systemic absorption is very high.

GAMOLENIC ACID

This is an essential fatty acid that is a component of evening primrose oil and has been used with limited success in the symptomatic relief of atopic eczema. It also has some anti-inflammatory activity in joint disease. Its use probably modifies the balance of inflammatory eicosanoids (prostaglandins and leukotrienes). It is taken as four to six 40 mg capsules twice daily. Adverse effects include headache, nausea and indigestion. Gamolenic acid is contra-indicated in patients with epilepsy or who are on drugs that lower the epileptic threshold.

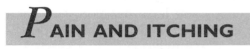

PAIN AND ITCHING

Some drugs are applied to the skin with varying efficacy to provide local analgesia including counterirritants (e.g. camphor and capsaicin), non-steroidal anti-inflammatory drugs (NSAIDs) and topical volatile aerosols (ethyl chloride spray). Topical capsaicin cream (0.075%) is an effective analgesic in patients with severe postherpetic neuralgia. The mechanism of its analgesic action is believed to be by depletion of substance P (and other neuroactive peptides) from C fibers. The major adverse effects are initial local hyperesthesiae and burning, and local irritation. Therapy is limited to 6–8 weeks.

The pathophysiology of itching is not clearly understood but probably involves the release of histamine and other mediators including serotonin, as well as local synthesis of prostaglandins and leukotrienes. The symptom of itching, which can be iatrogenic, often necessitates therapy. Scratching causes lichenification and should be discouraged. In young children with eczema this may necessitate the use of mittens. The key to management of pruritus is to identify the cause correctly before embarking on therapy. The sedative actions of antihistamines or phenothiazines may be helpful, especially at night. Local anesthetics are only of short-term use and commonly cause skin sensitization. Topical corticosteroids are most effective in local inflammatory conditions such as eczema. Cholestyramine (chapter 24) is of benefit in the intense pruritus that occurs with partial obstructive jaundice.

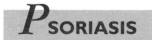

PSORIASIS

Psoriasis occurs in approximately 2% of the population. Its cause is unknown and no treatment is curative. The skin lesions are characterized by epidermal thickening and scaling due to increased epidermal undifferentiated cell proliferation with abnormal keratin. Therapy in mild cases consists of reassurance and a simple emollient cream (e.g. E45, Alpha Keri cream) or oil applied frequently to moisturize the skin. Such preparations should be continued even after improvement. More resistant cases are treated with salicylic acid, coal tar or dithranol, applied accurately to the lesions. Topical steroids are reserved for cases that do not respond to these simple remedies, and their use monitored by a specialist as they can worsen the diseases in some patients (notably precipitation of pustular psoriasis on stopping treatment). Calcitriol (a vitamin D analog) is effective topically. In some cases therapy with psoralens and ultraviolet A (UV-A) light (PUVA) (see below) is used in combination with good effect. Refractory cases are treated with oral retinoids, for example etretinate, 750 µg/kg/day.

Occasionally completely refractory cases justify immunosuppression with methotrexate (10–25 mg weekly; chapters 23 and 47), but chronic use can cause liver damage leading insidiously to cirrhosis. Potential recipients need to be warned of this and their liver function must be monitored meticulously. Cyclosporin (chapter 47), 3 mg/kg/day, is an alternative, but causes hypertension and nephrotoxocity. Regular monitoring of blood pressure and plasma cyclosporin concentrations is needed.

KERATOLYTICS

Keratolytics such as salicylic acid may help. Preparations of 2% salicylate are used initially, applied to the plaque, increasing gradually to 3–6% if necessary. Salicylic acid increases the rate of loss of surface epithelium. Side effects are few and include excessive drying, irritation, allergic contact sensitivity and, if used on large areas of skin, salicylism.

DITHRANOL

Dithranol is the most potent coal tar preparation against psoriasis. It may usefully be combined with ultraviolet B phototherapy. Short contact dithranol therapy is effective, and the use of high concentration dithranol (3–4%) formulated in a cream base and applied to lesions for 1 hour then washed off is more acceptable than older regimes. It

is convenient for use at home, is not so messy, less irritant and produces less stains on the skin or clothes than longer contact therapy.

CALCIPOTRIOL

Calcipotriol is used as a cream and applied twice daily onto mild to moderate psoriasis, maximum 100 g weekly for up to 6 weeks. It is an analog of calcitriol. Calcitriol receptors are present in keratinocytes, T and B lymphocytes and dermal fibroblasts; stimulation of these receptors on keratinocytes inhibits proliferation and differentiation. Adverse effects are local irritation, facial and perioral dermatitis and possible hypercalcemia and hypertriglyceridemia if used too extensively. It should not be used in pregnancy and is presently undergoing investigation as combination therapy with other therapies.

PHOTOCHEMOTHERAPY WITH UVA AND PSORALENS

Oral psoralen (usually 8-methoxypsoralen) and ultraviolet A light (PUVA) is now a well-established, albeit unlicensed, effective but somewhat inconvenient therapy for chronic plaque psoriasis. Psoralens intercalate DNA bases and when activated by light produce highly reactive oxygen species which sensitize the skin to the cytotoxic effects of long-wave UVA (320–400 nm wavelength) radiation. The usual course is 4–6 weeks. Psoralen is taken 2 hours before phototherapy. Skin burning and aging, cataracts and skin cancer are potential complications, especially with the higher total doses of UVA. Sun glasses are worn during UVA exposure to reduce the risk of cataract formation. Advances in psoralens and UVA light, notably optimization of dose regimen, reduce the risk of carcinogenicity. Combination therapy with retinoids or methotrexate, plus psoralens plus UVA is widely used. In Scandinavia, bathing with psoralens and UVA light has been in regular use for years. Photosensitivity is maximal immediately after the bath, and is about 15 times greater than with oral psoralens; it remains high for 15 min and then declines rapidly. Doses of UVA must be reduced accordingly and the minimum phototoxic dose assessed. Absorption of psoralen from the bath is low obviating the need to wear sunglasses.

Retinoids in psoriasis

ETRETINATE

See also therapy of acne above.

Use

This is an aromatic retinoid given orally for the treatment of severe resistant or complicated psoriasis and other disorders of keratinization. It should only be given under hospital supervision. A therapeutic effect occurs after 2–4 weeks with maximum benefit after 6 weeks. Treatment is limited to 6–9 months. The dose is 750 µg/kg/day as divided doses for 2–4 weeks, increased to 1000 µg/kg/day to induce response if necessary. The usual maintenance dose is 250–500 µg/kg/day. Relapse rates are high. Reliable contraception is essential for women of child-bearing potential.

Mechanism of action

The precise mechanism of retinoid action in psoriasis is unknown but it appears to affect gene expression in cell differentiation. Psoriatic mitoses are reduced, and acanthosis diminished.

Adverse effects

1. Mucocutaneous: cheilitis, dry mouth, epistaxis, dermatitis, desquamation, hair and nail loss.
2. Ophthalmological: papilloedema, night blindness, raised intracranial pressure.
3. Musculoskeletal: arthalgia, muscle stiffness, skeletal hyperostosis, premature fusion of epiphyses.
4. Teratogenicity.
5. Hepatotoxicity.
6. Hypertriglyceridemia.

Contraindications

Pregnant or breast-feeding women.

Pharmacokinetics

Etretinate is well absorbed (40%), but its absorption is improved when taken with a fatty meal as bile salts increase its solubility. It is 80–90% metabolized in the liver to its active metabolite acitretinin, the remaining 10–20% of the dose appears unchanged in the urine. The early plasma $t_{1/2}$ is 6–13 hours. Etretinate is deposited in adipose tissue and is eliminated from it very slowly with a terminal elimination half-life of 80–170 days. Because of its highly teratogenic effects, patients should take adequate contraceptive precautions for 2 years after stopping taking it.

Drug interactions

- Concomitant therapy with tetracycline and corticosteroids increases the risk of raised intracranial pressure.
- Caution should be exercised when prescribing other drugs that increase serum lipids, for example corticosteroids, thiazide diuretics.
- Phenobarbitone and phenytoin metabolism is impaired.
- Methotrexate plasma concentrations are increased.

ACITRETIN

Acitretin is available as an oral preparation, 25–50 mg, daily. Preliminary data suggest it to be as effective as etretinate, and perhaps less toxic because it is eliminated more rapidly from tissue stores. It is likely that it will replace etretinate.

Topical corticosteroids

Topical and systemic steroids should only be used in psoriasis under specialist supervision. Although corticosteroids may be effective, subsequent therapy becomes more difficult due to tachyphylaxis, and severe pustular psoriasis may occur during withdrawal of treatment.

Future therapies

There is considerable evidence to support a role for leukotrienes (LT) in the pathogenesis of psoriasis. The lipoxygenase product LTB_4 (a powerful neutrophil chemotaxin) has been found in psoriatic lesions, and probably synergizes with other inflammatory mediators. Fish oil concentrates rich in eicosapentaenoic acid and docosahexanoic acid alter the pathway of leukotriene biosynthesis, reducing LTB_4 and increasing LTB_5; there is some evidence of modest efficacy of fish oil consumption in psoriasis. Topical application of a selective inhibitor of 5-lipoxygenase reduces LTB_4 in chronic plaque psoriasis, and associated clinical improvement. Skin irritation is the major adverse effect. Prospects for other 5-lipoxygenase inhibitors with less topical irritation are promising.

*U*RTICARIA

Acute urticaria is usually due to a type 1 allergic reaction to an allergen. It may need therapy with adrenaline if associated with anaphylactic shock or laryngeal edema, but less severe cases respond to an oral antihistamine (e.g. chlorpheniramine, 4 mg, terfenadine, 60 mg, or cetirizine, 10 mg; chapter 47). Systemic corticosteroids are needed in refractory cases. Chronic urticaria usually responds to the combination of an oral antihistamine plus an oral β_2-agonist such as salbutamol, 4–8 mg, or terbutaline, 8–16 mg (chapter 30), or an H_2-blocker (cimetidine, 200 mg, or ranitidine, 150 mg, twice daily). Urticaria that is caused by cold temperature releasing histamine and local biosynthesis of prostaglandin D_2 responds to a combination of H_1- and H_2-blockers and sometimes also a cyclo-oxygenase inhibitor given prophylactically.

*S*UPERFICIAL BACTERIAL SKIN INFECTIONS

Skin infections are commonly due to staphylococci or streptococci. Impetigo or infected eczema are treated topically for no more than 2 weeks with antimicrobials. Suitable preparations are neomycin sulfate 0.5% or neomycin combined with bacitracin 2%. Mupirocin is an effective alternative especially for resistant organisms and particularly useful in eradicating the nasal carriage of staphylococci. It is best to limit the use of such topical agents to outside hospital and to give drugs that are not used systemically. Fucidin ointment 2% is also available. These topical agents may all cause skin irritation and sensitization.

*F*UNGAL SKIN AND NAIL INFECTIONS

See chapter 42 and Table 48.2 for drug
therapy of fungal skin and nail infections.

Table 48.2 Drug therapy of fungal skin and nail infections.

Fungal skin infection	Drug therapy	Comment
Candida infection of the skin, vulvovaginitis or balanitis	Topical antifungal therapy with nystatin cream (100 000 units/g) or ketoconazole 2%, clotrimazole 1% or miconazole 2% creams	Alternative topical agents are terbinafine 1% or amorolfine 0.25% creams. Systemic therapy may be necessary in refractory cases. Consider diabetes
Fungal nail infections, dermatophyte onychomycosis (T. rubrum)	Griseofulvin, 10 mg/kg, daily for 6–12 months	If systemic therapy is not tolerated, tioconazole 28% is applied daily for 6 months. Topical amorolfine 5% is another alternative
Pityriasis capitis, seborrheic dermatitis (dandruff)	Topical steroids – clobetasol propionate 0.05%, or betamethasone valerate 0.1%, with cetrimide shampoo	Severe cases may require additional topical ketoconazole 2% or clotrimazole 1%
Tinea capitis	Systemic therapy with fluconazole, itraconazole, miconazole or clotrimazole	–
Tinea corporis	Topical therapy with, e.g. ketoconazole 2% or clotrimazole 1% applied for 2–3 weeks	Systemic therapy is only necessary in refractory cases
Tinea pedis	As above	As above

*V*IRAL SKIN INFECTIONS

See chapter 42 and Table 48.3 for drug
therapy of viral skin infections.

Table 48.3 Drug therapy of viral skin infections.

Viral skin infection	Drug therapy	Comment
Initial or recurrent genital, labial, herpes simplex	Topical acyclovir cream 5% applied 4 hourly for 5 days. Systemic acyclovir therapy is required for buccal and vaginal herpes simplex	Idoxuridine 5% in dimethyl sulfoxide applied 4 hourly for 4–5 days has been used but is not as effective as acyclovir
Skin warts, papilloma virus infections	All treatments are destructive. Cryotherapy (solid CO_2, liquid nitrogen). Daily keratolytics such as 12% salicylic acid	For plantar warts use 1.5% formaldehyde or 10% glutaraldehyde. For anal warts use podophyllin resin 15% or podophyllotoxin 0.5% solution applied precisely on the lesions once or twice weekly

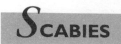CABIES

Scabies is due to infection with the louse *Sarcoptes scabei*. It is often transmitted during sexual intercouse and the possibility of other venereal infections needs consideration. Lindane (1% lotion applied topically, leave on for 24 hours, repeat if necessary after 7 days) and malathion (0.5% lotion applied to the hair, dry over 12 hours; scabies – apply to whole body omitting head and neck, leave for 24 hours) are effective, but should be avoided in children and pregnancy. Permethrin is an effective pyrethroid. Older preparations such as benzoyl benzoate (25% lotion) are still used, but should be avoided in children. The major adverse effect with all these therapies is skin irritation.

ICE

Head lice infection is caused by *Pediculus humanus capitis*. To prevent the emergence of resistant lice, preparations should be rotated every 3 years. Malathion and carbamyl are the recommended therapies as there is resistance to lindane. Carbamyl has recently been restricted to prescription only use following the demonstration that it is carcinogenic in rodents, although no cases of tumours in humans have been attributed to its use. Permethrin or phenothrin are effective. Recommended applications are malathion 0.5% in alcohol, carbamyl 0.5% in alcohol which are used for head lice. They are best used as lotions rather than shampoos, as the contact time with the head is longer and there is less dilution with water. Aqueous solutions are preferred for asthmatic and small children to minimize alcoholic fumes. The preparations are applied to the affected area and allowed to dry; a contact time of 12 hours or overnight is recommended. The hair is then washed and the nits removed with a special fine-toothed comb. Treatment for head lice should be repeated after 7 days to kill any lice emerging from eggs that might have survived the first application. Pubic lice should be treated with malathion 0.5% aqueous solution.

ADVERSE DRUG REACTIONS INVOLVING THE SKIN

Cutaneous drug reactions can arise from topically or systemicially administered drugs (chapter 11). Drug reactions to systemically administered drugs are typically erythematous and macular, like measles 'morbilliform'). They may be similar to those of viral infections or erythema multiforme and their appearance is seldom diagnostic. They usually occur within the first 1 to 2 weeks of therapy; however, some immunologically mediated reactions occur later, even months after starting drug therapy. Contact dermatitis is usually eczematous and is most commonly seen with antimicrobial drugs or antihistamines; the possibility that the vehicle in which the drug is applied could be the cause of such a reaction should always be considered.

The diagnosis of a drug-induced cutaneous reaction is obtained from an accurate drug

Table 48.4 Adverse effects of drugs on the skin.

Cutaneous eruption	Drugs commonly associated	Comment
Acne	Corticosteroids, androgens, anabolic steroids, phenytoin	
Alopecia	Cytotoxic chemotherapy, etretinate, gold, long-term heparin, oral contraceptives, sodium valproate	
Eczema	Cephalosporins, penicillins, phenothiazines	
Erythema multiforme	Barbiturates, allopurinol, sulfonamides, penicillins, NSAIDS, phenytoin	Inclusive of Stevens–Johnson syndrome
Erythema nodosum	Sulfonamides, antimicrobials, oral contraceptives	
Exfoliative dermatitis and erythroderma	Allopurinol, carbamazepine, gold, penicillins, phenothiazines	
Fixed eruptions	Barbiturates, laxatives, phenolphthalein, naproxen, nifedipine, penicillins, sulfonamides, tetracyclines, quinidine	These eruptions recur at the same site (often circumorally) with each administration of the drug, and may be purpuric or bullous
Lichenoid eruptions	Captopril, chloroquine, frusemide, gold, phenothiazines, thiazides	
Lupus erythematosus with butterfly rash	Hydralazine, isoniazid, phenytoin, procainamide	
Photosensitivity: systemic drugs	Amiodarone, chlorodiazepoxide, frusemide, griseofulvin, nalidixic acid, thiazides, tetracyclines, piroxicam	
Photosensitivity: topical drugs	Coal tar, hexachlorophane, p-aminobenzoic acid and its esters	
Pigmentation	Amiodarone, chloroquine, heavy metals, oral contraceptives, phenothiazines	AZT causes gray nails, chloroquine causes hair depigmentation
Pruritus	Oral contraceptives, phenothiazines, rifampicin	Without any rashes – rifampicin causes biliary stasis
Purpura	Thiazides, phenylbutazone, sulfonamides, sulfonylureas, quinine	May be thrombocytopenic or vasculitic
Toxic epidermal necrolysis	NSAIDs, penicillins, phenytoin, sulfonamides	
Toxic erythema	Ampicillin, sulfonamides, sulfonylureas, frusemide, thiazides	Usually occurs after 7–9 days of therapy or after 2–3 days in those previously exposed
Urticaria – chronic	Aspirin (NSAIDs), ACE inhibitors, gold, penicillins	
Vasculitis – allergic	Chlorpropamide, NSAIDs, phenytoin, sulfonamides, thiazides	

NSAIDs = non-steroidal anti-inflammatory drugs. ACE = angiotensin-converting enzyme.

history from the patient, especially the temporal relationship of the skin disorder to drug therapy. In milder cases and fixed drug eruptions readministration (rechallenge) with the suspect is sometimes justified. Patch testing is useful for contact dermatitis, reproducing the exposure and the causative process. Intradermal testing has so many confounding factors that it is seldom used. The treatment of drug-induced skin disorders is to remove the cause, apply cooling creams and antipruritics with topical steroids reserved for the most severe cases.

Table 48.4 describes commonly described drug reactions and possible culprits.

Photosensitivity

There are two forms of photosensitivity: phototoxicity and photoallergy. Phototoxicity is similar to drug toxicity, a predictable effect of too high a dose of UVB in a subject who has been exposed to a drug. The reaction is like severe sunburn and the threshold returns to normal when the drug is discontinued. Photoallergy is similar to drug allergy, a cell-mediated immune reaction that occurs only in some people and can be severe following even a small dose of drug. It is caused by a photochemical reaction caused by UVA where the drug combines with a tissue protein to form an antigen. Most commonly such reactions are eczematous, and may persist for months or years after the drug is withdrawn. For the common agents causing photosensitivty see Table 48.4.

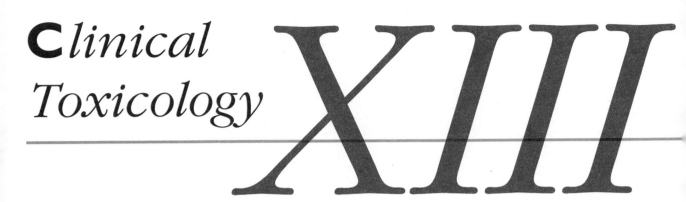

Clinical Toxicology XIII

Drug and Alcohol Abuse

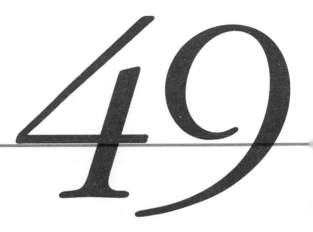

Definitions **668**

Opioid/narcotic analgesics **668**

Drugs that alter perception **672**

Central stimulants **673**

Central depressants **677**

Miscellaneous **683**

DEFINITIONS

The World Health Organization (WHO) (1969) definition of drug dependence is 'a state, psychic and sometimes physical, resulting from the interaction between a living organism and a drug characterized by behavioral and other responses that always include a compulsion to take the drug on a continuous or periodic basis in order to experience its psychic effects and sometimes to avoid the discomfort of its absence'. That is, drug dependence is always psychological and also sometimes physical. Tolerance may or may not be present.

The definition of drug addiction is a 'drive to seek out and consume your drug of choice as the priority in your life'.

The definition of drug abuse is 'the consumption of a drug apart from medical need or in unnecessary quantities'. 'Recreational drug use' describes the use of drugs for pleasure.

The harmful consequences of abuse include not only dependence and direct medical complications but also road traffic accidents and antisocial behavior. On a population basis non-illicit drugs such as alcohol and tobacco currently pose an even more important health problem than illicit drugs.

Up to 1961 most addicts of illicit drugs were middle-aged individuals who had initially experienced the drugs in a therapeutic situation or who handled drugs professionally. After this time the great increase in the number of addicts was due to the appearance of young, unstable, non-therapeutic addicts who belonged to a subculture in which drug taking was the norm. Those most at risk are young, immature, adventurous and easily led. Those with school, social or work problems are vulnerable as are those who would otherwise find difficulty in being accepted in social cliques. These addicts initially obtain drugs from other addicts and do not make their first contact with drugs because of pain or psychological disturbances. There is often a history of truancy, poor work record, inability to stand frustration or to plan for distant goals and an increased incidence of criminal behavior.

Although the number of drugs that are abused are legion they can be classified as shown in Table 49.1.

Table 49.1 Drugs of abuse and dependence.

Opioid/narcotic analgesics
Drugs that alter perception
Central stimulants
Central depressants
Miscellaneous

OPIOID/NARCOTIC ANALGESICS

The estimated number of opioid addicts in the UK is at least 100 000 and increasing. Although this is a relatively minor problem compared to the USA it is a major cause of crime and spread of human immunodeficiency virus (HIV) infection in the UK. Addicts may need more than £500 weekly to supply their addiction from the black market. 0.25 g heroin daily is common in a dependent addict. Often multiple drugs are used.

Table 49.2 Opioid drugs commonly abused.

Drugs	Comment
Diamorphine	Mainly obtained on the black market. It is of variable purity and cut with quinine, talc, lactose etc. It is usually mixed with water, heated until dissolved, and sometimes strained through cotton. It may be used intravenously (mainlining), subcutaneously (skin popping) or inhaled (snorted/chasing the dragon – heating up on foil and inhaling the smoke) ($t_{1/2}$ = 60–90 min)
Methadone	This is the mainstay of drug addiction clinics and is given as an elixir (long $t_{1/2}$ of 15–55 hours). It is very difficult to use elixir for injection
Dipipanone (+ cyclizine = 'diconal'®)	It was previously much used by non-clinic doctors treating addicts. It is easily crushed up and dissolved for i.v. use
Dextromoramide ('palfium')	It is similar in its abuse potential to dipipanone
Other opioids	All opioids including mixed agonists/antagonists, e.g. buprenorphine, have the potential to cause dependence

Diamorphine, dipipanone and cocaine (not an opioid) can only be prescribed to addicts for treatment of their addiction by doctors with a special license.

Heroin (diamorphine) is the drug of preference. It is often adulterated with other white powders such as quinine (which is bitter like opiates), caffeine, lactose and even chalks, starch and talc. Due to the variable purity the dose of black market heroin is always uncertain. The drug is taken intravenously, subcutaneously, orally and by inhalation ('chasing the dragon'). The latter method of use is more common amongst the 15–25-year-old age group. In addition to the illegal supply of heroin from the Middle East and Far East opioids are obtained from pharmacy thefts and the legal prescription of drugs for treatment of the addiction. Some of the drugs used are shown in Table 49.2.

The pharmacological actions of opioids are described in chapter 22 and the central nervous system (CNS) effects are summarized in Table 49.3.

Table 49.3 Central nervous system actions of opioids.

Analgesia
Euphoria
Drowsiness → sleep → coma
Decrease sensitivity of respiratory center to CO_2
Depress cough center
Stimulate chemoreceptor trigger zone – vomiting in 15%
Release antidiuretic hormone

Intoxication

For several seconds following intravenous injection heroin produces an intense euphoria (rush) which may be accompanied by nausea and vomiting but is nevertheless pleasurable. Over the next few hours the user may describe a warm sensation in the abdomen and chest, however, chronic users often state that the only effect they obtain is remission from abstinence symptoms.

On examination the patient may appear to be alternately dozing and waking. The patient may be hypotensive with a slow respiratory rate, the pupils pin point and speech infrequent and slurred. These signs can be reversed with naloxone. Hypothermia may be severe in a cold environment.

Overdose

This is commonly accidental due to unexpectedly potent heroin or waning tolerance. Severe overdose may cause immediate apnea, circulatory collapse, convulsions and cardiopulmonary arrest. Alternatively death may occur over a longer period of time usually due to hypoxia from direct respiratory center depression with mechanical asphyxia (tongue/vomit blocking airway).

A common complication of opioid poisoning is non-cardiogenic pulmonary edema. This is usually rapid in onset but may be delayed; therefore any patient admitted following heroin overdose should be hospitalized for at least 24 hours.

Naloxone reverses opioid poisoning. One should look for increase in pupil diameter, respiratory rate and depth of respiration during the intravenous injection. It may precipitate an acute abstinence syndrome in addicts and very rarely convulsions. This does **not** contraindicate its use in opioid overdoses in addicts. Severe hypoxia causes mydriasis.

Tolerance

This occurs when increasingly larger doses of drug must be administered to obtain the effects of the original dose. Tolerance affects the euphoric and analgesic effects so the addict requires more and more opioid for his 'buzz'. Changes in tolerance are much less apparent in the therapeutic use of opioids in the treatment of pain.

Medical complications

In addition to the social consequences of opioid addiction medical complications are common and some are listed in Table 49.4.

Withdrawal symptoms usually start at the time the next dose would usually be given and their intensity is related to the usual dose. For heroin, symptoms usually reach a maximum at 36–72 hours and gradually subside over the next 5–10 days. Table 49.5 lists features of the opioid abstinence syndrome.

Table 49.4 Medical complications of opioid addiction.

Infection	Endocarditis: bacterial, often tricuspid valve, staphyloccocal, fungal, e.g. *Candida* HIV/AIDS Abscesses Tetanus Septicemia Hepatitis
Pulmonary	Pneumonia: bacterial, fungal, aspiration Pulmonary edema: 'heroin lung' Embolism Atelectasis Fibrosis/granulomas
Skin	Injection scars Abscesses Cellulitis Lymphangitis Phlebitis Gangrene
Neurological	Cerebral edema Transverse myelitis Horner's syndrome Polyneuritis Crush injury Myopathy
Hepatic	Cirrhosis
Renal	Nephrotic syndrome with proliferative glomerulonephritis
Musculoskeletal	Osteomyelitis (usually lumbar vertebrae, *Pseudomonas, Staphylococcus, Candida*) Crush injury, myoglobinuria, rhabdomyolysis

Table 49.5 Opioid abstinence syndrome.

Early	Intermediate	Late
Yawning	Mydriasis	Involuntary muscle spasm
Lacrimation	Piloerection	Fever
Rhinorrhea	Flushing	Nausea and vomiting
Perspiration	Tachycardia	Abdominal cramps
	Twitching	Diarrhea
	Tremor	
	Restlessness	

Management of opioid addicts

Opioid addicts are best treated by specialized addiction clinics. A grossly simplified outline of the standard approach is summarized in Table 49.6. Success or failure depends largely on the self-motivation of the addict.

Opioid addicts rarely present to hospital asking for treatment of their addiction but more commonly present to physicians during routine medical or surgical treatment for a condition which may or may not be related to their addiction. Some patients will deny drug abuse and clinical examination should always include a search for signs of needle tracking and withdrawal. Acute abstinence in a casualty/general hospital setting is uncomfortable for the patient but most unlikely to be dangerous. Physicians are not allowed to prescribe diamorphine, cocaine or dipipanone to addicts for treatment of their addiction or abstinence unless they hold a special license. Likewise doctors must not treat unregistered addicts for their addiction; however, it is reasonable to treat a genuine opioid withdrawal syndrome with a low dose of opioid, for example oral codeine phosphate which will reduce some of the symptoms as well as being an effective antidiarrheal agent. If the patient requires an opioid for treatment of pain, for example myocardial infarction, then an opioid such as diamorphine may be administered. It is most probable the addict will require a larger dose than a non-addict patient. If a patient says they are being treated for their addiction it is always wise to confirm by telephoning their usual prescriber and/or the supplying pharmacist. If the patient is admitted to hospital one should obtain expert advice. Knowledge of local policies towards drug addicts is essential for anyone working in the accident and emergency department or who comes into contact with drug addicts.

The misuse of drugs regulations require that any doctor who attends a person whom that doctor considers or has reasonable grounds to suspect is addicted to any of the 14 notifiable drugs (see Appendix) shall, within 7 days of the attendance, furnish in writing particulars of that person to the Home Office. Patients should be referred to the local drug addiction clinic. General practitioners rarely like to manage addicts themselves. Some doctors treat addicts privately.

Concomitant illness or the medical complications of opioid addiction may be difficult to recognize because of the patient's extreme craving for their drug of addiction. Unfortunately this often leads to mistrust. One should always exclude a medical cause of pain before assuming the pain is related to the addict's desire for their drug of addiction. Atypical endocarditis and osteomyelitis are easy to miss. Drug addicts who share needles are at major risk of hepatitis B, hepatitis C and HIV infection.

Newborn children of addicted mothers may be born with an abstinence syndrome or less commonly features of drug overdose. Assisted ventilation is preferred to naloxone if apneic at birth. The abstinence syndrome is often treated with phenothiazines which may be required for 6 weeks.

Table 49.6 Management of opioid dependence.

- Assessment (to include two urines positive for opioids)
- Methadone mixture – maintenance and then gradual withdrawal – oral, or clonidine
- Counselling/social support
- Repeat urine testing to confirm use of methadone and not other drugs
- Contract system
- Avoid prescriptions of other opioids/sedatives
- Special 'drug free' centers – concentrate on psychological and social support through the acute and chronic abstinence phases

DRUGS THAT ALTER PERCEPTION

CANNABIS

Cannabis is Britain's most popular illicit drug. The most active constituent is tetrahydrocannabinol. It is most commonly mixed with tobacco and smoked, but it may be brewed into a drink or added to food. The pleasurable effects of cannabis include a sensation of relaxation, heightened perception of all the senses and euphoria. The nature and intensity of effects varies between individuals and is related to dose (the purity is often variable), the motivation and mood of the subject. The effects usually come on in minutes and last 1–2 hours. Conjunctival suffusion is common.

Acute adverse effects include dysphoric reactions such as anxiety or panic attacks, the impairment of performance of skilled tasks and sedation. This may lead to road traffic accidents. Chronic use has been associated with personality changes including 'amotivational syndrome' characterized by extreme lethargy. The association of chronic cannabis use with onset of schizophrenia is unproven.

Tetrahydrocannabinol and other cannabinoids are extremely lipid soluble and only slowly released from body fat. Although the acute effects wear off within hours of inhalation, cannabinoids are eliminated in the urine for weeks following ingestion.

LSD

Lysergic acid diethylamide is one of the most potent drugs known, the active oral dose being about 30 μg. The drug produces perceptual distortions and feelings of dissociation. Visual hallucinations are common and perception of time is lost. Some find the experiences pleasurable, others find them extremely frightening. Repeated use may lead to psychological dependence. Mode of action is unknown but is thought to be partly related to antagonism of 5-hydroxytryptamine (5HT) receptors. LSD is a dangerous drug which can lead to suicidal psychotic reactions.

Phencyclidine

Phencyclidine (PCP, 'angel dust') is another synthetic hallucinogen but its use is fortunately rare in the UK. Anesthesia, sedation or stimulation including violent physical reactions result from its use.

Psilocybin

Psilocybin is derived from 'magic mushrooms' and is related to LSD.

Mescaline

Mescaline, which is derived from a Mexican cactus, is also used for its hallucinogenic effects.

HALLUCINOGENIC AMPHETAMINES

Methylenedioxymethylamphetamine

Methylenedioxymethylamphetamine (MDMA) is structurally related to mescaline and amphetamine. It is generally known as 'ecstasy'. The use of this drug has increased dramatically in recent years. It has mixed hallucinogenic and stimulant properties and its use is associated with feelings of increased energy and euphoria and heightened perception; restlessness is common. Hyperpyrexia, dehydration, rhabdomyolysis, coma, hepatic damage and death have been reported. A principal danger associated with the use of MDMA is of abnormal behavior leading to road traffic accidents. Even more potent amphetamine analogs are also similarly abused. The dose of active ingredient in these illegal drugs is very variable which increases the hazard.

CENTRAL STIMULANTS

AMPHETAMINES

Amphetamines may cause dependence and psychotic states. Their therapeutic use is limited to specialist treatment of narcolepsy and possibly hyperactivity in children. They should not be prescribed in the management of depression or obesity. Amphetamines are abused for their stimulant properties. Acutely they may alleviate tiredness and induce a feeling of cheerfulness and confidence. With high doses, particularly after intravenous use, a sensation of intense exhilaration may occur. Users tend to become hyperactive at high doses, especially if repeated over a few days. Amphetamines can produce 'amphetamine psychosis' which is characterized by delirium, panic, hallucinations and feelings of persecution. Anxiety, irritability and restlessness are also common. The most common amphetamine used is amphetamine sulfate which is only available illegally. Prolonged use leads to psychological dependence, tolerance and hostility as well as irritation due to lack of sleep and food. Acutely amphetamines raise blood pressure.

COCAINE

Cocaine is derived from Andean coca shrub. It has powerful stimulant properties. 'Crack' is the free base of cocaine which is smoked or inhaled. Cocaine is relatively expensive. Regular users might consume 1–2 g a day and the cost can be £100 a gram. It is most commonly sniffed up the nose, although it can be injected or smoked. Acutely cocaine causes arousal, exhiliration, euphoria, indifference to pain and fatigue and the sensation of having great physical strength and mental capacity. Repeated large doses commonly precipitate an extreme surge of agitation and anxiety. Although tolerance and withdrawal symptoms are not as profound as with opiates, withdrawal after regular use is commonly associated with fatigue and mild depression. Frequent chronic use tends to be associated with more frequent adverse effects and so it is more commonly a drug of abuse than addiction. The adverse effects include anorexia, confused exhaustion, palpitations, damage to membranes lining the nostrils, and if injected, bloodborne infections. Use in pregnancy is associated with central nervous system damage of the fetus. 'Crack babies' can usually be cured of their 'addiction' by abstinence over a few weeks.

NICOTINE

Nicotine is an alkaloid present in the leaves of the tobacco plant, *Nicotiana tabacum*. There are no medical uses of nicotine but it is of very great importance in medicine because of its addictive properties and presence in tobacco.

Nicotine in low concentrations stimulates the nicotinic receptors of autonomic ganglia, and in higher concentrations is a ganglion blocker. Thus smoking can accelerate the heart via sympathetic stimulation, or slow it due to sympathetic block or parasympathetic stimulation. There is usually cutaneous and splanchnic vasoconstriction with an increased peripheral vascular resistance. Respiration is stimulated, partly via stimulation of chemoreceptors in the carotid body. Adrenaline and noradrenaline are secreted from the adrenal medulla. The motor end plate acetylcholine receptors are initially stimulated and then blocked, producing a paralysis of voluntary muscle.

The results of extensive central stimulation include wakefulness, tremor, fits, anorexia, nausea, vomiting, tachypnea and secretion of antidiuretic hormone (ADH). Nicotine is powerfully addicting, both psychologically and physically.

The percentage of nicotine in tobacco varies, but the smoke of a completely burned cigarette usually contains 1–6 mg and that of a cigar 15–40 mg. Acute administration of 60 mg nicotine, orally by ingestion, may be fatal.

Adverse effects of smoking

1. In men under 70 years of age the ratio of death rate among cigarette smokers to non-smokers is 2:1. Above the age of 70 years this ratio is 1.5:1. The principal causes are heart disease, lung cancer, chronic obstructive lung disease and peripheral vascular diseases. Some of the specific causes of death which are positively related with smoking are:

   - Ischemic heart disease (strongest correlation).
   - Cancers of lung, other respiratory sites and esophagus, lip and tongue.
   - Chronic bronchitis and emphysema, respiratory tuberculosis.
   - Pulmonary heart disease.
   - Aortic aneurysm.

   Cigarette smoking is a major risk factor for peptic ulcer recurrence. H_2-blockers appear less effective in smokers whilst sucralfate produces similar healing rates in smokers and non-smokers.

2. Smoking is pleasurable for confirmed smokers, and once the habit is established it is very difficult to eradicate. Even though the rituals of smoking can enhance sociability and provide tactile, gustatory and oro-labial gratification, it is difficult to discount the role of nicotine or some other chemical agent in tobacco as being active as a drug of dependence. Withdrawal can lead to an abstinence syndrome. This consists of craving, irritability, and sometimes physical features such as alimentary disturbances. The appetite for sugar is often increased during the withdrawal state.

3. Some of the metabolic disturbances of smoking, such as release of catecholamines and other amines from the adrenals, heart and platelets, and rises in blood fatty acids and glucose, predispose to cardiac arrhythmias, thrombosis and atherosclerosis. Further serious hazards from other products in smoke, in particular carbon monoxide, may also act as cardiotoxins and endanger ischemic tissues.

4. Buerger's disease (thromboangitis obliterans) is a disease of unknown etiology, but it is severely aggravated by smoking. The coronary vessels may show other changes in addition to atherosclerosis: hyaline thickening in the arterioles occurs almost exclusively in heavy smokers; fibrous intimal thickening of the coronary arteries is also characteristic of 'smoker's heart'. Although smoking usually increases cardiac output, in patients with impaired cardiac function, a fall in cardiac output can result.

5. Smoking accelerates aging changes in the lungs. These processes include increased residual volume, decreased vital capacity, increase in the closing volume and a progressive fall in arterial oxygen tension. The underlying degenerative changes appear to be loss of lung elasticity and loss of compliance of the chest wall. In addition, chronic obstructive airways disease and bronchitis are associated with smoking. The development of emphysema is markedly accelerated in cigarette smokers who have homozygous α_1-antitrypsin deficiency.

6. Smoking during pregnancy is associated with spontaneous abortion, premature delivery, small babies, increased perinatal mortality and an increased incidence of sudden infant death syndrome (cot death). In households where the parents smoke, there is an increased risk of pneumonia and bronchitis in preschool and schoolchildren, most marked during the first year of life.

Pharmacokinetics

Large amounts of tobacco taken by mouth result in delayed gastric emptying and the nicotine may provoke vomiting. Ninety per cent of nicotine from inhaled smoke is absorbed, whilst smoke taken into the mouth results in only 25–50% absorption. As well as via the gastrointestinal, buccal and respiratory epithelium, nicotine is also absorbed through the skin. A high concentration of nicotine may be present in the breast milk of smokers. Eighty to ninety per cent of circulating nicotine is metabolized in the liver, kidneys and lungs. Nicotine and its metabolites are excreted in the urine. Acidification of the urine accelerates excretion.

Each puff of cigarette smoke which is inhaled results in the absorption of 50–150 μg nicotine. Smoking cigarette butts results in a much higher yield per inhalation. Thus each inhalation is equivalent to an intravenous injection of 1–2 μg/kg nicotine. Smokers usually absorb 20–25% of the total nicotine in a cigarette. There is a rough correlation between the nicotine content of cigarettes and the peak plasma concentration of nicotine. The plasma elimination half-life is 25–40 min.

Peak plasma levels after smoking cigarettes (1.2 mg nicotine) are similar to those after chewing gum containing 4 mg nicotine. However, the rate of rise is much slower after chewing gum or applying transdermal patches. The use of such gums to wean smokers from cigarettes has been of limited success: perhaps because of this inability to mimic the nicotine pharmacokinetics of smoking. However, some patients find nicotine chewing gum or transdermal patches helpful. A high degree of motivation is always required if efforts to stop smoking are to be successful.

Effect of smoking on drug disposition and effects

The commonest effect of tobacco smoking on drug disposition is an increase in elimination consistent with induction of drug-metabolizing enzymes. Nicotine itself is metabolized more extensively by smokers than non-smokers and this is associated with an alteration in the rate of elimination of a number of other drugs. These effects are summarized in Table 49.7.

These changes in drug disposition may alter drug responses. Thus smokers require larger doses of pentazocine than non-smokers to achieve analgesia. The matter is complicated by the fact that smokers tend to have different sensory thresholds, psychosomatic characteristics and drug consumption histories compared to non-smokers. Thus

Table 49.7 Known effects of smoking on drug metabolism in humans.

Increased metabolism in smokers	Unaffected by smoking
Nicotine	Diazepam
Caffeine	Pethidine
Theophylline	Phenytoin
Imipramine	Nortriptyline
Pentazocine	Ethanol
	Warfarin

whilst no effect on diazepam metabolism due to smoking has been observed, the Boston Collaborative Drug Surveillance Program has clearly demonstrated that heavy smokers suffer less CNS depression after a standard dose of diazepam than non-smokers. Similar observations were also made for chlorpromazine and chlordiazepoxide. Whether these effects can be attributed to innate differences between smokers and non-smokers, to the presence of substances such as nicotine which exert their own pharmacological effects or to pharmacokinetic differences is unknown.

XANTHINES

This group of compounds includes caffeine (present in the seeds of the coffee plant, *Coffea arabica*, tea leaves from *Thea sinensis*, cocoa from the seeds of *Theobroma cacao* and in soft drinks derived from the cola nut of the *Cola acuminata* tree). Other members of the group are theobromine (in tea, coffee, cocoa and cola beverages) and theophylline (see chapter 30). Caffeine is undoubtedly the most widely ingested alkaloid: in the USA the average intake from coffee alone is about 200 mg/day for persons over 10 years of age. In addition caffeine is included in a number of proprietary and prescription medicines, particularly occurring in analgesic combinations. The major effects of these compounds are mediated by inhibition of phosphodiesterase, resulting in a raised intracellular cyclic adenosine monophosphate (AMP) concentration.

Adverse effects

1. A very wide range of behavior all the way from putting the shot to increased vigilance in boring tasks have been allegedly enhanced. These effects are less marked than with amphetamine and have been difficult to prove objectively. In large doses caffeine exerts an excitatory effect on the CNS manifested by tremor, anxiety, irritability and restlessness with interference with sleep. Such evidence as exists indicates that caffeine does not possess properties which lead to improved intellectual performance except perhaps when normal performance has been downgraded by fatigue or boredom. In animal experiments caffeine excites the CNS at all levels but the cerebral cortex is first affected, then the medulla, whilst the spinal cord is only affected by very large doses. The medullary respiratory, vagal and cardiovascular centers are all stimulated. Toxic doses result in convulsions but in humans the toxic dose (over 10 g) is so large that human fatality is unlikely. Theophylline shares these actions but theobromine is virtually inactive in this respect.
2. Circulatory effects include direct myocardial stimulation producing tachycardia, increased cardiac output, ectopic beats and palpitations. Direct effect on blood vessels result in dilatation of coronary, pulmonary and systemic vasculature but stimulation of the medullary vasomotor center tends to counter this so that the effect on blood pressure is unpredictable. Recently it has been suggested that patients with hypertension may be susceptible to increased blood pressure following caffeine. The cerebral circulation responds differently by constriction, hence the use of caffeine in migraine.
3. Bronchial smooth muscle relaxes producing bronchodilatation. Respiration is also stimulated centrally.
4. Mild diuresis occurs due to an increased glomerular filtration rate subsequent to dilatation of the afferent arterioles. Theophylline is the most powerful xanthine diuretic, theobromine has a more sustained effect but is less active whilst caffeine is the least powerful.
5. Caffeine increases gastric acid secretion via its action on cyclic AMP and xanthines in general may cause gastric irritation.

Pharmacokinetics

Caffeine is rapidly and completely absorbed after oral administration. Xanthines undergo a complex series of hepatic metabolic transformations by demethylation and oxidation as well as eventual ring cleavage to produce a series of methylxanthines and methylurates. The plasma half-life of caffeine is 2.5–12 hours. The plasma protein binding of caffeine is about 15%. Only 1–10% is excreted unchanged in the urine.

Caffeine dependence

This is exceedingly common and doubtless benign since caffeine imparts a relaxed sense of social acceptance and mild stimulation. Tolerance is low grade but definitely exists, but does not appear to develop uniformly to all the effects of caffeine. Heavy users are allegedly less sensitive than light users to the nervousness and wakefulness caused by coffee but are more sensitive to the euphoriant and stimulant actions. A mild withdrawal syndrome manifested by headache (possibly due to withdrawal of caffeine's vasoconstrictor effect), lethargy, nervousness, irritability and inefficiency occurs 12–16 hours after discontinuation. It is suggested that the breakfast cup of coffee wards off these dysphoric symptoms.

Adverse effects

These are few. It can cause extrasystoles and may be a cause of insomnia.

CENTRAL DEPRESSANTS

ALCOHOL AND ALCOHOLISM

Ethyl alcohol (alcohol) has few clinical uses when given systemically, but is of great medical importance because of its pathological and psychological effects when used as a beverage. The alcohol content of drinks ranges from 3.5 to 6% in beer, through 10% in wine and 20% in port to 40–55% in spirits (100° proof is 57% v/v). Most alcoholic beverages contain a number of congeneric substances formed as byproducts during the fermentation or distilling processes.

Alcohol is the most important drug of dependence, and in Western Europe and North America the incidence of alcoholism is about 5% in the adult population.

Pharmacokinetics

Ethyl alcohol is absorbed from the buccal, esophageal, gastric and intestinal mucosae: approximately 80% is absorbed from the small intestine. Alcohol delays gastric emptying and in high doses delays its own absorption by a negative feedback mediated via duodenal osmoreceptors. Large amounts of alcohol taken in dilute solution are also absorbed relatively slowly, possibly as a result of a volume effect on gastric emptying rate. Following oral administration alcohol can usually be detected in the blood within 5 min. Peak concentrations occur between 0.5 and 2 hours. Fats and carbohydrates delay absorption which follows zero-order kinetics. Individuals show great variation in speed of absorption and those habituated to alcohol often show a steeper rise and higher peak in blood concentration.

Alcohol is distributed throughout the body water. Alcohol penetrates the cerebrospinal fluid (CSF) (1.1 × blood concentration) and urine (1.3 × blood concentration). The maximum recommended weekly intake is 21 units for men and 14 for women (1 unit =

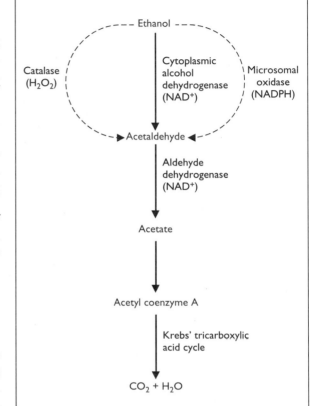

Fig. 49.1 Pathways of ethanol oxidation. $\longrightarrow$ major pathway. $---\!\!\!>$ minor pathways. NADP = nicotinamide diphosphate.

10 g ethanol = 1/2 pint normal strength beer, one glass of wine, 1 single measure of spirits). Ninety-five per cent is metabolized (mainly in the liver) and the remainder is excreted unchanged in the breath, urine and sweat. Hepatic oxidation to acetaldehyde is catalyzed by three parallel processes. The major pathway (Fig. 49.1) is rate limited by cytoplasmic alcohol dehydrogenase using nicotinamide adenine dinucleotide (NAD) as coenzyme. Large amounts of fructose (1–2 g/kg) accelerate alcohol metabolism but this has been found to be of minimal clinical value.

Although nutritional deficiencies may contribute to the toxicity of ethanol which is a source of calories but not vitamins or protein, it is now thought that it is the altered intracellular redox balance caused by an increased NADH/NAD$^+$ ratio that is responsible for the biochemical effects of acute and chronic alcohol abuse.

Increase in the relative concentration of NADH results in reduced metabolism and therefore accumulation of lactate, β-hydroxybutyrate, glutamate, malate, α-glycerophosphate and other substances requiring NAD$^+$ for elimination. The net effect of such changes includes impaired gluconeogenesis resulting in alcohol-induced hypoglycemia, and fatty infiltration of the liver due to impaired elimination of exogenous and endogenous fatty acids via the Krebs' cycle and enhanced triglyceride synthesis due to increased levels of α-glycerophosphate. Originally it was postulated that alcohol elimination obeys zero-order kinetics, i.e. is independent of the blood concentration above about 0.1 mg/ml. There is substantial evidence now that Michaelis–Menten kinetics more accurately describe the situation. The maximum reaction rate (V_m) and Michaelis–Menten constant (K_m) for the average man are approximately 25 mg/100 ml/hour and 10.5 mg/100 ml, respectively (chapter 3). It is, however, true to say that the average rate of alcohol elimination is approximately 10 ml/hour so that once an intoxicated state is reached an intake of 10 ml each hour will suffice to maintain it. The rate of metabolism is much more nearly the same in identical twins than in fraternal twins and genetic factors rather than environmental differences appear to control the overall rate. The rate of metabolism is much the same in young and old subjects, although the aged have a smaller apparent volume of distribution, probably due to decreased lean body mass, and so develop higher levels for a given dose. Similarly women, who have relatively more subcutaneous fat than men, also develop higher blood levels, which accounts for their liability to toxic damage from alcohol at lower levels of consumption.

Acute effects of alcohol

1. Nervous system
Decrease occurs in:

- Learning ability.
- Association formation.
- Attention span.
- Concentration.
- Versatility.
- Judgment and discrimination.
- Reasoning.

In individuals who are not heavy drinkers there is a rough correlation between blood alcohol concentrations and acute central nervous system effects:

- 20 mg/100 ml   sensation of relaxation.
- 30 mg/100 ml   mild euphoria.
- 50 mg/100 ml   mild incoordination.
- 100 mg/100 ml   obvious ataxia.
- 300 mg/100 ml   stupor.
- 400 mg/100 ml   deep anesthesia.

The rate of rise of concentration is also important. This list of blood alcohol concentrations is of no value in chronic alcoholics in whom a level of 200 mg/100 ml may produce little effect while at 400 mg/100 ml they may hold a coherent conversation. At high blood concentrations vomiting may occur and death may result from aspiration of gastric contents. The importance of alcohol as a factor in road traffic accidents is well known (Fig. 49.2). At present in the UK the legal limit for alcohol in the blood is 80 mg/100 ml. At this level of intoxication serious personal injuries or fatalities occur in some 10% of road accidents, which is more than double the rate occurring in accidents involving sober drivers.

The central depressant actions of alcohol greatly enhance the effects of other central depressant drugs.

In patients with organic brain damage alcohol may induce unusual aggression and destructiveness known as pathological intoxication. Death may also result from direct respiratory depression.

2. Circulatory system
Atrial fibrillation, cardiomyopathy, cutaneous vasodilatation, increased sweating (can

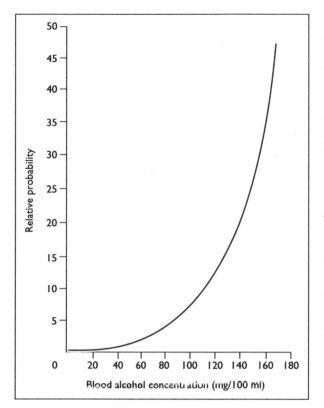

Fig. 49.2 Relative probability of causing a road accident at various blood alcohol concentrations. (From J.D.J. Harvard. *Hospital Update* 1975; **1**: 253.)

produce hypothermia) and splanchnic vasoconstriction occur.

Increased myocardial excitability produces:

- Increased heart rate.
- Raised cardiac output.
- Raised systolic blood pressure.
- Increased pulse pressure.

3. Other actions

Low concentrations of alcohol in the stomach increase acid and mucous secretion and produce congestion of the gastric mucosa. This is followed by a decrease in acid secretion and acute gastritis.

Alcohol suppresses ADH secretion and this is one of the reasons for polyuria following its ingestion.

Reduced gluconeogenesis leading to hypoglycemia may cause fits. Accumulation of lactate and other acids produces metabolic acidosis with excretion of an acid urine and stimulation of the respiratory center. In chronic alcoholics severe thiamine deficiency may also precipitate lactic acidosis and immediate treatment with intravenous thiamine is required.

Hyperuricemia may occur, resulting in acute gout in those predisposed to the condition, partly because of increased renal tubular excretion of organic acids, which compete with uric acid for secretion into the tubules.

Chronic effects of alcohol

Nervous system

Behavioral changes occur resulting in excessive alcohol intake with loss of control, i.e. the drinker can never be sure that he will be able to call a halt to his drinking once he has started to drink. This may lead to drinking with gradual loss of interest in normal activities resulting gradually in social disintegration with loss of job, friends and family. Some alcoholics make repeated attempts at abstinence but then go on a binge. Others are unable to abstain and do not get drunk frequently but top up intermittently day-in, day-out. In the confirmed alcoholic, periods of amnesia, emotional extremes (rage, depression, pathological jealousy), insomnia and seizures may occur. Acute withdrawal may result in:

- Tremor.
- Convulsions.
- Auditory hallucinations.
- Paranoid reactions.
- Delirium tremens (acute disorientation, autonomic hyperactivity, panic and unpleasant visual hallucinations) (see below).

Acute withdrawal symptoms reach a maximum 24–36 hours after the last drink, but the anorexia, nausea, vomiting, tremor, anxiety, malaise and inability to concentrate may last for 1–2 weeks.

Wernicke's encephalopathy (difficulty in concentrating, confusion, coma, nystagmus and ophthalmoplegia) and Korsakov's psychosis (gross memory defects with confabulation and disorientation in space and time) mainly due to the nutritional deficiency of thiamine associated with alcoholism. There is usually a partial response to thiamine which should initially be given intravenously, for example, 100 mg daily for 3 days. Some individuals inherit an abnormal form of the enzyme transketolase with reduced affinity for its coenzyme thiamine. Thus, if dietary thiamine intake falls, tissue transketolase activity is decreased which may result in neurological damage. This explains why only some alcoholics suffer these syndromes and demonstrates the general principle of a genetically determined variant being disclosed by an environmental stress or drug. Similarly peripheral neuropathy and retrobulbar neuritis are due to thiamine lack. A pellagra-like state may develop from nicotinic acid deficiency.

Chronic alcoholism can also produce:

- Chronic cerebral degeneration (leading to dementia) with or without diffuse cerebral atrophy.
- Marchiafava–Bignami syndrome (symmetrical demyelination of the corpus callosum leading to dementia, fits, paralysis and disturbance of motor skills).
- Central pontine myelinolysis (producing quadriplegia and pseudobulbar palsy).

Alimentary system

Chronic effects include:

- Morning nausea and vomiting.
- Abdominal pain, belching, gastritis.
- Peptic ulceration, hematemesis (including the Mallory–Weiss syndrome which is hematemesis due to esophageal tearing during forceful vomiting).
- Enlargement of the liver due to fatty infiltration in 70–80% alcoholics which is reversible.
- Pancreatitis (acute, subacute and chronic).
- Alcoholic hepatitis exhibits clinical features similar to other forms of toxic liver injury. The hypermetabolic state produced by alcohol produces maximal anoxia in the centrilobular hepatocytes which become necrotic.
- Cirrhosis.
- Poor dietary intake does not appear to be as important as was once believed. A direct hepatotoxic role for alcohol implies

that dietary supplements cannot counteract its effects on the liver and that the only way to reduce its toxicity is complete abstinence. Approximately 10% chronic alcoholics develop cirrhosis of variable severity. The level of alcohol intake at which the risk of liver disease becomes significant is contentious. Probably less than 60 g in men per day is innocuous but above this intake the risk of cirrhosis markedly increases. Predisposing factors for the development of cirrhosis include the female sex, histocompatibility antigens HLA B8, B13, B40 and the presence of hepatitis B markers. The rate of development of cirrhosis is independent of the duration of alcohol abuse and the amount consumed.

Alcohol stimulates secretin production which increases the flow of pancreatic enzymes. If these are retained in the pancreas due to edema of the sphincter of Oddi, then autodigestion can lead to pancreatic destruction and inflammation.

Cardiovascular system

Alcoholism is occasionally complicated by a myopathy affecting cardiac and/or skeletal muscle. A negative association between moderate alcohol intake and coronary disease has been demonstrated in several epidemiological studies. There is evidence of a correlation between chronic alcohol consumption and hypertension.

Hematological

Bone marrow suppression occurs, with consequent thrombocytopenia and inability to counter infections which are more common and serious in alcoholics. Macrocytic or hypochromic anemias, probably nutritional in origin, may develop and occasionally a hemolytic or sideroblastic anemia occurs.

Metabolism

1. Alcohol metabolism increases the intracellular $NADH/NAD^+$ ratio which inhibits the pyruvate carboxylase step in gluconeogenesis thus causing hypoglycemia.
2. Hypertriglyceridemia may occur in alcoholics with liver complications and also in

those with normal liver function. Zieve's syndrome comprises jaundice, hemolytic anemia and hyperlipidemia. Some patients with types III and IV hyperlipoproteinemia develop more severe triglyceridemia after alcohol.

3. Hyperuricemia, sometimes associated with acute gout, may occur.

In pregnancy

Alcoholic mothers produce babies exhibiting features of intrauterine growth retardation and mental deficiency, sometimes associated with motor deficits and failure to thrive. There are characteristic facial features which include microcephaly, micrognathia and a short upturned nose. This so-called fetal-alcohol syndrome is unlike that reported in severely undernourished women. Most obstetricians now recommend total abstinence.

Medical uses of alcohol

Apart from widespread use as a topical antiseptic and rubefacient systemic alcohol has other uses:

1. As a night sedative for individuals who habitually take alcohol and are deprived of their drug in hospital.
2. Intravenous alcohol is rarely used in obstetrics to suppress uterine contractions and delay premature labor. Given in moderate doses it may induce drowsiness: higher intravenous doses may produce anesthesia. Ethanol appears to be as effective as salbutamol in postponing preterm labor.
3. In methanol poisoning, the administration of large amounts of ethanol competes for oxidation, slowing the rate of metabolism of methanol to toxic formaldehyde. An ethanol infusion is also useful in the management of ethylene glycol poisoning.
4. Alcohol is included in oral opiate mixtures, for example of heroin and cocaine (Brompton mixture), for administration to the terminally ill patient. It may also improve appetite in such cases.
5. As a vasodilator in peripheral vascular disease (often a subjective but not an objective response).

6. One to two glasses of red wine daily to improve lipid profile – faith required!

Management of alcohol withdrawal

1. Seizures

Seizures during alcohol withdrawal generally develop within 12–24 hours of withdrawal. They are usually generalized and status epilepticus is rare. Benzodiazepines are commonly effective.

2. Delirium tremens

Delirium tremens is a medical emergency with a mortality of 5–10%. It occurs in less than 10% of patients withdrawing from alcohol. Management includes:

(a) Careful nursing in a quiet evenly illuminated room, if possible by the same staff on each shift.
(b) Sedation; either of the following agents are useful:

- Chlormethiazole is an effective sedative and anxiolytic but is potentially addictive. It may be given orally (2–4 capsules 8 hourly initially, reducing the dose to maintain light sedation) or as an intravenous infusion (0.8% solution, 40–100 ml initially over 10 min then reducing the rate to maintain sedation this must be titrated under direct medical supervision to avoid respiratory depression). Chlormethiazole undergoes substantial presystemic metabolism when given orally and bioavailability is markedly increased in patients with cirrhosis in whom the oral dose must be reduced.
- Benzodiazepines with a long half-life are suitable although cerebral sensitivity to these drugs is often decreased in alcoholics (cross-tolerance), so larger initial doses than usual are sometimes needed. Note that deep sedation is undesirable as respiratory depression will predispose the patient to hypostatic pneumonia and pressure sores.

(c) Correction of fluid and electrolyte balance.
(d) Vitamin replacement with adequate thiamine (e.g. 100 mg parenterally, daily for 3 days).
(e) Psychiatric referral.

Long-term management of the alcoholic

1. Psychotherapy
Individual psychotherapy and group therapy may be appropriate. Many clinicians skilled in the management of such patients feel that they should never take alcohol again, while others feel that in certain cases alcohol can be allowed so long as consumption is carefully controlled.

2. Alcohol-sensitizing drugs
These produce an unpleasant reaction when taken with alcohol. The only drug of this type used to treat alcoholics is disulfiram which inhibits aldehyde dehydrogenase leading to acetaldehyde accumulation if alcohol is taken causing flushing, sweating, nausea, headache, tachycardia and hypotension. Cardiac arrhythmias may occur with large amounts of alcohol. The small amounts of alcohol included in many medicines may be sufficient to produce a reaction and it is advisable for the patient to carry a card warning of the danger of alcohol administration. The oral dose is 800 mg on the first day reducing over a week to 100–200 mg daily. Subcutaneous disulfiram implants are not recommended. Disulfiram also inhibits phenytoin metabolism and can lead to phenytoin intoxication.

Evidence for the efficacy of disulfiram in the routine treatment of alcoholism is lacking, but if the patient is motivated may help during the first weeks of withdrawal when the craving for alcohol is strongest.

Interactions of alcohol with other drugs

1. Potentiation of effects of other CNS depressants, for example barbiturates, chloral, morphine, benzodiazepines.
2. Inhibition of metabolism of chloral via competition for alcohol dehydrogenase.
3. Acute alcohol ingestion may inhibit hepatic microsomal drug metabolizing enzymes probably by binding to cytochrome P_{450}.
4. Ethanol is a weak inducer of drug metabolism and its chronic administration results in increases in microsomal enzymes, cytochrome P_{450} and smooth endoplasmic reticulum. Increases in the rates of metabolism of warfarin, barbiturates, tolbutamide and phenytoin amongst others have been demonstrated. The evidence as to whether ethanol can induce its own metabolism is conflicting, and most of the increased tolerance to ethanol seen in alcoholics is due to central adaptation, for they do not appear to metabolize ethanol very differently from non-drinkers.
5. Enhancement of gastric irritation of aspirin, indomethacin and other gastric irritants.
6. Alterations in ethanol metabolism by other drugs is relatively unusual, since unlike most drugs it is predominantly metabolized in the cytoplasm. Chlorpromazine inhibits ethanol metabolism by direct inhibition of the dehydrogenase whilst phenobarbitone, clofibrate and fructose enhance its elimination.
7. Disulfiram-type reactions (flushing of the face, tachycardia, sweating, breathlessness, vomiting and hypotension) have been reported with metronidazole, sulfonylureas and trichloroethylene (industrial exposure).
8. Enhanced hypoglycemia produced by insulin and oral hypoglycemic agents.

BARBITURATES

With the significantly reduced prescription of barbiturates due to the introduction of the much safer benzodiazepines, the prevalence of barbiturate addiction has fallen dramatically. Some addicts are therapeutic addicts: barbiturates are 'downers' and are associated with tolerance and marked physical and psychological dependence. Barbiturates have similar effects on the CNS as alcohol but are more commonly associated with withdrawal convulsions. Overdoses are commonly fatal due to respiratory depression and/or asphyxia. Chloral hydrate and chlormethiazole have similar potential for dependence.

BENZODIAZEPINES

See chapter 15.

SOLVENTS

Solvent misuse is common in certain groups, predominantly in adolescents aged between 12 and 16. Solvents such as glues, paints, nail varnish removers, dry-cleaning fluids and 'Tippex' are sniffed, often with the aid of a plastic bag to increase the concentration of vapor. Inhaled solvent rapidly reaches the brain. The effect may be enhanced by reduced oxygen. Unlike drinking alcohol the effects come on almost instantly and usually resolve within half an hour. Disinhibition can lead to excessively gregarious, aggressive or emotional behavior. Some sniffers just vomit. In a stupor accidents are common and if overdose occurs, coma and asphyxiation may result. Some products may sensitize the heart and lead to cardiac arrhythmias. Most deaths are associated with aerosol inhalations or bags placed over the head.

Excessive chronic use, for example for 10 years, may lead to major organ failure as well as permanent brain damage.

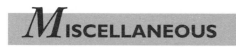

*M*ISCELLANEOUS

ANABOLIC STEROIDS

Anabolic steroids are abused by athletes to build up muscle tissue. Most synthetic anabolic steroids are derived from testosterone. They are particularly popular amongst body builders. Prevalence of anabolic steroid abuse by athletes is uncertain. If given by injection using unsterile equipment there is obviously risk of blood-borne disease as with other drugs of abuse. It is likely that chronic use is associated with hypertension, unusual hepatic and renal tumors, psychotic reactions and depression on withdrawal, and possibly sudden death from cardiac arrhythmias.

AMYL NITRATE AND BUTYL NITRATE

These inhaled drugs cause almost instant vasodilatation, hypotension, tachycardia and subjective 'rush'. They are claimed to enhance sexual pleasure and in addition dilate the anus. The hypotension can cause coma and frequent use is associated with methemoglobinemia.

Drug Overdose and Poisoning

50

Intentional self-poisoning **686**

Accidental poisoning **694**

Criminal poisoning **694**

*I*NTENTIONAL SELF-POISONING

Self-poisoning remains one of the commoner causes of acute medical admission in the UK. Carbon monoxide is the commonest agent implicated in fatal acute poisoning. Such patients seldom reach hospital alive. Co-proxamol (dextropropoxyphene plus paracetamol), paracetamol alone and tricyclic antidepressants are the commonest drugs used in fatal overdose (Table 50.1). Lithium, paraquat, salicylates, β-adrenoreceptor antagonists, digoxin and aminophylline continue to cause fatalities. This list of agents causing death from overdose does not reflect the commonest drugs on which individuals overdose. Benzodiazepines (often taken with alcohol) are the commonest group of drugs taken in an overdose, but are seldom fatal if taken in isolation. Eighty per cent of deaths from overdose occur outside hospital with a mortality of those treated in hospital being less than 1%. The vast majority of cases of self-poisoning fall into the psychological classification of suicidal gestures (or a cry for help). Relatively few are serious suicide attempts; however, the prescription of potent drugs with a low therapeutic ratio can cause death from an apparently trivial overdose.

Table 50.1 Top ten agents implicated in fatal suicides.

Agent	Number of deaths
1. Carbon monoxide	976
2. Co-proxamol	125
3. Dothiepin	69
4. Paracetamol	64
5. Amitriptyline	45
6. Temazepam	34
7. Aspirin	32
8. Insulin	16
9. Dextropropoxyphene	16
10. Chlormethiazole	13

Source: OPCS Mortality Statistics 1989. The numbers exclude those where more than one agent other than alcohol was taken.

Diagnosis

HISTORY

Self-poisoning may present as an unconscious patient being delivered to casualty or with a full history available from the patient or companions. Following an immediate assessment of vital functions, as full a history as possible should be obtained from the patient, relatives, companions and ambulance drivers as appropriate. A knowledge of the drugs or chemicals available is invaluable. Some patients in this situation give an unreliable history. A psychiatric history, particularly of depressive illness, previous suicide attempts or drug dependency, is relevant.

EXAMINATION

A meticulous, rapid but thorough clinical examination is essential not only to rule out other causes of coma or abnormal behavior, for example head injury, epilepsy, diabetes, hepatic encephalopathy, but also because the symptoms and signs may be characteristic of certain poisons. The clinical manifestations of some common poisons are summarized in Table 50.2.

Laboratory tests

Routine investigation of the comatose overdose patient should include blood glucose (rapidly determined by stick testing), biochemical determination of plasma electrolytes, urea, creatinine and arterial blood gases. Drug screens are often requested although rarely indicated as an emergency.

Table 50.3 indicates those drugs where the clinical state of a patient may be unhelpful in determining the severity of the overdose in

Table 50.2 Clinical manifestations of some common poisons.

Symptoms/signs of acute overdose	Common poisons
Coma, hypotension, flaccidity	Benzodiazepines and other hypnosedatives, alcohol
Coma, pin-point pupils, hypoventilation	Opioids
Coma, dilated pupils, hyperreflexia, tachycardia	Tricyclic antidepressants, phenothiazines; other drugs with anticholinergic properties
Restlessness, hypertonia, hyperreflexia, pyrexia	Amphetamines, MDMA, anticholinergic agents
Convulsions	Tricyclic antidepressants, phenothiazines, carbon monoxide, monoamine oxidase inhibitors, mefenamic acid, theophylline, hypoglycemic agents, lithium, cyanide
Tinnitus, overbreathing, pyrexia, sweating, flushing, usually alert	Salicylates
Burns in mouth, dysphagia, abdominal pain	Corrosives, caustics, paraquat

MDMA = Methylenedioxymethylamphetamine.

the acute stages. In each of these suspected overdoses emergency measurement of the plasma concentration can lead to life-saving treatment. For example, in the early stages patients with paracetamol overdoses are often asymptomatic and although it only rarely causes coma acutely, patients may have combined paracetamol with alcohol, a hypnosedative or opioid. As such an effective antidote (acetylcysteine) is available, it is recommended that the paracetamol concentration be measured in all unconscious patients who present as drug overdose.

When there is doubt as to the diagnosis, in particular in coma, samples of blood, urine and when available gastric aspirate should be collected. Subsequent toxicological screening may be necessary if the cause of the coma does not become apparent or recovery occur. Avoidable morbidity is more commonly due to a missed diagnosis such as head injury than failure to diagnose drug-induced coma.

Prevention of further absorption

Methods employed to reduce absorption are listed in Table 50.4.

Emesis can be achieved safely by stimulation of the pharynx (by fingers or other blunt instrument such as a teaspoon) or oral syrup of ipecacuanha. The former may be useful as first aid in the home but is often ineffective. Syrup of ipecacuanha is a plant extract whose most active ingredients are emetine and cephalin. These act as direct irritants to the gastrointestinal tract and stimulate the

Table 50.3 Common indications for emergency measurement of drug concentration.

Suspected overdose	Effect on management
Paracetamol	Administration of antidotes – acetylcysteine or methionine
Iron	Administration of antidote – desferrioxamine
Methanol/ethylene glycol	Administration of antidote – ethanol ± dialysis
Lithium	Dialysis
Salicylates	Simple rehydration or alkaline diuresis or dialysis
Theophylline	Necessity of ITU admission

Table 50.4 Methods of reducing absorption of poison.

Emesis
Gastric aspiration and lavage
Oral activated charcoal
Gut lavage and cathartics

medullary vomiting centre possibly through central $5HT_3$ receptors (the effect can be blocked by ondansetron, a $5HT_3$ receptor antagonist, chapter 30, p. 408). Syrup of ipecacuanha is effective at inducing vomiting in over 90% of patients within 30 min although there is much less evidence of its ability to empty the stomach, and for this reason it is now rarely recommended in the management of poisoning when more effective methods are available.

Gastric aspiration and lavage is the only acceptable method of emptying the stomach in a patient with impaired consciousness, having secured the airway with a cuffed endotracheal tube. If there is *any* suppression of the gag reflex a cuffed endotracheal tube is mandatory. Surprisingly the aspiration of tablet residues is often incomplete. Although the beneficial effect on outcome is difficult to prove, it is still common practice to perform a stomach washout if the patient presents within 4 hours of ingestion of a potentially toxic overdose. The sooner after ingestion this is performed the more likely significant recovery of drugs will occur. After ingestion of drugs which delay gastric emptying (e.g. tricyclic antidepressants) gastric lavage may be effective up to 10 hours after ingestion; after salicylate overdose gastric lavage is advised up to 24 hours after ingestion. Gastric lavage is unpleasant for the conscious patient and potentially hazardous. It should only be performed by experienced personnel with efficient suction apparatus close at hand (Table 50.5).

If the patient is uncooperative and refuses consent, this procedure cannot be performed. Gastric lavage is usually contraindicated following ingestion of corrosives and acids due to the risk of esophageal perforation. Following petroleum distillate ingestion the risk of aspiration pneumonia necessitates the use of a cuffed endotracheal tube.

An increasingly popular method to reduce drug/toxin absorption either after gastric lavage or in the uncooperative patient is oral activated charcoal which adsorbs drug in the gut. To be effective large amounts of charcoal are required, typically 10 times the amount of poison ingested and again timing is criti-

Table 50.5 Gastric aspiration and lavage.

1. If unconscious, protect airway with cuffed endotracheal tube.
   If semiconscious with effective gag reflex, place patient in head-down, left lateral position. An anesthetist with effective suction must be present.

2. Place the patient's head over the end/side of the bed so that the mouth is below the larynx.

3. Use a wide-bore lubricated orogastric tube.

4. Confirm the tube is in the stomach (not the tracheal) by auscultation of blowing air into the stomach; save the first sample of aspirate for possible future toxicological analysis (and possible direct identification of tablets/capsules).

5. Use 300–600 ml tap water for each wash, repeat 3 to 4 times. Continue if ingested tablets/capsules still present in the final aspirate.

6. Unless an oral antidote is to be administered leave 50 g of activated charcoal in the stomach.

cal with maximum effectiveness soon after ingestion. Its effectiveness is due to its large surface area (over 1000 m^2/g). Binding of charcoal to drug is by non-specific adsorption. Aspiration is a potential risk in a patient who subsequently loses consciousness or fits and vomits. Oral charcoal may also inactivate any oral antidote (e.g. methionine).

The use of repeated doses of activated charcoal may be indicated after ingestion of sustained release medications or after drugs with a small volume of distribution (such as salicylates, barbiturates or theophylline): the rationale is that these drugs will passively diffuse from the bloodstream if charcoal is present in sufficient amounts in the gut.

Whole gut lavage using large amounts of electrolyte solutions may be useful when large amounts of sustained release preparations, iron or lithium tablets or packets of smuggled narcotics have been taken. The use of cathartics although more easy to administer has not been shown to reduce morbidity.

Supportive therapy

Patients are generally managed with intensive supportive therapy whilst the drug is eliminated naturally by the body. After an initial assessment of vital signs and instigation of appropriate resuscitation, repeated observations are necessary as drugs may continue to be absorbed with a subsequent increase in plasma concentrations after admission. In the unconscious patient, repeated measurements of cardiovascular function including blood pressure, urine output and if possible continuous electrocardiographic (ECG) monitoring should be carried out. Plasma electrolytes and acid–base balance should be measured. Hypotension is the commonest cardiovascular complication of poisoning. This is usually due to peripheral vasodilatation but may be secondary to myocardial depression following, for example, β-blocker, tricyclic antidepressant or dextropropoxyphine poisoning. Hypotension can usually be managed with intravenous colloid. If this is inadequate positive inotropic agents (e.g. dobutamine) may be necessary. If arrhythmias occur any hypoxia or hypokalemia should be corrected, but antiarrhythmic drugs should only be administered in life-threatening situations. Respiratory function is best monitored using blood gas analysis: a $PaCO_2$ of greater than 6.5 is usually an indication for assisted ventilation. Serial minute volume measurements or continuous measurement of oxygen saturation using a pulse oximeter are also helpful to monitor deterioration or improvement in self-ventilation. Oxygen is not a substitute for inadequate ventilation. Respiratory stimulants increase mortality.

Enhancement of elimination

Methods to increase poison elimination are appropriate in less than 5% of overdose cases. Repeated oral doses of activated charcoal may enhance the elimination of a drug by 'gastrointestinal dialysis'. Several drugs are eliminated in bile and then reabsorbed in the small intestine. Activated charcoal can interrupt this enterohepatic

circulation by adsorbing drug in the gut lumen preventing reabsorption and enhancing fecal elimination. Cathartics such as magnesium sulfate can accelerate intestinal transit time which facilitates the process. Orally administered activated charcoal adsorbs drug in the gut lumen and effectively leaches drug from the intestinal circulation into the gut lumen down a diffusion gradient. Although studies in volunteers have shown this method to enhance the elimination of certain drugs its effectiveness in reducing morbidity in overdose is generally unproven. It is however extremely safe unless aspiration occurs. There are anecdotal reports of its value in the management of paracetamol, salicylate, digoxin, quinine, anticonvulsant and theophylline overdose. Forced diuresis is hazardous and is no longer recommmended. Alkaline diuresis should be considered in salicylate and phenobarbitone poisoning and acid diuresis may be helpful in phencyclidine and amphetamine/'ecstasy' poisoning.

Adjusting urinary pH is much more effective than causing massive urine output. Alkaline diuresis is particularly hazardous in the elderly due to sodium and water overload. Peritoneal dialysis, hemodialysis and, less commonly, charcoal hemoperfusion are sometimes used to enhance drug elimination. Table 50.6 summarizes the most important indications and methods for such

Table 50.6 Methods and indications for enhancement of poison elimination.

Method	Poison
Alkaline diuresis	Salicylates, phenobarbitone
Acid diuresis	Phencyclidine, ?amphetamine
Hemodialysis (peritoneal dialysis is also effective but two to three times less efficient)	Salicylates, methanol, ethylene glycol, lithium, phenobarbitone
Charcoal hemoperfusion	Barbiturates, theophylline, disopyramide
'Gastrointestinal dialysis' using activated charcoal	Salicylates, most anticonvulsants, digoxin, theophylline, quinine

elimination techniques. In addition exchange transfusion has been successfully used in the treatment of poisoning in some young children and infants. The risk of an elimination technique must be balanced against the possible benefit of enhanced elimination.

Specific antidotes

Antidotes are available for a small number of poisons and the most important are summarized in Table 50.7.

CHELATING AGENTS

Chelating agents possess two or more electron donor groups in a molecule that can coordinate with a polyvalent metal. The resulting coordination metal complex has a ring structure. For use in medicine the chelating agent and its metal complex must be non-toxic, soluble and readily excreted. Some recommended chelating agents are included in Table 50.7.

NALOXONE

Naloxone is a pure opioid antagonist at the μ-receptor with no intrinsic agonist activity (chapter 22). It rapidly reverses the effects of opioid drugs including morphine, diamorphine, pethidine, dextropropoxyphene, codeine and dipipanone. Injected intravenously, naloxone acts within 2 min and the plasma half-life is up to 1 hour. The half-life ($t_{1/2}$) of most opioid drugs is longer (e.g. dextropropoxyphene $t_{1/2}$ = 12–24 hours) and repeated doses or infusions of naloxone may be required. The usual dose is 0.8–1.2 mg although much higher doses may be required after massive opioid overdoses which are common in addicts and especially after a partial agonist (e.g. buprenorphine) overdose, because partial agonists must occupy a relatively large fraction of the receptors compared with full agonists like morphine in order to produce

Table 50.7 Antidotes and other specific measures.

Overdose drug	Antidote/other specific measures
Paracetamol	Acetylcysteine i.v. Methionine p.o.
Iron	Desferrioxamine
Cyanide	Oxygen, amyl nitrate (inhalation), dicobalt edetate i.v., sodium nitrite i.v. followed by sodium thiosulfate i.v.
Benzodiazepines	Flumazenil i.v.
β-Blockers	Atropine Isoprenaline Glucagon
Carbon monoxide	Oxygen Hyperbaric oxygen
Methanol/ethylene glycol	Ethanol
Lead (inorganic)	Sodium EDTA i.v. Penicillamine p.o. Dimercaptosuccinic acid (DMSA*) i.v. or p.o.
Mercury	Dimercaptopropane sulfonate (DMPS*) Dimercaptosuccinic acid (DMSA*) Dimercaprol Penicillamine
Opioids	Naloxone
Organophosphorus insecticides	Atropine, pralidoxime
Digoxin	Digoxin specific fab antibody fragments
Calcium channel blockers	Calcium chloride or gluconate i.v., glucagon
Insulin	50% dextrose i.v. Glucagon i.v. or i.m.

* N.B. DMSA and DMPS are not licensed in the UK.

even modest effects. Naloxone is not itself sedating, does not depress respiration and although it does not directly affect pupil size it does dilate a pupil constricted by an opiate. It has been given intramuscularly to achieve a longer duration of action. It can precipitate withdrawal reactions in narcotic addicts. This is not a contraindication, but it is wise to ensure that patients are appropriately restrained before administering naloxone.

Management of specific overdoses

PARACETAMOL

This over-the-counter mild analgesic is commonly taken in overdose. Although remarkably safe in therapeutic doses, overdoses of 7.5 g or more may cause hepatic failure, less commonly renal failure, and death (for discussion of mechanism see chapter 5). The patient is usually asymptomatic at the time of presentation but may complain of nausea and sweating. Right hypochondrial pain and anorexia may precede the development of hepatic failure. Coma is rare unless a hypnosedative or opioid (e.g. in the form of dextropropoxyphene in co-proxamol) has been taken as well.

If a potentially toxic overdose is suspected the stomach should be emptied if within 4 hours of ingestion. The antidote should be administered and blood taken for paracetamol concentration, prothrombin time, creatinine and liver enzymes. The decision to stop or continue the antidote can be made at a later time. The plasma paracetamol concentration should be obtained urgently and related to the graph shown in Fig. 50.1 which relates time from ingestion to plasma paracetamol concentration and probability of liver damage. If doubt exists concerning the time of ingestion it is better to err on the side of caution and give the antidote.

Intravenous acetylcysteine and/or oral methionine are potentially life-saving antidotes and are most effective if given within 8 hours of ingestion although benefit may be obtained from acetylcysteine up to 24 hours after ingestion. Acetylcysteine is administered as an intravenous infusion. The standard regimen is described in Table 50.8. In approximately 5% of patients pseudoallergic reactions occur. These are usually mild. If any hypotension or wheezing occur it is recommended the infusion is stopped and an antihistamine administered parenterally. If the reaction has completely resolved acetylcysteine may be restarted at a lower dose. Alternatively methionine may be used (see below).

Patients who are taking enzyme-inducing drugs (e.g. phenytoin, carbamazepine) or

Table 50.8 Administration of acetylcysteine (in 5% dextrose).

Dose	Diluent volume	Infusion period
150 mg/kg then	200 ml	15 minutes
50 mg/kg then	500 ml	4 hours
100 mg/kg	1000 ml	16 hours

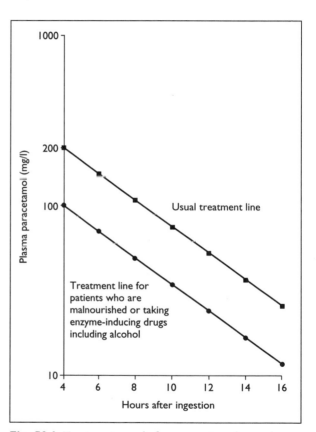

Fig. 50.1 Treatment graph for paracetamol overdose. The graph provides guidance as to the need for acetylcysteine treatment. The time in hours after ingestion is often uncertain: if in doubt – treat.

chronic alcoholics are at a higher risk of hepatic necrosis following paracetamol overdose. The prothrombin time is the first indicator of hepatic damage. If the prothrombin time and serum creatinine are normal when repeated at least 24 hours after the overdose, significant hepatic or renal damage is unlikely.

Methionine is an effective oral antidote in paracetamol poisoning. It has the advantages that it is very safe and cheap but has the disadvantage that absorption is delayed in comparison to i.v. acetylcysteine. Its efficacy has not been studied in late paracetamol overdoses.

SALICYLATE

Although also conscious, in contrast to paracetamol overdose, the patient usually feels ill after significant salicylate overdose, and presents with tinnitus and hyperventilation and is hot and sweating. Immediate management includes estimation of arterial blood gases, electrolytes, renal function and plasma salicylate concentration. The patient is usually dehydrated and requires intravenous fluids. Stomach washout is worthwhile up to 24 hours after ingestion. Activated charcoal should be administered after gastric lavage. Blood gases and arterial pH normally reveal a mixed metabolic acidosis and respiratory alkalosis. Respiratory alkalosis frequently predominates and is due to direct stimulation of the respiratory center. The metabolic acidosis is due to uncoupling of oxidative phosphorylation and lactic acidosis. If acidosis predominates the prognosis is grave. Absorption may be delayed and the plasma salicylate concentration can increase over many hours after ingestion. Depending on the salicylate concentration (Table 50.9) an alkaline diuresis should be commenced using sodium bicarbonate. This is, however, particularly hazardous in the elderly. Children metabolize aspirin less effectively than adults and are more likely to develop a metabolic acidosis and consequently are at higher risk of death. Plasma electrolytes, salicylate and arterial blood gases and pH must be measured regularly. Sodium bicarbonate may lead to hypokalemia which discourages formation of an alkaline urine. Hence supplemental intravenous potassium may have to be added to the bicarbonate. If the salicylate concentration reaches 800–1000 mg/l hemodialysis is likely to be necessary. Hemodialysis may also be life-saving at

Table 50.9 Urinary alkalinization regimen for aspirin.

Indicated in adults with a salicylate level in the range 600–800 mg/l and in elderly adults and children with levels in the range 450–750 mg/l.

Adults: 1 litre of 1.26% sodium bicarbonate (isotonic) + 40 mmol KCl i.v. over 4 hours, and/or 50 ml i.v. boluses of 8.5% sodium bicarbonate (NB Additional KCl will be required)

Children: 1 ml/kg of 8.4% sodium bicarbonate (= 1 mmol/kg) + 20 mmol KCl diluted in 0.5 litres dextrose saline infused at 2–3 ml/kg/hour

Source: National Poisons Information Service, Guy's Hospital, London.

lower salicylate concentrations if the patient's metabolic and clinical condition deteriorates.

TRICYCLIC ANTIDEPRESSANTS

Tricyclics cause death by arrhythmias, myocardial depression, convulsions or asphyxia. If the patient reaches hospital alive they may be conscious, confused, aggressive or in deep coma. Clinical signs include dilated pupils, hyperreflexia and tachycardia. Following immediate assessment of the patient including resuscitation and ECG monitoring as necessary blood should be taken for arterial blood gases and electrolytes. Gastric lavage should be performed up to 10 hours after ingestion. The patient must continue to be ECG monitored during this procedure and for 24 hours after clinical recovery.

The commonest arrhythmia is sinus tachycardia predominantly due to anticholinergic effects and does not require any intervention. Broadening of the QRS complex indicates a quinidine like effect (unless pre-existing bundle branch block is present) and is associated with poor prognosis. The only preventative antiarrhythmic therapy should be correction of any metabolic abnormalities, in particular hypokalemia, hypoxia and acidosis. Intravenous sodium bicarbonate (1–2 mmol/kg body weight) is the most effective treatment for the severely ill patient: its mode of action may involve a redistribution of the drug within the tissues. In extreme cases prolonged chest compressions may be required to maintain cardiac output. If life-threatening ventricular arrhythmias occur, phenytoin may be effective. Anticholinergic drugs should be avoided. If resistant ventricular tachycardia occurs intravenous magnesium, intravenous isoprenaline or overdrive pacing have been advocated. If ventricular tachycardia results in hypotension, DC shock is indicated. Convulsions should be treated with intravenous benzodiazepines.

Occasionally, assisted ventilation is necessary. The patient should be ECG monitored for at least 12 hours after the overdose and if arrhythmias occur then for longer.

Table 50.10 Poisons information.

Belfast	01232 240503
Birmingham	0121-554 3801
Cardiff	01222 709901
Dublin	Dublin 379964
	or Dublin 379964
Edinburgh	0131-229 2477
	0131-228 2441
	(Viewdata)
Leeds	0113 430715
	or 0113 316838
London	0171-635 9191
	or 0171-995 5095
Newcastle	0191-232 5131

Note: Some of these centres also advise on laboratory analytical services which may be of help in the diagnosis and management of a small number of cases.

CO-PROXAMOL

It is usually the dextropropoxyphene that causes death from overdose with this mixture of dextropropoxyphene and paracetamol. The patient may present with coma, hypoventilation and pin-point pupils. Immediate cardiopulmonary resuscitation and intravenous naloxone is indicated. The plasma paracetamol concentration should be measured and acetylcysteine administered according to Fig. 50.1.

OPIOID OVERDOSE

See chapter 22.

CARBON MONOXIDE

This is the commonest cause of fatal poisoning. Patients are usually male and die from carbon monoxide generated from car exhaust. (Catalytic convertors reduce the carbon monoxide emission and this may reduce the number of deaths.) Accidental carbon monoxide poisoning is also common and should be considered in the differential diagnosis of confusional states, headache and vomiting, particularly in winter as a result of inefficient heaters and inadequate ventilation. It may also be present in survivors of fires. The immediate management is removal from exposure and administration of oxygen. There is increasing evidence that hyperbaric oxygen speeds recovery and reduces neuropsychiatric complications.

NON-DRUG POISONS

There is a vast array of plants, garden preparations, pesticides, household products, cosmetics and industrial chemicals which may be ingested. Some substances such as paraquat and cyanides are extremely toxic whilst many are non-toxic unless enormous quantities are consumed. It is beyond the scope of this book to catalog and summarize the treatment of all poisons and the reader is strongly advised to contact one of the poisons information services (Table 50.10) whenever any doubt as to toxicity management exists.

Psychiatric assessment

It is important that selected overdose patients are reviewed by a psychiatrist. Although most patients take overdoses as a reaction to social/life events, some overdose patients are pathologically depressed. Tricyclic antidepressant drugs are potentially very toxic in overdose so the decision to treat is a balance between the efficacy of the drug and the risk of further overdose. Safer alternatives should be considered.

ACCIDENTAL POISONING

Accidental poisoning with drugs causes between 10 and 15 deaths per annum in children. Most commonly, tablets were prescribed to the parents and left insecure in the household or handbag. Unfortunately many drugs resemble sweets. Tricyclic antidepressants are commonly implicated. The use of child-proof containers and patient education should reduce the incidence of these unnecessary deaths. Non-drug substances that cause significant poisoning in children include antifreeze, cleaning liquids and pesticides.

In adults accidental poisoning most commonly occurs at work and is usually inhalation of noxious fumes. Factory and farm workers are at particular risk.

CRIMINAL POISONING

This is one mode of non-accidental injury to children. Homicidal poisoning is rare but possibly underdiagnosed. Suspicion is the key to diagnosis. Toxicological screens are invaluable.

Appendix

Legal Aspects of Prescribing

1. Misuse of Drugs Act 1971

Drugs controlled under this Act are divided into three classes: A, B and C in decreasing order of harmfulness. This division is solely for the purpose of determining penalties under the Act. Some commonly encountered drugs in each category are:

- Class A includes alfentanil, cocaine, dextromoramide, diamorphine (heroin), dipipanone, lysergide (LSD), methadone, morphine, opium, pethidine, phencyclidine and class B substances when prepared for injection.
- Class B includes oral amphetamines, barbiturates, cannabis, cannabis resin, codeine, ethylmorphine, glutethimide, pentazocine, phenmetrazine and pholcodine.
- Class C includes certain drugs related to the amphetamines such as benzphetamine and chlorphentermine, buprenorphine, diethylpropion, mazindol, meprobamate, pemoline, pipradrol and most benzodiazepines.

The Act gives powers to ministers to combat changes in drug abuse by amending these lists as seems necessary on advice from the Advisory Council on the Misuse of Drugs. This consists of not less than 20 members, with wide experience of the medical and social effects of drug abuse, whose function is to keep the national drug abuse situation under review. The Act prohibits import or export of controlled drugs without license and makes it an offense to produce a controlled drug or to supply or offer to supply one to another person. It is therefore illegal to knowingly grow cannabis in the garden. Similarly unlawful possession of a controlled drug is an offense as is allowing the use of premises for illegally producing a controlled drug, for smoking cannabis or opium or for preparing opium for smoking.

Doctors acting in a professional capacity may lawfully prescribe, administer, manufacture or supply a controlled drug but may be required to give information concerning quantities, number and frequency of occasions that the drug was prescribed, administered or supplied by him or her. It is an offense not to comply without reasonable excuse with this request or to give false information. There is no right of entry to a doctor's premises without a search warrant but the police may enter the premises and request the production of any documents relating to dealings with controlled drugs and inspect the stocks of such drugs.

2. Notification and Supply to Addicts Regulations 1973

These regulations imposed upon medical practitioners an obligation to notify the Home Office of addicts whom they believe to be taking any of the following drugs: cocaine, dextromoramide, diamorphine, dipipanone, hydrocodone, hydramorphone, levorphanol, methadone, morphine, opium, oxycodone, pethidine, phenazocine or piritramide. Notification must be made within 7 days to the Chief Medical Officer at the Home Office giving name, sex, date of birth, address and National Health Service number together with the drug involved, whether the patient injects any drug (whether or not notifiable) and the date of attendance. Notification is not necessary if the doctor believes that the drug is medically necessary or if the doctor of his partner (or colleague in hospital) has notified the patient within the preceding 12 months. Notification should be confirmed in writing if the patient is still being treated by the doctor. Except for the treatment of organic disease or injury a doctor must not administer or supply heroin, cocaine, dipipanone or any of their salts to an addict unless he has a special license from the Secretary of State to do so. This regulation effectively gives the treatment of these addicts over to specially designated physicians.

The index of addicts at the Home Office may be consulted by any doctor for information about a person under his care. It is sensible to check (by telephone) all new cases of addiction or suspected addiction against the index to prevent simultaneous prescriptions from two or more doctors.

Failure to notify an addict is an offense and can result in withdrawal of the doctor's authority to prescribe, administer, supply or authorize the supply of controlled drugs. Failure to comply with this direction is an offense and is treated in the same way as irresponsible prescribing of controlled drugs.

3. Misuse of Drugs Regulations 1973

Schedule 1 includes drugs such as cannabis and lysergide which are not used medicinally. Possession and supply are prohibited except in accordance with Home Office authority.

Schedule 2 includes drugs such as diamorphine (heroin), morphine, pethidine, quinalbarbitone, glutethimide, amphetamine and cocaine, and are subject to the full controlled drug requirements relating to prescriptions, safe custody, the need to keep registers etc. (unless exempted in schedule 5).

Schedule 3 includes the barbiturates (except quinalbarbitone, now schedule 2), buprenorphine and phentermine. They are subject to the special prescription requirements (except for phenobarbitone) but not to the safe custody requirements (except for buprenorphine and diethylpropion) or to the need to keep registers (although there are requirements for the retention of invoices for 2 years).

Schedule 4 includes 34 benzodiazepines and pemoline which are subject to minimal control. In particular, controlled drug prescription requirements do not apply and they are not subject to safe custody.

Schedule 5 includes those preparations which, because of their strength, are exempt from virtually all controlled drug requirements other than retention of invoices for 2 years.

4. Misuse of Drug (Safe Custody) Regulations 1973

These regulations require that any controlled drug other than those in schedule 1 must be kept in a locked receptacle which can only be opened by the doctor or somebody authorized by him or her to open it. A locked car or briefcase is not regarded as a locked receptacle for the purposes of the regulations.

5. Medicines Act 1968: Part III Medicines (Prescriptions Only) Order

These regulations became effective in February 1978, and replaced previous regulations restricting substances in schedule 4 of the poisons rules and part II of the Therapeutic Substances Act to prescription only. In place of these laws the Medicines Act categorizes drugs into:

(a) General Sales List: these may be purchased in any kind of shop or even from an automatic machine.
(b) Prescription Only Medicines (POMs): for which a prescription is required.
(c) Pharmacy Medicines: drugs not in category (a) or (b) but which can be supplied to a patient directly by a pharmacist without prescription.

In some cases it is the dosage which determines whether a drug is in a category (a) or (b). The pharmacist is also enabled to sell legally many ethical drugs previously limited to prescription provided the dosage is kept down. There is also provision made for the supply of emergency drugs at the request of a patient provided that only a small supply is given, that it has previously been prescribed by a doctor and that the substance requested is not in schedule 2 of the Misuse of Drugs Act 1971 (see above) or one of a number of other substances like barbiturates (except for epilepsy) or poisons like cyanide or strychnine.

Note that provisionally registered doctors cannot write prescriptions for POMs for dispensing outside of hospital.

Index

Note: users of the index should bear in mind that American English spelling is used throughout.

abortion
  spontaneous
    anesthesia and 78
    drug-induced 74
  therapeutic 503, 504
acetazolamide 444–5
acetylator status, effect on drug metabolism 120, 121–3
acetylcysteine 687, 691, 692, 693
6-acetylmorphine 240
acetylsalicylic acid *see* aspirin
acipimox 275
acitretin 659
acne 654–5
  drug-induced 102, 663
acquired immune deficiency syndrome (AIDS)
  antiretroviral therapy 567–71
  and tuberculosis therapy 547
  see also HIV-1 infection
acromegaly 510, 512
actinomycin D 588
activated partial thromboplastin time (APTT) 324, 328
acyclovir 521, 558–9, 575, 661
Addison's disease 486, 492, 547
adenosine 356, 364–5
adrenal hormones 486–95
adrenaline 368
  as antiarrhythmic 354, 355
  hypersensitivity disorders 643–4
adrenocortical insufficiency 489, 490, 492
adrenocorticotrophic hormone (ACTH) 514
  stimulation test 487
adrenoreceptors
  classification 12
  stimulation, pharmacological effects 346
adverse drug reactions (ADRs) 94–106
  allergic 100–4
  children 86
  classification 94
  elderly 86–7
  genetic factors 120
  hepatotoxicity 420–2
  minimization by use of drug combinations 110
  skin 662–4
  see also drug interactions, adverse
aerosols 36
  asthma 378, 380, 382–3, 385–6
  children 85
affective disorders *see* mood disorders
agonists 10, 14
  dose–response curve 11
  partial 16–17
  slow processes 17
agranulocytosis, drug-related 103
AIDS *see* acquired immune deficiency syndrome
akathisia, drug-induced 162, 189
albendazole 584
alclometasone 656

alcohol
  in drinks 677
  drug interactions 114, 682
  effects
    acute 678–9
    chronic 679–81
    on fetus 80
    on gout 128
  and hypertension 283
  medical uses 681
  pharmacokinetics 677–8
  poisoning 687
  withdrawal
    management 681–2
    symptoms 679
alcohol dehydrogenase, polymorphism 123
alcohol-sensitizing drugs 682
alcoholism 677, 679–81
  long-term management 682
aldosterone 488, 491–2
alginates, use in pregnancy 79
  in esophagitis 404
  in pregnancy 79
alkylating agents 596–9
  tumor resistance to 592
allergic reactions *see* hypersensitivity reactions
allergic rhinitis 644
allopurinol 128, 259, 583
almitrine 390–1
alopecia 655
  cancer chemotherapy 595
  drug-induced 102, 663
α-adrenoceptor antagonists (α-blockers) 296–7, 302, 344, 494
α-antitrypsin 390
alprostadil 504
alteplase 318, 319, 320
altitude sickness 445
aluminum salts 398–9
amantadine
  influenza prophylaxis 559
  Parkinsonism 185–6
  use in elderly 90
amebiasis, extraintestinal 579
Ames test 136
amikacin 521, 533–4, 574
  therapeutic monitoring 70
amiloride 305, 443–4
aminoglutethimide 608–9
aminoglycosides 533–4
  cancer chemotherapy 594
  fetal effects 75
  pregnancy 77
  therapeutic monitoring 70
aminophylline
  asthma 378, 383–4
  chronic bronchitis 380
  elimination, heart failure 58
  overdose 686
4-aminoquinolines 579
8-aminoquinolines 583

aminosalicylates 409–10
5-aminosalicylic acid (5ASA) 409–10
amiodarone 353, 355, 356, 357, 361–3
　therapeutic monitoring 72
amitriptyline 171, 172, 173, 179
　migraine prophylaxis 210
　overdose 686
amlodipine 34
　hypertension 294, 295, 296
　ischemic heart disease 315, 316
ammonia
ammonium chloride 451
amodiaquine 578
amorolfine 661
'amotivational syndrome' 672
amoxycillin 531
　use 519, 520, 522, 523, 524, 531
　　chronic bronchitis 379
　　infection in asthma 378
　　prophylactic 526, 530
amphetamines 673
　abuse 673
　as anorectics 423
　　obesity treatment 267–8
　overdose 687
amphotericin 552–3, 555, 595
　HIV-infected patients 574–5
ampicillin 531
　use 520, 521, 523, 524, 531
　　chronic bronchitis 379
　　prophylactic 526, 527, 528
amrinone 347
amyl nitrate 683
'amyotrophy' 459
anabolic steroids 505
　misuse 683
analeptics 390–1
analgesia, neuroleptanalgesia 219–20
analgesics
　combined tablets 236
　migraine 207
　mild/moderate pain 231–6
　postoperative pain 230–1
　potential sites of action 229
　severe pain 236–42
　terminal disease 229–30
　topical 657
　use in pregnancy 78
anaphylactic shock (acute anaphylaxis) 640–1
　treatment 644
anaphylactoid reaction 641
anayphylaxis, slow-reacting substance of 377
androgens 486, 504–6
anemia
　aplastic 623
　　drug-related 103
　chronic renal failure 624
　Diamond–Blackfan 626
　Fanconi's 623
　folic acid deficiency and 622
　hemolytic, drug-related 103

anemia (*cont.*)
　iron deficiency 616–20
　　pregnancy 622
　pernicious 620–1
anesthesia
　aspiration prevention 399, 401
　effects on fetus 75
　in pregnancy 78
anesthetics, general
　inhalation anesthetics 213–16
　　occupational hazards 216
　　uptake and distribution 212–13
　intravenous anesthetics 216–19
　malignant hyperthermia 120, 126
　mechanism of action 18, 212
　premedication 220
anesthetics, local 224–5
　intrathecal administration 39
'angel dust' 672
angina
　stable, management 309
　unstable 308
　　management 309–10
angiotensin II 292, 343, 495
angiotensin-converting enzyme (ACE) gene, polymorphism 125
angiotensin-converting enzyme (ACE) inhibitors 291–4, 342–4
　adverse effects 292–3, 343
　contraindications 292–3, 343
　drug interactions 294, 344
　mechanism of action 292, 342–3
　metabolism effects 292
　pharmacokinetics 293–4, 343–4
　use
　　elderly 90
　　heart failure 342–4
　　hypertension 291–2
　　pregnancy 80, 303
anion exchange resins 272–3
anistreplase (APSAC) 318, 319, 320
ankylosing spondylitis, NSAIDs 248, 250, 252
anorectic drugs 267, 422–3
antacids 398–9
　use in pregnancy 79
antagonists 10
　competitive 14–16
　dose–response curve 11
anthracyclines 606–7
anthranilic acids 251
antiandrogens 506
antiarrhythmic drugs 352–371
　classification 353–4
　therapeutic monitoring 71–2
antibacterial drugs 518–549
　asthma 377, 378
　cancer chemotherapy 594, 606–8
　choice 518
　chronic bronchitis 379–80, 388
　classification 518
　combination therapy 109, 525
　elderly 91

antibacterial drugs (*cont.*)
  hazards of inappropriate use 530
  hepatic encephalopathy 418–19
  infants and children 84
  interaction with oral contraceptives 115
  minimal inhibitory concentration (MIC) 519
  myobacterial infections 542–8
  in pregnancy 77–8
  prophylactic use 525–7
    in medicine 529–30
    pre-operative 527–9
  resistance to 524
  skin diseases 654, 660
antibacterial therapy, principles 518, 24
antibiotics *see* antibacterial drugs
antibodies, OKT3 637
anti-CD3 receptor antibodies 637
anticholinergic drugs
  asthma 377, 382
  irritable bowel syndrome 416
  overdose 687
anticholinesterases 191, 192, 452
anticoagulants 324–31
  oral 327–31
  in pregnancy and puerperium 79, 202, 334–5
  thyroid disease and 64–5
anticonvulsants 195–203
  drug interactions 198, 201
  mechanisms of action 194
  and osteomalacia 202
  skin reactions 102
  use in pregnancy 79, 202
  withdrawal 202–3
antidepressants 171–174
  effects on central nervous system, elderly 89–90
  non-tricyclic 173–4
  tricyclic 171, 172–3
    adverse effects 172
    anxiety treatment 157
    contraindications 172
    drug interactions 173
    in elderly 89
    mechanism of action 170, 172
    migraine prophylaxis 210
    overdose 686, 687, 692–3
    pharmacokinetics 172–3
    in pregnancy 80
    use 172
antidiuretic hormone (ADH)
  syndrome of inappropriate secretion 446
  otherwise see vasopressin
antidotes 690
antiemetics 405–9
  cancer chemotherapy 593
  classification 406
  migraine 207
  postoperative 231
  use in pregnancy 78
antiepileptics *see* anticonvulsants
antifungal drugs 552–7, 661
  immunocompromized host 552, 574–5

antigens 632
antihistamines (H_1) 642–3
  as antiemetics 406
  asthma 387
  interaction with alcohol 114
antihistamines (H_2)
  see histamine H_2 receptor antagonists
antihypertensive drugs 285–301
  choice 284
  diabetics 305
  drug interactions
    complementary 284, 287
    with NSAIDs 114, 284–5
  elderly 301–2
  pregnancy 302–3
  in renal impairment 305
anti-lymphocyte globulin (ALG) 636–7
antimetabolites 599–604
anti-Parkinsonian drugs 183–8
  in elderly 90
antiplatelet drugs 331–4
  see also aspirin
antiprogestagens 503
antipsychotics
  behavioral emergencies 167–8
  chorea 189
  dyskinesias and 189
  mechanism of action 160, 161–2
  schizophrenia management 160–7
antiretroviral drugs 568–71
antithyroid drugs 473–5
  use in pregnancy 80, 474
antiviral drugs 557–61, 661
  antiretroviral drugs 568–71
  use in pregnancy 78
anxiety, management 156–7
anxiolytics 156–7
aortic dissection, acute 304–5
aphrodisiacs 507
apomorphine 186, 187
appetite
  stimulation 424
  suppressants 267, 422–3
aprotinin 416
arachnidonic acid 433
arrhythmias *see* cardiac arrhythmias; *names of specific arrhythmias*
arteritis, giant cell 252, 490
arthritides, chronic, treatment
  drugs that suppress rheumatoid process 253–7
  NSAIDs 248–53
arthritis, psoriatic 248, 255, 256, 257
Arthus reaction 633
ascites 438
ascorbic acid *see* vitamin C
asparaginase, tumor resistance to 592
aspergillosis 552
aspirin 232–4
  children 84, 86
  drug interactions 234
    with warfarin 114, 330
    cardiovascular disease 316–17, 331–2

aspirin (*cont.*)
  overdose 686, 687, 692
  use
    anti-inflammatory 248
    cardiovascular disease 309, 310, 311, 316–17, 319, 331–2
    migraine 56, 207
    with oral anticoagulants 327
    pregnancy 78, 335
    with streptokinase 319
astemizole 642, 643, 644
asthma
  allergic 376
management
  acute severe asthma 377–8
  asthma with associated infection 377, 378
  chronic asthma 378–9
  drugs 380–7
  late-onset asthma 379
  principles 377–80
  non-allergic (late-onset) 376, 379
  pathophysiology 376–7
  prophylaxis 641
asystole 355
atenolol
  as antiarrhythmic 360, 361
  hypertension 287–291
    pregnancy 80, 303
  ischemic heart disease 314, 315
  migraine prophylaxis 209
atheroma
  and ischemic heart disease 308
  pathophysiology 264–6
  prevention 267–78
atopy 641
atovaquone 572, 573
atracurium 222
atrial fibrillation 351
  anticoagulation 327
  treatment 355–6
atrial flutter 351
  treatment 355–6
atrioventricular (AV) block 351
  treatment 357–8
atropine 367–8
  as antiarrhythmic 354, 357–8, 367
  asthma and bronchitis 382
auranofin
aurothiomalate 253, 254
autoimmune disease 632
azathioprine 256–7
  arthritic diseases 256
  hepatotoxicity 421
  immunosuppression 634
  inflammatory bowel disease 411
azelaic acid 654
azidothymidine (AZT) *see* zidovudine
azithromycin 535, 536, 573, 574
aztreonam 533

Bacille Calmette–Guérin (BCG) 573, 644, 645, 648
bacitracin 660
baclofen 188

bacterial infections
  diagnosis 518
  skin 660
  systemic 521
  treatment 519–24
  see also antibacterial drugs; mycobacterial infections; *names of specific infections*
bactericidal drugs 518
bacteriostatic drugs 518
barbiturates 682–3
  skin reactions 102
Barter's syndrome 449
BCG 644, 645, 648
BCNU 588, 593, 594
beclomethasone
  asthma 378, 385–6
  hay fever 641
  topical 656
behavioral emergencies 167–8
Behçet's disease 258
bendrofluazide 439–40
  heart failure 340
  hypertension 285, 286
  and impotence 506–7
benoxaprofen 97
benperidol 165
benserazide 183
benzathine penicillin 38
benzhexol 184
benzocaine 225
benzodiazepines 149–53
  adverse effects 150–1
    elderly 87–8
  dependence and withdrawal syndrome 151
  drug interactions 152–3
  interaction with alcohol 114
  mechanism of action 150
  overdose 686, 687, 690
  pharmacokinetics 151–2
  use 149–50
    acute psychotic episodes 167
    as antiemetic, cancer chemotherapy 409
    as anxiolytics 156–7
    delirium tremens 681
    epilepsy 199, 202
    as hypnotics 149–50
    intravenous anesthesia 218–19
    in pregnancy 80
benzothiazepines 315
benzoyl peroxide 654
benztropine 184
benzydamine, topical 235
benzyl benzoate 662
benzylpenicillin 531
  use 519, 520, 521, 522, 523, 531
    prophylatic 527, 528
bephenium 584
beri-beri 428, 429
β-adrenoceptor agonists
  asthma 377, 378, 380–2
  hypersensitivity disorders 642

β-adrenoceptor agonists (*cont.*)
  obesity treatment 268
  obstetrics 381
β-adrenoceptor antagonists (β-blockers) 287–91,
    313–15
  adverse effects 289–90, 314–15, 361
    skin 102
  cardioselective 288, 289
  classification 288–9
  combination with diuretics 291
  contraindications 289–90, 314–15, 361
  drug interactions 291, 361
    with calcium channel blockers 114, 316
    with lignocaine 117, 291
  mechanism of action 289, 313–14, 360–1
  overdose 686, 690
  partial agonists 288, 313–14
  pharmacokinetics 290, 315, 361
  pharmacological effects 314
  pheochromocytoma 494–5
  uses 313
    acute aortic dissection 304–5
    angina 310
    as antiarrhythmics 356–7, 360–1
    anxiety treatment 156
    diabetes 114, 288, 290, 305
    elderly 302
    hypertension 287–8, 291
    migraine prophylaxis 209
    myocardial infarction 310, 311
    pregnancy 303
    thyroid disease 474–5
  vascular 288, 289
  vasodilating 288–9
β-lactam antibiotics 530–3
betahistine 406
betamethasone 488, 661
bethanechol 452
bezafibrate 273, 274
biguanides 467–8
bile acid binding resins 272–3
bioavailability 31–2
bioequivalence 30–1, 32
biotechnology, drug development 134–5
biphosphonates 479, 482–3
  bone pain in terminally ill 230
bisacodyl 414
bismuth chelate 403
bisodium etidronate 483
bisulphan 588, 597
bladder, drugs affecting 452, 452–3
blastomycosis 552, 553, 555, 556
bleomycin 607–8
  adverse effects 593
  cancer chemotherapy 587, 607
blood–brain barrier
  renal disease 59
  infants and children 84
blood dyscrasias, drug-related 103
blood flukes 584

blood pressure
  diastolic, relationship with risks of stroke and
      coronary heart disease 280
  measurement 282–3
  see also hypertension
body mass index (BMI) 268
bone
  metabolic diseases 478
bone marrow suppression, cancer chemotherapy 594
botulinum toxin A 190
botulinum toxin F 190
bradycardia(s) 351, 357
bran 412–13
brand names 31, 32
breast feeding 85
  drugs to avoid 85
breast milk, drugs in 85
breathlessness 378
bretylium 355, 370–1
British National Formulary (BNF) 6
bromocriptine 186, 510, 511–12
bronchiolitis 561
bronchitis
  acute 379
  chronic 379–80
bronchodilators
  asthma 377, 378, 379, 380–5
  chronic bronchitis 380
budesonide
  asthma 378, 385–6
  hay fever 641
  topical 656
Buerger's disease 674
bullae, drug-induced 102
bumetanide 342, 441
bupivacaine 224–5
buprenorphine 16, 17, 242
  sublingual administration 35
buserelin 513–14
  intranasal administration 37
  tolerance induction 17
buspirone 156, 157
butyl nitrate 683
butyrophenones 161, 165, 408

caffeine 675–6
α calcidol 479
calciferol 480, 481
calcipotriol 658
calcitonin 479, 481–2
calcitrol 479, 480
calcium
  excretion, increasing 479
  metabolism 478–83
calcium carbonate 398, 481, 483
calcium channel blockers 294–6, 315–16
  overdose 690
    migraine prophylaxis 210
    myocardial infarction management 311
calcium chloride 369
calcium gluconate 450

calcium lactate 481
cancer
  management 586
  metastases 592–3
  pathophysiology 586
cancer cells 586
  effect of cytotoxic drugs 587–90
  total eradication 590
cancer chemotherapy 586–611
  adjuvant chemotherapy 592–3
  combination therapy 587, 591
  complications 593–6
  general principles 587
  see also cytotoxic drugs
Candida infections, drug treatment 552, 553–4, 555,
    556, 557
  cancer chemotherapy patients 595
  HIV-infected patients 568, 574
cannabinoids 408
cannabis 507, 672
capreomycin 548
capsaicin, topical 657
captopril 291–3, 342, 343
carbachol 452
carbamazepine 198–9
  therapeutic monitoring 70–1
  use in pregnancy 79
carbamyl 662
carbenicillin 532
carbenoxolone 404
carbidopa 183
carbimazole 473–4
carbon monoxide poisoning 686, 687, 690, 693
carbonic anhydrase inhibitors 444–5
carboplatin 610
carboprost 504
carcinogenicity testing 136
cardiac arrest, advanced life support 354–5
cardiac arrhythmias
  digoxin-induced 366
  management 355–8
    in cardiac arrest 354–5
    drug treatment 355–71
    general principles 352–3
  pathophysiology 350
  supraventricular 351–2
  ventricular 352
  see also names of specific arrhythmias
cardiac failure, pharmacokinetic effects 57–9
cardiac glycosides 344–5, 356
cardiopulmonary resuscitation 354
cardioversion, DC 355, 356, 357, 366
carmustine (BCNU) 588
carotene 427
cataracts, diabetics 459
catechol-O-methyltransferase 45
catecholamine metabolism 45
CCNU 588, 593, 594
cefaclor 532
cefadroxil 520, 532
cefotaxime 519, 522, 532

ceftazidime 532
cefuroxime 521, 532
  chronic bronchitis 379
  prophylactic use 527, 528
celiac disease, effects on drug absorption 56
celiprolol 289
cephalexin 57, 532
cephalosporins 532
  use in pregnancy 77
cetirizine 642, 643, 644
cetrimide 661
charcoal, oral activated 688, 689
chelating agents 18, 690
chemoreceptor trigger zone (CTZ) 406
chenodeoxcycholic acid 422
children, drugs in 84–6
  hyperlipidemia treatment 277–8
  hypnotics 156
  pharmacodynamics 84–5
  pharmacokinetics 84
  poisoning 694
  route of drug administration 85–6
  see also infants
chloral 155
  derivatives 155
chloral hydrate 683
chlorambucil 588, 594, 597
  adverse effects 593
chloramphenicol 534–5
  metabolism, infants and children 84
  use 519, 524, 534
chlordiazepoxide
  allergic reactions 150
  pharmacokinetics 151, 152
chlormethiazole 153–4, 200, 681, 683
  overdose 686
chloroquine 255–6, 579–80
chlorpheniramine 642, 644
chlorpromazine 160–7
  hepatotoxicity 421
  as antiemetic 408
  use in terminally ill 230
chlorpropamide
  hepatotoxicity 421
  skin 102
  diabetes mellitus 465, 466
  use in elderly 91
cholecalciferol 479, 480
cholesterol
  and atherogenesis 264, 266
  biosynthesis 264
  plasma levels 269–70
    lowering 268–9, 270–8
    screening 269
    see also hypercholesterolemia
cholestyramine 33, 272
cholinergic crisis 192
chorea 189
chorioncarcinoma 599
cilastatin 533

cimetidine 399–400, 401
  distribution, effect of renal disease 59
  use in elderly 88
cinchonism 357, 359
cinnarizine 406
ciprofloxacin 524, 530, 539
  asthma 378
  HIV-infected patients 574
  prophylactic use 529
  use in pregnancy 77
cisapride 405
cisplatin 593, 609–10
citric acid/potassium citrate 451
clarithromycin 378, 535, 536, 573, 574
clavulanic acid 531
clemstine 642
clindamycin
  HIV-infected patients 573
  Pneumocystis carinii pneumonia 572
  prophylactic use 526
  skin diseases 654
clinical trials 7–8, 132–143
  adverse drug reactions 95–6
clobetasol 661
  topical 656
clobetasone 656
clofazimine 548, 574
clofibrate 273
clomiphene 499, 513
clonazepam 149, 199
clonidine 301
clonidine suppression test 493
Clonorchis sinensis infestations 579
clorazepate 151
Clostridium botulinum toxin A-hemagglutinin complex
  190
clotrimazole 552, 556, 661
clozapine 161–2, 166–7
coagulation factors and hemophilias A and B 627–8
coagulation process 322–3
coal tar 658
co-amilofruse 443
co-amilozide 444
co-amoxiclav 531–2
  asthma 377
  chronic bronchitis 379
  prophylactic use 529
co-beneldopa 183
cocaine 669, 673
  effects on fetus 75, 81
  local anesthesia 225
co-careldopa 183
coccidiomycosis 552, 553
  HIV-infected patients 575
co-danthramer 414
codeine 241–2
  diarrhea 415
  skin reactions 102
cod liver oil 277
colchicine 258–9
colestipol 272

colfosceril palmitate 389–90
colitis, ulcerative 409, 410
coma
  diabetic 464
  myxedema 471–2
combination drug therapy 109–10
Committee on Safety of Medicines (CSM) 132, 133,
  142–3
compliance
  children 85
  elderly 88–9
concentration 22
  see also drug concentration
condylomata acuminata 562
congenital malformations, drug-induced 74–5
conjugation reactions, drug metabolism 42, 44–5
Conn's syndrome 443, 492
constipation 411–414
  in pregnancy 79
contact dermatitis 101, 662, 663
contraception
  combined oral contraceptive 500–2
    progestogen only 502–3
  postcoital 501
convulsions
  alcohol withdrawal 681
  epileptic *see* epilepsy
  febrile 203
copper 433–4
  deficiency 433–4
co-proxamol 236
  overdose 686, 693
coronary heart disease
  risk factors 264–5
    modification 267–9
    see also hyperlipidemia; hypertension
  see also ischemic heart disease
corticosteroids 486–92
  adverse effects, children 86
  asthma 378, 385–6
  cancer chemotherapy 609
  chronic bronchitis 380
  with cytotoxic drugs 409
  effects on fetus 80
  inflammatory bowel disease 409
  inhaled 378, 385–6
  percutaneous 35
  topical 656–7, 658, 659–60
  tuberculosis therapy 547
  see also glucocorticoids; mineralocorticoids
cortisol *see* hydrocortisone
cortisone acetate 488, 490
co-triamterzide 444
co-trimoxazole 109, 524, 538
  absorption, effect of Crohn's disease 56–7
  cancer chemotherapy 595
  Pneumocystis carinii pneumonia 568, 571
cough suppressants 388–9
'crack' 673
cretinism 471, 476

Crohn's disease 409, 410
  effects on drug absorption 56–7
cromoglycate 378, 379, 386–7
cromokalim 297
cryptococcosis 553, 554, 555, 556
  immunocompromised host 552, 574–5
Cushing's syndrome 486, 487, 488, 491
cyanide poisoning 690
cyanocobalamin 620
cyclic adenosine monophosphate 13
cyclizine 406, 642, 643
  use in pregnancy 78
cyclo-oxygenase inhibition by NSAIDs 248–50
cyclophosphamide 598
  adverse effects 593
  cancer chemotherapy 588, 597, 598
  immunosuppression 635
cycloserine 548
cyclosporin, psoriasis 658
cyclosporin 637–9
  therapeutic monitoring 72
cyproheptadine 424
cyproterone acetate 506, 654, 655
cystic fibrosis, effect on cephalexin absorption 57
cysticercosis 584
cystosine arabinoside
  cancer chemotherapy 588
  tumor resistance 592
cytarabine 602–3
  adverse effects 593
cytochrome P_{450} 43
  enzyme induction 46
  enzyme inhibition 47
  isoenzymes 43
  in liver disease 63
cytomegalovirus (CMV) infections 558, 559
  immunocompromised hosts 559, 560, 575
cytosine arabinoside 602–3
cytotoxic drugs 596–611
  action 587–90
    combination chemotherapy 591
    cycle non-specific 587–8
    phase specific 588
  adverse effects 593–5
    skin 102
  predictive toxicity tests 592
  resistance to 591–2
  use
    adjuvant chemotherapy 592–3
    combination therapy 587, 591
    general principles 587–90
    intermittent 590

dacarbazine 588
  adverse effects 593
dalteparin 326
danazol 505, 513
dantrolene 188
  hepatotoxicity 421
DAO see diamine oxidase
dapsone 548–9, 572

daunomycin 588
daunorubicin 607
DC cardioversion 355, 356, 357, 366
DDAVP see desmopressin
debrisoquine, defective hydroxylation 120, 123
decosahexanoic acid 433
dehydration 447–8
3-dehydroretinol 426
delirium tremens 681
demeclocycline 446
dental treatment, antibacterial prophylaxis 525–6
depression 170
  drug treatment 170–9
  elderly 89, 179
  management 170–1
  pathophysiology 170
dermatitis
  contact 101, 662, 663
  exfoliative 102, 663
dermatomyositis 252
dermatophyte infections 554, 556, 557
desalkylfurazem 152
desamino-D-arginine vasopressin (DDAVP see desmopressin
desbutylhalofantrine 582
desensitization
  drug allergy 106
  receptors 17
desflurane 216
desipramine 173
desmethyldiazepam 151, 152
desmopressin (DDAVP) 448, 627
  intranasal administration 37
desogestrel 499, 500
dexamethasone 488, 491
dexfenfluramine 268
dextromoramide 669
  use in terminally ill 230
dextropropoxyphene 236, 331
  overdose 686
diabetes insipidus 440, 446, 448
diabetes mellitus
  effects of corticosteroids 488
  hypertension and 305
  impotence 507
  insulin-dependent (IDDM; type I diabetes; juvenile
    onset diabetes) 458, 459
    management 459–62
  insulin-requiring, use of β-blockers 114, 288, 290
    elderly 90–1
    surgery 462
  non-insulin-dependent (NIDDM; type II diabetes;
    maturity onset diabetes) 458–9
    management 460–2
  pathophysiology 458–9
diamine oxidase (DAO) 43, 44
diamorphine 229, 230, 240
  abuse 668–9
diarrhea 415
  traveler's 415–16

diazepam 150–2
  intravenous 149, 205
    anesthesia 218–19
    status elepticus 199
  rectal 35, 199, 202, 203
  for sleep disturbance 149
  spasticity treatment 188
diazoxide 297, 298
dichloralphenazone 155
diclofenac 251, 452
'diconal' 669
didanosine (DDI) *see* dideoxyinosine
didehydrodideoxythymidine (D4T) 570
dideoxycytidine (DDC) 568, 569, 570
dideoxyinosine 567–8, 569, 570
diet
  and cardiovascular risk 268
  cirrhosis of liver 439
  diabetes mellitus 460–1, 465
  fiber in 412–13
  hypercholesterolemia 270–1
  and hypertension 283
  weight reduction 268
  see also vitamins; *names of specific nutrients*
diethylcarbamazine 584
diethylpropion 268, 423
diethylstilbestrol 499
  effects on fetus 76
diflucortolone 656
digitalis 344
digoxin
  adverse effects 345, 366
  contraindications 345, 366
  drug interactions 117, 345, 367
    with diuretics 115
    with quinidine 359
  formulations, non-equivalence 31, 367
  mechanism of action 344–5, 365–6
  overdose 686, 690
  pharmacokinetics 345, 366–7
    effect of renal disease 59
  therapeutic monitoring 70
  thyroid disease and 64
  use
    as antiarrhythmic 355–7, 365–6
    in elderly 90
    heart failure 344
dihydrocodeine 241
dihydrofolate 579
dihydropyridines 294, 295, 296, 315, 316
dihydrotestosterone 504, 505
1,25-dihydroxycholecalciferol 479
dihydroxypropoxymethylguanine (DHPG) *see* ganciclovir
diltiazem 294, 295, 315, 316
dinoprostone 504
dioctyl sodium sulfosuccinate 413
diphenhydramine 642
diphenoxylate 415
diphenybutyl piperidines 161, 15
dipipanone 669

dipropylacetate *see* sodium valproate
dipyridamole 333
disease, effects on drug disposition 56–65
disopyramide 353, 357, 359–60
distigmine 452
disulfiram 47
  alcoholism 682
dithranol 658
diuresis, drug elimination 53
diuretics 285–7, 340–2, 439–46
  effects on
    elderly 90
    gout 128
  use as anorectics 423
  use in elderly 302
  use in pregnancy 80, 303
dobutamine 346–7
domperidone 187, 407
dopa decarboxylase inhibitors 183
dopamine 346–7
  endogenous release 185–8
  heart failure 346
  receptor agonists 186–7
dopamine antagonists, as antiemetics 407–8
dopaminergic drugs, Parkinsonism 184–8
dosages
  clinical trials 140–1
  constant rate infusion 21
  effect of non-linear kinetics 27–8
  elderly 88
  infants and children 86
  loading doses 25
  preclinical studies 135–6
  single bolus administration 23
dose ratio 14, 15
dose–response curves 11, 15
  drug interactions and 111
dothiepin 172
  overdose 686
Down's syndrome, drug sensitivity 128
doxapram 390, 391
doxazosin 34, 296, 297
doxepin 172
doxorubicin 606–7
  adverse effects 593, 594, 595
  cancer chemotherapy 588 606–7
doxycycline 519, 520, 536
  chronic bronchitis 379
  malaria 581
  traveler's diarrhea 415
droperidol
  as antiemetic 408
  behavioral emergencies 168
  neuroleptanalgesia 219
drug absorption 30–9
  drug interactions and 115
  effect of renal disease 59
  effects of cardiac failure 57
  effects of gastrointestinal disease 56
  effects of liver disease 63
  elderly 87

drug absorption (*cont.*)
  infants and children 84
  pregnancy 76
  prevention, in poisoning 687–8
  sustained release preparations 34
drug abuse 668
  definition 668
  law and 696–7
drug addiction 668–71
  definition 668
  management of addicts 671
  notification of addicts 696–7
drug administration
  constant rate infusion 20–2
  repeated (multiple) dosing 24–5
  routes of *see* routes of administration
  single bolus dose 22–4
drug clearance 21–4
drug concentration, plasma 20–32
  and drug response, pharmacokinetic factors 69
  monitoring 68–72
drug dependence 668
  definition 668
drug disposition, effect of smoking 675
drug distribution 20–6
  drug interactions and 115
  effect of cardiac failure 57–8
  effect of liver disease 63
  effect of non-linear kinetics 26–8
  effect of renal impairment 59
  elderly 87
  enterohepatic circulation and 28
  infants and children 84
  pregnancy 76
  volume of 22–3
    effect of cardiac failure 57
    effect of liver disease 63
    pregnancy 76
drug elimination 20–7
  by liver, effects of cardiac failure 58
  dialysis in 23–4
  drug interactions and 117–18
  effects of cardiac failure 58–9
  elderly 88
  enhancement in overdose 689
  infants and children 84
  pregnancy 77
  renal *see* renal excretion of drugs
drug history 5–6
drug interactions 108–18
drug metabolism 42–8
  by intestinal organisms 34, 44
  drug interactions and 115–17
  effect of liver disease 62, 63
  effect of renal failure 59
  effect of thyroid disease 64–5
  elderly 87–8
  enzyme induction 46
    interactions due to 46, 115–16
  enzyme inhibition 47
    interactions due to 47, 116–17

drug metabolism (*cont.*)
  genetic factors 120–4
    polygenic influences 128–9
  infants and children 84
  phase I 42–4
  phase II (conjugation reactions) 42, 44–5
  pregnancy 76–7
  presystemic ('first-pass' effect) 47–9
drug overdose 686–93
  opioids 670, 687, 690
drug reactions, adverse *see* adverse drug reactions;
    drug interactions, adverse
drugs
  design 134
  development 7–8, 132–143
  generic 142
  law and 696–7
  mechanisms of action 10–18
  multiple use 108
    see also drug interactions
  potency 11
  recreational use 668
  research, codes of practice 133–4
  safety 132
    regulation 132–3, 140–1
  sources of information 6, 8
  use of 4, 5
    scientific basis 7–8
  see also pharmacodynamics; pharmacogenetics;
      pharmacokinetics
DTIC 588
duodenal ulcer 397–403
dynorphins 237
dyschezia 412
dyskinesia
  drug-induced 162, 189
  tardive 162, 189–90
    drug-induced 162, 189
dyslipidemia 268–9, 270
dyspepsia, management in pregnancy 78–9
dysthymia 171
dystonia, drug-induced 162, 189

eclampsia, management 302–3
'ecstasy' 672, 687, 689
eczema 656–7
  drug-induced 663
  infected 660
edema 438–445
edrophonium 191, 192
eflomithine 583
eicosapentanoic acid 433
elderly, drugs in 86–91
  antihypertensive treatment 301–2
  depression treatment 179
  hyperlipidemia treatment 277
  hypnotics 156
electrolyte balance *see* fluid and electrolyte balance
electromechanical dissociation 355
emphysema 379–80
enalapril 291, 292, 293, 342
encainide 353

encephalins 237
encephalitis, herpes simplex 558
encephalopathy
    hepatic 417–19
    hypertensive 304
endocarditis, infective *see* infective endocarditis
endoplasmic reticulum, hepatic, drug metabolism 42–3
endorphins 237
enflurane 214
enoxaparin 326
enoximone 347
enteric fever 524
enuresis, nocturnal 448, 452
enzyme induction 46
    drug interactions and 46, 115–16
    tests for 46
enzyme inhibition 47
    drug interactions and 47, 116–17
eosinophilia, pulmonary 391
epidermal necrolysis 102
epilepsy 194
    management, in pregnancy 79
    treatment
        drugs 195–20
        pregnancy 202
        principles 194–5
    use of antidepressants 179
epirubicin 606
epoetin 624
epoprostenol (prostacyclin) 332–3
Epsom salts 413
ergocalciferol 479, 480
ergometrine 503
ergotamine 208
    rectal administration 35
erythema multiforme 102, 663
erythema nodosa 102
erythroderma 663
erythromycin 519–23, 535, 535–6
    chronic bronchitis 379
    prophylactic use 526, 528–530
    skin diseases 654
    use in pregnancy 77
erythropoietin, recombinant human 624
esmolol 290, 360
esophageal disorders 404–5
esophageal varices 419
esophagitis 399, 401
    reflux 404
essential fatty acids 433
estradiol, metabolism by intestinal organisms 44
estradiol-17β 498, 499
estrogen antagonists 499
estrogens 498–9
    cancer chemotherapy 608
    in oral contraceptives 500–2
    synthetic, hepatotoxicity 421
    use in pregnancy 80
estrone 498
ethambutol 542–3, 545, 546
    HIV-infected patients 574

ethanol *see* alcohol
ethics committees 142–3
ethinylestradiol 498, 499, 500, 501
ethionamide 548
ethosuximide 195–6
etridronate 483
etoposide 605–6
    adverse effects 593, 595
    cancer chemotherapy 588
etretinate 428, 659
European Union, drug regulation 133–4
exercise, benefits 268
expectorants 389
eye drops 37
    steroid 120, 124

factor VIII 627–8
    deficiency 627
factor IX 628
    deficiency 627, 628
familial hypercholesterolemia (FH), effect on drug
        action 124
fansidar 579, 580–1
fascioliasis 579, 584
fats, dietary 268
fatty acids, essential 433
febrile convulsions 203
felbinac, topical 235
fenfluramine 268, 423
fenofibrate 273
fenoterol 380
fentanyl 219–20
ferritin 616
ferrous fumarate 617, 618
ferrous gluconate 617, 618
ferrous sulfate 617, 618
fetal alcohol syndrome 80–1, 681
fetus, effects of drugs 74–6
    cytotoxic 595
fever, drug-related 104
fiber, dietary 412–13
fibrates 273–4
fibrinolytic drugs 318–20, 322
filgrastim 624–5
finasteride 504, 506
fish oils 276–7
    psoriasis 659
    vitamin supplement 427
FK 506 639
flecainide 353, 360
fluandrolene 656
fluclorolone 656
flucloxacillin 520, 521, 522, 523, 531
    prophylactic use 527, 528, 530
fluconazole 524, 556–7, 595, 661
    immunocompromised host 552, 568, 574–5
fluconcinolone 656
flucytosine (5-fluorocytosine) 554–5
    HIV-infected patients 574
fludrocortisone 488, 492

fluid and electrolyte balance, alterations, and drug
  interactions 114–15
fluid and electrolyte disorders
  diabetics 463
  overhydration 446
  potassium disorders 449–51
  volume depletion 447–8
  volume overload 438–9
    diuretic treatment 439–46
fluid replacement 447–8
flukes 584
flumazenil 153, 219
flunarizine, migraine prophylaxis 210
flunisolide 641
flunitrazepam 149
fluocinonide 656
5-fluorouracil 554, 588, 603–4
  adverse effects 593
  tumor resistance to 592
fluoxetine 174, 175
flupenthixol 161, 166, 171
fluphenazine 161
flurazepam 149, 152
fluroquinolones, use in pregnancy 77
fluspirilene 161, 165
fluticasone 385–6, 641
fluvoxamine 174, 175
folic acid 621–2
  cellular mechanism of action 622
  deficiency 621–2
  pharmacokinetics 622
  use 620, 621
    in pregnancy 622
folinic acid 573, 579, 599, 600
follicle-stimulating hormone (FSH) 498, 504, 512
food, effect on drug absorption 34
Food and Drug Administration (FDA) 133
formaldehyde 661
formularies 6
foscarnet 559–60, 570, 575
fosinopril 293
frusemide 441–2
  heart failure 340–1
  hypertension 304, 305
fusidic acid, hepatotoxicity 421
fucidin 660
fungal infections
  cancer chemotherapy patients 595
  immunocompromised hosts 552, 574–5
  skin and nails 661
  see also antifungal drugs

G-proteins see guanosine triphosphate- (GTP) binding
  proteins
gabapentin 201
galactorrhea 511–12
gallstones 422
  drug-related 104
gamolenic acid 657
ganciclovir 560, 575
ganglion blockers 300–1

gastric aspiration and lavage 688
gastric cancer, anti-secretory drugs and 402
gastric emptying
  and drug absorption 56
  pathological factors affecting 56
gastric ulcer 388, 397, 401–4
gastritis, antral 397
gastrointestinal disorders
  effect on drug absorption 34
  effects on drug disposition 56–7
  infections 523–4
  oral drug administration 33
gastrointestinal tract
  drug absorption 33–4
  flora, drug metabolism by 34, 44
gemeprost 503
gemfibrozil 273, 274
genetic diseases, effect on drug action/toxicity 124,
  125–8
genetic polymorphisms, effects
  drug metabolism 120, 121–4, 129
  drug response 120m 124–8
  polygenic influences 128–9
genitourinary infections, antibacterial therapy 520–1
genitourinary system, drugs affecting 452–3
gentamicin
  therapeutic monitoring 70
  use 520–4, 533–4
    prophylactic 526, 527, 528
gestodene 499, 500
giardiasis 579, 583
gigantism 510
Gilbert's disease 128
glaucoma 445, 446
  pilocarpine 'Ocusert' treatment system 37
  steroid eye drops and 124
glibenclamide
  diabetes mellitus 465, 466
  use in elderly 91
gliclazide, diabetes mellitus 465, 466
glomerular filtration of drugs 52
glomerular filtration rate (GFR)
  effect of aging 88
  estimation 60
glucagon test, pheochromocytoma 494
glucocorticoids 486–91
  actions 486, 487
  adverse effects 486–9
  arthritic diseases 252–3
  asthma 377, 378
  hypersensitivity disorders 641
  immunosuppression 635–6
  mechanism of action 636
  thyroid disease and 65
  tuberculosis 547
  under- and oversecretion 487
  use, hypercalcemia 479
  withdrawal 486–7
gluconate 481
glucose 6–phosphatase dehydrogenase (G6PD)
  deficiency 120, 125–6

glucuronidation, drug metabolism 44
glutamine, in conjugation reactions 44
glutaraldehyde 661
glutathione conjugates 45
glycerol suppositories 414
glyceryl trinitrate (GTN) 309–10, 312–13
  sublingual administration 35
glycine, in conjugation reactions 44
glycosuria, diabetes 459
glycylxylidide (GX) 358
goiter 470
gold, skin reactions 102
gold salts 253–4
gonadorelin analogs 513–14
gonadotrophin-releasing hormone (GnRH) 498, 513
  see also gonadorelin
gonadotrophins 512–13
goserelin 513–14
gout 258–60
  aggravation by drugs 128
graft rejection, prevention 489, 491, 634, 636, 637
granisetron 408
granulocyte colony-stimulating factor (G-CSF) 624–5
granulocyte macrophage colony-stimulating factor
  (GM-CSF) 625, 626
Graves' disease 470
gray baby syndrome 46, 84, 535
griseofulvin 554, 661
  skin reactions 102
growth factors, hematopoietic 619, 623–7
growth hormone 510
growth retardation 510
guanosine triphosphate (GTP)-binding proteins (G-
  proteins) 13, 17
guinea worm 584
Guthrie test 471

hair loss, cancer chemotherapy 595
halcinonide 656
half-life of drugs 21–4
halibut liver oil 427
halides, skin reactions 102
hallucinogenic drugs 672
halofantrine 582
haloperidol 165, 167
halothane 213–14
hayfever 644
headache 207
  see also migraine
heart arrhythmias see cardiac arrhythmias
heart disease see coronary heart disease; ischemic
  heart disease
heart failure 338
  pathophysiology 338–9
  treatment
    drugs 340–7
    general measures 339–40
    objectives 339
    shock 340
heart valves, prosthetic, anticoagulation 327
heart see also cardiac

Helicobacter pylori 397, 403
helminthic infections 584
hematinics 616–22
hematopoiesis 619
hematopoietic growth factors 619, 623–7
hemolysis, drug-induced, inherited diseases and 120,
  125–6
hemophilias A and B 627–8
hemosiderin 616
heparin 324–6
  use in angina 310
    myocardial infarction 310
    pregnancy and puerperium 79, 334–5
hepatitis
  drug-related 104
  viral 419–20
    immunoglobulin therapy 648–9
    vaccines 646
heroin addiction 668–71
herpes simplex infections 558, 661
  immunocompromised hosts 559, 575
herpes virus infections 558, 559, 560–1
herpes zoster infections 558, 561
hirudin analogs 326–7
histamine 640–1
  and hypersensitivity reactions 640–1
  receptors 640–1
histamine H_1-receptor antagonists see antihistamines
histamine H_2-receptor antagonists 399–401
  use in pregnancy 79
histoplasmosis 552, 553, 555, 556
  HIV-infected patients 575
HIV-1
  life cycle 566, 567
  nucleoside analog resistance 570
  structure 567
HIV-1 infection
  immunopathogenesis 566–7
  infective complications 568, 571–5
  pathophysiology 566–7
  treatment
    antiretroviral drugs 567–71
    general guidelines 567–8
HMGCoA reductase inhibitors 274–5
  adverse effects, hepatotoxicity 421
  effect of familial hypercholesterolemia on 124
Hodgkin's disease 597, 610
hookworm 584
hormone replacement therapy 498–9
hormones
  acne therapy 655
  adrenal 486–95
  cancer chemotherapy 608–9
  effects on fetus 80
  pituitary 510–14
  sex 498–506
  thyroid 470
human chorionic gonadotrophin (HCG) 512
human immunodeficiency virus see HIV
human menopausal gonadotrophin (HMG) 512
Huntington's chorea 189

hydatid disease 584
hydralazine 299–300, 344
   eclampsia/pre-eclampsia 302
   metabolism, acetylator status and 122
   use in pregnancy 80
hydrochlorothiazide 285, 439–40
hydrocortisone 486, 488, 489–90
   actions 487
   intravenous 489
     asthma 377, 385
   pharmacokinetics 490
   topical 656
   under- and oversecretion 487
   use 488–9
     inflammatory bowel disease 409
hydrolysis, drug metabolism
   endoplasmic reticulum 43
   non-endoplasmic reticulum 44
hydroxocobalamin 620
β-hydroxy-β-methylglutaryl co-enzyme A *see* HMGCoA
hydroxychloroquine 255
1-α-hydroxycholecalciferol 479–81
hydroxylation, defective 120, 123
7-hydroxymethotrexate 601
hydroxyprogesterone 609
4-hydroxypropranolol 290
5-hydroxytryptamine (5HT; serotonin)
   asthma 376
   receptor antagonists 408
   reuptake inhibitors 171, 174–5
     use in pregnancy 80
5-hydroxytryptamine syndrome 175, 176
hyoscine 406, 416
hyperaldosteronism 443
   primary *see* Conn's syndrome
hypercalcemia
   diuretic-induced 286
   of malignancy 478, 482, 483
   treatment 478–9, 482–3
hypercholesterolemia
   diuretic-induced 286
   familial 124, 276, 277
     heterozygous 274, 275, 278
     homozygous 275, 276
   screening 269
   secondary 270
   treatment
     dietary 270–1
     drug 271–8
hyperglycemia
   diabetics 461, 463, 464
     treatment 463
   diuretic-induced 286, 341
   insulin-induced posthypoglycemic 464
hyperkalemia 450–1
   drug-induced 93, 115, 294
hyperlipidemia
   and thrombosis 266
   treatment
     approaches to 269–71
     children 277–8

hyperlipidemia (*cont.*)
   treatment (*cont.*)
     drugs 271–7
     elderly 277
     in pregnancy 278
hyperprolactinemia 511–12
hypersensitivity reactions 632–3
   asthma 376
   involving histamine release 640–1
   to drugs 100–5
hypertension 280–305
   accelerated 303–4
   acute aortic dissection 304–5
   'benign' intracranial 445
   malignant 303–4
   portal 419
   pregnancy 80, 299, 301–3
   and renal failure 305
hyperthermia, malignant 120, 126, 223
hyperthyroidism 470
   drug treatment 473
   neonatal 475
hypertriglyceridemia 270, 271, 277
hyperuricemia 258–9
   diuretic-induced 286, 441
hypervitaminosis A 427
hypnotics 148–56
   effects on central nervous system, elderly 89
hypoglycemia
   β-blockers and 290
   insulin therapy and 461–2, 464
   oral hypoglycemic drugs 465–8
hypoglycemic agents
   oral 465–8
     use in elderly 90–1
   overdose 687
hypokalemia 449–50
   diuretic-induced 115, 286, 287, 341, 342, 441
hypomagnesemia, diuretic-induced 286, 287, 341, 441
hyponatremia 446
   diuretic-induced 286, 341, 441
hypoparathyroidism 480, 481
hyposensitization, drug allergy 106
hypotension
   in poisoning 689
   postural, drug-induced, in elderly 88
hypothyroidism 470
   congenital 476
   treatment 471–2

ibuprofen 234–5, 249, 251
   topical 235
   use in pregnancy 78
idarubicin 606
idiopathic thrombocytopenic purpura (ITP) 623
idoxuridine (IDU) 560–1
ifosfamide 597, 598
   adverse effects 593, 595
   cancer chemotherapy 588
imidazoles 555–6
imipenem–cilastatin 533

imipramine 172, 173
immune response 632
    chemical mediators 640–1
        blockade 641–3
    enhancement 644–5
    suppression 633–9
    to drugs 100
    vaccines and 645–8
immunoglobulins
    prophylactic 563
    as therapy 648–9
immunostimulants 644–5
immunosuppressant therapy 633
immunosuppressive drugs 634–9
    adverse effects 639
    arthritis 256–7
    inflammatory bowel disease 411
    sites of action 634
impetigo 660
impotence 453
    drug-induced 506–7
    treatment 505, 507
incontinence, urge 452
indoleacetic acid 250–1
indomethacin 250
    rectal administration 35
infants, drugs in 84–6
    see also children
infections see bacterial/fungal/mycobacterial/
        parasitic/viral infections; names of specific
        infections
infective endocarditis
    antibacterial prophylaxis 525–7
    antibacterial therapy 522
infertility
    anovulatory 513
    cancer chemotherapy 595
inflammatory bowel disease 409–11
influenza
    prophylaxis 559
    treatment 559, 561
    vaccine 646, 647
infusion, constant rate 20–2
    plasma drug concentration 20–1
inhalation anesthetics see under anesthetics, general
inhalation of drugs 36
    asthma 380, 382, 385–7
    children 85
injections
    intramuscular 37–8
        children 85
        depot 38
    intrathecal 39
    intravenous 38–9
        children 85–6
    subcutaneous 38
insecticides 690, 693
insomnia
    drug treatment 148–55
    elderly 89

insulin 458–465
    diabetes treatment 461–5
        types of insulin 461–2
    overdose 686, 690
    secretion 458
    subcutaneous injection 38
intensive care units, sedation 220
interferons 420
    cancer chemotherapy 611
    HIV-1 infection 571
    viral hepatitis 420
    viral infections 561–3
interleukin-2 611, 645
interleukin-3 626
interleukin-6 626
international normalized ration (INR), oral
        anticoagulants 327–9
intraocular pressure, raised, glucorticoid-induced 120,
        124
iodine
    effects on fetus 80
    radioactive 475–6
5-iodo-2–deoxyuridine 560–1
ion exchange resins, hyperkalemia 451
ionamide 548
ipecacuanha, syrup of 687–8
ipratropium 36, 377, 382–3
iprindole 173–4
iron 616
    deficiency 616–17
        pregnancy 622
        treatment 617–20
    disposition 616
    overdose 687, 690
    pharmacokinetics 616
    pysiology and biochemistry 616
iron preparations
    children 617–18
    iron dextran, 618–19
    iron sorbitol citric acid 619–20
    oral 617–18
    parenteral 618–20
irritable bowel syndrome 416
ischemic heart disease
    drug treatment 312–20
    pathophysiology 308
    see also coronary heart disease
isocarboxazid 175
isoflurane 214–15
isoniazid 542–4, 546, 547
    hepatotoxicity 421
    HIV-infected patients 573–4
    metabolism, acetylator status and 121–2
isonicotinic acid hydrazide (INH) see isoniazid
isoprenaline 368–9
    use in elderly 88
isosorbide dinitrate 312
isosorbide mononitrate 312
isotretinoin 428, 654, 655
itching 657
    drug-induced 663

itraconazole 556, 661
  immunocompromized host 552, 574–5
ivermectin 584

jet lag 155–6

kaolin cephalin clotting time (KCCT) 324
kaolin compound powder BPC 415
Kaposi's sarcoma 611
keratitis, herpetic 558, 561
keratolytics 658
kernicterus 46, 84, 112
ketamine 218
ketoacidosis, diabetics 462, 463
ketoconazole 555–6, 595, 661
  cancer chemotherapy 609
  immunocompromized host 552, 574
kidneys
  and blood pressure/hypertension 281
  effects of methotrexate 601
  see also renal

labetalol 288, 303
  pheochromocytoma 494
  use in pregnancy 80
lactation, suppression 511
lactulose 413
  oral 418
lamotrigine 201
Lanoxin 31
Lassa fever 561
law and drugs 696–7
laxatives 412–14
  abuse 414
  use in pregnancy 79
lead poisoning 690
Legionnaire's disease 544
leishmaniasis 583
lemakalim 297
leprosy 548–9
leu-encephalin 237
leukemias 587, 588, 589, 598
  acute 602, 606, 607
  acute lymphatic 599
  acute lymphoblastic 605
leukotrienes 233
  asthma 376–7
levamisole 584, 645
levodopa 183, 185
  use in elderly 90
levonorgestrel 499, 500, 501
libido, drugs affecting 507
lice 662
lichenoid eruptions 102, 663
lignocaine
  adverse effects 224, 358
  drug interactions 358–9
    with β-blockers 117
  mechanism of action 358
  metabolism, route of administration and 48

lignocaine (*cont.*)
  pharmacokinetics 358
    effect of heart failure 57, 58, 358
  use
    as antiarrhythmic 353, 354, 357, 358–9
    local anesthesia 224
lindane 662
linoleic acid 433
linolenic acid 433
lipocortin 486
lipoproteins
  low density 264–6
  transport 265
liquid paraffin 413
lisinopril 293
lithium 167, 177–8
  effects on fetus 80
  interaction with NSAIDs 249
  overdose 686, 687
  therapeutic monitoring 70
liver
  adverse drug effects 104
  drug metabolism 42–9
    elderly 87–8
    indices 62
  drug reactions in 420–2
liver disease
  alcohol and 680
  cirrhosis 438–9, 680
  drug-induced 420–2
  effects on drug disposition 63–4
  encephalopathy/liver failure 417–19
  esophageal varices 419
  portal hypertension 419
  prescription in 63–4
  viral hepatitis 419–20
liver flukes 584
'locked-in syndrome' 446
lofepramine 174, 175, 179
Lomotil 415
lomustine (CCNU) 588
long-term oxygen therapy (LTOT) 380
loop diuretics 285, 340, 341, 441–3
loperamide 415, 416
loprazolam 149–50
loratadine 642, 643
lorazepam 151, 167
lormetazepam 149–50
low density lipoproteins (LDL) and atherogenesis
  264–6
Lown–Ganong–Levine syndrome 352
loxapine 161, 162, 166
LSD 672
lungs
  adverse effects of drugs 391
  drug administration 36
lupus erythematosus 102, 663
luteinizing hormone (LH) 498, 504
  synthetic 512–13
lymphadenopathy, drug-related 103
lymphocytes 632

lymphomas, drug treatment 587, 588, 590, 610, 611
  alkylating agents 598
  antibiotics 606, 607
  antimetabolites 599, 603
  hormones 609
  see also Hodkin's disease
lysergic acid diethylamide 672
lysuride 186

macrolides 535–6
magnesium 369–70
  as antiarrhythmic 369–70
  myocardial infarction 310–11
magnesium salts 398–9
magnesium sulfate 302, 413
malaria 578–83
malathion 662
malgramostim 625, 626
malignancy *see* cancer
malignant hyperthermia 120, 126, 223
maloprim 579
mania 167
mannitol 445, 446
maprotiline 171, 173–4
mazindol 423
MDMA 672, 687
mebendazole 584
mebeverine 416
meclozine 406
  use in pregnancy 78
Medicines Act (1968) 133
  Part II Medicines (Prescriptions Only) Order 697
Medicines Commission 133
Medicines Control Agency (MCA) 133
Mediterranean fever, familial 258
medroxyprogesterone 502, 609
mefenamic acid 251
  overdose 687
mefloquine 579, 581–2
megestrol 609
melanosis coli 414
melasoprol 583
melphalan 588, 594, 597
Mendelson's syndrome 399
meningitis
  bacterial 522
  cryptococcal 555, 568
  route of drug administration 39
  tuberculous 546
meningoencephalitis, herpetic 558
2-mercaptoethane sulfonate sodium 598–9
6-mercaptopurine 256, 257, 588, 602
  tumor resistance to 592
mercapturic acid formation, drug metabolism 45
mercury poisoning 690
mesalazine 33, 410
mescaline 672
mesna 598–9
mesterolone 505
metabolic acidosis, diabetic 463

metal chelating agents 18, 690
met-encephalin 237
metformin 467–8
methadone 241, 669
methanol/ethylene glycol, overdose 687, 690
methemoglobinemia 120, 125, 126
methimazole 65, 473–4
methionine 687, 691, 692
methotrexate 257
  adverse effects 593
    hepatotoxicity 421
  cancer chemotherapy 588, 599–602
  immunosuppression 257, 635
  psoriasis 658
  therapeutic monitoring 71
  tumor resistance to 592
methotrimeprazine 161
1-methyl-4-phenyl-1, 2, 5, 6-tetrahydropyridine (MPTP) 183
methylation, drug metabolism 45
methylcellulose 267, 413, 423
methyldopa
  eclampsia/pre-eclampsia 302
  hepatotoxicity 421
  hypertension 301
    pregnancy 303
  use in pregnancy 80
methylenedioxymethylamphetamine (MDMA; 'ectasy') 672
  overdose/poisoning 687, 689
methylprednisolone 488
  topical 656
methyltestosterone 505
methylxanthines 383–5
methysergide 209–10
metoclopramide 407
  migraine 207
  use in pregnancy 78, 79
metolazone 439–40
metoprolol 287, 288, 290, 303
  ischemic heart disease 314, 315
  migraine prophylaxis 209
  use, as antiarrhythmic 360, 361
metriphonate 584
metronidazole 537–8, 584
  rectal administration 35
  use 521, 523, 524, 537
    in pregnancy 77–8
    prophylactic 527, 528, 530
mianserin 171, 173, 179
Michaelis–Menten equation 26–7
miconazole 552, 556, 661
micturition, increased frequency 452
midazolam 149
  intravenous anesthesia 219
  pharmacokinetics 151
mifepristone 501, 503
migraine 206–10
  effect on aspirin absorption 56
  oral contraceptives and 501
milk–alkali syndrome 398
milrinone 347

mineralocorticoids 486, 488, 491–2
minimum alveolar concentration (MAC) 212
minocycline 536
  skin diseases 654
minoxidil 297–8
minoxidil sulfate 655
misoprostol 402
  use in pregnancy 79
Misuse of Drugs Act 1971 696
Misuse of Drugs Regulations 1973 697
Misuse of Drugs (Safe Custody) Regulations 1973 697
mithramycin 479
mitomycin C 588, 593
mitozantrone 607
  adverse effects 593
  cancer chemotherapy 588
moclobamide 175
moniliasis see candidiasis
monitoring
  adverse drug reactions 94–106
  drug therapy 68–72
    pharmacokinetic factors and drug response 69
    practical aspects 69–70
monoamine oxidase (MAO) 43–4, 187
monoamine oxidase inhibitors (MAOI) 171, 175–7
  anxiety treatment 157
  overdose 687
  type B inhibitors 187–8
monobactams 533
monoethyl-glycylxylidide (MEGX) 358
mood disorders 170–9
morphine 237–40
  ureteric colic 452
    diarrhea 415
    terminal disease 229, 230
morphine-6–glucuronide 239–40
motion sickness 406
mountain sickness 445
movement disorders 182–203
mucolytics 389
mupirocin 660
muscarinic agonists 452
muscarinic receptor antagonists 183–4
  as antiemetics 406
  asthma 382–3
  peptic ulceration 402–3
muscle relaxants 221
  depolarizing agents 222–3
  non-depolarizing agents 221–2
mustine 596, 597–8
  adverse effects 593, 594
mutagenicity testing 136
myasthenia gravis 190–2
myasthenic crisis 192
mycobacterial infections 542–9
  HIV-infected patients 547, 573–4
  see also leprosy; tuberculosis
Mycobacterium avium intracellulare complex therapy
    574
myeloma 598

myelosuppression, cancer chemotherapy 594
myocardial infarction 308–11
  combined drug treatment 109
  effect on drug distribution 57–8
    fibrinolytic drugs 318–19
myositis 252
myxedema coma 471–2

nabilone 408
nail infections, fungal 557, 661
nails, drug reactions 102
nalidixic acid 539
naloxone 237, 242–3, 670
  as antidote 690
  use in pregnancy 78
naltrexone 243
nandrolone 505
naproxen 251
narcotics see opioids
natriuresis, diuretics 439–46
nausea 405
  antiemetics 406–9
  cytotoxic drugs and 409, 593–4
  pregnancy 406
nebivolol 289
nedocromil 386–7, 641
nefopam 235–6
nematodes 584
neomycin 418, 660
neostigmine 191–2
nephritis, interstitial, drug-related 104
nephropathy, diabetic 459
nephrotic syndrome 438, 635
  drug-related 104
  effects on drug disposition 61
netilmicin 533
netilmicin, therapeutic monitoring 70
neuralgia, trigeminal 228
neuroleptanalgesia 219–20
neuroleptanalgesia 219–20
neuroleptics see antipsychotics
neuropathy, diabetic 459
niacin 430
  deficiency 430
nicardipine 294–6, 315
niclosamide 584
nicotinamide 430
nicotine 673–5
nicotine patches 267
nicotine acid 430
  deficiency 430
nicotinic acid derivatives 275–6
nifedipine
  hypertension 294–6, 304
  ischemic heart disease 315, 316
nifurtimox 583
nimodipine 295
nitrates, organic 344
  ischemic heart disease 312

nitrazepam 149, 150
nitric oxide 312–13
nitrofurantoin 521
  hepatotoxicity 421
nitrofurazone 583
nitrogen mustard 588
nitroimidazoles 556
nitroprusside 298–9, 304, 305, 312, 495
nitrous oxide 215
nitrous oxide/oxygen mixture 231
nivarabine 570
nociception 228
non-steroidal anti-inflammatory drugs (NSAIDs)
    230–35, 248–53
      with antihypertensives 114, 284–5
      with warfarin 330–1
    and peptic ulceration 397, 398
noradrenaline 346
nordiazepam 151, 152
norethisterone 499, 500, 502, 609
norgestimate 499, 500
norgestrel 502
norpethidine 241
nortestosterone 499–500
nortriptyline 172, 173
nose, drug administration 37
Notification and Supply to Addicts Regulations 1973
    696–7
nucleoside reverse transcriptase inhibitors 568–70
  resistance to 570
nystatin 552, 552, 553–4, 574, 595, 61

obesity 422
  and cardiovascular risk 267
  treatment 267–8, 422–3
occulomucocutaneous syndrome 314–15
octreotide 510–12
  liver disease 417, 419
ointments 36
OKT3 antibodies 637
olsalazine 33, 410
omeprazole 399, 401–2, 405
  use in pregnancy 79
onchocerciasis 584
oncogenes 586
ondansetron 408
opioid antagonists 242–3, see naloxone
opioids
  addiction 668–71
  analgesia 236–42
  anesthesia 219
  central nervous system actions 669
  diarrhea 415
  effects on fetus 75
  overdose 670, 687
    antidote 690
  in pregnancy 78
  receptors 237
  thyroid disease and 65
  ureteric colic 452
opium 236

oral contraceptives
  combined 500–2
  drug interactions
    with antibiotics 115
    with antiepileptics 201
  progestogen only 502–3
organ transplantation 489, 491
  immunosuppressive therapy 634, 637, 639
oropharyngeal infections 522
orphenadrine 184
osmotic agents 413
osteoarthritis, NSAIDs 248, 253
osteomalacia 479
  anticonvulsant 202
  prevention and treatment 480, 481
osteomyelitis, antibacterial therapy 523
osteoporosis
  glucocorticoids and 488
  postmenopausal 482
  vertebral 483
ouabain 344, 356
overdone see poisoning
ovulation induction 513
oxamniquine 584
oxazepam, pharmacokinetics 152
oxicams 252
oxidation, drug metabolism
  endoplasmic reticulum 43
  genetic polymorphisms 123
  non-endoplasmic reticulum 43–4
oxitropium 383
oxpertine 161, 166
oxprenolol 16, 288, 290, 291, 360
oxygen therapy
  long-term, chronic bronchitis 380
  mechanism of action 18
  myocardial infarction 310
  respiratory failure 388
oxyphenbutazone 252
oxytetracycline 654
oxytocic drugs 503–4
oxytocin 503, 514

Paget's disease 482, 483
pain
  angina 308
  bone 230
  management see analgesics
  mechanism 228
  perception 228
  urological 452
pamidronate 483
pancreatic disease, effects on drug absorption 57
pancreatic insufficiency 417
pancreatitis 416–17
  drugs associated with 417
pancuronium 222
panic attacks 156–7
papaverine 236, 453, 507
papilloma virus infections 661
para-aminohippuric acid (PAH), clearance 53

paracetamol 231–2
  hepatotoxicity 421
  migraine 207
  overdose 686, 687, 690, 691–2
  use in pregnancy 78
Paragonimiasus infestations 579
paraquat poisoning 686, 687, 693
parasitic infections 578–84
parathyroid hormone (PTH) 478
pargyline 187
Parkinsonism 182–8
  drug-induced 189
  treatment
    elderly 90
paroxetine 174, 175
patches
  drug administration 36
  GTN 312, 313
  hormone replacement therapy 498
  nicotine 267
pellagra 430
penicillamine 254–5
penicillin
  allergic reaction 101
  meningitis, route of administration 39
penicillin G *see* benzylpenicillin
penicillin V 519, 522
  prophylactic 529, 530
penicillins 531
  antipseudomonal 532
  combination with probenecid 110
  extended range 531–2
  skin reactions 102
  use 519 24, 531
    in pregnancy 77
    prophylactic 527–30
pentamidine 572
  Pneumocystis carinii pneumonia 572, 595
  trypanosomal infection 583
pentapeptides 237
pentazocine 242
pentolinium 300
pentolinium suppression test 493
peppermint oil 416
peptic ulceration 396–404
  glucocorticoids and 488–9
  management in pregnancy 79
pergolide 186–7
pericyazine 161
permethrin 662
perphenazine 161, 408
pessaries 37
pesticides 690, 693
pethidine 231, 241
  fetal effects 75, 78
  ureteric colic 452
pharmacodynamics 7, 10–18
  clinical trials 140
  drug interactions 114–15
  elderly 88
  genetic factors 120
  infants and children 84–5

pharmacogenetics 120–9
pharmacokinetics 7, 20–8
  clinical trials 140
  drug interactions 115–18
  effects of disease 65–65
  elderly 87
  genetic factors 120
  infants and children 84
  non-linear (dose-dependent) 26–8
  one-compartment model with first order elimination 20–5
  in pregnancy 76–7
  two-compartment model 25–6
pharmacology 7
  animal 7
  clinical 7
phencyclidine (PCP) 218, 672
phenelzine 175, 176
phenformin 468
phenindamine 643
phenindione 327, 329
phenobarbitone 198
  metabolism, infants and children 84
phenolphthalein, skin reactions 102
phenothiazines 162–4, 189
  skin reaction 102
  overdose 687
  use as antiemetics 407–8
  use in pregnancy 80
phenothrin 662
phenoxybenzamine 15, 296, 494–5
phenoxymethylpenicillin 530, 531
phentermine 423
phentolamine 453, 494, 495, 507
phenylacetic acids 251
phenylalkylamines 315
phenylbutazone 252
  interaction with warfarin 330
  skin reactions 102
phenylethanolamine *N*-methyltransferase 45
phenytoin 194–203
  hepatotoxicity 421
  drug interactions 116, 117, 197, 198
    bioavailability differences 31, 197
    effect of liver disease 59, 198
    effect of renal disease 59, 198
  therapeutic monitoring 70–1, 198–9
    use as antiarrhythmic 353
    use in pregnancy 79, 196
pheochromocytoma 492–5
  diagnosis 300, 492–4
  intraoperative medication 495
  pre-operative management 494–5
phosphate enema 414
3'-phosphoadenosine 5'-phosphosulfate (PAPS) 45
phosphodiesterase (PDE) inhibitors 347
phospholipase enzymes 13
photochemotherapy 658–9
photosensitivity 101, 102, 663, 664
pilocarpine, glaucoma treatment 37
  'Ocusert' system 37
pimozide 161, 165
pinacidil 297

pindolol 16, 288, 360
piperazine 584
pipercaillin 521, 532
pipothiazine 161
pirenzepine 402, 403, 416
piroxicam 252
   topical 235
   transdermal administration 36
pituitary hormone
   anterior 510–15
   posterior 514
pityriasis rosea 556
pityriasis versicolor 557
pizotifen 209, 424
placenta 74
plant fiber 412–13
Plasmodium life cycle 578
platelet activating factor (PAF) 13, 376
platinum compounds 609–10
Pneumocystis carinii infection 583
   pneumonia 571–2, 595
pneumonia
   antibacterial therapy 520
   Pneumocystis carinii 571–2, 595
podophyllin derivatives 605–6
podophyllin resin 661
podophyllinotoxin 661
poisoning 686–94
poisons information centers 693
polyarteritis nodosa 252
polydipsia 448
   diabetes 459
polyenes 552–4
polymyalgia rheumatica 252
polypharmacy 108
   see also drug interactions
polyuria 448
   diabetes 459
porphyria 102, 120, 126–8
portal hypertension 419
potassium
   deficiency 449–50
   excess 450–1
   replacement 449, 450
potassium channel activators 297–8
potassium perchlorate 474
potency of drugs 11
practolol 314
pravastatin 274–5
praziquantel 584
prazosin 296, 297, 494
pre-eclampsia
   management 302–3
prednisolone 488, 490–1
   arthritic diseases 252
   asthma 378, 385
   chronic bronchitis 380
   inflammatory bowel disease 409
   Pneumocystis carinii pneumonia 571
prednisolone 488, 490–1

pregnancy
   alcoholism and 681
   drugs in 74–81
      antithyroid drugs 474
   eclampsia/pre-eclampsia 302–3
   folic acid supplementation 622
   hyperlipidemia treatment 278
   hypertension 80, 299, 301–3
   iron supplementation 622
   malaria prophylaxis 579
   nausea/sickness 406
   use of anticoagulants 334–5
   vitamin A 427
prescription 5, 6
   elderly 91
   generic versus proprietary 31, 32
   legal aspects 696–7
prilocaine 225
primaquine 579, 582
   Pneumocystis carinii pneumonia 572
probenecid 259–60
   combination with
      penicillins 110
      zidovudine 110
probucol 268, 276
procainamide metabolism, acetylator status and 122
procaine penicillin 531
procarbazine 593, 610–11
procarbazine methyl 588
prochlorperazine 161, 408
   pregnancy 78
   terminally ill 230
procyclidine 167, 184
prodrugs 32
progesterone 498, 499, 500
   analogs 499
progestogens 499–503
   cancer chemotherapy 609
   effects on fetus 80
proguanil 579, 583
proinsulin 458
promazine 161
promethazine 154, 642
propafenone 353
propionic acids 251
propofol 217–18, 220
propranolol 288–91, 303
   ischemic heart disease 314, 315
   liver disease 419
   metabolism, route of administration and 48
   migraine prophylaxis 209
propylthiouracil 65, 474
prostacyclin 332–3
prostaglandin analogs 402
prostaglandins 503–4
   asthma 376
   use 504
prostatic obstruction 452–3
protamine sulfate 326
prothionamide 548
proton pump inhibitor 401–2

protozoal infection 583
protriptyline 172
provocation tests, allergic reactions 105
pruritus 657
    drug-induced 663
Pseudoallecheria boydii 556
pseudogout 258
pseudohypoparathyroidism 474, 481
pseudoparathyroidism 13
psilocybin 672
psoralen with ultraviolet a (PUVA) 658–9
psoriasis 657–60
psoriatic arthritis 248, 255, 256, 257
psychiatric disorders, depot intramuscular injections 38
psychosis, acute episodes 167–8
puerperium, use of anticoagulants 334–5
pulmonary disease, drug-induced 391
pulmonary embolism 324, 327
puromycin 583
purpura
    drug-induced 102, 663
    idiopathic thrombocytopenia 623
pyloric stenosis, effects on drug absorption 56
pyrantel 584
pyrazinamide 542–3, 545–6
    hepatotoxicity 421
    HIV-infected patients 573–4
pyrazolone compounds 252
pyridostigmine 191
pyridoxal 430
pyridoxamine 430
pyridoxine 430–1
    deficiency 431
pyrimethamine 573, 579, 580–1, 583
pyrimethamine/sulfadiazine 583

quinapril 291, 292, 293
quinidine 357, 359
    volume of distribution, in heart failure 57
quinine 580–1
    in pregnancy 78
    volume of distribution, in heart failure 57
quinolones 539

radiation sickness 407, 408
ranitidine 399, 400–1, 419
rashes, drug-induced 101–3
receptors
    abnormalities 10
    classification 12
    desensitization 17
    and drug action 10
    and signal transduction 11–13
    up-regulation 17
    see also adrenoreceptors
record linkage, adverse drug reactions 99
recreational drug use 668
rectum, drug administration 35
    children 86
reduction, drug metabolism
    endoplasmic reticulum 43
    non-endoplasmic reticulum 44

remoxipride 161, 167
renal dialysis, blood pressure control 305
renal disease
    drug-related 104
    drugs to be used with caution/avoided 60–1
    hypertension and 281, 305
    pharmacokinetic effects 59–61
    prescription in 60–11, 62
    renal hemodynamics and 61
renal excretion of drugs 52–4
    drug interactions 116–17
    effect of cardiac failure 58–9
    effect of renal impairment 59–61
    elderly 88
    infants 84
    pregnancy 77
renal tubules
    drug reabsorption
        active 54
        passive distal 53–4
    drug secretion 52–3
reproductive endocrinology
    female 498–504
    male 504–7
reproductive testing of drugs 136
resins, plasma cholesterol lowering 271–3
respiratory distress syndrome 389
respiratory failure 387–8, 391
respiratory stimulants 390–1
respiratory surfactant 389–90
respiratory tract infections, antibacterial therapy 519
resuscitation, cardiopulmonary 354
retinoic acid *see* vitamin A
retinoids 428
    acne 654, 655
    and cancer 428
    psoriasis 659
retinol 426–8
retinopathy, diabetic 459
reverse transcriptase (RT) inhibitors, HIV 568–71
Reye's syndrome 86, 233, 318
rheumatoid arthritis treatment
    drugs that suppress rheumatoid process 253–7
    NSAIDs 248–53
riboflavin 429
    deficiency 429
rickets 479
    prevention and treatment 479, 480–1
rifabutin 574
rifampicin 520, 544–5
    hepatotoxicity 421
    HIV-infected patients 573–4
    leprosy 548
    prophylactic use 529
    tuberculosis 542–7, 573–4
    tuberculous meningitis 546
ringworm 554, 556, 557
Ro-24-7429 571
Ro-31-8959 571
roundworms 584

routes of administration
  and absorption 30, 32
  buccal 34–5
  children 85–6
  and drug metabolism 47–8
  ear 37
  eye 37
  intramuscular injection 37–8
  intrathecal injection 39
  intravenous injection 38–9
  lungs 36
  nose 37
  oral 30–34
    sustained release preparations 34
    for systemic effects 33–4
  rectal 35
  skin 35–6
  subcutaneous injection 38
  sublingual 34–5
  vagina 37

salbutamol
  asthma 377, 380–1, 382
  inhaled 36
  metabolism, route of administration and 48
  obstetrics 381
salicylates 233–4, 317
  hepatotoxicity 421
  overdose 686, 687, 692
  skin reactions 102
salicylic acid 232, 658
salicylism 318
salmeterol 382
salt and water depletion 447–8
salt and water overload 438–9
  diuretic treatment 438, 439–46
sarcomas 606
  Kaposi's 611
  osteogenic 599
saturated vapor pressure (SVP) 212
scabies 662
Schildt plot 15, 16
Schilling test 620
schistosomiasis 584
schizophrenia
  drug treatment 161–7
  management 160–1
  pathophysiology 160
scurvy 431
seasonal affective disorder 179
sedation, night, elderly 89
seizures *see* convulsions; epilepsy
selective serotonin reuptake inhibitors (SSRI) 174–5, 179
selegiline 183, 187–8
selenium 434
senna 414
septicemia 521
serotonin *see* 5-hydroxytryptamine
sertraline 174
serum sickness 101, 103, 641

sevoflurane 216
sex hormones 608
  female 498–504
  male 504–6
sexual performance, male, drugs affecting 506–7
shingles 558, 561
shock 340, 345
  anaphylactic 640–1
    treatment 644
  cardiogenic 340, 345, 346
shock lung 388
sick sinus syndrome 351, 357
sickness 405–6
  antiemetics 406–9
  mountain (altitude) 445
  pregnancy 406
  radiation 407, 408
  travel 406
signal transduction processes 13
simvastatin 274–5
sinus arrhythmias 351
skin
  analgesia 657
  drug absorption 35–6
  drug reactions 101–3, 662–4
  patches 36
skin creams
  absorption 36
  vehicle 36
skin diseases/disorders 654–62
  infections 523
    fungal 553, 554
    herpes 558, 561
  topical drugs, absorption 35–6
skin testing, allergic reactions 105
sleep 148
  disturbances
    drug treatment 149–55
    elderly 89
    jet lag 155–6
    management 148–9
    night work and 156
slow-reacting substance of analyphylaxis (SRS-A) 377
smoking
  adverse effects 674
  and atheroma formation 267
  central stimulation 673
  effects on drug metabolism 675
  effects on fetus 81
  nicotine absorption 674–5
  stopping 267, 675
sodium aurothiomalate 253, 254
sodium bicarbonate 398, 450, 451
sodium clodronate 483
sodium cromoglycate 378, 379, 386–7, 641
sodium fusidate 537
  use 520, 522, 523, 537
    skin 660
sodium nitroprusside 298–9, 304, 305, 312, 495
sodium sulfate 413
sodium thiopentone 216–17

sodium valproate 79, 199–200
soft tissue infections, antibacterial therapy 523
solvent misuse 683
somatostatin 510
somatotropin 510
Somogyi effect 464
sotalol 290, 353, 356, 357, 363
spasticity 188
spironolactone 443
sporotrichosis 553
stanozolol 505
statistics, clinical trials 138–9
status epilepticus 202
stavudine 570
stem cell factor 626–7
steroids, skin reactions 102
stilbestrol 498, 499, 500
stomach washout 688
streptokinase 318–20
streptomycin 102, 542–3, 546
stroke
    anticoagulation 327
    risk, relationship to coronary heart disease 280
sucralfate 403
    use in pregnancy 79
suicide 179, 686
sulfadiazine 573, 583
sulfadimidine 538
sulfadoxine 538, 579, 580–1
sulfamethoxazole 538
sulfamethoxazole/trimethoprim 583
sulfapyridine 410
sulfasalazine 33, 256, 410
sulfation, drug metabolism 45
sulfinpyrazone 34, 259–60, 317
sulfonamides 538
    skin reactions 102
sulfonylureas 465–7
    adverse effects 466
    drug interactions 467
    mechanism of action 466
    pharmacokinetics 466
    use 465
sulfoxidation, polymorphism 123
sulindac 249, 250–1
sulpiride 161, 167
sumatriptan 207–8
supraventricular tachycardias *see* tachycardias, supraventricular
suramin 583
surfactant, respiratory 389–90
suxamethonium 222–3
    sensitivity to 120, 123–4
sympathomimetic amines 345–7
synacthen test 487
synergy 109
systemic lupus erythematosis
    azathioprine 256
    chloroquine/hydroxychloroquine 255
    drug-induced 300
    NSAIDs 252

systemic lupus syndrome 101, 104

tachycardia–bradycardia syndrome (sick sinus syndrome) 351, 357
tachycardi(s)
    sinus 351
    supraventricular 351–2, 355–7
    ventricular 352, 357
tacrolimus 639
tamoxifen 499
tapeworms 584
tat inhibitor, HIV 570–1
teicoplanin 522, 537
temazepam 150
    overdose 686
    pharmacokinetics 152
teratogenesis 74–5
    cancer chemotherapy 595
teratogenic drugs 74–5
    recognition 75–6
terazosin 34, 296, 297
terbinafine 557, 661
terbutaline 380, 382
terfenadine 387, 642, 643, 644
terminal disease, pain relief 229–30
testosterone 486, 504, 505–6
tetany, hypoglycemic 481
tetracosactrin 514
tetracycline
    effects on fetus 75
    hepatotoxicity 421
    use 519, 520, 536
tetracyclines 536
    adverse effects
        children 86
        skin 102
    chronic bronchitis 379
    skin diseases 654
tetrahydrocannabinol 672
thalidomide 75, 132–3
theobromines 675, 676
theophylline 347, 675, 383–5
    adverse effects 384, 676
    asthma 378, 383–5
    drug interactions 384–5
    elimination, heart failure 58
    overdose 687
    therapeutic monitoring 71
therapeutics
    drug history 5–6
    drug monitoring 68–72
    planning 6
    prescribing errors
    risk/benefit ratio 4–5
    use of drugs 4, 5
thiabendazole 584
thiamin *see* vitamin B
thiazides 285–7, 340, 341, 439–41
    skin reactions 102
6-thioguanine 588
thiopentone 216–17
thioridazine 161, 164

thiouracils, skin reactions 102
thioxanthines 161, 166
threadworm 584
thromboangitis obliterans 674
thrombocytopenia, drug-related 103
thrombocytopenic purpura, idiopathic 623
thrombolysis, myocardial infarction 310
thrombosis
    pathophysiology 322–3
    treatment and prevention 324
        anticoagulants 324–31
        antiplatelet drugs 331–4
        warfarin-induced 329
thromboxane receptors antagonists 332
thromboxane synthase inhibitors 332
thromboxane synthesis 331
    effect of aspirin 316–17, 331–2
thrombus
    red 322
    white 322
thyroid 470
thyroid crisis 475
thyroid disease
    effects on drug disposition 64–5
    pathophysiology 470
    treatment 470–5
thyrotrophin *see* thyroid-stimulating hormone
thyrotrophin-releasing hormone (TRH) 470, 472–3
thyroxine 470
    as anorectic 423
        obesity treatment 268
    effects of thyroid disease on 65
    treatment of thyroid disease 471–2, 475
tiaconazole 557, 661
ticlopidine 333–4
timestin 532
tinea *see* ringworm
tobramycin 533, 534
    therapeutic monitoring 70
tocopherol *see* vitamin E
tolbutamide
    diabetes mellitus 465, 466
    distribution, effect of liver disease 63
    hepatotoxicity 421
    slow metabolism 123
tolerance induction, therapeutic effects by 17
toxicity of drugs, preclinical studies 135–6
toxicokinetics 136
toxoplasmosis 583
    HIV-infected patients 573
trace elements 433–4
tranquillizers
    effects on central nervous system, elderly 89
    use in pregnancy 80
transferrin 616, 617
transketolase deficiency 128
transplantation *see* organ transplantation
tranylcypromine 175
travel sickness 406
trazodone 171, 174, 175
tretinoin 654, 655

triamcinolone 253, 488
triamterene 250, 305, 341, 342, 444
triazolam 150
triazoles 556–7
tribavirin 561
trichinosis 584
trichloracetic acid 155
trichlorethanol 155
triclofos 155
trifluoperazine 161
trifluoperidol 165
triglycerides, marine 276–7
triiodothyronine (TS) 470
    treatment of thyroid disease 471–2
trimelarsan 583
trimetaphan 300, 304
trimethoprim 538
    absorption, effect of Crohn's disease 56–7
    pregnancy 77
    use 519, 520, 521, 539
        chronic bronchitis 379
        infection in asthma 378
        Pneumocystis carinii pneumonia 572
        prophylactic 529
        trypanosomal infection 583
triplopen 530
triprolidine 642
trisodium phosphonoformate *see* foscarnet
trypanosomal infection 583
tryparsamide 583
L-tryptophan 178–9
tuberculosis 542
    treatment
        AIDS/HIV infection 547, 573–4
        in cancer chemotherapy patients 595
        chemoprophylaxis 547
        combined drug treatment 109
        drugs 542
tuberculous meningitis, treatment 546
tubocurarine 221–2
tumor markers 590

ulcerative colitis 409, 410
ultraviolet A, psoriasis 658–9
United Kingdom, drug regulation 132–4, 142–3
United States, Food and Drug Administration 133
urea
    enterohepatic circulation 417–18
    hepatic encephalopathy 417–18
ureteric colic 452
uric acid production 258–9
uricosuric drugs 259–60
urine
    acidification 451
    alkalinization 451–2
    retention 452
urokinase 318
ursodeoxycholic acid 422
urticaria 659
    drug-induced 102, 663

vaccines 645–8
vagina, drug administration 35
valproate 79, 199–200
vancomycin 522, 523, 537
  prophylactic 526
vanillyl mandelic acid (VMA) measurement 492–3
vasculitis
  allergic 63
  drug-related 104
vasopressin 447, 514
  and diabetes insipidus 447–8
vecuronium 222
ventilatory failure 387–8, 391
ventricular ectopic beats 352
  treatment 357
ventricular fibrillation 355, 357
ventricular tachycardia 352
  treatment 357
verapamil 364
  use
    as antiarrhythmic 353–4, 355, 356, 363–4
    hypertension 294, 295, 296
    ischemic heart disease 315–16
    migraine prophylaxis 210
vigabatrin 100–2
viloxazine 173–4
vinblastine 589, 594, 604–5
vinca alkaloids 588–9
  adverse effects 593
vincristine 594, 604–5
vindesine 604, 605
viral infections
  drug therapy 557–61
    immunoglobulin prophylaxis 563
    interferons 561–3
  skin 661
  see also antiviral drugs; HIV-1 infection; names of
    specific infections
viral protease inhibitor, HIV 571
vitamin A 426–8
  deficiency 427–8
  derivatives 428
vitamin B$_1$ 428–9
  alcoholism 680
  deficiency 428–9
vitamin B$_2$ 429
  deficiency 429
vitamin B$_6$ 430–1
  deficiency 431
vitamin B$_{12}$ 620
  cellular mechanism of action 620–1
  deficiency 620–1, 622
  pharmacokinetics 621
  use 620
vitamin C 431–2
  deficiency 431
  urine acidification 451

vitamin D 479
  and calcium metabolism 479
  deficiency 479–80
  metabolic pathway 479, 480
  preparations of 479–81
vitamin E 432
  deficiency 432
vitamin K, liver disease 419
vitamins 426
  deficiency 426
  physiology 426
volume of distribution see under drug distribution
vomiting 405–6
  antiemetics 406–9
  cytotoxic drugs and 409, 593, 593–4
  induction 687–8
  pregnancy 406
von Willebrand factor 627

Ward–Romano syndrome 643
warfarin 327–31
  adverse effects
    fetus 75, 329, 334
  drug interactions 116, 117, 330–1
    with aspirin 114, 330
    with NSAIDs 330–1
  resistance to 124–5
  use in elderly 88
  use in pregnancy and puerperium 79, 334–5
warts 661
water
  depletion 447–8
  overload 446
    along with salt excess 438–46
Wegener's granulomatosis 257
weight
  gain 424
  ideal 268
  reduction 267–8
    diabetes 461
Wernicke–Korsakov syndrome 128
whipworm 584
Wolff–Parkinson–White (WPW) syndrome 352, 356,
  364, 365, 366
wound infections, antibacterial therapy 523

xanthine alkaloids 347
xanthine oxidase 44
xanthines 675–6

yeasts, nail infections 557

zidovudine 567–8, 570, 575
  combination with probenecid 110
zinc 433
  deficiency 433
Zollinger–Ellison syndrome 397, 401
zopiclone 154–5
zuclopenthixol 161, 166